Recent Advances in
BLOOD COAGULATION

EDITED BY

L. POLLER

NUMBER THREE

CHURCHILL LIVINGSTONE
EDINBURGH LONDON MELBOURNE AND NEW YORK 1981

CHURCHILL LIVINGSTONE
Medical Division of Longman Group Limited

Distributed in the United States of America by
Churchill Livingstone Inc., 19 West 44th Street,
New York, N.Y. 10036, and by associated companies,
branches and representatives throughout
the world.

First published 1981

ISBN 0 443 02182 1
ISSN 0143-6740

British Library Cataloguing in Publication Data
Recent advances in blood coagulation. – No. 3
   1. Blood – Coagulation, Disorders of
   616.1'57'005   RC647.C55   76-42237

Printed in Great Britain at The Pitman Press, Bath

Recent Advances in
BLOOD COAGULATION

L. POLLER DSc(Manch) MD FRCPath

Honorary Lecturer, University of Manchester. Director of National (UK) Reference Laboratory for Anticoagulant Reagents and Control. Consultant Haematologist, Withington Hospital, University Hospital of South Manchester.

Preface

The pace of research and development in blood coagulation has prompted a further volume in this series at a shorter time interval. The success of the previous volumes, necessitating reprinting, has been gratifying and appears to have firmly established the series in the blood coagulation literature.

The view of all the contributors has always been that the theme of topicality should prevail with emphasis throughout on recent developments. The subjects for review in this volume are those which were felt to be important and in which there have been major recent advances.

The editor is again extremely indebted to the individual chapter authors, not only for the high quality of their contributions but also for the great care with which they prepared their manuscripts and compiled their references. This again made editing a relatively light and pleasant duty.

Manchester, 1981   L.P.

Contributors

ULRICH ABILDGAARD
Consultant Haematologist, Aker Hospital, Oslo, Norway

R. K. ARCHER
Senior Pathologist, Medical Research Council Laboratory Animals Centre, Carshalton, Surrey, UK

ROBERT F. BAUGH
Assistant Research Biochemist, Department of Pathology, University of California School of Medicine, San Diego, USA

MICHAEL A. BETTMAN
Assistant Professor of Radiology, Harvard Medical School; Scholar of the James Picker Foundation; and Cardiovascular Radiologist, Brigham and Women's Hospital, Boston, Massachusetts, USA

PIETER BRAKMAN
Director, Gaubius Institute TNO, Leiden, the Netherlands

EMILE J. P. BROMMER
Consultant Haematologist, Gaubius Institute TNO, Leiden and University Hospital, Leiden, the Netherlands

PAUL DIDISHEIM
Professor of Laboratory Medicine, Mayo Medical School, Rochester, Minnesota, USA

M. B. DONATI
Head of Laboratory for Haemostasis and Thrombosis Research, Istituto di Ricerche Farmacologiche Mario Negri, Milan, Italy

MICHAEL GENT
Associate Dean (Research) and Professor of Clinical Epidemiology and Biostatistics, Faculty of Health Sciences, McMaster University, Hamilton, Ontario, Canada

JONATHAN M. GERRARD
Assistant Professor, Department of Pediatrics, University of Manitoba Health Sciences Center, Winnipeg, Manitoba, Canada

FRITS HAVERKATE
Biochemist, Gaubius Institute TNO, Leiden, the Netherlands

CECIL HOUGIE
Professor of Pathology, University of California Medical Center, San Diego, School of
Medicine, and Director of Clinical Coagulation Laboratory, University of California
Medical Center, San Diego, USA

CORNELIS KLUFT
Biochemist, Gaubius Institute TNO, Leiden, the Netherlands

Z. S. LATTALO
Associate Professor, Department of Radiobiology, Institute of Nuclear Research,
Warsaw, Poland

P. M. MANNUCCI
Professor of Medicine, Universita Degli Studi di Milano, Milan, Italy

WILLIAM L. NICHOLS
Consultant in Hematology and Internal Medicine, Mayo Clinic, Rochester, Minnesota, USA

DEREK OGSTON
Regius Professor of Physiology, University of Aberdeen, Aberdeen Teaching Hospitals, Aberdeen, UK

A. POGGI
Research Assistant, Laboratory of Haemostasis and Thrombosis Research, Istituto di
Ricerche Farmacologiche Mario Negri, Milan, Italy

EDWIN W. SALZMAN
Associate Director of Surgery, Beth Israel Hospital and Professor of Surgery, Harvard
Medical School, Boston, Massachusetts, USA

N. SEMERARO
Associate Professor, Department of Microbiology, University of Bari, Bari, Italy

JAN J. SIXMA
Professor of Haematology, Division of Haemostasis, University Hospital, Utrecht,
the Netherlands

DAAN W. TRAAS
Biochemist, Gaubius Institute TNO, Leiden, the Netherlands

GERRIT WIJNGAARDS
Biochemist, Gaubius Institute TNO, Leiden, the Netherlands

Contents

1. Platelet structure, biochemistry and physiology

William L. Nichols   Jonathan M. Gerrard   Paul Didisheim

All this taken together makes it more apparent that blood coagulation is under the direct influence of the blood platelet. Thus, in the future in studying the function and changes of blood, this constant and well represented new constituent must always be taken into account.

*Giulio Bizzozero, 1882**

During the nearly 100 years since Bizzozero distinguished the blood platelets and their involvement in blood clotting, much has been learned about these cells and their functions. Qualitative platelet defects are now increasingly recognized in patients with bleeding or thrombotic problems. The study of such platelets has provided new understanding of platelet function and of the molecular mechanisms of hemostasis.

In this chapter we review major recent advances in platelet ultrastructure, biochemistry and physiology, and then in Chapter 2 we focus on the pathophysiology and diagnosis of the congenital and acquired qualitative platelet disorders, as these are understood at the beginning of the 1980s.

The burgeoning literature on platelets has become vast. In reviewing this literature, we have selectively synthesized that which we think contributes importantly toward a mechanistic understanding of processes important in platelet hemostatic function and dysfunction. Limitations of space and time preclude extensive bibliographic citations, and also preclude review of such topics as megakaryopoiesis and thrombopoiesis, platelet kinetics, blood rheology and platelet interactions with other formed elements of the blood, quantitative disorders of platelets (e.g. 'pure' thrombocytopenias unassociated with recognized qualitative abnormalities), platelet storage and transfusion, or platelet involvement in immune, inflammatory or neoplastic processes.

PLATELET STRUCTURE, BIOCHEMISTRY AND PHYSIOLOGY

General structure and function of blood platelets

The resting cell

Blood platelets in the quiescent state are small, anucleate discoid cells, much like miniature versions of discuses thrown by athletes (Fig. 1.1). In human blood, the platelets normally number 130 000 to 400 000 per microliter, have an average diameter of 2–3 microns and an average volume of about 8 cubic microns (Karpatkin, 1977; Stahl et al, 1978). The outside cell surface is generally smooth, with occasional pockmarked indentations where channels of the surface connected canalicular system (SCCS) exit. Inside the cell, organelles including dense granules, alpha granules,

---

* Quoted by Henry (1977)

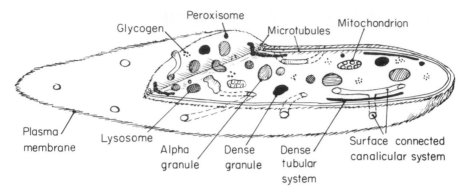

Fig. 1.1   Diagrammatic representation of an unactivated human platelet. In the resting cell, shown sectioned through the sagittal and equatorial planes, granules including dense granules, α-granules, lysosomes and peroxisomes are randomly distributed throughout the cell. Mitochondria and glycogen particles can also be seen. A microtubule band encircles the cell just beneath the plasma membrane. The surface-connected canalicular system and the dense tubular system are prominent in the region near the microtubule band.

lysosomes, peroxisomes, and mitochondria are randomly distributed. Also scattered throughout the cell cytoplasm are glycogen granules. In the plane of the largest diameter, a bundle of microtubules curves around just beneath the cell membrane, travelling the entire circumference of the cell. Two membrane systems weave throughout the cell interior. The SCCS, an invagination of the plasma membrane, contains channels which are continuous with the extracellular space. The dense tubular system (DTS), a smooth endoplasmic reticulum, occurs particularly in close association with the SCCS, and with the circumferential microtubule band. Contractile proteins exist in the cell cytoplasm, but these proteins are not easily seen in the resting cell, in part because of a dense intracellular matrix, and probably also because they exist to a considerable degree in a depolymerized, non-filamentous form. Resting or unactivated platelets are normally nonadherent to each other or to endothelialized vascular surfaces, but can be easily excited by a variety of stimuli to become sticky and activated.

Nomenclature of platelet activation phenomena
Platelet '*activation*' is a loosely defined term implying significant functional, bio-chemical and/or structural alteration of platelets, not found in the unstimulated and unexcited state. Such activation ordinarily requires metabolically intact platelets, and is usually defined operationally by one or more of the following terms. *Adhesion* refers to platelet attachment to the wall of a blood vessel or foreign surface. *Shape change* or viscous metamorphosis represents loss of the resting discoid shape with spherical transformation of the platelet followed by pseudopodial extension. *Aggregation* indicates non-immunologic cohesion of activated, sticky platelets to one another, while *agglutination* is a term reserved for immunologic clumping. *Release reaction* refers to the secretion by platelets of certain substances stored in intracellular organelles. This reaction usually follows one or more of the activation processes noted above, and has been subclassified by Holmsen (1975) into sequential stages (release I and II) in which with increasing stimulus strength, the contents of different storage

organelles (α-granules and dense granules, then lysosomes) are progressively extruded. Platelet *procoagulant activities* are mostly latent in resting platelets, but become manifest with platelet activation processes, serving ultimately to accelerate the generation of thrombin, and the conversion of fibrinogen to fibrin. *Primary hemostasis* encompasses the interaction of platelets with blood vessels and certain coagulation factors to form a *hemostatic plug* (reviewed in the chapter by Sixma), and is sometimes conceptually distinguished from 'secondary hemostasis' which mainly involves plasmatic coagulation and fibrin clot formation. *Platelet retention* reflects the progressive numerical diminution of the platelet content of whole blood exuding from a small wound or passing across a foreign surface. This phenomenon is thought to result from several platelet activation processes including adhesion, shape change, aggregation and release reactions.

Structural changes with cell activation
Major activation processes in platelets include: (1) adhesion of these cells to sites of vessel wall injury; (2) cohesion of platelets into cell aggregates (aggregation); (3) changes in cell shape with extension of pseudopods and centralization of granules; and (4) labilization of granule contents by fusion of granule and plasma membranes so as to connect the granule interior to the channels of the SCCS. These four processes can occur separately from one another, although usually one or more occur together. Thus, platelets initially adhering to sites of vessel wall injury are frequently discoid, but later shape change occurs and cell aggregates form (Baumgartner and Muggli, 1976). Platelet-platelet stickiness of discoid cells can occur during the first wave of epinephrine-induced aggregation. Usually shape change precedes aggregation as when ADP, thrombin, collagen or arachidonic acid is stirred with these cells to stimulate them.

With a change in cell shape and granule centralization (Fig. 1.2a), considerable polymerization of actin occurs, and microfilaments are visible principally in three locations in the cell: in the pseudopods, surrounding the centralized granules in close association with the microtubules, and as a central contractile gel in degranulated platelets (Gerrard & White, 1976). In cell aggregates (Fig. 1.2b), granules move to the center of the aggregate more often than to the center of the individual cells (Gerrard et al, 1979a). Thus a coordination exists between proteins involved in platelet stickiness and aggregation, and those involved in granule centralization. Granule secretion appears to involve both labilization of granules and granule centralization (Gerrard et al, 1977a).

The platelet plasma membrane
The plasma membrane represents the site of platelet interactions with the external environment, and is intimately involved in the control or generation of the many specialized functional properties of platelets. Unique morphologic features of the platelet plasma membrane, noted in the previous section, include numerous 'intracellular' invaginations through pores to form the SCCS, effectively providing for a relative excess of membrane surface, and for close apposition of internal organelles to the external surface. Techniques for isolating platelet plasma membranes have been the subject of reviews (Barber et al, 1971; Crawford & Taylor, 1977; Sixma & Lips, 1978), and it should be noted that most platelet plasma membrane preparations may

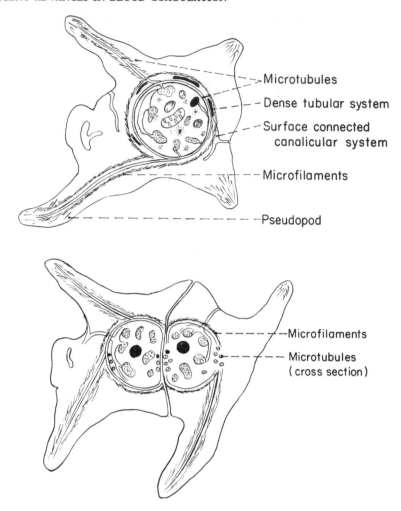

Fig. 1.2(a) A single activated platelet. In an activated cell which is not attached to other cells, pseudopods containing microfilaments are visible, and granules are centralized. Surrounding the centralized granules are microfilaments and microtubules. The surface connected canalicular system and dense tubular system continue a close association with the microtubules and centralizing granules.

(b) Two attached activated platelets. When activated cells are attached to one another, granule centralization now occurs toward the center of the small aggregate.

also contain some components from intraplatelet structures. Recent studies have discerned a number of unique molecular features of the platelet plasma membrane systems, and elucidate some biochemical mechanisms important for specific platelet functions.

Lipids

Human platelet membrane preparations contain about 35 per cent lipids, 8 per cent carbohydrates, and 57 per cent proteins by weight (Crawford & Taylor, 1977; Shattil & Cooper, 1978). The bulk of the membrane lipid bilayer is composed of phospholipids (65 to 75 per cent by weight), while cholesterol comprises most of the neutral lipids (20 to 25 per cent), and glycolipids (2 to 5 per cent) account for almost all the remainder. On a molar basis membrane cholesterol is about half the phospholipid content. Cholesterol is not synthesized by human platelets, but can be readily incorporated into platelet membranes in vitro and probably in vivo from plasma lipoproteins (Colman, 1978; Shattil & Cooper, 1978; Stuart et al, 1980). Increased membrane cholesterol content renders the lipid bilayer more rigid (less fluid), and seems associated with the hyperreactivity of such platelets to various stimuli.

Membrane glycerophospholipids can be synthesized by platelets, using glycerol to form a three carbon backbone to which are attached (in most cases) one phosphate ester and two fatty acids:

$$R—CO—O—CH_2$$
$$R'—CO—O—CH \qquad O$$
$$CH_2—O—P—O—X$$
$$\|$$
$$O$$

Phosphatidylcholine: X = Choline
Phosphatidylserine: X = Serine
Phosphatidylinositol: X = Inositol
Phosphatidylethanolamine: X = Ethanolamine
Phosphatidic Acid: X = Hydrogen

R, R': = Hydrocarbon chain of fatty acid

Lysophospholipids lack one of the two fatty acid side chains.

The fatty acid moieties of membrane phospholipids can be saturated with hydrogen or unsaturated, the latter being mainly derived from essential fatty acids in the diet. The polyunsaturated fatty acid, arachidonic acid (20 carbons and 4 double bonds, $20:4$), is one of the most abundant fatty acids in platelet membranes (Marcus, 1978). In non-activated platelets this fatty acid exists almost exclusively esterified into the phospholipids; phosphatidylethanolamine (PE), phosphatidylserine (PS), phosphatidylinositol (PI), and phosphatidylcholine (PC) mainly attached to the middle carbon of the glycerol backbone (Marcus, 1978; Shattil & Cooper, 1978). Liberation of free arachidonic acid from platelet membrane phospholipids by specific lipases is believed to be a major control point of the platelet prostaglandin metabolic pathways, ultimately accelerating or limiting the generation of thromboxanes, potent mediators of platelet activation. (Prostaglandin metabolism is reviewed more fully in a subsequent section.)

There is reasonable evidence for asymmetric distribution of certain phospholipid species on the two sides of platelet membrane lipid bilayers (Shattil & Cooper, 1978; Zwaal, 1978; Schick, 1979). The preferential inside surface exposure of the acidic phospholipids PE, PS and PI in membrane systems of non-activated platelets is thought to be relevant to platelet prostaglandin metabolism. With platelet activation, PE and PS may become more externally exposed (Shattil & Cooper, 1978; Bevers et al, 1979; Schick, 1979) thus providing a catalytically important lipid surface (platelet procoagulant activity) for the generation of activated plasmatic coagulation factors.

Glycolipids contain about one-third of the platelet membrane carbohydrates (Glöckner et al, 1978; Schick, 1979), and probably are largely exposed on the external membrane surface, as are the glycoproteins. Because many glycolipids contain sialic acid, it is likely that they contribute significantly to the relatively large negative surface charge of the platelet. Other functions of platelet membrane glycolipids are unknown, but some components might serve as membrane antigens in a fashion analogous to the erythrocyte ABH and Ii systems (Dejter-Juszynski et al, 1978; Watanabe et al, 1979).

Carbohydrates

The platelet glycocalyx or external plasma membrane coat is rich in carbohydrates which, in addition to the glycolipid contributions, are also provided by glycosamino-glycans or mucopolysaccharides, and by glycoproteins. The principal platelet glyco-saminoglycan is chondroitin 4-sulfate (Hagen, 1972; Ward & Packham, 1979), a releasable surface component of both platelet plasma membranes and storage granule membranes. Functions of cell surface glycosaminoglycans are largely unknown, but they are thought to be important in cell-cell and cell-surface interactions (Lindahl & Höök, 1978). Most glycosaminoglycans are found to be covalently associated with a specific core protein to form a proteoglycan complex. A platelet-derived proteoglycan carrier of platelet factor 4 (PF4) has been shown to consist of four chondroitin sulfate chains and a core protein (Barber et al, 1972), and is probably important in the interaction of PF4 with heparin, another glycosaminoglycan (Niewiarowski & Levine, 1979; Lindahl & Höök, 1978).

Glycoproteins

The externally exposed plasma membrane proteins of platelets are largely, if not exclusively, glycoproteins, and generally are intrinsically bound in the lipid bilayer. Current analytical techniques have permitted identification of up to seven 'major' or relatively abundant externally exposed platelet membrane glycoproteins. Other 'minor' or less abundant surface glycoproteins are now recognized (Phillips & Agin, 1977b; Andersson & Gahmberg, 1978; McGregor et al, 1979; Nichols et al, 1979), so that in total, there are at least 15 discernible human platelet membrane glyco-protein species. These cell surface glycoproteins are believed to play important and diverse roles in platelet function, including mediation of cell-cell and cell-surface interactions, generation of surface specificity and antigenicity, activities as message receptors and transducers, and functions in membrane transport phenomena. In addition, loss of surface sialic acids or glycoproteins appears to be a principal mechanism of platelet senescence in vivo (Greenberg et al, 1979b).

Table 1.1 outlines some characteristics of the major platelet membrane glyco-proteins. It should be noted that, as yet, there is no universally employed nomencla-ture for these glycoproteins. This reflects that relatively few platelet membrane glycoproteins have been isolated in sufficient quantity and homogeneity to permit comprehensive biochemical identification and characterization.

Among the components of the glycoprotein I (GP I) group, a readily solubilized or proteolytically liberated component, 'glycocalicin' or GP Is (Okumura & Jamieson, 1976; Nurden & Caen, 1978), has been isolated and partially characterized. It is rich in sialic acid, and seems implicated in platelet interaction with thrombin (Ganguly & Gould, 1979; Okumura et al, 1978), and in Willebrand factor-mediated adhesion of platelets to each other and to subendothelial surfaces (Okumura & Jamieson, 1976; Baumgartner et al, 1977). Glycocalicin shares some structural and functional charac-teristics with the integral membrane protein GP Ib, but recent studies suggest that these proteins are non-identical (Cooper et al, 1979; Moroi et al, 1979; Nachman et al, 1979; Solum et al, 1979). Both GP Is and GP Ib are quantitatively decreased in

Table 1.1   Major human platelet membrane glycoproteins.

Nomenclature[1]	Apparent Molecular Weight[2,3]	Comments
Ia	167 000	
Ib	143 000	Decreased in Bernard-Soulier disease
Is	148 000[4]	'Glycocalicin'; Decreased in Bernard-Soulier disease
Ic[3]	134 000	Minor component; ? Glycosylated
IIa	157 000	
IIb	132 000	Decreased in Glanzmann's thrombasthenia
IIc[5]	110 000[5]	
IIIa (III)[3,4]	114 000	α-actinin; Decreased in Glanzmann's thrombasthenia
IIIb (IV)[3,4]	97 000	

[1] Nurden & Caen, 1979.
[2] Electrophoretic estimate; reduced glycopeptide.
[3] Phillips & Agin, 1977a.
[4] Okumura & Jamieson, 1976
[5] George, 1978.

platelets of patients with Bernard-Soulier disease. These platelets display defects in adhesion to the subendothelium, do not aggregate in response to ristocetin and Willebrand factor, and show diminished responsiveness to thrombin (Weiss et al, 1974; Caen et al, 1976; Okumura et al, 1978; Jamieson & Okumura, 1978). Elucidation of the biochemical and functional relationships of GP Is and GP Ib awaits isolation and characterization of the membrane bound form.

Glycoproteins IIb and IIIa are quantitatively decreased in platelets of patients with Glanzmann's thrombasthenia (Phillips & Agin, 1977c; Nurden & Caen, 1978; Jamieson et al, 1979), and the platelet-specific alloantigen Pl[A1] is also deficient (Kunicki & Aster, 1978). Glycoprotein IIIa has recently been tentatively identified as platelet alpha-actinin (Gerrard et al, 1979a) and as the structural carrier of Pl[A1] activity (Kunicki & Aster, 1979). Gerrard et al (1979a) have suggested that membrane bound alpha-actinin (GP IIIa) may serve as an anchor point for attachment of actin filaments to the inside of the platelet membrane, thus linking the platelet contractile apparatus to the membrane in a fashion analogous to skeletal muscle Z-band attachment sites for actin. Phillips et al (1979) have provided evidence that GP IIb and GP IIIa are involved in the direct interaction of platelets with each other during aggregation.

Alloantibodies directed against specific surface antigens missing in Bernard-Soulier platelets (GP I) or in thrombasthenic platelets (GP II or III) confer the corresponding functional defects when incubated with normal platelets (Nurden & Caen, 1978). There is, therefore, abundant evidence that platelet membrane glycoproteins are critical for certain platelet functions.

Proteins

Analysis of detergent solubilized platelet membranes by high resolution electrophoretic techniques has permitted the recognition of a large number of different protein and glycoprotein components. Some represent membrane associated components of platelet contractile proteins (actin, myosin, tropomyosin). Functional identities of most of the remainder are currently unknown, but it is likely that a substantial portion of the different species are enzymes. Among the tentatively identified membrane

Table 1.2   Platelet receptors

Ligand	Sites/Platelet[a]	Affinity (M^{-1})[a,b]	Notes[c]	Reference
ADP	1×10^5	6×10^6	HM	Nachman & Ferris, 1974
ADP	1×10^5	5×10^5	HP	Born & Feinberg, 1975
ADP	- - - - - -	5×10^6	HM	Legrand & Caen, 1976
ADP	- - - - - -	3×10^6	HM	Adler & Handin, 1979
Epinephrine	1×10^5	- - - - - -	HP	McMillan et al, 1979
Dihydroergocryptine	2×10^2	1×10^9	HP	Newman et al, 1978
Dihydroergocryptine	5×10^2	2×10^8	HP	Kaywin et al, 1978
Clonidine	1×10^2	5×10^7	HP	Shattil et al, 1979b
Serotonin	7×10^3 (2×10^3)	4×10^7 (7×10^6)	RP	Drummond & Gordon, 1975
Serotonin	1×10^3 (7×10^3)	6×10^{10} (7×10^9)	HP	Boullin et al, 1977
Collagen $\alpha1$ chain	2×10^5	2×10^6	HM	Chiang & Kang, 1976
PGD_2	2×10^2	2×10^7	HP	Cooper & Ahern, 1979
PGE_1	4×10^2 (- - - - - -)	2×10^8 (5×10^5)	HP	Schafer et al, 1979
PGI_2	1×10^2 (3×10^3)	8×10^7 (1×10^6)	HP	Siegel et al, 1979
Fibrinogen	5×10^3	1×10^7	H-HP	Marguerie et al, 1979
Fibrinogen	4×10^4	1×10^7	H-HP	Bennett & Vilaire, 1979
Thrombin	3×10^2 (3×10^3)	5×10^8 (8×10^6)	H-HP	Martin et al, 1976
Thrombin	7×10^2 (6×10^4)	3×10^8 (2×10^6)	H-HM	Tam & Detwiler, 1979
Thrombin	5×10^2 (4×10^4)	3×10^8 (2×10^6)	H-HP	Tam & Detwiler, 1979
Factor V	8×10^2	3×10^8	B-BP	Tracy et al, 1979
Factor Va	9×10^2 (4×10^3)	3×10^9 (3×10^8)	B-BP	Tracy et al, 1979
Factor Xa	2×10^2	3×10^{10}	H-HP	Miletich et al, 1978
Factor Xa	4×10^2	1×10^{10}	B-BP	Dahlbäck & Stenflo, 1978
Factor VIII R:Ag	3×10^5	2×10^9	H-HP	Kao et al, 1979a

[a] Estimated to one significant digit. Lower affinity sites in parentheses.
[b] Expressed as the association or affinity constant (Ka) of the equilibrium binding of ligand to receptor. Larger values imply greater affinity.
[c] Abbreviations: HM = human platelet membranes; HP = human platelets; RP = rat platelets; H-HP = human factor and human platelets; H-HM = human factor and human platelet membranes; B-BP = bovine factor and bovine platelets.

endoenzymes, those of particular interest relate to cyclic AMP metabolism (adenylate cyclase, cAMP dependent protein kinases: Smith & Damus, 1977; Steer & Wood, 1979), prostaglandin metabolism (diglyceride lipase, phospholipase A_2: Schoene, 1978; Bell et al, 1979), and membrane transport (calcium and magnesium dependent ATPases: Crawford & Taylor, 1977). Platelet collagen-glycosyl transferases are thought to be ectoenzymes, and may be of importance in the interaction of platelet surface glycoproteins with collagen (Michaeli & Orloff, 1976; Crawford & Taylor, 1977).

Receptors
A number of platelet 'receptors' for ligands of biologic or pharmacologic importance have been identified. Table 1.2 outlines properties of the more well defined platelet receptor activities. In most cases some, but not all of the usually accepted criteria for designation of membrane binding as a 'receptor' (Cuatrecasas & Hollenberg, 1976; Mills & MacFarlane, 1976; Ryan & Lee, 1976) have been met. These platelet receptor functions are probably largely mediated by membrane proteins, as evidenced by the marked reduction of binding sites observed in several studies following partial

proteolysis of the platelet surface. With few exceptions, the binding proteins are structurally unidentified.

Although fibrinogen is required for ADP-induced platelet aggregation (Mustard et al, 1978), ADP binding to the platelet membrane does not require fibrinogen. Adenine nucleotides are thought to be of major importance in the platelet activation process, and work is in progress to isolate receptor proteins from platelet membranes (Bennett et al, 1978; Adler & Handin, 1979).

Platelet membranes actively transport serotonin, and it has been suggested that the high affinity membrane binding of serotonin may represent a receptor site, while lower affinity sites may represent the transport component (Drummond & Gordon, 1975; Boullin et al, 1977). The physiological significance of alpha-adrenergic membrane receptors is unknown, despite the high membrane affinity and potent ability of such agonists to activate platelets in vitro.

Collagen fibrils, structural components of the vascular subendothelium and wall, are clearly important in primary hemostasis, but the complexity of these structures has compounded the difficulty of understanding the biochemical mechanisms of platelet-collagen interaction. Both the primary and the quaternary structures of collagen species seem important in platelet adhesion and subsequent aggregation (Chiang & Kang, 1976; Santoro & Cunningham, 1977; Fauvel et al, 1978; Fauvel et al, 1979; Brown et al, 1980).

Prostacyclin (PGI_2), produced by endothelial cells, exerts a profound inhibitory influence on platelets and is thought to represent a major mechanism for the non-thrombogenicity of intact, endothelialized vascular surfaces (Moncada & Vane, 1979). Characterization of platelet receptors for this endothelial 'hormone' will allow investigation of the possible role of platelet PGI_2 receptor abnormalities in patients with thrombotic diatheses (Siegel et al, 1979). Platelet PGI_2 receptors appear to be distinct from those for PGD_2, the major inhibitory prostaglandin produced by platelets (Cooper & Ahern, 1979).

Platelet receptors for immunoglobulin (Fc) and for complement components exist, but are biochemically less well defined. Cheng and Hawiger (1979) have reported isolation of a platelet Fc receptor which is a surface glycoprotein. Insulin receptors have also been demonstrated (Hajek et al, 1979), as have specific receptors for dipyridamole (Subbarao et al, 1977). Receptors for plasmatic coagulation factors are discussed in a subsequent section.

Antigens
Structural components of the platelet HLA antigen system have been solubilized and purified (Bernier et al, 1974; Gockerman & Jacob, 1979), and the protein structural components appear similar, but not identical to those isolated from lymphocytes (Springer et al, 1977). The probable glycolipid structure of platelet ABH antigens, and the glycoprotein structure of the Pl[A1] antigen have been noted above. The structural basis for other platelet antigen systems such as Pl[E] and Ko is unknown.

Internal membrane systems

Surface Connected Canalicular System (SCCS)
The SCCS, an invagination of the plasma membrane, serves as a conduit through

which secreted granule contents pass to the cell exterior (White, 1974). In addition, the SCCS has been suggested, analogous to skeletal muscle t-tubules, as having a role in transmission of activating stimuli to the cell interior by means of propagated depolarization. The demonstration of divalent cation-stimulated ATPase activity as well as calcium (Cutler et al, 1978) in the membranes of the SCCS could also allow for local calcium release or flux from these membranes.

Dense Tubular System (DTS)

The DTS, a smooth endoplasmic reticulum, is strongly implicated as the major site of sequestration of calcium used for initiation of platelet activation processes such as shape change, granule centralization, and secretion (Robblee et al, 1973; Käser-Glanzmann et al, 1977; Cutler et al, 1978; White & Gerrard, 1980). It is thus analogous to skeletal muscle sarcotubules which sequester or release calcium to control muscle contraction. The close connections inside the platelet between DTS and SCCS support an interaction between these two membrane systems in control of cell activation. The DTS is also the major site of platelet prostaglandin and thromboxane synthesis (Gerrard et al, 1976; Hammarström & Falardeau, 1977). In addition, adenylate cyclase and divalent cation-activated ATPase activities have been demonstrated in the DTS (Cutler et al, 1978). Platelet calcium, prostaglandin and cyclic nucleotide metabolism is outlined more fully in subsequent sections.

Organelles

Dense granules

Human dense granules (dense bodies) contain calcium, pyrophosphate, ADP, ATP, serotonin and possibly antiplasmin (Holmsen, 1975; Joist et al, 1976). In human granules, the electron dense material which gives the granules their name is calcium (Skaer et al, 1974; Gerrard et al, 1977b). About 65 per cent of human platelet ADP and ATP is stored in dense granules ('storage pool') and may be secreted during platelet activation, but does not exchange readily with the remaining 35 per cent of adenine nucleotides which form the cytoplasmic 'metabolic pool' (Holmsen & Weiss, 1979). Functionally the granules make an important contribution to the aggregability of platelets, as indicated by deficient aggregation in patients with Hermansky-Pudlak syndrome whose platelets lack these organelles (Rendu et al, 1978; Weiss et al, 1979b). In this regard, ADP secreted from these granules appears to be of prime importance since the amount of ADP releasable from granules is more than enough to cause full aggregation if added to the cell exterior.

The role of other dense granule components in platelet activation is less clear, although secreted calcium may provide a high local concentration immediately extracellullarly to facilitate platelet-platelet cohesion which requires calcium. Platelets do not synthesize serotonin, but actively scavenge it from plasma. Secreted serotonin, in addition to its platelet aggregating and smooth muscle constricting effects, may potentiate immune mediated endothelial cell injury (Boogaerts et al, 1979). ATP and serotonin are frequently used to monitor platelet secretion, as labelled serotonin is rapidly taken up into these granules, and a modified aggregometer is now available which measures the continuous release of ATP (Feinman et al, 1977). Recent studies suggest an acidic pH within the dense granules may facilitate amine (serotonin) accumulation, providing a novel understanding of granule function (Johnson et al, 1978).

Alpha granules
Alpha granules contain a variety of proteins, some platelet specific (Table 1.3). The

Table 1.3   Contents of platelet granules.

Dense granule	α-granule	Lysosome	Peroxisome
ADP	Platelet factor 4	Acid hydrolases	Catalase
ATP	β-thromboglobulin	Cathepsins D, E	
Calcium	Platelet-derived		
Serotonin	growth factor		
Pyrophosphate	Permeability factor		
Antiplasmin?	Chemotactic factor		
	Bactericidal factor		
	Thrombospondin (TSP)		
	Fibrinogen		
	Factor V		
	Factor VIII R:Ag		
	Fibronectin		
	Albumin		

importance of these secreted proteins in platelet function is uncertain, though moderate dysfunction of platelets deficient in alpha granules (Gray Platelet Syndrome: White, 1979; Gerrard et al, 1979b; Nurden et al, 1979) suggests that they do contribute. Platelet α-granules may be heterogeneous with respect to their capabilities to store different proteins (Holmsen & Weiss, 1979).

Platelet factor four (PF4), and to a lesser extent beta-thromboglobulin (βTG) and low affinity PF4, have antiheparin activity. The low molecular weight protein subunits mediating these activities have been extensively characterized and are structurally similar (Fukami et al, 1979; Niewiarowski & Levine, 1979; Rucinski et al, 1979). The role of these secretable antiheparin proteins in hemostasis is largely unknown, but Walsh et al (1974) have suggested they might promote plasmatic coagulation around platelet hemostatic plugs by neutralizing heparin locally.

Platelet derived growth factor (PDGF) is a heat stable basic protein which can stimulate DNA synthesis and proliferation of a variety of confluent cells in tissue culture, including fibroblasts and arterial smooth muscle cells (Ross et al, 1974; Antoniades et al, 1979; Heldin et al, 1979; Kaplan et al, 1979a, 1979b). This low molecular weight platelet protein has been implicated as causative in promoting arterial smooth muscle proliferation in response to endothelial injury, and may be of importance in the development of atherosclerosis (Ross et al, 1974; Friedman & Burns, 1978; Fuster et al, 1978; Harker et al, 1978). Other cationic proteins of α-granules are less well characterized, and include a vascular permeability factor, a chemotactic factor, and a bactericidal factor (Holmsen & Weiss, 1979; Niewiarowski & Levine, 1979).

Thrombospondin or thrombin sensitive protein is a high molecular weight glycoprotein composed of three disulfide-bonded subunits (Lawler et al, 1978). It is the major glycoprotein (GP Ig) of platelet α-granules (Solum et al, 1977; Nurden et al,

1979), but as yet its function is unknown. Small amounts of fibronectin (cold-insoluble globulin), another large protein, have also been localized to α-granules (Zucker et al, 1979b; Plow et al, 1979a). The role of fibronectin in platelet adhesion to subendothelial collagen fibrils is uncertain (Bensusan et al, 1978; Santoro & Cunningham, 1979).

Certain platelet-derived coagulation factors are also found in α-granules. These include platelet fibrinogen, and probably also platelet factor V and platelet factor VIII-related antigen (James et al, 1977; Pifer et al, 1977; Gerrard et al, 1979b; Nurden et al, 1979; Zucker et al, 1979a). Platelet coagulant factors and activities are discussed in a subsequent section.

Lysosomes

With special cytochemical staining techniques (Bentfield & Bainton, 1975), platelet lysosomes can be distinguished from α-granules, and are found to make up only a small proportion of the platelet organelle population. Platelet lysosomes contain a number of degradative enzymes including cathepsins and other proteases and hydrolases (Bentfield & Bainton, 1975; Da Prada et al, 1976; Ehrlich & Gordon, 1976; Niewiarowski, 1977). Lysosomal enzymes are secreted but only with very strong stimuli. These degradative enzymes may be of importance in platelet phagocytic processes, and perhaps also in platelet interactions with subendothelial surfaces (Ehrlich & Gordon, 1976; Niewiarowski, 1977).

Peroxisomes

Platelet peroxisomes contain catalase, and appear similar to peroxisomes in other cells (Breton-Gorius & Guichard, 1975). No specific function for platelet peroxisomes is known, though they may protect the cell by scavenging hydrogen peroxide.

Mitochondria

Platelet mitochondria help in providing synthesis of ATP which is essential for most platelet functions (Holmsen, 1977). Platelets in plasma can readily utilize glycolysis to compensate for defective mitochondrial function (Holmsen et al, 1974). Thus mitochondria provide a supplementary source of ATP. The burst of oxygen consumption occurring with platelet stimulation is mainly due to oxygenation of liberated arachidonic acid, forming prostaglandin endoperoxides (Bressler et al, 1979). Glycogen is a major component of platelets, providing a stored energy source (Akkerman, 1978).

Cytoskeleton and contractile apparatus

Microtubules

In the resting cell, considerable evidence suggests that the circumferential micro-tubule band is a flexible cytoskeleton exerting tension outward, producing the discoid shape of the platelet (White & Gerrard, 1979). Consistent with this, selective depolymerization of microtubules converts the cell to a more spherical form.

Microtubules account for about 3 per cent of the total platelet protein and are predominantly composed of heterodimers of α and β tubulin subunits, noncovalently polymerized to form hollow tubular cylinders (Castle & Crawford, 1977; Steiner &

Ikeda, 1979; White & Gerrard, 1979). Microtubule assembly, although incompletely characterized in platelets or other cells, requires divalent cations, GTP or ATP, and microtubule-associated proteins, and is associated with phosphorylation of tubulin (Ikeda & Steiner, 1979; Sloboda & Rosenbaum, 1979). Antimitotic drugs such as colchicine, vincristine, vinblastine, podophylotoxins, anthracyclines (daunorubicin) and griseofulvin bind to tubulin and inhibit polymerization (David-Pfeuty et al, 1979). Interestingly, most platelet functions are not greatly inhibited when vincristine is administered to humans (Steinherz et al, 1976). Exposure of platelets to cold temperatures also disassembles microtubules.

In resting platelets it is estimated that the majority of tubulin is polymerized as microtubules (Steiner & Ikeda, 1979). On stimulation transient depolymerization of microtubules occurs, followed by repolymerization. With platelet activation the peripheral microtubule band becomes constricted, and microtubules can also be seen to enter pseudopods (White & Gerrard, 1979).

Microfilaments
The microfilamentous platelet contractile and cytoskeletal apparatus contributes importantly to most aspects of platelet function including megakaryopoiesis and thrombopoiesis, and in activation processes such as pseudopod formation, internal contraction, granule labilization and secretion, and clot retraction (Cohen et al, 1979b). Structural and regulatory components of the cytoskeletal contractile apparatus are outlined in Table 1.4, and account for a substantial proportion of total platelet

Table 1.4 Platelet cytoskeletal and contractile proteins.

Protein	Subunits/Isomers	Molecular weight	Polymers
Tubulin		110 000 dimer	Microtubule
	$\alpha\,\beta$	55 000	
G-actin	$\beta\,\gamma$	42 000 isomers	Microfilament (F-actin)
Profilin		16 000	
Filamin (ABP)		240 000–270 000	Forms dimer or ? multimer
α-Actinin		90 000–110 000	Forms dimer or ? multimer
Myosin		460 000–500 000	Bipolar filament
	H chain	194 000–212 000	
	L chain$_1$	20 000	
	L chain$_2$	16 000	
Tropomyosin		60 000 dimer	Filaments
	$\alpha\,\beta$	29 000	

proteins. Knowledge of the interaction of these proteins is far from complete, but recent studies provide improved understanding.

Actin is the most abundant of platelet proteins and is structurally slightly different from the predominantly α isoactin form of skeletal muscle actin (Hunter & Garrels, 1977; Landon et al, 1977). In addition to platelet actin β and γ isoelectric forms, there is also evidence for other heterogeneity of platelet actins (Gallagher et al, 1976; Cohen, 1979). The actin concentration in platelets is less than in skeletal muscle, yet far surpasses the critical concentration usually necessary for polymerization of globular G-actin subunits to form filamentous or fibrous F-actin (Adelstein & Pollard, 1978).

In contrast to the mostly polymerized actin of skeletal muscle, in the resting platelet evidence now shows that actin exists to a considerable degree in a non-filamentous form (profilamentous actin or profilactin) perhaps associated with profilin, a small protein which maintains actin in this form (Harris & Weeds, 1978; Markey et al, 1978; Markey & Lindberg, 1979). Profilin seems to bind to both the β and γ isoelectric forms of G-actin, indicating that these forms may not be different functionally (Kendrick-Jones et al, 1979). Thus, in resting platelets there is probably a fairly large cytoplasmic 'storage pool' of non-filamentous actin ready to participate in activation processes.

With platelet stimulation actin polymerization and organization occur, forming thin actin filaments (Fig. 1.3). This structural gelling is facilitated by actin-binding protein

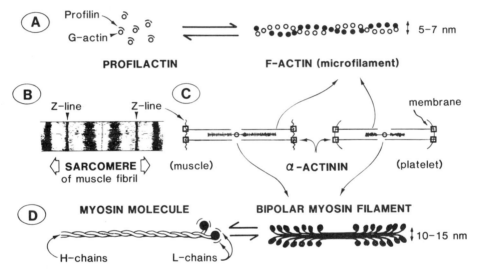

Fig. 1.3 Molecular and ultrastructural components of the platelet contractile apparatus. (a) Profilin binds to globular actin molecules, forming a profilactin complex, causing actin to remain depolymerized. With platelet activation, microfilamentous double helical polymers of actin then form. (b) Ultrastructure of a skeletal muscle fibril sarcomere, bounded at each end by a Z-line. (c) To the left, macromolecular structure of a portion of a skeletal muscle fibril sarcomere. To the right, a macromolecular analogy of the platelet contractile apparatus, showing the proposed function of α-actinin which anchors actin microfilaments to the Z-line in skeletal muscle fibril sarcomeres, and which is believed to anchor platelet actin microfilaments to the platelet membrane. (d) Platelet myosin molecules are composed of two noncovalently-linked heavy chains, each of which binds two different myosin light chains at its globular end. During platelet activation processes, myosin molecules can polymerize to form bipolar myosin filaments.

(ABP, filamin) and by α-actinin (Schollmeyer et al, 1978; Phillips et al, 1979). In the absence of these actin-gelling proteins, purified actin can be polymerized in vitro to form randomly oriented thin microfilaments of six to seven nanometer diameter, while in the presence of either gelling protein the thin actin filaments form crossmeshed bundles. When both gelling proteins are present, additional actin organization into parallel arrays of microfilaments is seen, similar to those observed in the pseudopodia of activated platelets. Alpha-actinin is now thought to be an integral membrane glycoprotein (GP IIIa), and seems implicated in linking microfilaments to the platelet membrane, and platelet membranes to each other (Gerrard et al, 1979a; Phillips et al, 1979). Actin-binding protein (ABP) does not seem to be membrane bound in resting platelets. There is some evidence suggesting ABP may require phosphorylation for its actin crosslinking activity (Wallach et al, 1978; Lucas et al, 1979).

The concentration of myosin in platelets is much less than in skeletal muscle. Consequently there is a significantly greater molar excess of actin over myosin in platelets (100:1) than in skeletal muscle (6:1) (Adelstein & Pollard, 1978). Because of the relative excess of actin in platelets, it has been suggested that platelet actomyosin contractile filaments might be capable of extreme shortening, and that actin may serve not only in formation of a platelet actomyosin contractile apparatus, but may also contribute to formation of a platelet cytoskeleton (Pollard et al, 1977; Lucas et al, 1979). While myosin contributes to the contractile apparatus, it may not be a structural component of the labile platelet cytoskeleton (Lucas et al, 1979).

Platelet myosin is structurally somewhat different from skeletal muscle myosin. Two different myosin light chains are bound noncovalently to the globular 'head' region of one myosin heavy chain, two sets of each of the three polypeptides forming the dimerized platelet myosin molecule by noncovalent bonding (Pollard et al, 1977; Adelstein & Pollard, 1978). During platelet activation bipolar filaments of myosin form from soluble myosin so that globular myosin heads are exposed near each end of the filaments. The 'head' domains of myosin are responsible for binding to actin filaments, and for the myosin ATPase activity that is seen concomitantly, generating contractile force and movement.

A series of regulatory proteins has been recently recognized in platelets, providing a biochemical basis for calcium dependent regulation of the actin-activated myosin ATPase contractile activity described above. It is now believed that phosphorylation of the larger of the two light chains of myosin significantly increases both actin-activated myosin ATPase activity and the contractile force generated by platelet actomyosin (Adelstein & Conti, 1975; Lebowitz & Cooke, 1978). Phosphorylation of platelet myosin light chain is mediated, in the presence of magnesium and ATP, by a myosin light chain kinase which requires calcium and a calcium dependent regulatory protein (CDR, calmodulin) for its activity (Adelstein & Pollard, 1978; Dabrowska & Hartshorne, 1978; Hathaway & Adelstein, 1979). Once phosphorylated, myosin interacts with actin and ATP to produce contractile force proportional to the extent of phosphorylation (Lebowitz & Cooke, 1978). Thus platelet myosin can be 'switched on' by calcium. Platelet myosin light chain phosphatase may be able to 'switch off' myosin (Barylko et al, 1977). Evidence for the importance of this phosphorylation in platelet function comes from studies showing that phosphorylation occurs during activation of platelets induced by thrombin, collagen, or the calcium ionophore, A23187 (Daniel et al, 1977; Haslam & Lynham, 1976, 1977). Other platelet proteins which might also regulate myosin include a myosin phosphorylation factor (Hadgian & Feinstein, 1979) and a calcium-independent myosin light chain kinase (Daniel & Adelstein, 1976).

In skeletal muscle the tropomyosin-troponin complex provides for the calcium dependent regulation of actin, shielding the myosin binding sites of filamentous actin when calcium is not present (Smillie, 1979). Platelets contain tropomyosin (Cohen &

Cohen, 1972; Côté et al, 1978), but platelet troponin has not been identified with certainty (Cohen et al, 1973; Adelstein & Pollard, 1978).

Intermediate or ten nanometer filaments are cytoskeletal structures found in a variety of mammalian cell types, but these or their protein components have not yet been identified in platelets (Lazarides, 1980).

The retraction of blood clots by platelets is a remarkable feat, considering that clot volume can be reduced nearly 50 per cent by cells which, in their resting state, would comprise less than 1 per cent of the initial clot volume (Adelstein & Pollard, 1978). This phenomenon can probably be accounted for by the binding of platelet surfaces to fibrin and to each other, by the long filaments of actin observed in the extended pseudopodia of activated platelets, and by the hypothesized extreme shortening provided by the platelet contractile apparatus.

Prostaglandins

Prostaglandins and thromboxanes are a group of lipids with major regulatory effects on platelets. The production of these compounds by platelets and the vessel wall is outlined in Figure 1.4.

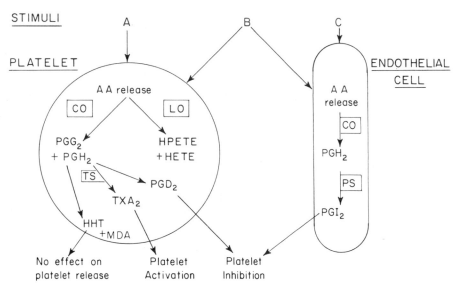

Fig. 1.4   Metabolism of arachidonic acid in platelets and endothelial cells. Various stimuli (A, B or C), can effect a release of arachidonic acid in either one or both locations. Abbreviations used include: AA = arachidonic acid; PG = prostaglandin; CO = fatty acid cyclooxygenase; LO = lipoxygenase; TS = thromboxane synthetase; PS = prostacyclin synthetase; TXA_2 = thromboxane A_2; HPETE = 12L-hydroperoxy-5,8,10,14 eicosatetraenoic acid; HETE = 12L-hydroxy-5,8,10,14-eicosatetraenoic acid; HHT = 12L-hydroxy-5,8,10-heptadecatrienoic acid; MDA = malondialdehyde. PGD_2, a relatively minor product of platelet arachidonic acid metabolism, is included as it can inhibit platelet function and may be important in some circumstances. Not included are PGE_2 and $PGF_{2\alpha}$, two minor products with little effect on platelet function.

Arachidonic acid, the usual substrate for platelet prostaglandin synthesis, is made available when a stimulus acts on platelets, liberating this unsaturated fatty acid from the 2-position of platelet glycerophospholipids. Labelling studies (Bills et al, 1976) suggest arachidonic acid is released from phosphatidylcholine and phosphatidylinositol (PI), while direct measurement of fatty acids shows a decrease only in PI-released arachidonic acid (Broekman et al, 1979; Lapetina & Cuatrecasas, 1979).

Two pathways have been proposed for fatty acid release. A phospholipase A_2 enzyme was first proposed. However, numerous attempts to isolate a sufficiently active and specific enzyme from platelets have so far failed (Apitz-Castro et al, 1979; Trugnan et al, 1979; Jesse & Franson, 1979). This may be due to a failure to reconstitute the enzyme with critical components or activators. The alternate pathway involves an initial phospholipase C enzyme which cleaves PI, specifically producing diglyceride (Rittenhouse-Simmons, 1979; Mauco et al, 1979). Since PI in platelets contains almost solely arachidonic acid and stearic acid, the observed specificity for arachidonic acid could be controlled. The second step in this pathway could be a diglyceride lipase which attacks the diglyceride, releasing arachidonic acid (Bell et al, 1979; Bry et al, 1979). An argument against this pathway is that the diglyceride released by the phospholipase C may be almost entirely converted to phosphatidic acid (Lapetina & Cuatrecasas, 1979). At the present time, evidence supports the initial event being activation of phospholipase C, but whether arachidonic acid is released from the diglyceride or secondarily by activation of phospholipase A_2 remains to be determined.

Following arachidonic acid release, the fatty acid is converted by a cyclo-oxygenase enzyme to two labile endoperoxides, PGG_2 and PGH_2, or by a lipoxygenase enzyme to HPETE and HETE (Fig. 1.4) (Hamberg & Samuelsson, 1974). The endoperoxides are converted primarily to thromboxane A_2 by a thromboxane synthetase, or spontaneously to the degradation products HHT and MDA, with small amounts being converted to PGD_2, PGE_2, and $PGF_{2\alpha}$ by specific synthetases. Thromboxane A_2, a very potent aggregating agent, has a short half-life and is degraded to thromboxane B_2 (Hamberg et al, 1975), although in plasma thromboxane A_2 is more stable and has a half-life of several minutes (Smith et al, 1976). Addition of thromboxane A_2 to platelets causes shape change with pseudopod formation and granule centralization (Gerrard & White, 1978). It can directly (without ADP release) cause stickiness of platelets to form aggregates, and it can also cause granule secretion (Hamberg et al, 1975; Charo et al, 1977; Gerrard & White, 1978). Some evidence implicates a flux of calcium triggered by this agent as being critically involved (Gerrard & White, 1978). Controversy exists as to whether PGG_2 and PGH_2 must be converted to thromboxane A_2 or whether they have some activating effect on their own. In the absence of specific inhibitors, the endoperoxides are rapidly metabolized to thromboxane A_2, so that in the usual situation thromboxane A_2 is the major active agent.

Prostaglandin I_2 (PGI_2, PGX, prostacyclin), produced by the vessel wall from prostaglandin endoperoxides, potently inhibits platelet activation by elevating cyclic AMP levels in platelets (Moncada et al, 1976; Gorman et al, 1977; Tateson et al, 1977). Prostaglandin D_2, produced by platelets, acts similarly but is less potent, and since less is produced it is probably much less significant (Oelz et al, 1977). It is uncertain whether endoperoxides from platelets are used by cells in the vessel wall, as suggested by Moncada and Vane (1979). It would appear that usually platelet endoperoxides are rapidly converted in platelets, so little escapes (Needleman et al, 1979b). Where thromboxane synthetase is specifically inhibited conversion of platelet endoperoxides to PGI_2 by the vessel wall may be important.

The production of prostaglandins and thromboxanes with activating and inhibitory actions has led to the concept that a balance in production of these compounds may be critical in overall hemostatic function, with alterations in disease states contributing to bleeding or thrombotic tendencies (Moncada et al, 1976; Gerrard & White, 1978). Of particular interest in this regard are studies of eicosapentaenoic acid, a fatty acid found in certain fish which can be an alternate substance for prostaglandin synthesis (Dyerberg & Bang, 1978; Culp et al, 1979; Needleman et al, 1979a). Some controversy exists concerning the exact metabolism of this fatty acid in vivo but it would appear that it is a relatively poor substrate for cyclo-oxygenase, and acts primarily as an inhibitor of arachidonic acid conversion (Needleman et al, 1979a). The result is that platelets enriched in this fatty acid function less well than normal platelets (Dyerberg & Bang, 1978). Eskimos with a diet rich in this fatty acid may have a mild bleeding disorder, and may be protected against atherosclerosis (Dyerberg & Bang, 1978, 1979).

Another dietary factor which has been shown to influence prostaglandin and thromboxane synthesis is cholesterol. Enrichment of platelet membranes with cholesterol enhances production of thromboxane A_2 in response to thrombin (Stuart et al, 1980). In addition to the effects of dietary manipulations, the potential for using drugs to alter prostaglandin and thromboxane synthesis has also been an area of considerable recent study. These are discussed more fully in Chapter 2 in the section on acquired platelet disorders.

Calcium

An increasing body of evidence assigns calcium important roles both extracellularly and intracellularly in platelet function. Extracellular calcium is required for cell-cell attachment during the aggregation process, perhaps because it is needed to facilitate fibrinogen binding (Bennett & Vilaire, 1979). Calcium levels in plasma are more than sufficient for this function, although secretion of calcium from dense granules during platelet activation may provide additional calcium for the local area near the cell membrane.

Intracellularly, cytoplasmic calcium plays a pivotal role during platelet activation. In the resting cell, cytoplasmic calcium is believed to be maintained at a very low concentration (10^{-7} to 10^{-8} M). Many lines of evidence support the concept that a flux of calcium occurs on cell stimulation, raising cytoplasmic calcium levels and causing a change in platelet shape leading to pseudopod extension, granule centralization, secretion, and an alteration in the external surface membrane rendering it sticky so that cell-cell attachment or aggregation can occur (Massini, 1977; Detwiler et al, 1978). At a biochemical level calcium has been shown to regulate actin-myosin interaction, and the activity of platelet phospholipases C and A_2. Calcium activation of these processes may require the calcium-dependent regulatory protein, calmodulin (Dabrowska & Hartshorne, 1978; Hathaway & Adelstein, 1979; Wong & Cheung, 1979).

It appears that there are at least two mechanisms involved in producing the flux of calcium which stimulates platelet shape change and granule centralization, the first dependent on production of prostaglandin endoperoxides and thromboxane A_2, the second independent of such production (Gerrard & White, 1978). The dense tubular system (DTS) seems to be the critical calcium storage reservoir utilized as a source of this cation, although small amounts may also be released from the plasma membrane, and some extracellular calcium may be recruited during the late stages of platelet activation by thrombin (Massini, 1977). The demonstration that thromboxane A_2 was synthesized in the DTS has led to the concept that thromboxane A_2 might mediate calcium release from the DTS by serving as a calcium ionophore (Gerrard & White, 1978). Some evidence supports this concept, but additional studies are needed to better understand this mechanism and its control.

Other evidence implicates phosphatidylinositol turnover as an important component of the thromboxane A_2-independent mechanism for producing calcium flux (Gerrard et al, 1979c). Phosphatidic acid and lysophosphatidic acid, produced as a result of the breakdown of phosphatidylinositol, can under some circumstances act as calcium ionophores and may be directly involved in mediating calcium flux. A lysophospholipid, 'platelet activating factor', may also be involved in a thromboxane-independent mechanism (Chignard et al, 1979).

An intriguing aspect of the platelet phosphatidylinositoi response is that the arachidonic acid used for synthesis of thromboxane A_2 may in certain circumstances be released from the diacylglycerol produced during phosphatidylinositol degradation by phospholipase C (Bell et al, 1979). This suggests a close interrelationship between thromboxane A_2-independent and -dependent mechanisms, as might be expected from results showing that strong platelet stimuli like thrombin usually activate both mechanisms. Evidence that calcium is involved both in steps (phospholipase C and A_2) leading to release of arachidonic acid (the precursor of thromboxane A_2) as well as in the effects of thromboxane A_2 has led to the concept that a series of two interrelated calcium fluxes may occur during platelet activation (Gerrard & White, 1978). This concept may be supported by recent studies differentiating calcium fluxes induced by epinephrine and by arachidonic acid (Johnson et al, 1979; Owen & Le Breton, 1979).

Cyclic nucleotides
Cyclic AMP appears to be very important as a second messenger mediating the inhibition of a variety of platelet functions including the inhibition of shape change, granule centralization, secretion, aggregation, fibrinogen binding and phospholipase C activation (Haslam et al, 1978; Hawiger et al, 1980; Lapetina et al, 1980). Increased cyclic AMP levels may be produced by such agents as prostaglandins D_2, E_1 and I_2 or adenosine which activate adenylate cyclase to cause synthesis of cyclic AMP, and by dipyridamole or theophylline which inhibit the phosphodiesterase responsible for degradation of cyclic AMP. The major inhibitory effect of cyclic AMP is currently believed to be through its action on a protein kinase to phosphorylate a 24 000 molecular weight protein which facilitates the removal of calcium from the cytoplasm and the storage of this cation in the dense tubular system (Käser-Glanzmann et al, 1977; Fox et al, 1979). In view of the widespread effects of calcium on platelet function, it is certainly possible that the major inhibitory effects of cyclic AMP are exerted primarily through this effect on calcium sequestration. Further study of this mechanism is needed, as the magnitude of the effect on calcium sequestration so far demonstrated is less than might be predicted from knowledge of the potency of cyclic AMP as an inhibitory agent.

Guanylate cyclase, the enzyme which synthesizes cyclic GMP, is stimulated during platelet activation induced by many agents, resulting in a raised level of cyclic GMP and perhaps a considerable increase in the turnover of this nucleotide (Goldberg & Haddox, 1977). The function of cyclic GMP is unclear as addition of it or analogs to platelets has no effect, and agents such as ascorbic acid can markedly elevate platelet cyclic GMP levels without producing an effect on the platelets themselves. One recent suggestion is that cyclic GMP may provide a localized energy source.

Platelet interactions with coagulation proteins
It has long been recognized that platelets contribute to plasmatic coagulation, in addition to or as part of their functions in primary hemostasis. Recent investigations amplify these aspects of platelet function, underscoring a major role for platelets in generating various coagulant activities and in directing or localizing such activities within the vascular system so as to form a platelet-fibrin hemostatic plug. Furthermore, there is increasing evidence that coagulation proteins (such as fibrinogen and fibrin, prothrombin and thrombin, von Willebrand factor, and probably factor V/Va and factor X/Xa) are essential for normal platelet hemostatic function. Additionally, significant amounts of certain coagulation proteins are found in platelets and may be secreted or otherwise made available during platelet activation. Finally, platelets may avidly bind some coagulation proteins, thereby providing for: (1) platelet adhesion to surfaces (e.g. by binding von Willebrand factor); or (2) a catalytic mechanism for the ultimate, localized generation of thrombin and fibrin (e.g. by binding factors Xa and Va to form the prothrombinase complex); or (3) platelet activation as a consequence of such binding (e.g. by binding thrombin); or (4) platelet aggregation as a consequence of such binding (e.g. binding of fibrinogen or fibrin).

The association of coagulation proteins with platelets is outlined in Table 1.5, while

Table 1.5   Platelet association of coagulation factors[a]

Platelet association[b]	Clotting factors
Loosely adsorbed	Plasma Fibrinogen Prothrombin Factor VII Factor IX Factor X
Less readily eluted	Factor VIII:C Plasma Factor XI Plasma Factor XII
Not eluted	Platelet Fibrinogen Platelet Factor XIII Factor V Factor VIII R:Ag Platelet Factor XI-like activity
Bound to platelet membranes	Fibrinogen[c] Thrombin Factor V and Va Factor Xa Factor VIII R:Ag Factor IXa? Factor XI/XIa?

[a] Modified from Walsh (1979)
[b] Non-activated platelets
[c] Requires platelet activation

Table 1.2 contains information about platelet membrane receptors for coagulation proteins, and Table 1.3 notes the localization of certain coagulation factors within platelet organelles.

Fibrinogen

In addition to plasma fibrinogen loosely adsorbed to non-activated platelets, intracellular fibrinogen represents 2 to 6 per cent of total platelet proteins and is stored in platelet α-granules (James et al, 1977; Kaplan et al, 1979b). Platelet factor 5 is platelet fibrinogen (Owen et al, 1975; Ulutin, 1976). Characterization of fibrinogens from the platelets and the plasma of patients with congenital dysfibrinogenemias indicates that platelet fibrinogen may be structurally and functionally different from plasma fibrinogen (Soria et al, 1976; James et al, 1977; Jandrot-Perres et al, 1979). Other studies, demonstrating lack of exchange between platelet and plasma fibrinogen pools, support a possible uniqueness of intraplatelet fibrinogen (Castaldi & Caen, 1965; Nachman & Marcus, 1968; James et al, 1977). Conversely, Doolittle et al (1974) maintain that platelet and plasma fibrinogens are identical. The intraplatelet fibrinogen content is reduced but apparently not absent in congenital afibrinogenemia (Castaldi & Caen, 1965; Nachman & Marcus, 1968; Weiss & Rogers, 1971), and is greatly reduced in most, but not all cases of Glanzmann's thrombasthenia (Castaldi & Caen, 1965; Caen et al, 1966; Peterson et al, 1979).

A third mechanism of fibrinogen association with platelets has been recently recognized by the demonstration of specific platelet receptors for plasmatic fibrinogen (Bennett & Vilaire, 1979; Marguerie et al, 1979; Plow et al, 1979b; Hawiger et al, 1980). These high affinity binding sites (Table 1.2) are not expressed in resting platelets, but can be readily induced by exogenous ADP, epinephrine or thrombin. Platelet fibrinogen binding activity is supported by divalent cations and occurs concomitantly with the initial shape change of platelet activation induced by ADP. Prostacyclin and PGD_2 potently inhibit the expression of these stimulus-induced fibrinogen binding sites on platelets (Hawiger et al, 1980), probably as a consequence of increased platelet cyclic AMP levels induced by these prostaglandins.

Fibrinogen plays an essential role in platelet hemostatic plug formation, as indicated by several lines of evidence. Afibrinogenemic patients frequently have prolonged bleeding times (Weiss & Rogers, 1971; Owen et al, 1975), and moderate deficiencies of platelet aggregation in these patients support a role for fibrinogen in the development of such aggregates (Inceman et al, 1966; Weiss & Rogers, 1971). The relatively mild deficiencies of platelet function may be explained by the requirement for only very small amounts of membrane-bound fibrinogen for platelet aggregation (Mustard et al, 1978, 1979), and the avidity of platelet membrane binding sites for available fibrinogen (Bennett & Vilaire, 1979). Platelets from patients with Glanzmann's thrombasthenia lack membrane binding sites for fibrinogen, and cannot form aggregates in response to ADP, epinephrine, collagen or thrombin (Bennett & Vilaire, 1979; Mustard et al, 1979; Peerschke et al, 1979; Coller, 1980).

The essential role of fibrinogen in platelet-platelet attachment is substantiated by studies on washed normal cells which show that fibrinogen is necessary for the primary wave of platelet aggregation induced by ADP or epinephrine (Mustard et al, 1978, 1979). When the surfaces of washed normal platelets are treated with proteolytic enzymes, fibrinogen receptors become available; exogenous fibrinogen can then bind to these receptors and induce platelet-platelet attachment (Greenberg et al, 1979a; Mustard et al, 1979). Miller et al (1975) and Tollefsen and Majerus (1975), studying the inhibition of thrombin-induced aggregation of washed platelets by plasmin or by antifibrinogen antibody, have provided evidence that platelets may secrete the fibrinogen necessary for thrombin-induced platelet aggregation. Collagen-induced platelet aggregation proceeds readily in washed suspensions of normal platelets (Huzoor-Akbar & Ardlie, 1976), but mildly deficient collagen-induced aggregation of afibrinogenemic platelets (Weiss & Rogers, 1971) and delayed collagen-induced aggregation of gel filtered platelets together with acceleration of clumping when fibrinogen is added (Fine et al, 1976) suggest that plasmatic or platelet fibrinogen are probably involved in collagen-induced platelet aggregation.

Polymerizing or polymerized fibrin can activate platelets (Niewiarowski et al, 1972; Michaeli & Orloff, 1976; Orloff & Michaeli, 1976). Chao et al (1980) have shown that fibrinogen can be secreted relatively rapidly from washed platelets following thrombin stimulation, and that the secreted fibrinogen is subsequently found, immunologically and ultrastructurally, as fibrin deposited on the membrane surfaces of aggregated platelets. Other ultrastructural studies also support a bridging role for fibrin in platelet-platelet attachment (Shirasawa et al, 1972).

Fibrinogen seems of lesser importance for platelet adhesion to subendothelial surfaces since such adhesion is essentially normal in Glanzmann's thrombasthenia (Baumgartner et al, 1977) in which platelet fibrinogen binding is absent. The adhesion of platelets to foreign surfaces is enhanced by fibrinogen (Mason et al, 1976; Michaeli & Orloff, 1976; Salzman et al, 1977; Coller, 1980).

Factor XIII

Plasma factor XIII (fibrin stabilizing factor) consists of two subunits noncovalently associated to form a tetrameric complex, a_2b_2 (Rider et al, 1978). Platelet and megakaryocyte cytoplasm contains only the potentially catalytic factor XIII subunit, a_2 which is structurally, immunologically and functionally identical with the plasma a_2 subunit. Platelet factor XIII contributes substantially to total factor XIII activity found in blood. Thrombocytopenia significantly decreases plasma factor XIII activity, suggesting a major role for platelets in the generation of this activity (Rider et al, 1978). Cohen and associates (1979a, 1979c) and Mui and Ganguly (1977) have implicated activated factor XIII or a factor XIIIa-like platelet transamidase in the calcium dependent cross-linking of platelet contractile proteins, membrane glycoproteins and fibrin. Depletion of platelet nucleotides, as a consequence of platelet activation and secretion, may be important in the facilitation of factor XIIIa-catalyzed cross-linking of these proteins (Cohen et al, 1979c). The relatively large amount of factor XIII in platelets may also allow for a high local concentration of this fibrin stabilizing enzyme in platelet-fibrin hemostatic plugs, although there is evidence that platelet factor XIII may not be secreted during platelet activation (Joist & Niewiarowski, 1973).

Thrombin

Thrombin is one of the most potent activators of platelets. Interaction of thrombin with the platelet surface is thought to represent the initial event in platelet activation by thrombin. Several investigators have characterized thrombin binding to platelets

(Table 1.2), noting high and low affinity binding. Evidence suggests the differing affinities may represent two classes of thrombin binding sites, the higher affinity sites being probably more important (Workman et al, 1977; Tam et al, 1979). The binding of thrombin to the platelet surface can be distinguished from its platelet activating effects, as modified and inactivated thrombin binds normally to platelets, but does not activate them (Tollefsen et al, 1974; Mohammed et al, 1976; Workman et al, 1977; Tam & Detwiler, 1978). Only catalytically active thrombin, able to convert fibrinogen to fibrin, seems capable both of binding to platelets and of producing platelet aggregation or secretion.

There is a variety of evidence (reviewed by Okumura et al, 1978 and by Ganguly & Gould, 1979) implicating components of the platelet membrane GP I complex in thrombin binding, but their role as the putative thrombin receptor is not firmly established. Photoaffinity labelling (Larsen & Simons, 1979) suggests other platelet glycoproteins might serve as thrombin receptors, while another membrane glycoprotein (GP V) may be a proteolytic substrate for thrombin (Phillips & Agin, 1977b; Berndt & Phillips, 1979; Mosher et al, 1979). The latter 'thrombin sensitive protein' of the platelet membrane is distinct from the α-granule major glycoprotein, thrombospondin or TSP, secreted from thrombin stimulated platelets (Phillips & Agin, 1977b; Lawler et al, 1978). Since catalytically active thrombin seems necessary for platelet activation, it has been thought that a proteolytic event may be essential for thrombin-induced platelet activation. This concept remains conjectural.

Once membrane bound, thrombin potently induces platelet secretion or aggregation or both, apparently by diverse mechanisms. When stirred with platelets, thrombin causes platelet aggregation and secretion of granule contents, while in the absence of stirring, secretion still occurs (Mills & MacFarlane, 1976). Aggregation-independent platelet secretion can also be induced by collagen, but not by ADP or epinephrine (Charo et al, 1977). At low concentrations of thrombin, platelet secretion can be mediated by prostaglandin endoperoxides and thromboxanes, while higher thrombin concentrations can elicit secretion even when cyclooxygenase is blocked and cyclic AMP levels are elevated by PGI_2 (Charo et al, 1977; Shuman et al, 1979). The biochemical basis of this latter platelet activation pathway is not known, but could involve translocation of calcium (Kinlough-Rathbone et al, 1977) or release of lysophospholipid from membranes (Chignard et al, 1979; Gerrard et al, 1979d). There is some evidence to suggest that thrombin, perhaps generated on platelet surfaces, may be important in the mediation of collagen-induced platelet aggregation in plasma (Huzoor-Akbar & Ardlie, 1977c; Nichols et al, 1980).

Prothrombinase complex
Thrombin is most effectively generated from its zymogen precursor, prothrombin, by the participation of several components to form the 'prothrombinase complex' (Nesheim et al, 1980). These components include factor Xa, factor V/Va, ionic calcium, and phospholipid vesicles or membranes. Although artificial lipid bilayers or membranes from other blood cells can serve as a source of phospholipid for the prothrombinase complex, there is reasonable evidence that platelets normally are the major source, serving to localize thrombin generation in the vascular system. As this important topic is treated in some detail in Chapter 3, only the major points are noted here, and depicted schematically in Figure 1.5.

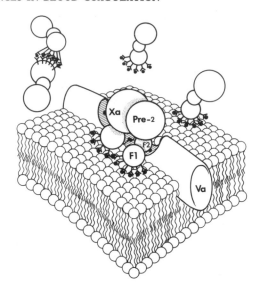

Fig. 1.5   Model of the activation of prothrombin, catalyzed by the prothrombinase complex, as it might occur on the surface of the platelet membrane lipid bilayer. A molecule of factor Va is embedded in the lipid surface and is in 1:1 stoichiometry with factor Xa, activation of the factor Va cofactor through proteolytic cleavage being suggested by a fissure in the model. Molecules of prothrombin, with the prothrombin fragment 1, prothrombin fragment 2 and prethrombin 2 domains, are shown both in solution and bound to the lipid surface, the latter accomplished through calcium ion bridging mediated by the γ-carboxyglutamate residues of the fragment 1 domain. Reprinted by permission of M. E. Nesheim and K. G. Mann, and Elsevier/North-Holland, New York (Nesheim et al, 1980).

Platelet factor 3 (PF 3) activity generally refers to the ability of platelets to accelerate prothrombin consumption, thrombin generation and fibrin formation in plasma (Owen et al, 1975; Ulutin, 1976; Shattil & Cooper, 1978). Though there is little doubt that platelets accelerate clotting by providing a phospholipo(glyco)protein surface, this general procoagulant activity of platelets remains poorly defined functionally and structurally. As there is now reasonable evidence that a number of apparently different platelet procoagulant activities may contribute to PF 3 activity (e.g., platelet participation in the prothrombinase and 'tenase' complexes, other factor X-converting activities of platelets, platelet contact or collagen-induced coagulant activities), this term is probably best avoided except in a general sense. Prothrombin consumption, one measure of PF 3 activity, remains of some use as a screening test of platelet function.

Both *factor V and factor Va* (produced by thrombin cleavage of factor V) can bind with high affinity to specific sites on the platelet surface, evidence suggesting that two different membrane binding sites may be involved (Table 1.2) (Tracy et al, 1979, 1980). Although phospholipids, particularly the acidic phospholipids, are probably vital in such binding (Bloom et al, 1979), the participation of membrane protein and the structural organization of the platelet membrane binding sites for these coagulation proteins is not known. It is thought that in plasma the factor V binding sites of platelet membranes are mostly saturated with factor V (Tracy et al, 1980), perhaps thereby providing a catalytic surface for initial generation of small amounts of thrombin from prothrombin when factor Xa is present (Nesheim et al, 1980; Tracy et al, 1980). One may speculate that such thrombin might activate both platelets and certain coagulation proteins (e.g. factor V), greatly accelerating the local production of thrombin on the platelet surface. Binding of factor Va to platelet surfaces apparently does not require platelet activation (Tracy et al, 1979; Kane et al, 1980). In addition to the surface localization of factor V on platelets, it is thought that this protein is also localized intracellularly (Breederveld et al, 1975; Østerud et al, 1977; Kane et al, 1980), perhaps in α-granules (Pifer et al, 1977) from which it might be secreted.

The specific, high affinity binding of *factor Xa* to platelets is mediated through the receptor function generated by factor Va and its membrane binding site (Miletich et al, 1978; Dahlbäck & Stenflo, 1978; Kane et al, 1980) in conjunction with ionic calcium, so as to form the prothrombinase complex (Fig. 1.5). Additional evidence that factor Va forms a major component of the factor Xa receptor site on platelets comes from studies showing deficient binding of factor Xa to platelets in the presence of alloantibodies to factor V or in patients congenitally deficient in factor V (Majerus et al, 1980). Severe deficiency of factor V, though rare, produces a significant hemorrhagic diathesis, frequently associated with prolongation of the bleeding time (Owen et al, 1975). A patient lacking platelet factor Xa (and presumably factor Va) binding sites has a bleeding disorder characterized by deficient platelet procoagulant activity and abnormal prothrombin consumption, but normal bleeding times, normal plasmatic coagulation proteins, and apparently normal platelet lipid and protein composition (Miletich et al, 1979; Weiss et al, 1979a).

Once assembled, the *prothrombinase complex* can rapidly generate thrombin from prothrombin (Nesheim et al, 1980), evidence indicating that thrombin formation may occur early in the initial stages of blood clotting (Jensen et al, 1976; Shuman & Majerus, 1976; Majerus et al, 1980), perhaps thereby providing small amounts of thrombin sufficient for the activation of platelets and some coagulation proteins. Binding of factor Xa to platelets is thought to protect this factor against inactivation by antithrombin III (Miletich et al, 1978), while the factor Va on the platelet surface may, by binding factor Xa to form the prothrombinase complex, be protected from inactivation by activated protein C, a vitamin K-dependent protease (Comp & Esmon, 1979; Nesheim et al, 1980). It is not yet clear whether factor V or factor Va on platelet surfaces participates in the thrombin formation seen early in blood clotting, but it is apparent from information available that platelets contribute significantly to the localized generation of thrombin in the vascular system.

Factor X activation
Activation of factor X to form factor Xa is believed to be a critical step in the hemostatic mechanism, allowing formation of the prothrombinase complex and the ultimate generation of thrombin. There appear to be several catalytic mechanisms available for the activation of factor X in blood (Seegers, 1976; Semeraro & Vermylen, 1977; Seegers & Ghosh, 1980), some probably of more importance than others for hemostasis in vivo. Evidence indicates that platelets participate in at least two of these factor X activation mechanisms, perhaps thereby allowing for the local generation of factor Xa on platelet surfaces.

Platelet '*intrinsic factor Xa-forming activity*' refers to the ability of platelets to catalyze the activation of factor X in the presence of factor IXa, factor VIII/VIIIa and ionic calcium which, with platelets, are thought to form a *'tenase complex'* (Zwaal, 1978; Walsh, 1979) possibly analogous organizationally to the prothrombinase complex (Fig. 1.5). The structural features of the platelet membrane which mediate this activity are largely unknown, but it is thought that the phospholipid requirements for the tenase complex may be different from those mediating the prothrombinase complex (Walsh, 1978).

Semeraro and Vermylen (1977) have described an apparently *'direct' factor X activator activity* of platelets which seems independent of factors VII, VIII or IX, and of exogenous platelet stimulation. Direct activation of factor X has also been observed by van Wijk et al (1979), using purified human factor X and washed human platelets. Neither the mechanism nor the relative importance of this means of factor X activation is clear, but investigations by Semeraro et al (1979) suggest this platelet activity may often be deficient in those patients with chronic myeloproliferative disorders who have a bleeding diathesis.

Willebrand factor
In addition to its presence in plasma and in or on vascular surfaces, von Willebrand factor [factor VIII-related antigen (VIIIR:Ag) and activity (VIIIR:WF)] is also found in megakaryocytes and in platelets (Howard et al, 1974; Nachman & Jaffe, 1975; Nachman et al, 1977b; Piovella et al, 1978; Slot et al, 1978) apparently partly localized in α-granules from which it can be secreted during platelet activation processes (Koutts et al, 1978; Sultan et al, 1979; Zucker et al, 1979a). Specific binding of Willebrand factor to platelets has been identified (Kao et al, 1979a, b; Schneider-Trip et al, 1979). The extent of such binding in vitro seems to depend on the presence and concentration of ristocetin in the human test system, the values cited in Table 1.2 being obtained at 1 mg/ml ristocetin. These platelet membrane binding sites may preferentially bind the higher molecular weight, more active forms of Willebrand factor (Doucet de Bruïne et al, 1978; Koutts & Zimmerman, 1979), the nature and extent of glycosylation of Willebrand factor being perhaps also of importance for its platelet binding and aggregation-promoting properties (De Marco et al, 1979; Gralnick & Morisato, 1979). The physiological counterpart of ristocetin remains unknown, but recent reports suggest that treatment of platelets with small amounts of thrombin (which might be generated early in the hemostatic process in vivo) can induce binding sites for Willebrand factor, similar to those expressed in the presence of ristocetin (Koutts & Zimmerman, 1979; Ohara & Hawiger, 1979).

Binding of Willebrand factor to platelets is thought to be of major importance for platelet adhesion to subendothelial vascular surfaces although other mechanisms, Willebrand factor-independent and poorly defined, also contribute to platelet-vessel wall adhesion which may be mediated via 'multiple interactions' (Santoro & Cunningham, 1979). Willebrand factor-dependent adhesion of platelets to the vascular wall is mainly operative in ex vivo systems at high wall-shear-rate flow conditions (which allow only brief contacts of platelets with vessel walls), such as those found in small blood vessels and capillaries (Baumgartner et al, 1977; Tschopp & Baumgartner, 1980). Platelet adhesion to the subendothelium is deficient not only in von Willebrand's disease (vWD), but also in the Bernard-Soulier syndrome (Weiss et al, 1974; Caen et al, 1976; Baumgartner et al, 1977) in which platelets lack components of the membrane glycoprotein I (GP I) complex (Caen et al, 1976;

Nurden & Caen, 1979), do not aggregate in response to ristocetin and Willebrand factor (Nurden & Caen, 1978), and are deficient in membrane binding sites for Willebrand factor (Ando et al, 1979; Moake et al, 1979). Antibodies directed against components of the membrane GP I complex inhibit platelet aggregation induced by ristocetin and factor VIIIR:WF, and also inhibit platelet adhesion to subendothelial surfaces (Tobelem et al, 1976; Nachman et al, 1977a). These studies indicate that platelet membrane binding of Willebrand factor is probably important for platelet-vessel adhesion, and that certain membrane glycoproteins are essential for such binding. The origins, structural and functional differences, and the relative contributions of intra-platelet, membrane-bound, plasmatic, endothelial or subendothelial Willebrand factor in platelet-vessel hemostatic interaction are not yet clear. Recent studies suggest that intra-platelet VIIIR:Ag may be decreased or absent in some patients with von Willebrand's disease, and that the intra-platelet VIIIR:Ag in other patients with vWD may sometimes be structurally or functionally abnormal, or not secreted in response to platelet stimulation (Meucci et al, 1978; Ruggeri et al, 1978; Holmberg & Nilsson, 1979; Sultan et al, 1979). These differing anomalies of intra-platelet Willebrand factor may reflect the several variant types of von Willebrand's disease thought to exist, including a recently described variant in which platelet binding of VIIIR:Ag and platelet aggregation are increased in the presence of ristocetin (Ruggeri & Zimmerman, 1980).

Other platelet coagulant activities

A number of platelet coagulant or anticoagulant activities have been described, in addition to those already reviewed. The mechanisms and importance of these additional platelet activities in the hemostatic process are less well defined.

Platelet *factor XI-like activities* may apparently result either from an endogenous factor XI-like protein present in or on platelet membranes, or from platelet mediated activation of membrane-associated plasmatic factor XI (Lipscomb & Walsh, 1979; Connellan et al, 1980; Walsh & Tuszynski, 1980). These platelet activities can be promoted by collagen or thrombin, and have also been called 'collagen-induced coagulant activity'. It has been proposed that such platelet procoagulant activities may be specifically deficient in the Bernard-Soulier syndrome (Lipscomb & Walsh, 1979), in some patients with Glanzmann's thrombasthenia (Walsh, 1979), or in some patients with Hemophilia A (Walsh, 1979) and may be increased in certain patients with plasmatic factor XI deficiency (Walsh & Tuszynski, 1980), or with chronic myeloproliferative disorders (Walsh et al, 1977b). Such variability in platelet procoagulant activity in these disorders might account for the observed differences in clinical severity among patients with these disorders. Other investigators have not confirmed platelet factor XI-like activities (Schiffman et al, 1977; Giddings et al, 1978), perhaps because of differing assay systems. Interactions of platelets with components of the contact activation system are further reviewed in the chapter by Ogston.

Additional coagulant and anticoagulant activities reported to be associated with platelets include: platelet factor 6 or platelet *antiplasmins* (Owen et al, 1975; Joist et al, 1976; Ulutin, 1976; Joist, 1977); platelet *plasminogen activators and anti-activators* (Joist, 1977; Lockhart et al, 1979); platelet factor 2 or *fibrinogen activating factor* (Owen et al, 1975; Ulutin, 1976); platelet factor 7 or platelet *cothromboplastin* (Owen et al, 1975; Ulutin, 1976); platelet *antithrombin activities* (Tullis & Watanabe, 1978);

platelet α_2-*macroglobulin* and α_1-*antitrypsin* (Nachman & Harpel, 1976; Bagdasarian & Colman, 1978). *Platelet factor 4* is discussed in the section on α-granules, while *platelet factor 1* (platelet factor V/Va), *platelet factor 5* (platelet fibrinogen) and *platelet factor 3* are discussed in preceding paragraphs of this section.

Summary

During the decade since the first volume in this series, improved techniques in cell biology and biochemistry, coupled with an increasing interest by an expanding variety of investigators, have resulted in several significant advances in the recognition and understanding of platelet functions and their regulatory mechanisms.

In the hemostatic interaction of platelets with blood vessels and plasmatic coagulation proteins, the development of platelet 'stickiness' in response to a variety of specific stimuli is a crucial step, allowing adhesion of platelets to surfaces, cohesion of platelets to each other, and the ultimate generation of a properly localized platelet-fibrin plug. Several of the biochemical and structural processes mediating the genesis of platelet activation, stickiness and hemostatic plug formation have been identified and partially characterized. Recent studies emphasize that these processes are quite complex and probably finely tuned.

Structural features and receptor functions of the platelet plasma membrane, crucial both for platelet stimulation and for platelet responses, have been recognized. The identity, localization and possible roles of a number of cellular biochemical mediators and inhibitors of platelet activation (including cyclic nucleotides, certain lipids and prostaglandins, cytoskeletal and contractile proteins, calcium and calcium regulatory processes, and substances secreted during platelet activation) are now known, but imperfectly understood. The intimate and specific interaction of certain plasmatic coagulation proteins with the platelet plasma membrane is better understood, providing partial comprehension of the mechanisms mediating platelet activation, stickiness, adhesion, cohesion and procoagulant activities. Specific chemical substances (such as thromboxanes, calcium, adenine nucleotides and platelet-specific proteins), secreted or liberated externally during platelet activation processes, interact importantly both with platelets and with blood vessels so as to secure hemostasis and healing.

The study of patients whose platelets are defective in one or more of these many physiological processes has contributed importantly to current understanding of the relative importance of these processes for hemostasis in vivo. In Chapter 2 we review these platelet defects, particularly as they reflect the normal hemostatic mechanism.

BIBLIOGRAPHY

Adelstein R S, Conti M A 1975 Phosphorylation of platelet myosin increases actin-associated myosin ATPase activity. Nature 256: 597–598

Adelstein R S, Pollard T D 1978 Platelet contractile proteins. In: Spaet T H (ed) Progress in Hemostasis and Thrombosis, Grune & Stratton, New York, Vol 4, p 37–58

Adler, J R, Handin R I 1979 Solubilization and characterization of a platelet membrane ADP-binding protein. Journal of Biological Chemistry 254: 3866–3872

Akkerman J W H 1978 Regulation of carbohydrate metabolism in platelets: a review. Thrombosis and Haemostasis 39: 712–724

Andersson L C, Gahmberg C G 1978 Surface glycoproteins of human white blood cells: analysis by surface labelling. Blood 52: 57–67

Ando Y, Yamamoto M, Watanabe K, Ikeda Y, Toyama K, Yamada K 1979 Defective ^{125}I-factor VIII binding to platelets in patients with Bernard-Soulier syndrome and von Willebrand's disease. Thrombosis and Haemostasis 42: 374

Antoniades H N, Scher C D, Stiles C D 1979 Purification of human platelet-derived growth factor. Proceedings of the National Academy of Sciences, USA 76: 1809–1813

Aptiz-Castro R J, Mas M A, Crus M R, Jain M K 1979 Isolation of homogeneous phospholipase A$_2$ from human platelets. Biochemical and Biophysical Research Communications 91: 63–71

Bagdasarian A, Colman R W 1978 Subcellular localization and purification of platelet α_1-antitrypsin. Blood 51: 139–156

Barber A J, Käser-Glanzmann R, Jákabova M, Lüscher E F 1972 Characterization of a chondroitin 4-sulfate proteoglycan carrier for heparin neutralizing activity (platelet factor 4) released from human blood platelets. Biochimica et Biophysica Acta 286: 312–329

Barber A J, Pepper D S, Jamieson G A 1971 A comparison of methods for platelet lysis and the isolation of platelet membranes. Thrombosis et Diathesis Haemorrhagica 26: 38–57

Barylko B, Conti M A, Adelstein R S 1977 Properties of platelet myosin light chain phosphatase. Biophysical Journal 17: 270a

Baumgartner H R, Muggli R 1976 Adhesion and aggregation: morphological demonstration and quantitation in vivo and in vitro. In: Gordon J L (ed) Platelets in Biology and Pathology, Research Monographs in Cell and Tissue Physiology, Elsevier, Amsterdam, p 23–60

Baumgartner H R, Tschopp T B, Meyer D 1980 Shear rate dependent inhibition of platelet adhesion and aggregation on collagenous surfaces by antibodies to human factor VIII/vonWillebrand factor. British Journal of Haematology 44: 127–139

Baumgartner H R, Tschopp T B, Weiss H J 1977 Platelet interaction with collagen fibrils in flowing blood: II. Impaired adhesion-aggregation and bleeding disorders. Thrombosis and Haemostasis 37: 17–28

Bell R L, Kennerly D A, Stanford N, Majerus P W 1979 Diglyceride lipase: a pathway for arachidonate release from platelets. Proceedings of the National Academy of Sciences, USA 76: 3238–3241

Bennett J S, Vilaire G 1979 Exposure of platelet fibrinogen receptors by ADP and epinephrine. Journal of Clinical Investigation 64: 1393–1401

Bennett J S, Colman R F, Colman R W 1978 Identification of adenine nucleotide binding proteins in human platelet membranes by affinity labelling with 5'-p-fluorosulfonylbenzoyl adenosine. Journal of Biological Chemistry 253: 7346–7354

Bensusan H B, Koh R O, Henry K G, Murray B A, Culp L A 1978 Evidence that fibronectin is the collagen receptor on platelet membranes. Proceedings of the National Academy of Sciences, USA 75: 5864–5868

Bentfield M E, Bainton D F 1975 Cytochemical localization of lysosomal enzymes in rat megakaryocytes and platelets. Journal of Clinical Investigation 56: 1635–1639

Berndt M C, Phillips D R 1979 Purification of glycoprotein V, the thrombin substrate on platelet membranes. Blood 54 (Supplement 1): 233a

Bernier I, Dautigny A, Colombani J, Jolles P 1974 Detergent-solubilized HLA antigens from human platelets: a comparative study of various purification techniques. Biochimica et Biophysica Acta 356: 82–90

Bevers E M, Comfurius P C, Zwaal R F A 1979 Activation of platelet factor 3. Thrombosis and Haemostasis 42: 211

Bills T K, Smith J B, Silver M J 1976 Metabolism of (^{14}C) arachidonic acid by human platelets. Biochimica et Biophysica Acta 424: 303–314

Bloom J W, Nesheim M E, Mann K G 1979 Phospholipid-binding properties of bovine factor V and factor Va. Biochemistry 18: 4419–4425

Boogaerts M A, Moldow C F, Yamada O, Frischberg B, Jacob H S 1979 Platelets and their products potentiate immune endothelial cell injury. Blood 54 (Supplement 1): 235a

Born G V R, Feinberg H 1975 Binding of adenosine diphosphate to intact human platelets. Journal of Physiology 251: 803–816

Boullin D J, Glenton P A M, Molyneaux D, Peters J R, Roach B 1977 Binding of 5-hydroxytryptamine to human blood platelets. British Journal of Pharmacology 61: 453p

Breederveld K, Giddings J C, ten Cate J W, Bloom A L 1975 The localization of factor V within normal human platelets and the demonstration of a platelet-factor V antigen in congenital factor V deficiency. British Journal of Haematology 29: 405–412

Bressler N M, Broekman M J, Marcus A J 1979 Concurrent studies of oxygen consumption and aggregation in stimulated human platelets. Blood 53: 167–178

Breton-Gorius J, Guichard J 1975 Two different types of granules in megakaryocytes and platelets as revealed by the diaminobenzidine reaction. Journal de Microscopie et de Biologie Cellulaire 23: 197–202

Broekman M J, Ward J W, Marcus A J 1979 Endogenous phospholipid metabolism in stimulated human platelets is limited to phosphatidylinositol and phosphatidic acid. Clinical Research 27: 459a

Brown J A, Jimenez S A, Colman R W 1980 Collagen-induced platelet shape change: the role of collagen quaternary structure. Journal of Laboratory and Clinical Medicine 95: 90–98

Bry K, Andersson L C, Kuusi T, Kinnunen P K J 1979 Monoacylglycerol hydrolase in human platelets. Biochimica et Biophysica Acta 575: 121–127

Caen J P, Castaldi P A, Leclerc J C, Inceman S, Larrieu M J, Probst M, Bernard J 1966 Congenital bleeding disorders with long bleeding time and normal platelet count: I. Glanzmann's thrombasthenia (report of 15 patients). American Journal of Medicine 1: 4–26

Caen J P, Nurden A T, Jeanneau C, Michel H, Tobelem G, Levy-Toledano S, Sultan Y, Valenci F, Bernard J 1976 Bernard-Soulier syndrome: a new platelet glycoprotein abnormality. Journal of Laboratory and Clinical Medicine 87: 586–596

Castaldi P A, Caen J 1965 Platelet fibrinogen. Journal of Clinical Pathology 18: 579–585

Castle A G, Crawford N 1977 The isolation and characterization of platelet microtubule proteins. Biochimica et Biophysica Acta 494: 76–91

Chao F C, Campo S R, Kenney D M 1980 Localization of fibrin converted by thrombin from released platelet fibrinogen. Blood 55: 187–194

Charo I F, Feinman R D, Detwiler T C 1977 Interrelations of platelet aggregation and secretion. Journal of Clinical Investigation 60: 866–873

Cheng C M, Hawiger J 1979 Affinity isolation and characterization of immunoglobulin G Fc fragment-binding glycoprotein from human blood platelets. Journal of Biological Chemistry 254: 2165–2167

Chiang T M, Kang A H 1976 Binding of chick skin collagen $\alpha 1$ chain by isolated membranes from human platelets. Journal of Biological Chemistry 254: 6347–6351

Chignard M, Le Couedic J-P, Tencé M, Vargaftig B B, Benveniste J 1979 The role of platelet-activating factor in platelet aggregation. Nature 279: 799–800

Cohen I 1979 The contractile system of blood platelets and its function. Methods and Achievements in Experimental Pathology 9: 40–86

Cohen I, Cohen C 1972 A tropomyosin-like protein from human platelets. Journal of Molecular Biology 68: 383–387

Cohen I, Glaser T 1979a Calcium-dependent cross-linking processes in platelets. Thrombosis and Haemostasis 42: 378

Cohen I, Kaminski E, DeVries A 1973 Actin-linked regulation of the human platelet contractile system. Federation of the European Biological Societies Letters 34: 315–317

Cohen I, Blankenberg T A, Borden D, Veis A 1979c Factor XIIIa-catalyzed cross-linking of platelet and muscle actin: regulation by adenosine triphosphate. Thrombosis and Haemostasis 42: 395

Cohen I, Gerrard J M, Bergman R N, White J G 1979b The role of contractile filaments in platelet activation. In: Peeters H (ed) Protides of the Biological Fluids, Pergamon Press, Oxford, p 555–556

Coller B S 1979 Asialofibrinogen supports platelet aggregation and adhesion to glass. Blood 53: 326–332

Coller B S 1980 Interaction of normal, thrombasthenic, and Bernard-Soulier platelets with immobilized fibrinogen: defective platelet-fibrinogen interaction in thrombasthenia. Blood 55: 169–178

Colman R W 1978 Platelet function in hyperbetalipoproteinemia. Thrombosis and Haemostasis 39: 284–293

Comp P C, Esmon C T 1979 Activated protein C inhibits platelet prothrombin-converting activity. Blood 54: 1272–1281

Connellan J M, Bowden D S, Smith I, Castaldi P A 1980 The use of antibodies to investigate the role of factor XI in platelets. Thrombosis Research 17: 225–238

Cooper B, Ahern D 1979 Characterization of the platelet prostaglandin D_2 receptor. Journal of Clinical Investigation 64: 586–590

Cooper H A, Clemetson K J, Lüscher E F 1979 Human platelet membrane receptor for bovine von Willebrand factor (platelet aggregating factor): an integral membrane glycoprotein. Proceedings of the National Academy of Sciences, USA 76: 1069–1073

Côté G P, Lewis W G, Pato M D, Smillie L B 1978 Platelet tropomyosin: lack of binding to skeletal muscle troponin and correlation with sequence. Federation of the European Biological Societies Letters 94: 131–135

Crawford N, Taylor D G 1977 Biochemical aspects of platelet behaviour associated with surface membrane reactivity. British Medical Bulletin 33: 199–206

Cuatrecasas P, Hollenberg M D 1976 Membrane receptors and hormone action. Advances in Protein Chemistry 30: 251–451

Culp B R, Titus B G, Lands W E M 1979 Inhibition of prostaglandin biosynthesis by eicosapentaenoic acid. Prostaglandins and Medicine 3: 269–278

Cutler L, Rodan G, Feinstein M B 1978 Cytochemical localization of adenylate cyclase and of calcium ion, magnesium ion-activated ATPases in the dense tubular system of human blood platelets. Biochimica et Biophysica Acta 542: 357–371

Dabrowska R, Hartshorne D J 1978 A Ca^{2+} and modulator dependent myosin light chain kinase from non-muscle cells. Biochemical and Biophysical Research Communications 85: 1352–1359

Dahlbäck B, Stenflo J 1978 Binding of bovine coagulation factor Xa to platelets. Biochemistry 17: 4938–4945

Daniel J L, Adelstein R S 1976 Isolation and properties of platelet myosin light chain kinase. Biochemistry 15: 2370–2377

Daniel J L, Holmsen H, Adelstein R S 1977 Thrombin-stimulated myosin phosphorylation in intact platelets and its possible involvement in secretion. Thrombosis et Diathesis Haemorrhagica 38: 984–989

Da Prada M, Jákabova R, Lüscher E F, Pletscher A, Richards F G 1976 Subcellular localization of the heparin-neutralizing factor in blood platelets. Physiology 257: 495–501

David-Pfeuty T, Simon C, Pantaloni D 1979 Effect of antimitotic drugs on tubulin GTPase activity and self-assembly. Journal of Biological Chemistry 254: 11696–11702

Dejter-Juszynski M, Harpaz N, Flowers H M, Sharon N 1978 Blood group ABH-specific macroglycolipids of human erythrocytes: isolation in high yield from a crude membrane glycoprotein fraction. European Journal of Biochemistry 83: 363–373

De Marco L, Shapiro S S, Ingerman C M 1979 Human asialo-factor VIII: a ristocetin-independent aggregating agent. Blood 54 (Supplement 1): 237a

Detwiler T C, Charo I F, Feinman R D 1978 Evidence that calcium regulates platelet function. Thrombosis and Haemostasis 40: 207–211

Doolittle R F, Takagi T, Cottrell B A 1974 Platelet and plasma fibrinogens are identical gene products. Science 185: 368–370

Doucet-de Bruïne M H M, Sixma J J, Over J, Beeser-Visser N H 1978 Heterogeneity of human factor VIII: II. Characterization of forms of factor VIII binding to platelets in the presence of ristocetin. Journal of Laboratory and Clinical Medicine 92: 96–107

Drummond A H, Gordon J L 1975 Specific binding sites for 5-hydroxytryptamine on rat blood platelets. Biochemical Journal 150: 129–130

Dyerberg J, Bang H O 1978 Dietary fat and thrombosis. Lancet 1: 152–154

Dyerberg, J, Bang H O 1979 Lipid metabolism, atherogenesis, and haemostasis in Eskimos: the role of the prostaglandin-3 family. Haemostasis 8: 227–233

Ehrlich H P, Gordon J L 1976 Proteinases in platelets. In: Gordon J L (ed) Platelets in Biology and Pathology, Research Monographs in Cell and Tissue Physiology, Elsevier, Amsterdam, p 353–372

Fauvel, F, Legrand Y J, Bentz H, Fietzek P P, Kuhn K, Caen J P 1978 Platelet-collagen interaction: adhesion of human blood platelets to purified (CB4) peptide from type III collagen. Thrombosis Research 12: 841–850

Fauvel F, Legrand Y J, Bentz H, Pignaud G, Kuhn K, Caen J P 1979 Aminoacid sequence of a peptide from type III collagen involved in platelet adhesion. Thrombosis and Haemostasis 42: 162

Feinman R D, Lubowsky J, Charo I, Detwiler T D 1977 The lumi-aggregometer: a new instrument for simultaneous measurement of secretion and aggregation by platelets. Journal of Laboratory and Clinical Medicine 90: 125–129

Fine K M, Ashbrook P C, Brigden L P, Maldonado J E, Didisheim P 1976 Gel-filtered human platelets: ultrastructure, function, and role of proteins in inhibition of aggregation by aspirin. American Journal of Pathology 84: 11–24

Fox J E B, Smith A, Haslam R J 1979 Possible role of a membrane phosphopolypeptide in the inhibition of platelet function by cyclic AMP. Thrombosis and Haemostasis 42: 80

Friedman R J, Burns E R 1978 Role of platelets in the proliferative response of the injured artery. In: Spaet T H (ed) Progress in Hemostasis and Thrombosis, Grune & Stratton, New York, Volume 4, p 249–278

Fukami M H, Niewiarowski S, Rucinski B, Salganicoff L 1979 Subcellular localization of human platelet antiheparin proteins. Thrombosis Research 14: 433–443

Fuster V, Bowie E J W, Lewis J C, Fass D N, Owen C A, Brown A L 1978 Resistance to arteriosclerosis in pigs with von Willebrand's disease. Journal of Clinical Investigation 61: 722–730

Gallagher M, Detwiler T C, Stracher A 1976 Two forms of platelet actin that may differ from skeletal muscle actin. In: Goldman R, Pollard T, Rosenbaum J (eds) Cell Motility (Cold Spring Harbor Conferences on Cell Proliferation) Cold Spring Harbor Laboratory, Massachusetts, Vol 3 p 475–485

Ganguly P, Gould M L 1979 Thrombin receptors of human platelets: thrombin bindings and antithrombin properties of glycoprotein I. British Journal of Haematology 42: 137–145

George J N 1978 Studies on platelet plasma membranes: IV. Quantitative analysis of platelet membrane glycoproteins by (^{125}I)-diazotized diiodosulfanilic acid labelling and SDS-polyacrylamide gel electrophoresis. Journal of Laboratory and Clinical Medicine 92: 430–446

Gerrard J M, White J G 1976 the structure and function of platelets with emphasis on their contractile nature. Pathobiology Annual 6: 31–58

Gerrard J M, White J G 1978 Prostaglandins and thromboxanes: 'middlemen' modulating platelet function in hemostasis and thrombosis. In: Spaet T H (ed) Progress in Hemostasis and Thrombosis, Grune & Stratton, New York, Vol 4, p 87–125

Gerrard J M, Rao G H R, White J G 1977b The influence of reserpine and ethylenediaminetetraacetic acid (EDTA) on serotonin storage organelles of blood platelets. American Journal of Pathology 87: 633–646

Gerrard J M, Kindom S E, Peterson D A, White J G 1979c Lysophosphatidic acids: II. Interaction of the effects of adenosine diphosphate and lysophosphatidic acids in dog, rabbit and human platelets. American Journal of Pathology 97: 531–547

Gerrard J M, Schollmeyer J V, Phillips D R, White J G 1979a Alpha-actinin deficiency in thrombasthenia: possible identity of a-actinin and glycoprotein III. American Journal of Pathology 94: 509–528

Gerrard J M, White J G, Rao G H R, Townsend D 1976 Localization of platelet prostaglandin production in the platelet dense tubular system. American Journal of Pathology 82: 283–298

Gerrard J M, Townsend D, Stoddard S, Witkop C J, White J G 1977a The influence of prostaglandin G_2 on platelet ultrastructure and platelet secretion. American Journal of Pathology 86: 99–116

Gerrard J M, Kindom S E, Peterson D A, Peller J, Krautz K E, White J G 1979d Lysophosphatidic acids: influence on platelet aggregation and intracellular calcium flux. American Journal of Pathology 96: 423–438

Gerrard J M, Phillips D R, Rao G H R, Plow E F, Walz D W, Ross R, Harker L A, White J G 1979b The role of a-granules and their contents in platelet function: studies of the gray platelet syndrome, a selective deficiency of these organelles. Blood 54 (Supplement 1): 241a

Giddings J C, Shearn S A M, Bloom A L 1978 Platelet-associated coagulation factors: immunological detection and the effect of calcium. British Journal of Haematology 39: 569–577

Glöckner W M, Kaulen H D, Uhlenbruck G 1978 Immunochemical detection of the Thomsen-Friedenreich antigen (T-antigen) on platelet plasma membranes. Thrombosis and Haemostasis 39: 186–192

Gockerman J P, Jacob W 1979 Purification and characterization of papain-solubilized HLA antigens from human platelets. Blood 53: 838–850

Goldberg N D, Haddox M K 1977 Cyclic GMP metabolism and involvement in biological regulation. Annual Review of Biochemistry 46: 823–896

Gorman R R, Bunting S, Miller O V 1977 Modulation of human platelet adenylate cyclase by prostacyclin (PGX). Prostaglandins 13: 377–388

Gralnick H R, Morisato D R 1979 The importance of the carbohydrate moiety of the factor VIII/von Willebrand factor protein in the binding to and agglutination of human platelets. Thrombosis and Haemostasis 42: 372

Greenberg J P, Packham M A, Guccione M A, Rand M L, Reimers H J, Mustad J F 1979b Survival of blood platelets treated in vitro with chymotrypsin, plasmin, trypsin, or neuraminidase. Blood 53: 916–927

Greenberg J P, Packham M A, Guccione M A, Harfenist E J, Orr J L, Kinlough-Rathbone R L, Perry D W, Mustard J F 1979a The effect of pretreatment of human or rabbit platelets with chymotrypsin on their responses to human fibrinogen and aggregating agents. Blood 54: 753–765

Hadgian R A, Feinstein M B 1979 Platelet myosin phosphorylation factor (MPF). Thrombosis and Haemostasis 42: 11

Hagen I 1972 The release of glycosaminoglycans during exposure of human platelets to thrombin and polystyrene latex particles. Biochimica et Biophysica Acta 273: 141–148

Hajek A S, Joist J H, Baker R K, Jarett L, Daughaday W H 1979 Demonstration and partial characterization of insulin receptors in human platelets. Journal of Clinical Investigation 63: 1060–1065

Hamberg M, Samuelsson B 1974 Prostaglandin endoperoxides: novel transformations of arachidonic acid in human platelets. Proceedings of the National Academy of Sciences, USA 71: 345–349

Hamberg M, Svensson J, Samuelsson B 1975 Thromboxanes: a new group of biologically active compounds derived from prostaglandin endoperoxides. Proceedings of the National Academy of Sciences, USA 72: 2994–2998

Hammarström S, Falardeau P 1977 Resolution of prostaglandin endoperoxide synthase and thromboxane synthase of human platelets. Proceedings of the National Academy of Sciences, USA 74: 3691–3695

Harker L A, Ross R, Glomsett J A 1978 The role of endothelial cell injury and platelet response in atherogenesis. Thrombosis and Haemostasis 39: 312–321

Harris H E, Weeds A G 1978 Platelet actin: subcellular distribution and association with profilin. Federation of the European Biological Societies Letters 90: 84–88

Haslam R J, Lynham J A 1976 Increased phosphorylation of specific blood platelet proteins in association with the release reaction. Biochemical Society Transactions 4: 694–697

Haslam R J, Lynham J A 1977 Relationship between phosphorylation of blood platelet proteins and secretion of granule constituents: I. Effects of different aggregating agents. Biochemical and Biophysical Research Communications 77: 714–722

Haslam R J, Davidson M M L, Davies T, Lynham J A, McClenaghan M D 1978 Regulation of blood platelet function by cyclic nucleotides. Advances in Cyclic Nucleotide Research 9: 533–552

Hathaway D R, Adelstein R S 1979 Human platelet myosin light chain kinase requires the calcium binding protein calmodulin for activity. Proceedings of the National Academy of Sciences, USA 76: 1653–1657

Hawiger J, Parkinson S, Timmons S 1980 Prostacyclin inhibits mobilization of fibrinogen-binding sites on human ADP- and thrombin-treated platelets. Nature 283: 195–197

Heldin C H, Westermark B, Wasteson A 1979 Platelet-derived growth factor: purification and partial characterization. Proceedings of the National Academy of Sciences, USA 76: 3722–3726

Henry R L 1977 Platelet function. Seminars in Thrombosis and Hemostasis 4: 93–122

Holmberg L, Nilsson I M 1979 VIIIR:Ag in platelets from patients with various forms of von Willebrand's disease. Thrombosis and Haemostasis 42: 1033–1038

Holmsen H 1975 Biochemistry of the platelet release reaction. In: CIBA Foundation Symposium, Biochemistry and Pharmacology of Platelets, Elsevier, Amsterdam, p 175–205

Holmsen H 1977 Platelet energy metabolism in relation to function. In: Mills D C B, Paretti F I (eds) Platelets and Thrombosis, Academic Press, London, p 45–62

Holmsen H, Weiss H J 1979 Secretable storage pools in platelets. Annual Review of Medicine 30: 119–134

Holmsen H, Setkowsky C A, Day H J 1974 Effects of antimycin and 2-deoxyglucose on adenine nucleotides in human platelets. Role of metabolic adenosine triphosphate in primary aggregation, secondary aggregation and shape change of platelets. Biochemical Journal 144: 385–396

Howard M A, Montgomery D C, Hardisty R M 1974 Factor VIII-related antigen in platelets. Thrombosis Research 4: 617–624

Hunter T, Garrels J I 1977 Characterization of the mRNAs for α-β- and γ-actin. Cell 12: 767–781

Huzoor-Akbar, Ardlie N G 1976 Evidence that collagen releases human platelet constituents by two different mechanisms. British Journal of Haematology 34: 137–146

Huzoor-Akbar, Ardlie N G 1977c Platelet activation in haemostasis: role of thrombin and other clotting factors in platelet-collagen interaction. Haemostasis 6: 59–71

Ikeda Y, Steiner M 1979 Phosphorylation and protein kinase activity of platelet tubulin. Journal of Biological Chemistry 254: 66–74

Inceman S, Caen J, Bernard J 1966 Aggregation, adhesion, and viscous metamorphosis of platelets in congenital fibrinogen deficiencies. Journal of Laboratory and Clinical Medicine 68: 21–32

James H L, Ganguly P, Jackson C W 1977 Characterization and origin of fibrinogen in blood platelets: a review with recent data. Thrombosis and Haemostasis 38: 939–954

Jamieson G A, Okumura T 1978 Reduced thrombin binding and aggregation in Bernard-Soulier platelets. Journal of Clinical Investigation 60: 861–864

Jamieson G A, Okumura T, Fishback B, Johnson M M, Egan J J, Weiss H J 1979 Platelet membrane glycoproteins in thrombasthenia, Bernard-Soulier syndrome, and storage pool disease. Journal of Laboratory and Clinical Medicine 93: 652–660

Jandrot-Perres M, Mosesson M W, Denninger M H, Ménaché D 1979 Studies of platelet fibrinogen from a subject with a congenital plasma fibrinogen abnormality (fibrinogen Paris I). Blood 54: 1109–1116

Jensen A H-B, Beguin S, Josso F 1976 Factor V and VIII activation 'in vivo' during bleeding: evidence of thrombin formation at the early stage. Pathologie Biologie 24 (Supplement): 6–10

Jesse R L, Franson R C 1979 Modulation of purified phospholipase A_2 activity from human platelets by calcium and indomethacin. Biochimica et Biophysica Acta 575: 467–470

Johnson G J, Leis L A, Rao G H R, White J G 1979 Arachidonate-induced platelet aggregation in the dog. Thrombosis Research 14: 147–154

Johnson R G, Scarpa A, Salganicoff L 1978 Internal pH of isolated serotonin containing granules of pig platelets. Journal of Biological Chemistry 253: 7061–7068

Joist J H 1977 Platelets and fibrinolysis. Thrombosis and Haemostasis 38: 955–962

Joist J H, Niewiarowski S 1973 Retention of platelet fibrin stabilizing factor during the platelet release reaction and clot retraction. Thrombosis et Diathesis Haemorrhagica 29: 679–683

Joist J H, Niewiarowski S, Nath N, Mustard J F 1976 Platelet antiplasmin: its extrusion during the release reaction, subcellular localization, characterization and relationship to antiheparin in pig platelets. Journal of Laboratory and Clinical Medicine 87: 659–669

Kane W H, Lindhout M J, Jackson C M, Majerus P W 1980 Factor Va-dependent binding of factor Xa to human platelets. Journal of Biological Chemistry 255: 1170–1174

Kao K-J, Pizzo S V, McKee P A 1979a Demonstration and characterization of specific binding sites for factor VIII/von Willebrand factor on human platelets. Journal of Clinical Investigation 63: 656–664

Kao K-J, Pizzo S V, McKee P A 1979b Platelet receptors for human factor VIII/von Willebrand protein: functional correlation of receptor occupancy and ristocetin-induced platelet aggregation. Proceedings of the National Academy of Sciences, USA 76: 5317–5320

Kaplan D R, Chao F C, Stiles C D, Antoniades H N, Scher C D 1979a Platelet α-granules contain a growth factor for fibroblasts. Blood 53: 1043–1052

Kaplan K L, Broekman M J, Chernoff A, Lesnik G R, Drillings M 1979b Platelet α-granule proteins: studies on release and subcellular localization. Blood 53: 604–618

Karpatkin S 1977 Composition of platelets: In: Williams W J, Beutler E, Erslev A J, Rundles R W (eds) Hematology, Second Edition, McGraw-Hill, New York, Chapter 129, p 1176–1187

Käser-Glanzmann R, Jákabova M, George J N, Lüscher E F 1977 Stimulation of calcium uptake in platelet membrane vesicles by adenosine 3'5'-cyclic monophosphate and protein kinase. Biochimica et Biophysica Acta 466: 429–440

34 RECENT ADVANCES IN BLOOD COAGULATION

Kaywin P, McDonough M, Insel P A, Shattil S J 1978 Platelet function in essential thrombocythemia: decreased epinephrine responsiveness associated with a deficiency of platelet α-adrenergic receptors. New England Journal of Medicine 299: 505–509

Kendrick-Jones J, Jakes R, Nyström L E, Lindberg U 1979 Chemical characterization of actin and profilin from calf spleen profilactin. In: Peters H (ed) Protides of the Biological Fluids, Pergamon Press, Oxford, p 493–498

Kinlough-Rathbone R L, Packham M A, Reimers H-J, Cazenave J-P, Mustard J F 1977 Mechanisms of platelet shape change, aggregation and release induced by collagen, thrombin, or A23187. Journal of Laboratory and Clinical Medicine 90: 707–719

Koutts, J, Zimmerman T S 1979 Selective binding of different molecular species of factor VIII to isolated platelet membranes and to intact thrombin stimulated platelets. Thrombosis and Haemostasis 42: 373

Koutts J, Walsh P N, Plow E F, Fenton J W, Zimmerman T S 1978 Active release of human platelet factor VIII-related antigen by adenosine diphosphate, collagen and thrombin. Journal of Clinical Investigation 62: 1255–1263

Kunicki T J, Aster R H 1978 Deletion of the platelet-specific allo-antigen Pl^{A1} from platelets in Glanzmann's thrombasthenia. Journal of Clinical Investigation 61: 1225–1231

Kunicki T J, Aster R H 1979 Association of the platelet-specific alloantigen Pl^{A1} (Zu^a) with the platelet membrane glycoprotein IIIa. Thrombosis and Haemostasis 42: 422

Landon F, Huc C, Thomé F, Oriol C, Olomucki A 1977 Human platelet actin: evidence of β and γ forms and similarity of properties with sarcomeric actin. European Journal of Biochemistry 81: 571–577

Lapetina E G, Cuatrecasas P 1979 Stimulation of phosphatidic acid production in platelets precedes the formation of arachidonate and parallels the release of serotonin. Biochemica et Biophysica Acta 573: 394–402

Lapetina E G, Billah M M, Cuatrecasas P 1980 Stimulation of the phosphatidylinositol-specific phospholipase C and the release of arachidonic acid in activated platelets. In: Mann K G, Taylor F B (eds) The Regulation of Coagulation, Elsevier/North Holland, New York, p 491–497

Larsen N E, Simons E R 1979 Isolation and investigation of the platelet thrombin receptor. Blood 54 (Supplement 1): 250a

Lawler J W, Slayter H S, Coligan J E 1978 Isolation and characterization of a high molecular weight protein from human blood platelets. Journal of Biological Chemistry 253: 8609–8616

Lazarides E 1980 Intermediate filaments as mechanical integrators of cellular space. Nature 283: 249–256

Lebowitz E A, Cooke R 1978 Contractile properties of actomyosin from human blood platelets. Journal of Biological Chemistry 253: 5443–5447

Legrand C, Caen J P 1976 Binding of ^{14}C-ADP by thrombasthenic platelet membranes. Haemostasis 5: 231–238

Lindahl U, Höök M 1978 Glycosaminoglycans and their binding to biological macromolecules. Annual Review of Biochemistry 47: 385–417

Lipscomb M S, Walsh P N 1979 Human platelets and factor XI: localization in platelet membranes of factor XI-like activity and its functional distinction from plasma factor XI. Journal of Clinical Investigation 63: 1006–1014

Lockhart M S, Comp P C, Taylor F B 1979 Role of platelets in lysis of dilute clots. Journal of Laboratory and Clinical Medicine 94: 285–294

Lucas R C, Rosenberg S, Shafiq S, Stracher A, Lawrence J 1979 The isolation and characterization of a cytoskeleton and a contractile apparatus from human platelets. In: Peters H (ed) Protides of the Biological Fluids, Pergamon Press, Oxford, p 465–470

Majerus P W, Miletich J P, Kane W H, Hofmann S L, Stanford N, Jackson C M 1980 The formation of thrombin on the platelet surface. In: Mann K G, Taylor F B (eds) The Regulation of Coagulation, Elsevier/North Holland, New York, p 215–224

Marcus A J 1978 The role of lipids in platelet function: with particular reference to the arachidonic acid pathway. Journal of Lipid Research 19: 793–826

Marguerie G A, Plow E F, Edgington T S 1979 Human platelets possess an inducible and saturable receptor specific for fibrinogen. Journal of Biological Chemistry 254: 5357–5363

Markey F, Lindberg U 1979 Biochemical evidence for actin filament formation as a primary response in stimulation of platelets with thrombin: the possible role of the profilin-actin complex. In: Peters H, (ed) Protides of the Biological Fluids, Pergamon Press, Oxford, p 487–492

Markey F, Lindberg U, Eriksson L 1978 Human platelets contain profilin, a potential regulator of actin polymerizability. Federation of the European Biological Societies letters 88: 75–79

Martin B M, Wasiewski W W, Fenton J W, Detwiler T C 1976 Equilibrium binding of thrombin to platelets. Biochemistry 15: 4886–4893

Mason R G, Mohammed S F, Chuang H Y K, Richardson T D 1976 The adhesion of platelets to subendothelium, collagen and artificial surfaces. Seminars in Thrombosis and Haemostasis 3: 98–116

Massini P 1977 The role of calcium in the stimulation of platelets. In: Mills D C B, Pareti F I (eds) Platelets and Thrombosis, Academic Press, New York, p 33–43

Mauco G, Chap H, Douste-Blazy L 1979 Characterization and properties of a phosphatidylinositol phosphodiesterase (phospholipase C) from platelet cytosol. Federation of the European Biological Societies Letters 100: 367–370

McGregor J L, Clemetson K J, James E, Dechavanne M 1979 A comparison of techniques used to study externally oriented proteins and glycoproteins of human blood platelets. Thrombosis Research 16: 437–452

McMillan R, Bakich N J, Yelenosky R J 1979 The adrenalin binding site on human platelets. British Journal of Haematology 41: 597–604

Meucci P, Peake I R, Bloom A L 1978 Factor VIII-related activities in normal, haemophiliac and von Willebrand's disease platelet fractions. Thrombosis and Haemostasis 40: 288–301

Michaeli D, Orloff K G 1976 Molecular considerations of platelet adhesion. In: Spaet T H (ed) Progress in Hemostasis and Thrombosis, Grune and Stratton, New York, Vol 3, p 29–59

Miletich J P, Jackson C M, Majerus P W 1978 Properties of the factor Xa binding site on human platelets. Journal of Biology Chemistry 253: 6908–6916

Miletich J P, Kane W H, Hofmann S L, Stanford N, Majerus P W 1979 Deficiency of factor Xa-factor Va binding sites on the platelets of a patient with a bleeding disorder. Blood 54: 1015–1022

Miller J L, Katz A J, Feinstein M B 1975 Plasmin inhibition of thrombin-induced platelet aggregation. Thrombosis et Diathesis Hemorrhagica 3: 286–309

Mills D C B, MacFarlane D E 1976 Platelet receptors. In: Gordon J L (ed) Platelets in Biology and Pathology, Research Monographs in Cell and Tissue Physiology, Elsevier, Amsterdam, Chapter 7, p 159–202

Moake J, Olson J, Troll J, Peterson D, Cimo P, Weinger R 1979 Defective binding of ^{125}I-von Willebrand factor (vWF) to Bernard-Soulier platelets. Blood 54 (Supplement 1): 253a

Mohammed S F, Whitworth C, Chuang H Y K, Lundblad R L, Mason R G 1976 Multiple active forms of thrombin: binding to platelets and effects on platelet function. Proceedings of the National Academy of Sciences, USA 73: 1660–1663

Moncada S, Vane J R 1979 Arachidonic acid metabolites and the interactions between platelets and blood-vessel walls. New England Journal of Medicine 300: 1142–1147

Moncada S, Flower R J, Russels N 1978 Dipyridamole and platelet function. Lancet 2: 1257–1258

Moncada S, Gryglewski R, Bunting S, Vane J R 1976 An enzyme isolated from arteries transforms prostaglandin endoperoxides to an unstable substance that inhibits platelet aggregation. Nature 263: 663–665

Moroi M, Dubay E, Jamieson G A 1979 Purification of platelet glycocalicin and glycoprotein I by affinity techniques. Thrombosis and Haemostasis 42: 421

Mosher D F, Vaheri A, Choate J J, Gahmberg C G 1979 Action of thrombin on surface glycoproteins of human platelets. Blood 53: 437–445

Mui P T K, Ganguly P 1977 Cross-linking of actin and fibrin by fibrin-stabilizing factor. American Journal of Physiology 233: H346–H349

Mustard J F, Packham M A, Kinlough-Rathbone R L, Perry D W, Regoeczi E 1978 Fibrinogen and ADP-induced platelet aggregation. Blood 57: 453–466

Mustard J F, Kinlough-Rathbone R L, Packham M A, Perry D W, Harfenist E J, Pai K R N 1979 Comparison of fibrinogen association with normal and thrombasthenic platelets on exposure to ADP or chymotrypsin. Blood 54: 987–993

Nachman R L, Ferris B 1974 Binding of adenosine diphosphate by isolated membranes from human platelets. Journal of Biological Chemistry 249: 704–710

Nachman R L, Harpel P C 1976 Platelet α_2-macroglobulin and α_1-anti-trypsin. Journal of Biological Chemistry 251: 4514–4521

Nachman R L, Jaffe E 1975 Subcellular platelet factor VIII antigen and von Willebrand factor. Journal of Experimental Medicine 141: 1101–1113

Nachman R L., Marcus A J 1968 Immunological studies of proteins associated with the subcellular fractions of thrombasthenic and afibrinogenemic platelets. British Journal of Haematology 15: 181–189

Nachman R L, Jaffe E A, Weksler B B 1977a Immunoinhibition of ristocetin-induced aggregation. Journal of Clinical Investigation 59: 143–148

Nachman R L, Kinoshita T, Ferris B 1979 Structural analysis of human platelet membrane glycoprotein I complex. Proceedings of the National Academy of Sciences, USA 76: 2952–2954

Nachman R L, Levine R, Jaffe E A 1977b Synthesis of factor VIII antigen by cultured guinea pig megakaryocytes. Journal of Clinical Investigation 60: 914–921

Needleman P, Wyche A, Raz A 1979b Platelet and blood vessel arachidonate metabolism and interactions. Journal of Clinical Investigation 63: 345–349

Needleman P, Raz A, Minkes M S, Ferrendelli J A, Sprecher H 1979a Triene prostaglandins: prostacyclin and thromboxane biosynthesis and unique biological properties. Proceedings of the National Academy of Sciences, USA 76: 944–948

Nesheim M E, Hibbard L S, Tracy P B, Bloom J W, Myrmel K H, Mann K G 1980 Participation of factor

Va in prothrombinase. In: Mann K G, Taylor F B (eds) The regulation of coagulation. Elsevier/North Holland, New York, p 145–160

Newman K D, Williams L T, Bishopric H, Lefkowitz R J 1978 Identification of α-adrenergic receptors in human platelets by (^{3}H) dihydroergocryptine binding. Journal of Clinical Investigation 61: 395–402

Nichols W L, Gastineau D A, Mann K G 1979 Isolation of human platelet and red blood cell plasma membrane proteins by preparative detergent electrophoresis. Biochimica et Biophysica Acta 554: 293–308

Nichols W L, Tracy P B, Nesheim M E, Mann K G 1980 DAPA inhibition of collagen-induced platelet aggregation. Seegers Symposium: 'Contributions to Hemostasis', Detroit

Niewiarowski S 1977 Proteins secreted by the platelet. Thrombosis and Haemostasis 38: 924–938

Niewiarowski S, Levine S P 1979 Characterization and assay of platelet secretory proteins. In: Schmidt R M (ed) CRC Handbook Series in Clinical Laboratory Science, Section I: Hematology, CRC Press, Boca Raton, FL Volume 1, p 435–446

Niewiarowski S, Regoeczi E, Stewart G J, Senyi A F, Mustard J F 1972 Platelet interaction with polymerizing fibrin. Journal of Clinical Investigation 51: 685–700

Nurden A T, Caen J P 1978 Membrane glycoproteins and human platelet function. British Journal of Haematology 38: 155–160

Nurden A T, Caen J P 1979 The different glycoprotein abnormalities in thrombasthenic and Bernard-Soulier platelets. Seminars in Hematology 16: 234:250

Nurden A T, Rendu F, Kunicki T, Caen J P 1979 Characterization of the molecular defects of the platelets of two patients with the gray platelet syndrome. Blood 54 (Supplement 1): 254a

Oelz O, Oelz R, Knapp H R 1977 Biosynthesis of prostaglandin D_2: I. Formation of prostaglandin D_2 by human platelets. Prostaglandins 9: 109–121

Ohara S, Hawiger J 1979 Interaction of factor VIII–VWF with human platelets is stimulated by thrombin. Blood 54 (Supplement 1): 294a

Okuma M, Uchino H 1979 Altered arachidonate metabolism by platelets in patients with myeloproliferative disorders. Blood 54: 1258–1271

Okumura T, Jamieson G A 1976 Platelet glycocalicin. Journal of Biological Chemistry 251: 5944–5949, 5950–5955

Okumura T, Hasitz M, Jamieson G A 1978 Platelet glycocalicin: interaction with thrombin and role as thrombin receptor of the platelet surface. Journal of Biological Chemistry 253: 3435–3443

Orloff K G, Michaeli D 1976 Fibrin-induced release of platelet serotonin. American Journal of Physiology 231: 344–350

Østerud B, Rapaport S I, Lavine K K 1977 Factor V activity of platelets: evidence for an activated factor V molecule and for a platelet activator. Blood 49: 819–834

Owen C A Jr, Bowie E J W, Thompson J H Jr 1975 The Diagnosis of Bleeding Disorders 2d ed. Little, Brown & Co., Boston

Owen N E, LeBreton G C 1979 Alterations in intraplatelet Ca^{2+} binding induced by epinephrine, A23187, U46619, prostaglandin E or prostacyclin. Blood 54 (Supplement 1): 254a

Peerschke E I, Grant R A, Zucker M B 1979 Relationship between aggregation and binding of ^{125}I-fibrinogen and ^{45} calcium to human platelets. Thrombosis and Haemostasis 42: 358

Peterson D M, Wehring B, Yu S H, Moake J L 1979 Correlation of abnormal membrane glycoproteins with decreased amounts of fibrinogen in thrombasthenic platelets as demonstrated by two-dimensional gel electrophoresis. Blood 54 (Supplement 1): 256a

Phillips D R, Agin P P 1977a Platelet plasma membrane glycoproteins: evidence for the presence of nonequivalent disulfide bonds using nonreduced-reduced two-dimensional gel electrophoresis. Journal of Biological Chemistry 252: 2121–2126

Phillips D R, Agin P P 1977b Platelet plasma membrane glycoproteins: identification of a proteolytic substrate for thrombin. Biochemical and Biophysical Research Communications 75: 940–947

Phillips D R, Agin P P 1977c Platelet membrane defects in Glanzmann's thrombasthenia. Journal of Clinical Investigation 60: 535–545

Phillips D R, Jennings L K, Edwards H H 1979 Platelet glycoproteins in platelet aggregation. Thrombosis and Haemostasis 42: 431

Pifer D D, Colman R W, Chesney C M 1977 Subcellular localization and secretion of factor V by human platelets. Thrombosis and Haemostasis 38: 126

Piovella F, Nalli G, Malamani G D, Majolino I, Frassoni F, Sitar G M, Ruggeri A, Dell'Orbo C, Ascari E 1978 The ultrastructural localization of factor VIII-antigen in human platelets, megakaryocytes and endothelial cells using a ferritin-labelled antibody. British Journal of Haematology 30: 209–213

Plow E F, Birdwell C, Ginsberg M H 1979a Identification and quantitation of platelet-associated fibronectin antigen. Journal of Clinical Investigation 63: 540–543

Plow E F, Marguerie B A, Edgington T S 1979b Induction of the fibrinogen receptor on human platelets by epinephrine. Blood 54 (Supplement 1): 257a

Pollard T D, Fujiwara K, Handin R, Weiss G 1977 Contractile proteins in platelet activation and contraction. Annals of the New York Academy of Sciences 283: 218–236

Rendu F, Breton-Gorius J, Trugnan G, Castro-Malaspina H, Andrieu J-M, Bereziat G, Lebret M, Caen J P 1978 Studies on a new variant of the Hermansky-Pudlak syndrome: qualitative, ultrastructural, and functional abnormalities of the platelet dense bodies associated with phospholipase A defect. American Journal of Hematology 4: 387–399

Rider D M, McDonough R P, McDonough J 1978 A possible contributory role of the platelet in the formation of plasma factor XIII. British Journal of Haematology 39: 579–588

Rittenhouse-Simmons S 1979 Production of diglyceride from phosphatidylinositol in activated human platelets. Journal of Clinical Investigation 63: 580–587

Robblee L S, Shepro D, Belamarich F A 1973 Calcium uptake and associated adenosine triphosphatase activity of isolated platelet membranes. Journal of General Physiology 61: 462–481

Ross R, Glomset J, Kariya B, Harker L A 1974 A platelet-dependent serum factor that stimulates the proliferation of arterial smooth muscle cells in vitro. Proceedings of the National Academy of Sciences, USA 71: 1207–1210

Rucinski B, Niewiarowski S, James P, Walz D A, Budzynski A Z 1979 Antiheparin proteins secreted by human platelets: purification, characterization and radioimmunoassay. Blood 53: 47–62

Ruggeri Z M, Zimmerman T S 1980 Heightened ristocetin-induced factor VIII/von Willebrand factor-platelet interaction in a new subtype of von Willebrand's disease: implications for the measurement of 'von Willebrand factor'. In: Mann K G, Taylor F B (eds) The Regulation of Coagulation, Elsevier/North Holland, New York, p 327–330

Ruggeri Z M, Mannucci P M, Bader R, Barbui T 1978 Factor VIII-related properties in platelets from patients with von Willebrand's disease. Journal of Laboratory and Clinical Medicine 91: 132–140

Ryan R J, Lee C Y 1976 The role of membrane bound receptors. Biology of Reproduction 14: 16–29

Salzman E W, Lindon J, Brier D, Merrill E W 1977 Surface-induced platelet adhesion, aggregation and release. Annals of the New York Academy of Sciences 283: 114–127

Santoro S A, Cunningham L W 1977 Collagen-mediated platelet aggregation. Journal of Clinical Investigation 60: 1054–1060

Santoro S A, Cunningham L W 1979 Fibronectin and the multiple interaction model for platelet-collagen adhesion. Proceedings of the National Academy of Sciences, USA 76: 2644–2648

Schafer A I, Cooper B, O'Hara D, Handin R I 1979 Identification of platelet receptors for prostaglandin I_2 and D_2. Journal of Biological Chemistry 254: 2914–2917

Schick P K 1979 The role of platelet membrane lipids in platelet hemostatic activities. Seminars in Hematology 16: 221–233

Schiffman S, Rimon A, Rapaport S I 1977 Factor XI and platelets: evidence that platelets contain only minimal factor XI activity and antigen. British Journal of Haematology 35: 429–436

Schneider-Trip M D, Jenkins C S P, Kahlé L H, Sturk A, ten Cate J W 1979 Studies on the mechanism of ristocetin-induced platelet aggregation: binding of factor VIII to platelets. British Journal of Haematology 43: 99–112

Schoene N W 1978 Properties of platelet phospholipase A_2. Advances in Prostaglandin and Thromboxane Research 3: 121–126

Schollmeyer J V, Rao G H R, White J G 1978 An actin-binding protein in human platelets: interactions with α-actinin on gelation of actin and the influence of cytochalasin. American Journal of Pathology 93: 433–446

Seegers W H 1976 Role of platelets in blood coagulation. In: Ulutin O N, The Platelets: Fundamentals and Clinical Applications, Kagit ve Basin Isleri A G, Istanbul, Chapter 5, p 90–105

Seegers W H, Ghosh A 1980 The activation of factor X and factor $X\beta$ with factor VII or protein M. Thrombosis Research 17: 501–506

Semeraro N, Vermylen J 1977 Evidence that washed human platelets possess factor X-activator activity. British Journal of Haematology 36: 107–115

Semeraro N, Cortellazzo S, Colucci M, Barbui T 1979 A hitherto undescribed defect of platelet coagulant activity in polycythaemia vera and essential thrombocythaemia. Thrombosis Research 16: 795–802

Shattil S J, Cooper R A 1978 Role of membrane lipid composition, organization, and fluidity in human platelet function. In: Spaet T H (ed) Progress in Hemostasis and Thrombosis, Grune & Stratton, New York, Vol 4, p 59–86

Shattil S J, McDonough M, Turnbull J, Insel P A 1979b Identification of α-adrenergic receptors on human platelets using ^{3}H-clonidine. Blood 54 (Supplement 1): 260a

Shirasawa K, Barton B P, Chandler A B 1972 Localization of ferritin-conjugated anti-fibrin/fibrinogen in platelet aggregates produced in vitro. American Journal of Pathology 66: 379–405

Shuman M A, Majerus P W 1976 The measurement of thrombin in clotting blood by radioimmunoassay. Journal of Clinical Investigation 58: 1249–1258

Shuman M A, Botney M, Fenton J W 1979 Thrombin-induced platelet secretion: further evidence for a specific pathway. Journal of Clinical Investigation 63: 1211–1218

Siegel A M, Smith J B, Silver M J, Nicolaou K C, Ahern D 1979 Selective binding site for

(^{3}H)-prostacyclin on platelets. Journal of Clinical Investigation 63: 215–220

Sixma J J, Lips J P N 1978 Isolation of platelet membranes: a review. Thrombosis and Haemostasis 39: 328–337

Skaer R J, Peters P D, Emmines J P 1974 The localization of calcium and phosphorus in human platelets. Journal of Cell Science 15: 679–692

Sloboda R D, Rosenbaum J L 1979 Decoration and stabilization of intact, smooth-walled microtubules with microtuble-associated proteins. Biochemistry 18: 48–55

Slot J W, Bouma B N, Montgomery R, Zimmerman T W 1978 Platelet factor VIII-related antigen: immunofluorescent localization. Thrombosis Research 13: 871–878

Smillie L B 1979 Structure and functions of tropomyosins from muscle and non-muscle sources. Trends in Biological Sciences 4: 151–154

Smith D, Damus P S 1977 Effect of thrombin and ADP on a membrane bound cyclic AMP dependent kinase of human platelets. Thrombosis Research 10: 301–308

Smith J B, Ingerman C, Silver M J 1976 Persistence of thromboxane A_2-like material and platelet release inducing activity in plasma. Journal of Clinical Investigation 58: 1119–1122

Solum N O, Hagen I, Peterka M 1977 Human platelet glycoproteins: further evidence that the 'GP I band' from whole platelets contains three different polypeptides. Thrombosis Research 10: 71–82

Solum N O, Hagen I, Filion-Myklebust C, Stabaek T 1979 On the membrane association of platelet glycocalicin. Thrombosis and Haemostasis 42: 421

Soria J, Soria C, Samama M, Poirot E, Kling C 1976 Human platelet fibrinogen: a protein different from plasma fibrinogen. Pathologie Biologie 24 (Supplement): 15–17

Springer T A, Kaufman J F, Siddoway L A, Mann D L, Strominger J L 1977 Purification of HLA-linked B lymphocyte alloantigens in immunologically active form by preparative sodium dodecylsulfate-gel electrophoresis and studies on their subunit association. Journal of Biological Chemistry 252: 6201–6207

Stahl K, Thermann H, Dame W R 1978 Ultrastructural morphometric investigations on normal human platelets. Haemostasis 7: 242–251

Steer M L, Wood A 1979 Regulation of human platelet adenylate cyclase by epinephrine, prostaglandin E_1 and guanine nucleotides. Journal of Biological Chemistry 254: 10791–10797

Steiner M, Ikeda Y 1979 Quantitative assessment of polymerized and depolymerized platelet microtubules: changes caused by aggregating agents. Journal of Clinical Investigation 63: 443–448

Steinherz P G, Miller D R, Hilgartner M W, Schmalzer E A 1976 Platelet dysfunction in vincristine treated patients. British Journal of Haematology 32: 439–450

Stuart M J, Gerrard J M, White J G 1980 Effect of cholesterol on production of thromboxane B_2 by platelets in vitro. New England Journal of Medicine 302: 6–10

Subbarao K, Rucinski B, Rausch M A, Schmid K, Niewiarowski S 1977 Binding of dipyridamole to human platelets and to α_1 acid glycoprotein and its significance for the inhibition of adenosine uptake. Journal of Clinical Investigation 60: 936–943

Sultan Y, Maisonneuve P, Angeles-Cano E 1979 Release of VIIIR:Ag and VIIIR:WF during thrombin and collagen induced aggregation. Thrombosis Research 15: 415–419

Tam S W, Detwiler T C 1978 Binding of thrombin to human platelet plasma membranes. Biochimica et Biophysica Acta 543: 194–201

Tam S W, Fenton J W, Detwiler T C 1979 Dissociation of thrombin from platelets by hirudin: evidence for receptor processing. Journal of Biological Chemistry 254: 8723–8725

Tateson J E, Moncada S, Vane J R 1977 Effects of prostacyclin (PGX) on cyclic AMP concentrations in human platelets. Prostaglandins 13: 389–398

Tobelem G, Levy-Toledano S, Bredoux R, Michel H, Nurden A, Caen J, Degos L 1976 New approach to determination of specific functions of platelet membrane sites. Nature 263: 427–429

Tollefsen D M, Majerus P W 1975 Inhibition of human platelet aggregation by monovalent antifibrinogen antibody fragments. Journal of Clinical Investigation 55: 1259–1268

Tollefsen D M, Feagler J R, Majerus P W 1974 The binding of thrombin to the surface of human platelets. Journal of Biological Chemistry 249: 2646–2654

Tracy P B, Peterson J M, Nesheim M E, McDuffie F C, Mann K G 1979 Interaction of coagulation factor V and factor Va with platelets. Journal of Biological Chemistry 254: 10354–10361

Tracy P B, Peterson J M, Nesheim M E, McDuffie F C, Mann K G 1980 Platelet interaction with bovine coagulation factor V and factor Va. In: Mann K G, Taylor F B (eds) The Regulation of Coagulation, Elsevier/North Holland, New York, p 237–243

Trugnan G, Bereziat G, Manier M-C, Polonovski J 1979 Phospholipase activities in subcellular fractions of human platelets. Biochimica et Biophysica Acta 573: 61–72

Tschopp T B, Baumgartner H R 1980 Platelet-subendothelium interaction in hereditary and experimental von Willebrand's disease. In: Mann K G, Taylor F B (eds) The Regulation of Coagulation, Elsevier/North Holland, New York, p 317–325

Tullis J L, Watanabe K 1978 Platelet antithrombin deficiency: a new clinical entity. American Journal of Medicine 65: 472–478

Ulutin O N 1976 The platelets: fundamentals and clinical applications. Kagit ve Basin Isleri A. S., Istanbul

van Wijk E M, Kahlé L N, ten Cate J W 1979 Factor X activation by washed human platelets. Thrombosis and Haemostasis 42: 56

Wallach D, Davies P G A, Pastan I 1978 Purification of mammalian filamin. Journal of Biological Chemistry 253: 3328–3335

Walsh P N 1978 Different requirements for intrinsic factor-Xa forming activity and platelet factor 3 activity and their relationship to platelet aggregation and secretion. British Journal of Haematology 40: 311–331

Walsh P N 1979 Contributions of platelets to intrinsic coagulation. In: Schmidt R N (ed) CRC Handbook Series in Clinical Laboratory Science, CRC Press, Boca Raton, Florida, Section I: Hematology, Vol 1, p 351–359

Walsh P N, Tuszynski G P 1980 Factor XI, platelets and hemostatic control. In: Mann K G, Taylor F B (eds) The Regulation of Coagulation, Elsevier/North Holland, New York, p 251–257

Walsh P N, Biggs R, Gagnatelli G 1974 Platelet antiheparin activity. British Journal of Haematology 26: 405–419

Walsh P N, Murphy S, Barry W E 1977b The role of platelets in the pathogenesis of thrombosis and hemorrhage in patients with thrombocytosis. Thrombosis and Haemostasis 38: 1085–1096

Walsh P N, Goldberg R E, Tax R L, Magargal L E 1977a Platelet coagulant activities and retinal vein thrombosis. Thrombosis and Haemostasis 38: 399–406

Ward J V, Packham M A 1979 Characterization of the sulfated glycosaminoglycan on the surface and in the storage granules of rabbit platelets. Biochimica et Biophysica Acta 583: 196–207

Watanabe K, Hakomori S, Childs R A, Feizi T 1979 Characterization of a blood group I-active ganglioside. Journal of Biological Chemistry 254: 3221–3228

Weiss H J, Rogers J 1971 Fibrinogen and platelets in the primary arrest of bleeding: studies in two patients with congenital afibrinogenemia. New England Journal of Medicine 285: 369–374

Weiss H J, Vicic W J, Lages B A, Rogers J 1979a Isolated deficiency of platelet procoagulant activity. American Journal of Medicine 67: 206–213

Weiss H J, Tschopp T B, Baumgartner H R, Sussman I I, Johnson M M, Egan J J 1974 Decreased adhesion of giant (Bernard-Soulier) platelets to subendothelium. American Journal of Medicine 57: 920–925

Weiss H J, Witte L D, Kaplan K L, Lages B A, Chernoff A, Nossel H L, Goodman D S, Baumgartner H R 1979b Heterogeneity in storage pool deficiency: studies on granule-bound substances in 18 patients including variants deficient in α-granules, platelet factor 4, β-thromboglobulin and platelet derived growth factor. Blood 54: 1296–1319

White J G 1974 Electron microscopic studies of platelet secretion. In: Spaet T H (ed) Progress in Hemostasis and Thrombosis, Grune & Stratton, Vol 2, p 49–98

White J G 1979 Ultrastructural studies of the gray platelet syndrome. American Journal of Pathology 95: 445–462

White J G, Gerrard J M 1979 Interaction of microtubules and microfilaments in platelet contractile physiology. Methods and Achievements in Experimental Pathology 9: 1–39

White J G, Gerrard J M 1980 The cell biology of platelets. In: Weissman G (ed) The Cell Biology of Inflammation, Elsevier/North Holland, Amsterdam/New York, 83–143

Wong P Y K, Cheung W Y 1979 Calmodulin stimulates human platelet phospholipase A_2. Biochemical and Biophysical Research Communications 90: 473–480

Workman E F, White G C, Lundblad R L 1977 Structure-function relationships in the interaction of α-thrombin with blood platelets. Journal of Biological Chemistry 252: 7118–7123

Zucker M B, Broekman M J, Kaplan K L 1979a Factor VIII-related antigen in human blood platelets: localization and release by thrombin and collagen. Journal of Laboratory and Clinical Medicine 94: 675–682

Zucker M B, Mosesson M W, Broekman M J, Kaplan K L 1979b Release of platelet fibronectin (cold-insoluble globulin) from α-granules induced by thrombin or collagen: lack of requirement for plasma fibronectin in ADP-induced platelet aggregation. Blood 54: 8–12

Zwaal R F A 1978 Membrane and lipid involvement in blood coagulation. Biochimica et Biophysica Acta 515: 163–205

2. Qualitative platelet disorders

William L. Nichols   Paul Didisheim   Jonathan M. Gerrard

In Chapter 1 we reviewed recent advances in the understanding of platelet ultrastructure, biochemistry and physiology, focusing on the mechanisms of platelet participation in the hemostatic process. Advances in the comprehension and analysis of platelet function and dysfunction have allowed recognition and detailed study of increasing numbers of patients whose hemostatic defects can be attributed to congenital or acquired abnormalities of platelet function (thrombocytopathies). Such study of patients with dysfunctional platelets has contributed importantly to current concepts of platelet function and of the molecular mechanisms of platelet participation in the hemostatic process. In this Chapter we review recent advances in knowledge of the pathophysiology and diagnosis of the congenital and acquired qualitative platelet disorders.

CONGENITAL QUALITATIVE PLATELET DISORDERS

A great variety of these uncommon disorders has been described but only a few are relatively well defined in terms of specific abnormalities of platelet function and in fewer are the defective mechanisms even partially characterized. This review will focus mainly on the latter, emphasizing the disordered physiology as it mirrors normal platelet function.

Glanzmann's thrombasthenia

This autosomal recessive disorder, though rare, is one of the more commonly recognized congenital qualitative platelet defects, perhaps in part because the afflicted patients have significant bleeding problems, and in part because laboratory testing yields a distinctive pattern of abnormalities. Another much rarer congenital platelet disorder, 'essential athrombia', is said to mimic Glanzmann's thrombasthenia in that platelet aggregation is defective (Ulutin, 1976), but normal clot retraction and only partially defective platelet aggregation in the former condition suggest it is distinct from the latter. Currently recognized features of Glanzmann's thrombasthenia are outlined in Table 2.1, and referenced in this section and in Chapter 1. Those features of major significance for unequivocal diagnosis are specifically noted in Table 2.1.

Although most patients with Glanzmann's thrombasthenia display all of the tabulated features to a rather uniform degree, variations in intraplatelet fibrinogen content, or in the clot retraction defect ('thrombasthenia') or of the expression of other abnormalities suggest the disorder may be microheterogencous (Caen et al, 1966; Caen, 1972). Additionally, polytransfused patients can develop thrombocytopenia, presumably due to antiplatelet antibodies. Glanzmann's thrombasthenia is the principal congenital platelet disorder in which platelet aggregation is severely

Table 2.1   Features of Glanzmann's thrombasthenia

Abnormal	Normal
Long bleeding time*	Normal platelet count*
No platelet clumps on native blood smear*	Normal platelet morphology*
No aggregation (ADP, epinephrine, collagen, thrombin, arachidonate)*	Normal shape change (ADP, thrombin collagen, arachidonate)†
Decreased clot retraction*	'Aggregate' with ristocetin/VIII R:WF†
Decreased platelet retention on glass surfaces and in glass bead columns†	Normal receptor binding (ADP, thrombin)
Decreased/abnormal membrane GP IIb & IIIa†	Adhere to subendothelium
Decreased Pl^{A1} antigen†	Normal prostaglandin metabolism
Absent fibrinogen receptors†	Normal 'release' induced by thrombin, arachidonate, ionophores
Absent 'lectin-aggregation receptor'	Normal quinidine-antibody receptor
Decreased α-actinin	Normal platelet life-span
Decreased 'release' induced by ADP, epinephrine, collagen	
Decreased intraplatelet fibrinogen	
Variable prothrombin consumption	
Decreased contact- or collagen-induced coagulant activity	

* Features of major significance for diagnosis.
† Additional fetures of diagnostic importance.

defective (absent) in response to almost all stimuli. An exception among these stimuli is the response of thrombasthenic platelets to bovine or porcine VIII R:WF ('platelet aggregating factor') or to ristocetin and human VIII R:WF (Cooper et al, 1979). These substances can induce cohesion or aggregation of normal or thrombasthenic platelets, but when stirred in an aggregometer with ristocetin and human plasma the clumped thrombasthenic platelets can undergo cyclical de-clumping which can be inhibited by aspirin (Chediak et al, 1979), perhaps because ADP and ATP secretion is prevented by the latter maneuver. Neither the mechanisms of this peculiar response of thrombasthenic platelets, nor of the ability of ristocetin and ATP to restore the defective clot retraction in thrombasthenia (Chediak et al, 1978) are known. One possibility is that human Willebrand factor, by binding to platelet receptors in the presence of ristocetin, may be able to mediate platelet-platelet bridging by partially substituting for the aggregation-promoting functions of the membrane glycoproteins deficient in thrombasthenia (see below).

There is some evidence to suggest that asymptomatic heterozygote carriers of this disorder may sometimes be detected by the discovery of a slightly prolonged bleeding time or of abnormal platelet retention in glass bead columns (Cronberg et al, 1967), despite normal aggregation and clot retraction (Friedman et al, 1964; Pittman & Graham, 1964; Cronberg et al, 1967). Quantitative determination of platelet Pl^{A1} antigen expression (Kunicki & Aster, 1978), or quantitative gel electrophoretic analysis of platelet proteins may prove to be more sensitive techniques for investigation of suspected heterozygotes.

Since Nurden and Caen's observation (1974) of platelet membrane glycoprotein abnormalities in Glanzmann's thrombasthenia, the deficiencies of glycoproteins IIb and IIIa and the apparent normality of other platelet membrane proteins have been confirmed in a number of other laboratories. Subsequent to this fundamental observation, several other apparently interrelated defects of the thrombasthenic platelet membrane have been discovered. Deficiency of the PlAl antigen (present on the platelets in about 98 per cent of normal subjects: Kunicki and Aster, 1978) and deficiency of α-actinin (Gerrard et al, 1979a) in thrombasthenic platelets are both thought to reflect the deficiency of membrane GP IIIa. Deficiencies of fibrinogen binding sites or of a thrombin-induced 'lectin-aggregation receptor' function (Gartner et al, 1978, 1979) on thrombasthenic platelet membranes seem likely to be related to the observed glycoprotein deficiencies, but this relationship is not yet established. Studies by Kinlough-Rathbone et al (1979) support a close relationship between platelet fibrinogen receptor sites and the platelet lectin activity reported by Gartner et al (1979). One hypothesis which could account for many of the observed normalities and abnormalities of platelet function in Glanzmann's thrombasthenia is outlined in Figure 2.1.

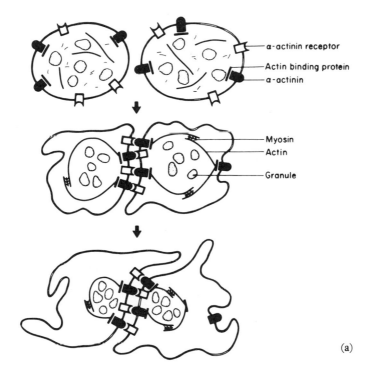

(a)

Fig. 2.1 (a) A proposed model for the interaction of contractile proteins in normal platelets. Following activation of the resting platelet (top), shape change and adherence to adjacent platelets occur (middle). At sites of cell-cell adhesion, α-actinin is shown interacting with a receptor to hold platelets together. As contraction progresses, α-actinin anchors an actin-binding protein and actin to the membrane at the site of cell-cell attachment so that the contraction pulls the granules toward the center of the two platelets. The use of the term 'actin binding protein' is not necessarily meant to imply that this is Filamin (ABP), but rather that there must be a type of actin-binding protein which binds the tails of the actin filaments in order for force to be generated during the contraction. (b) A proposed model for the interaction of platelet contractile filaments in thrombasthenic platelets. Following stimulation, the resting cell (top) undergoes shape change (middle). Actin polymerizes and, in the presence of calcium, actin-myosin interaction takes place. Actin-binding protein anchors filaments of actin so that contraction can occur. As contraction progresses (bottom), the actin-binding protein, lacking a membrane binding site (α-actinin), is pulled away from the membrane and granules are pulled to the center of the cell. Concomitantly, cell-cell adhesion (aggregation)

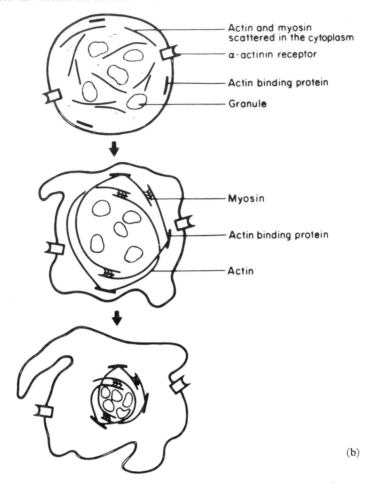

(b)

does not occur, due to the absence of α-actinin (GP IIIa) on the platelet surface. It is not yet known whether this glycoprotein (GP IIIa) or GP IIb might also act as fibrinogen receptors, further accounting for the absence of such activity, and of platelet aggregation in thrombasthenic platelets. Either or both of these glycoproteins might also mediate the 'lectin-aggregation receptor' activity which is also deficient in thrombasthenic platelets. Reprinted with permission of J. M. Gerrard and The American Journal of Pathology (Gerrard et al, 1979a).

Bernard-Soulier syndrome

In contrast to the defective aggregation and normal subendothelial adhesion of platelets in Glanzmann's thrombasthenia, the converse is found in the Bernard-Soulier syndrome where platelet aggregation is relatively normal in response to most stimuli, but the platelets are severely defective in their ability to adhere to subendothelial surfaces (Weiss et al, 1974; Baumgartner et al, 1977). As in Glanzmann's thrombasthenia, bleeding problems can be severe in Bernard-Soulier disease, emphasizing the importance of both platelet-platelet cohesion (aggregation) and of platelet-vessel adhesion in hemostatic plug formation. Table 2.2 outlines the features currently recognized as characteristic of this rare autosomal recessive disorder. The

Bernard-Soulier syndrome is distinct from other congenital macrothrombocytopathic thrombocytopenias (Table 2.6; see below), and those features of particular importance for unequivocal diagnosis of Bernard-Soulier syndrome are specifically noted in Table 2.2.

Table 2.2   Features of Bernard-Soulier syndrome

Abnormal	Normal
Long bleeding time*	Platelets clump on native blood smear*
Thrombocytopenia*	Aggregation (ADP, epinephrine, thrombin,
Giant platelets*	collagen, arachidonate)*
Absent aggregation (ristocetin + VIII R:WF)*	Normal clot retraction*
Decreased/abnormal membrane GP Ib & Is*	Normal prostaglandin metabolism
Decreased sialic acid and negative surface charge	Normal 'release' induced by ADP, epinephrine
Reduced receptor binding (VIII R:AG, thrombin)	collagen, arachidonate
Decreased quinidine-antibody receptors	Normal Pl^{Al} antigen
Decreased subendothelial adhesion	
Variable shape change (ADP)	
Decreased 'release' (thrombin, VIII R:WF)	
Decreased platelet retention in glass bead columns	
Abnormal collagen-induced coagulant activity	
Abnormal prothrombin consumption	
Decreased platelet life span	
Nonspecific morphologic abnormalities	

* Features of major significance for diagnosis.

Asymptomatic heterozygous carriers of this disorder usually have normal platelet counts and bleeding times, but may have an increased percentage of macrothrombocytes, compared to normal subjects (Bithell et al, 1972). Heterozygote detection might also be possible by means of ristocetin/VIII R:WF platelet aggregation, or by quantitative gel electrophoresis of platelet proteins, or by measuring platelet quinidine-antibody receptors (which are apparently present on all normal platelets: Kunicki et al, 1978), but such studies of obligate carriers have not been reported. Deficiency of the latter membrane receptors is apparently not due to the deficiency of membrane glycoproteins Ib and Is in Bernard-Soulier platelets (Kunicki et al, 1978).

The recent demonstrations of various defects in Bernard-Soulier platelet structure and function support the concept (Nurden & Caen, 1975) of a major role for the interaction of specific platelet membrane proteins (components of the GP I 'complex') with specific plasmatic proteins (Willebrand factor) in the mediation of specific platelet functions (platelet-vessel adhesion). In the Bernard-Soulier syndrome these supporting observations include: decreased platelet sialic acid and surface charge (membrane defect: Gröttum & Solum, 1969); absent platelet aggregation in response to bovine Willebrand factor (Bithell et al, 1972; Howard et al, 1973); decreased platelet adhesion to subendothelial surfaces (Weiss et al, 1974; Caen et al, 1976; Baumgartner et al, 1977); abnormalities of platelet membrane glycoproteins (Nurden & Caen, 1975; Caen et al, 1976; Jenkins et al, 1976; Jamieson et al, 1979); and diminished membrane binding of Willebrand factor (Ando, 1979; Moake et al, 1979). The platelet dysfunction resulting from the abnormal interaction of specific platelet proteins with specific plasmatic proteins is summarized in Table 2.3.

Table 2.3 Abnormal proteins and platelet dysfunction

Disorder	Platelet dysfunction	Defective protein
von Willebrand's Disease	Adhesion	VIII R:WF
Bernard-Soulier Syndrome	Adhesion	GP Ib, Is
Glanzmann's Thrombasthenia	Aggregation	GP IIb, IIIa
Afibrinogenemia	Aggregation	Fibrinogen

Platelet storage and secretion disorders

Formerly included under the general rubric of 'thrombocytopathy' or 'thrombo-pathy', these disorders were distinguished following the introduction of the platelet aggregometer into clinical practice (Hardisty & Hutton, 1967; O'Brien, 1967; Weiss, 1967). At about the same time, aspirin ingestion was observed to cause an apparently identical defect (inhibition of ADP release, defective collagen-induced platelet aggregation, and absence of 'secondary aggregation' in response to ADP or epinephrine: Weiss & Aledort, 1967; Evans et al, 1968; O'Brien, 1968; Zucker & Peterson, 1968). Platelet aggregometry remains the chief means of identifying these disorders which may be due either to defective storage by platelet secretory granules ('*storage pool deficiencies*') or to defective mechanisms of granular secretion ('*release defects*'). Both types of disorders can be associated with variable bleeding tendencies (mild to moderately severe), and often but not always display similar aggregometric patterns. Differentiation of defects of storage from those of release can be made by morphologic observation and quantitation of platelet storage granules, and by measurement of the intraplatelet content and the secretion of stored substances such as those of dense granules (adenine nucleotides, serotonin, calcium) or of α-granules (platelet factor 4, β-thromboglobulin, platelet derived growth factor, platelet fibri-nogen) or of lysosomes (acid hydrolases). Recent studies re-emphasize the clinical heterogeneity of these disorders (Table 2.4), and provide improved understanding of the several mechanisms which may be involved.

Granule storage disorders

Defective granule storage is now recognized in a wide variety of congenital and acquired qualitative platelet disorders. In a few of these disorders storage pool

Table 2.4 Heterogeneity of platelet storage/release defects

Congenital disorders	Acquired disorders
Hermansky-Pudlak syndrome[a]	Drugs
Chédiak-Higashi syndrome[a]	Myeloproliferative syndromes
Wiskott-Aldrich syndrome[a]	Autoimmune disorders
Gray platelet syndrome[a]	Consumptive thrombocytopenias
Thrombocytopenia-absent radius syndrome[a]	Other
Alport's syndrome	
Down's syndrome	
Enzyme deficiencies	
cyclooxygenase	
thromboxane synthetase	
Other thrombocytopathies	

[a] Abnormal granule storage. Other listed disorders can have defective release of granule contents, which may or may not be due to abnormal storage.

deficiency represents the major currently recognized platelet defect, while in the remainder other functional defects may also occur. Biochemically confirmed storage pool deficiencies have usually been associated with decreased numbers of storage organelles (dense granules or α-granules or both). Weiss et al (1979b) have proposed a classification of these disorders, based upon differing deficiencies of dense or α-granules and their contents (Table 2.5).

Table 2.5 Platelet storage deficiencies

Nomenclature[a]	Affected Organelle	Example
α	α-granule	Gray platelet syndrome
δ	dense granule	Hermansky-Pudlak syndrome
αδ	α-and dense granules	Heterogeneous
λ	lysosome	None described

[a] Weiss et al (1979b).

ALPHA GRANULE DISORDERS

Isolated deficiency of α-granules and their contents appears to be exceedingly rare, as only four cases have so far been described (Gerrard et al, 1979b; Nurden et al, 1979), all of patients with mild bleeding disorders and 'gray platelets.' The *gray platelet syndrome* was described by Raccuglia in 1971, the affected patient displaying hypogranular platelets, mild to moderate thrombocytopenia, marked prolongation of the bleeding time, a mild bleeding tendency, and nearly normal platelet aggregation in response to ADP, epinephrine or collagen. The more recently reported studies, including those of White (1979), have confirmed a specific deficiency of α-granules and their contents (PF4, β-thromboglobulin, platelet derived growth factor, thrombospondin, platelet fibrinogen) in these patients. This syndrome appears to be clinically heterogeneous. Deficiency of α-granules may occur more frequently in combination with dense granule deficiency (see below).

DENSE GRANULE DISORDERS

Unique deficiencies of dense granules and their contents are much more commonly recognized than are deficiences of only α-granules, and appear to be frequently associated with mild to moderately severe bleeding syndromes. Many of these patients have been recognized as albinos or partial albinos (Logan et al, 1971; Hardisty et al, 1972; Maurer et al, 1972), although non-albinos may also have isolated dense granule defects (Weiss et al, 1979b) while other albinos apparently have neither defective platelets nor bleeding tendencies (Logan et al, 1971; Hardisty et al, 1972). It now seems apparent that those albinos with a bleeding disorder and a deficiency of platelet dense granules represent examples of the *Hermansky-Pudlak syndrome*, described by these authors in 1959 and charcterized by tyrosinase-positive oculo-cutaneous albinism, ceroid-like pigment deposition in reticuloendothelial cells, and a significant hemorrhagic diathesis associated with a prolonged bleeding time. More recent studies (White et al, 1971; White & Witkop, 1972; Hermansky & Cieslar, 1976; Rendu et al,

1978; Weiss et al, 1979b) have documented a deficiency of platelet dense granules and their contents in this autosomal recessive syndrome. Gerritsen et al (1977) observed that heterozygous carriers of this disorder are phenotypically normal, but have defective storage of serotonin in their platelets. A recent report (Garay et al, 1979) emphasizes the occurrence of pulmonary interstitial fibrosis or an inflammatory-like bowel syndrome in these patients, associated with tissue deposition of the ceroid-like material. Although the basic biochemical disturbances underlying this disorder are not clear, several studies (Hermanksy & Cieslar, 1976; Malmsten et al, 1977; Rendu et al, 1978) suggest that defective phospholipid metabolism, perhaps resulting from an impairment of arachidonic acid incorporation or release, may be involved.

The *Chédiak-Higashi syndrome* represents another phenotypically recognizable autosomal recessive disorder (partial or psuedo-albinism, giant inclusion granules in leukocytes and platelets, propensity for pyogenic infections, hemorrhagic tendency) in which the bleeding disorder and platelet functional defect are now thought to result mainly from a deficiency of dense granules and their contents (Bell et al, 1976a; Buchanan & Handin, 1976; Boxer et al, 1977; Meyers et al, 1979a). Other congenital syndromes in which deficient or defective platelet dense granule storage may occur include the sex-linked *Wiskott-Aldrich syndrome* (Gröttum et al, 1969), some cases of the autosomal recessive *thrombocytopenia-absent radius (TAR) syndrome* (Day & Holmsen, 1972), and patients with *Down's syndrome* (McCoy & Enns, 1978). In the latter disorder there is no hemorrhagic diathesis and the defective platelet storage of serotonin is thought to reflect an abnormality of serotonin uptake by the platelet membrane rather than a defect of dense granule function.

Isolated congenital deficiencies of dense granules and their contents can also occur in the absence of other phenotypically apparent abnormalities, and result in mild to moderate bleeding tendencies. These disorders are genetically and clinically hetero-geneous, and their incidence probably exceeds that of the albino-associated dense granule defects (Lorez et al, 1979; Weiss et al, 1979b). Recent studies indicate that, while platelet aggregation induced by ADP, epinephrine or collagen is usually abnormal in disorders with dense granule deficiency, arachidonate-induced platelet aggregation is often normal (White & Witkop, 1972; Gerrard et al, 1975; Weiss et al, 1976; Ingerman et al, 1978; Meyers et al, 1979b; Minkes et al, 1979). These investigations support the concept that secretion of dense granule substances is important for the 'secondary wave' of platelet aggregation in response to weak stimuli, and also indicate that secreted dense granule substances are not essential for platelet aggregation which can be mediated by prostaglandin endoperoxides or by other mechanisms. The observation of normal arachidonate-induced platelet aggregation in the presence of partially impaired aggregation induced by ADP, epinephrine and collagen may be helpful in identifying patients with deficiencies of dense granules. Correction of the abnormal aggregation of these platelets by mixing them with equal portions of aspirin-treated platelets (White & Witkop, 1972; Gerrard et al, 1975) is another means for identifying dense granule deficiency. Thromboxane A_2, generated upon stimulation of dense granule-deficient platelets, can be released and can act as an intercellular messenger effecting aggregation and secretion of the aspirin-treated normal platelets. ADP secreted from the latter platelets may, in turn, promote aggregation of the dense granule-deficient platelets. These and other observations (Minkes et al, 1979) also support the concept of multiple mechanisms mediating platelet aggregation (thromboxanes, secreted ADP, and other thromboxane- and ADP-independent pathways). In addition to moderate defects of platelet aggregation, dense granule-deficient platelets may display mildly decreased adhesion to subendothelial surfaces, the latter function being normal in aspirin-treated platelets (Weiss et al, 1975; Baumgartner et al, 1977).

It has been reported that infusion of cryoprecipitate preparations (Gerritsen et al, 1978) may temporarily ameliorate the hemostatic defect in patients with dense granule deficiencies. Neither the mechanisms nor the general efficacy of such treatment are yet known. Platelet storage pool or secretion deficiency syndromes may also occur on an acquired basis (Table 2.4). These acquired platelet defects are discussed in the section on acquired qualitative platelet disorders.

COMBINED DENSE AND ALPHA GRANULE DEFICIENCIES

Combined deficiencies of platelet dense and α-granules have been recently recognized in a few patients with congenital storage pool deficiency syndromes (Weiss et al, 1979b). Although they have a significant bleeding tendency, the patients reported appear to have no other clinically evident stigmata suggesting deficiency of both types of storage organelles. The few cases reported thus far do not allow conclusions as to whether clinical bleeding may be more severe in patients with combined storage pool deficiencies than in patients with only defects of dense granules. Another study (Pareti et al, 1979a) suggests that combined storage deficiency syndromes may be considerably less common than isolated dense granule deficiency syndromes. Deficiencies of lysosomal granules and their contents have not been reported.

Secretion or release defects

These congenital disorders, like the granule storage (storage pool) thrombocytopathies, are associated with deficient secretion of granular contents such that platelet aggregation is partially defective in response to ADP, epinephrine or collagen. In contrast to the granule storage deficiencies, in the syndromes of defective release, platelet storage granules and their contents are quantitatively normal, but the stored substances are inadequately secreted in response to stimuli. These maladies have been associated with minimal to moderate bleeding, and are probably more common, and even more heterogeneous in origin, than the defects of granular storage. In only a few of these disorders are the defective mechanisms of secretion partially understood.

The acquired platelet secretion defect associated with aspirin ingestion ('*aspirin defect*') closely mimics the functional abnormalities characteristic of some congenital platelet release disorders (i.e., normal platelet subendothelial adhesion, but defective collagen-induced aggregation, lack of 'secondary aggregation' in response to ADP or epinephrine, and totally absent platelet aggregation following addition of arachidonic acid). While in the case of aspirin ingestion these functional defects are now thought to result from an inability of platelets to generate thromboxanes from arachidonic acid, due to inactivation of the platelet cyclo-oxygenase enzyme by aspirin (see section on acquired qualitative platelet disorders), a few patients with similar defects of platelet function and a lifelong mild bleeding tendency have been found to have an apparently congenital *deficiency of cyclo-oxygenase enzyme function* (Malmsten et al, 1975; Weiss & Lages, 1977; Lagarde et al, 1978; Pareti et al, 1979b; Nyman et al, 1979). Another patient with a similar bleeding disorder and platelet functional defects may have a *deficiency of platelet thromboxane synthetase enzyme function* (Weiss & Lages, 1977). These patients apparently have no other phenotypic abnormalities.

A large variety of patients with bleeding syndromes and platelet secretion defects have been described. A few of these patients may display phenotypic syndromes such as the autosomal dominantly inherited *Alport's syndrome* (macrothrombocytopathia, deafness, nephritis: Epstein et al, 1972; Clare et al, 1979). Some may have structurally abnormal platelets, such as '*Swiss-cheese*' *platelets* (Smith et al, 1973; Maldonado, 1974a) or *microthrombocytes* (Maurer et al, 1974). Others may have an associated defect of plasmatic proteins such as *Hemophilia A* (Chesney et al, 1974) or *von Willebrand's disease* (Dowling et al, 1976). Most have no additionally recognized clinical features, other than a bleeding disorder (Sahud & Aggeler, 1969; Weiss et al, 1969; Weiss & Rogers, 1972; Kubisz, 1973; Pareti et al, 1974; Chesney et al, 1977; Wu et al, 1979). While some of these patients might have defects of platelet prostaglandin metabolism, in none are the biochemical defects known.

Other studies suggest that mild abnormalities of platelet function, manifest by deficient platelet secretion and/or deficient platelet aggregation, particularly in response to epinephrine or collagen, might not be uncommon (Lackner & Karpatkin, 1975; Czapek et al, 1978). These individuals, otherwise hemostatically normal, may be particularly sensitive to the 'antiplatelet' effects of aspirin which can greatly prolong the bleeding time ('*aspirin tolerance test*': Quick, 1966; Stuart et al, 1979), and result in 'oozing and bruising'' (Zucker et al, 1972; Czapek et al, 1978).

Congenital thrombocytopathic thrombocytopenia
The congenital thrombocytopathic thrombocytopenias (Table 2.6) comprise another

Table 2.6   Congenital thrombocytopathic thrombocytopenia

Macrothrombocytic thrombocytopenias
   Bernard-Soulier syndrome
   'Montreal platelet syndrome'
   Alport's syndrome (macrothrombocytopathia, deafness, nephritis)
   'Swiss cheese platelet' syndromes
   May-Hegglin anomaly
   Other macrothrombocytic thrombocytopathies

Microthrombocytic thrombocytopenias
   Wiskott-Aldrich syndrome
   TAR syndrome (some cases)
   Other microthrombocytic thrombocytopathies

Miscellaneous thrombocytopathic thrombocytopenias
   Sex-linked inheritance
   Autosomal recessive inheritance
   Autosomal dominant inheritance
   'Sporadic'

---

large category of bleeding syndromes due to qualitative platelet disorders, all characterized by thrombocytopenia of variable degree, in addition to platelet function defects. Determination of platelet size or volume by morphometric or electronic particle sizing techniques (Murphy, 1972; Milton & Frojmovic, 1979) may be of help in differentiating these disorders, some of which may have an increased proportion of macrothrombocytes or microthrombocytes. A few of these disorders may have other distinguishing features such as the Döhle bodies found in the granulocytes and monocytes of patients with the *May-Hegglin anomaly* (Lusher et al, 1968; Gausis et al, 1969; Goudemand & Parquet-Gernez, 1973; Godwin & Ginsburg, 1974). Other recognizable syndromes in patients with these disorders are noted in Table 2.6, and referenced in this and preceding sections.

It is now appreciated that a number of individuals with congenital thrombocyto-pathic thrombocytopenia may have no other phenotypical abnormalities, but have a hereditary disorder. In the majority of reported families the inheritance has been autosomal dominant or codominant, and much less often sex-linked or recessive (Bithell et al, 1965; Quick, 1965; Kurstjens et al, 1968; Vossen et al, 1968; Murphy, 1972; Sultan et al, 1974; Ardlie et al, 1976). Platelet survival and bone marrow megakaryocytes have often been normal, but abnormalities of platelet function have been commonly noted, in addition to thrombocytopenia. The biochemical defects in these disorders are not known. As these types of disorders may closely resemble the more frequently observed acquired thrombocytopenias (e.g., immune-mediated thrombocytopenias), and as corticosteroid therapy or splenectomy is usually not indicated for treatment of the congenital disorders (Murphy, 1972), it is particularly important to be aware of their existence. Testing for the presence of antiplatelet antibodies may be of some additional help in distinguishing the acquired immune-mediated thrombocytopenias from the congenital thrombocytopenias.

Significance of congenital platelet dysfunction

Congenital qualitative platelet disorders, including the hereditary thrombocytopenias, are probably at least as common as the hereditary abnormalities of plasmatic coagulation factors. Though congenital platelet dysfunction may often result in only mild bleeding symptoms, and therefore be often overlooked, improved recognition and detailed study of patients with these disorders should be of benefit not only to the afflicted patients, but also for the impetus such study provides for improved understanding of the normal mechanisms of platelet participation in the hemostatic process.

ACQUIRED QUALITATIVE PLATELET DISORDERS

Acquired platelet dysfunction is probably second only to thrombocytopenia as the major cause of clinical bleeding disorders. In addition, several acquired qualitative platelet disorders have been associated with thrombotic tendencies.

Myeloproliferative disorders (MPD)

Bleeding or thrombotic tendencies in association with myeloproliferative disorders have long been recognized. Abnormal bleeding has been characterized by easy bruising, epistaxes, and gastrointestinal hemorrhage in the face of a normal or elevated platelet count and little or no abnormality in the plasma coagulation factor or fibrinolytic mechanisms. Frequent prolongation of the bleeding time led to suspicion of a qualitative platelet defect. Paradoxically, thrombosis also is common, such that abnormal bleeding or clotting contributes significantly to morbidity and mortality. Recent evidence suggests that this puzzling clinical spectrum may on occasion be explained by a process of disseminated intravascular platelet aggregation and an acquired platelet storage pool defect (see below).

Primary hemorrhagic thrombocythemia (essential thrombocythemia, ET)

In 1955 Hardisty and Wolff described abnormalities of platelet function in five patients with this disorder; these included defective platelet coagulant activity as measured in the thromboplastin generation test in five, and reduced platelet serotonin in three. Platelet coagulant activity was not reduced in patients with other MPD without bleeding; however platelet serotonin level was not correlated with bleeding. Although hemorrhagic manifestations usually dominate, thrombotic events may occur. In one series of nine patients, aged 46 to 83, incipient gangrene of the toes was especially common (Hussain et al, 1978). Decreased epinephrine-induced platelet aggregation was the commonest platelet function abnormality noted in these patients. ADP-induced aggregation was usually normal and platelet factor 3 availability was normal in all patients. In a report of six patients with ET under 30 years of age (Hoagland & Silverstein, 1978), abnormal epinephrine aggregation and variable ADP aggregation occurred in six, abnormal collagen aggregation in none, abnormal platelet retention in two, spontaneous platelet aggregation and variable prothrombin consumption in one. No hemorrhagic or thrombotic complications were observed in a 14-month to 10-year followup without treatment. The clinical contrast between these two latter studies may be reconciled by the concept that the frequency of thrombotic or hemorrhagic manifestations in ET is governed largely by the presence of vascular disease (which increases with age) and less by the nature of the platelet defect. Platelet function testing may be of value in distinguishing ET from secondary thrombocytosis (see below). In the latter, platelet function tests are usually normal or nearly so. Such testing may be of particular diagnostic help in the patient with thrombocytosis who lacks other clinical or laboratory features typical of MPD.

Polycythemia vera (PV)

Patients with poorly controlled polycythemia vera are at increased risk for hemorrhage or thrombotic complications. The incidence of abnormal platelet function in PV may approach 80 per cent (Berger et al, 1973), being especially increased in those patients with elevated hematocrits and platelet counts or with 'spent' PV. No relation has been found between the observed abnormalities of platelet function and the hemorrhagic or thrombotic tendency.

Myelofibrosis (MF) and agnogenic myeloid metaplasia (AMM)

A bleeding tendency associated with this disorder has been recognized since the condition was first decribed. Hepatic or portal vein thrombosis is not rare, and other thrombotic events account for a substantial proportion of deaths (Silverstein, 1975). In 1966 Didisheim and Bunting investigated ten patients with MF and a normal platelet count, and found evidence of a qualitative platelet disorder in most of these. A prolonged bleeding time was seen in nine of ten, abnormal prothrombin consumption in four of nine, reduced platelet factor 3 in three of eight, and diminished adhesion to the lips of a bleeding-time wound in three of the six patients examined.

Chronic granulocytic leukemia (CGL)

Gerrard et al (1978) examined platelet function in eight patients. Seven had an absent second wave of epinephrine-induced aggregation, and five had impaired collagen aggregation. The platelets of all seven with abnormal epinephrine responses aggregated with arachidonic acid, thus excluding a cyclo-oxygenase deficiency. In five patients evaluated, a marked decrease in ADP, serotonin, and number of dense granules in platelets was found. Mixing platelets of CGL patients with platelets of normal subjects who had ingested aspirin led to normal malondialdehyde production. These findings suggest that CGL platelets have an acquired storage pool deficiency, but have intact prostaglandin and thromboxane synthetic pathways.

Paroxysmal nocturnal hemoglobinuria (PNH)
In this disorder, sometimes considered as a myeloproliferative syndrome (Dameshek, 1969), a membrane defect of erythrocytes, granulocytes and platelets renders these cells unusually susceptible to the lytic actions of plasma complement components (Rosse, 1977). Dixon and Rosse (1977) have implicated the complement-induced hyperactivatability of PNH platelets in the thrombotic complications frequently seen in PNH.

General observations
Major structural abnormalities were observed in the platelets of 15 of 16 patients with myelomonocytic leukemia or 'preleukemia' (Maldonado et al, 1974; Maldonado & Pierre, 1975). In most cases there were two platelet populations, one morphologically normal and one abnormal. The most salient changes included giant forms (up to 10 μm in diameter), rounded forms, decrease or absence of microtubules, and increase in immature elements. There was a striking variation in size and shape of granules, some being up to 2.5 μm in diameter. There was no correlation between the chromosomal changes observed by cytogenetic analysis and the platelet structural anomalies. Similar major structural abnormalities, including paucity of granules, were noted in patients with chronic MPD (Maldonado, 1974b).

The ultrastructure and adenine nucleotide metabolism of platelets from nine patients with leukemia were investigated (Cowan et al, 1975). These leukemias included CGL in blast crisis, acute myeloblastic leukemia, acute monocytic leukemia, and hairy cell leukemia (leukemic reticuloendotheliosis). Structural alterations, similar to those noted in the paragraph above, were observed. Intracellular ATP and ADP concentrations were significantly reduced; addition of ADP or collagen to platelets resulted in delayed and incomplete shape change and impaired centripetal migration of organelles and degranulation; addition of collagen resulted in release of subnormal amounts of ADP and ATP. Rendu et al (1979) found reduced numbers of dense bodies in platelets of patients with MPD. Patients with AMM had few or no dense bodies, and had platelet aggregation anomalies like those mentioned above as well as diminished thrombin-induced serotonin release. These findings taken together suggest that the disorder in many patients with MPD may be classified as an acquired *storage pool deficiency* (SPD). Zuzel et al (1979) arrived at a similar conclusion in studies of patients with hairy cell leukemia (leukemic reticuloendotheliosis).

Keenan et al (1977) found abnormal platelet lipid peroxidation in ten patients with differing MPD, suggesting *abnormal prostaglandin metabolism*. Platelet lipoxygenase and cyclo-oxygenase pathways were investigated in 33 patients with various MPD (Okuma & Uchino, 1979). Decreased lipoxygenase was observed in three of three patients with MF, eight of 14 with CGL, six of 12 with PV, and one of four with ET. Cyclo-oxygenase activity was decreased in only three of the 33 patients: one with

CGL, one with PV, and one with ET. In four of 10 patients with a selective lipoxygenase deficiency, platelets were aggregated by lower concentrations of arachidonic acid than were normal platelets, suggesting increased generation of thromboxane A_2 via the cyclo-oxygenase pathway. It was postulated that this latter defect might contribute to the thrombotic tendency which may exist in some patients with these disorders, although the incidence of bleeding and thrombosis in this series was too low to test that hypothesis. On the other hand in two patients with preleukemia, Russell et al (1979) found evidence for production of TXA_2 of normal quantity but low biological activity. Cooper et al (1978) found platelet resistance to the inhibitory effects of PGD_2 in 20 of 23 patients with MPD, and suggested such resistance may contribute to a thrombotic diathesis.

A number of studies have suggested that *platelet aggregometry* is of value in distinguishing patients with elevated platelet counts associated with MPD from patients with reactive thrombocytosis (McClure et al, 1966; Spaet et al, 1969; Sultan & Jeanneau, 1971; Cardamone et al, 1972; Inceman & Tangün, 1972; Neemeh et al, 1972; Zucker & Mielke, 1972; Berger et al, 1973; Ginsburg, 1975; Hagedorn et al, 1979; Nishimura et al, 1979; Pareti et al, 1979c). These tests were usually normal in patients with reactive thrombocytosis. Absent or decreased aggregation with epinephrine or collagen seem to be the most common changes seen in MPD. Bleeding time and platelet aggregation with collagen may correlate best with hemorrhagic manifestations. In some of these studies ATP and ADP were reduced in the platelets of patients with abnormal aggregation, as was release of these nucleotides following platelet stimulation. In contrast, platelets of the patients with normal functions contained near-normal nucleotide levels. The data suggest that these platelet defects may often be attributable to reduction of releasable ADP in the platelets of patients with MPD. Wu et al (1978) investigated 28 patients with thrombocythemia due to MPD and 11 with reactive thrombocytosis. None of the latter had thrombotic or hemorrhagic complications, but thrombosis was noted in seven and bleeding in two of those with thrombocythemia. All seven who had thrombotic complications had *circulating platelet aggregates*, and six had *spontaneous platelet aggregation*.

Elevated plasma *β-thromboglobulin* (β-TG) and reduced platelet β-TG were found in 16 patients with MPD (Boughton et al, 1978). In thrombocytosis related to other causes, similar but less marked changes were found. The abnormalities were increased during episodes of clinical thrombosis and could be suppressed in four of six patients by aspirin therapy, providing further evidence of an acquired storage pool defect in MPD (Boughton et al, 1977).

Alterations of *platelet coagulant activities* were studied by Walsh et al (1977b) in 22 patients with thrombocytosis. Two of 16 patients with MPD had thrombotic complications, and their platelets had increased coagulant activities concerned with the early phases of intrinsic coagulation (collagen-induced coagulant activity). Semeraro et al (1979) found a reduction in platelet factor X-activating activity in six of 12 patients with ET or PV. This reduction seemed to be related to bleeding or thrombotic complications. In both of these studies platelet factor 3 activities, measured by Stypven time, were normal.

Platelet membrane glycoproteins have been analyzed in patients with MPD (Vainer & Bussel, 1976 and 1977; Bolin et al, 1977; Fujimura et al, 1979). In all studies, quantitative abnormalities of various major membrane glycoproteins were found, most commonly an apparent increase or decrease in the GP I group. Qualitative abnormalities frequently noted include altered electrophoretic migration or abnormal heterogeneity of the major membrane glycoprotein species. Bolin et al (1977) could not correlate glycoprotein alterations with diagnosis, platelet counts or platelet aggregation responses, though patients with increased numbers of large platelets seemed to have similar alterations of one glycoprotein species. A reduced number of *membrane binding sites* for thrombin, PGD_2 or dihydroergocryptine has been observed in patients with MPD (Cooper & Ahern, 1979; Ganguly et al, 1978; Kaywin et al, 1978; Vainer & Bussel, 1979). Such alterations in plasma membrane structure or function seem analogous to those generally seen in malignant or transformed cells. In platelets these membrane alterations are likely to be significant in the pathogenesis of thrombohemorrhagic phenomena. *Platelet survival* is often decreased in chronic MPD (Weinfeld et al, 1975). An inverse correlation between splenic size and platelet survival has been noted. It is not known whether the observed abnormalities of certain platelet membrane glycoproteins may also contribute to decreased platelet survival.

The paradoxical occurrence of thrombosis and hemorrhage in some patients with MPD may be explained by the unifying concept of *disseminated intravascular platelet release and aggregation* with the circulation of disaggregated platelets which have acquired a *storage pool defect*. In some patients, depending upon the type and clinical severity of MPD, platelets are probably structurally and functionally abnormal from the time they are released into the circulation, and so are 'born' with a storage or release defect. Megakaryocytes in patients with MPD are commonly abnormal structurally, supporting this concept (Maldonado, 1974b; Maldonado & Pierre, 1975; Cowan et al, 1975). It is tempting to speculate that those patients who have predominantly the latter kind of platelets are particularly prone to have bleeding complications, whereas those whose platelets undergo release, aggregation and disaggregation in the circulation are more likely to be have thromboembolic problems.

Despite numerous studies of platelet structure and function in MPD, several of which show prognostic promise, it is not yet possible by laboratory means to identify clearly which patients are at greater risk for hemorrhage or thrombosis. Further study seems warranted, both for this purpose, and for improved understanding of the mechanisms of platelet dysfunction, hemorrhage and thrombosis in these disorders.

Acquired storage pool or release defects

These types of defects have also been observed in conditions other than MPD. Like the congenital platelet storage pool or release disorders, the acquired defects are heterogeneous in origin. Regan et al (1974) studied platelet function in 19 patients with *systemic lupus erythematosus*. Impaired platelet function, consistent with a storage pool or release defect, was observed in half of the patients, all of whom had normal platelet counts, and some of whom had antiplatelet globulins in their sera. Clancy et al (1972) found similar platelet function abnormalities in nine of 11 patients with *chronic idiopathic thrombocytopenic purpura* at a time when their platelet counts were normal. Zahavi and Marder (1974) described a patient with an antiplatelet antibody and other autoimmune phenomena in addition to thrombophlebitis; platelet studies showed aggregation patterns and alterations of stored substances consistent with storage pool defect. Platelet functions returned to normal and platelet antibody disappeared following steroid therapy. The thrombophlebitis might have resulted from the intravascular release of thrombogenic platelet components (i.e. ADP, TXA_2).

The platelet disorder in patients with *cyanotic congenital heart disease* (Ekert & Sheers, 1974) may be another example of storage or release defects. Delayed or absent platelet aggregation with epinephrine, and defective serotonin release in response to ADP have been observed. Corrective surgery usually restored platelet function to normal. It must be kept in mind that, because of their severe polycythemia, the platelet rich plasma of these patients has a higher than normal citrate anticoagulant concentration, which may contribute in part to the in vitro abnormalities of platelet function reported.

The hemostatic defect induced by *cardiopulmonary bypass* is complex but includes thrombocytopenia and qualitative platelet disorder. McKenna et al (1975) examined 13 patients undergoing open-heart surgery. At the end of bypass, reductions in platelet adhesiveness to glass beads and in platelet aggregation to ADP, as well as elevated fibrin degradation products and reduced fibrinogen and platelet count were observed. Platelet total and releasable ADP and ATP dropped significantly when comparing pre- and post-operative specimens (Beurling-Harbury & Galvan, 1978). The decrease in secretory ADP was significantly correlated with postoperative bleeding and with duration of bypass. Patients with severe valvular heart disease had lower releasable platelet ADP and ATP levels than did controls, and also had reduced total platelet ADP (Beurling-Harbury & Galvan, 1978). The releasable ADP levels were correlated with the severity of surgical and postoperative bleeding. Although the surgery itself may contribute to this complex hemostatic disorder, platelet injury caused by the bypass is probably the major factor. Holcomb et al (1979) have observed that infusion of prostacyclin (PGI_2) during cardiopulmonary bypass improves platelet function and survival, reducing intra- and post-operative bleeding. Use of this agent may prove to be important in reducing the morbidity and mortality associated with cardiopulmonary bypass surgery.

Renal disease

Platelet dysfunction plays a role in the bleeding tendency associated with *uremia*. Abnormalities have included reductions in in vivo platelet adhesiveness, retention by glass beads, coagulant activity (in TGT), factor-3 availability, and clot retraction (Lewis et al, 1956; Castaldi et al, 1966; Horowitz et al, 1967; Eknoyan et al, 1969). Eknoyan et al found a significant inverse correlation between the serum urea nitrogen and creatinine levels and platelet adhesiveness. Ingestion of urea prolonged the bleeding time in five of 10 normal subjects, and decreased platelet adhesiveness to pathological levels in eight. The pattern of aggregation defect suggests inhibition of the release reaction (Hutton & O'Shea, 1968). These abnormalities as well as the bleeding tendency are correctable by hemodialysis or peritoneal dialysis (Stewart & Castaldi, 1967), implying that they are caused by metabolites retained in the plasma. Horowitz et al (1970) provided evidence that the inhibitory substance is neither urea nor creatinine but guanidinosuccinic acid; Davis et al (1972) however found urea to be inhibitory. Rabiner and Molinas (1970) implicated the increased plasma levels of phenolic acids. The mechanism of inhibition of platelet function by these classes of compounds may differ (Rabiner, 1972). Remuzzi et al (1977) found elevated prostacyclin-like activity in venous tissues from three uremic patients with prolonged bleeding times, suggesting this platelet inhibitory compound might contribute to uremic bleeding.

Children with nonuremic *active glomerular disease* have *enhanced* platelet aggregation (Bang et al, 1972). This may be caused by loss in the urine of plasma proteins normally responsible for inhibition of platelet aggregation. A reduction in the mean threshhold concentration of ADP or arachidonic acid required to induce platelet aggregation was found in 19 patients with *nephrotic syndrome* (Remuzzi et al, 1979). All had low serum levels of albumin, the level correlating significantly with aggregation threshold. Restitution of normal albumin levels in vitro or in vivo resulted in return of the arachidonic aggregation thresholds to normal. While albumin might act by altering platelet prostaglandin metabolism, other mechanisms such as hypercholesterolemia-induced platelet hyperfunction (see section on lipid alterations) could be more significant. These observations may have relevance to the thrombotic tendency in this disorder.

Dysproteinemias
Vigliano and Horowitz (1967) reported that IgA myeloma protein interferes with fibrinogen polymerization and also coats collagen; the latter action could explain the prolonged bleeding time despite a normal platelet count which may be seen in patients with multiple myeloma. Platelet aggregation may also be suppressed, possibly by coating of platelets by the abnormal protein (Bang et al, 1972). Kasturi & Saraya (1978), noting decreased platelet factor 3 availability in dysproteinemic patients, hypothesized that high plasma concentrations of these abnormal globulins may produce intravascular platelet activation resulting in impaired platelet function.

Fibrinogen and fibrin degradation products (FDP)
FDP inhibit platelet aggregation, contributing in this way (as well as by their effects on the coagulation mechanism) to the hemostatic failure seen with disseminated intravascular coagulation (DIC) (Sharp, 1977). Jerushalmy & Zucker (1966) suggested that FDP inhibit platelet activation and release induced by thrombin, collagen, or ADP. Low molecular weight (dialysable) FDP seem most potent in inhibiting platelet aggregation (Stachurska et al, 1979). Acquired storage pool deficiency of platelets may also be seen in DIC (Pareti et al, 1976), suggesting that intravascular platelet aggregation may contribute to platelet hemostatic failure in this disorder, in addition to contributions from thrombocytopenia and from the inhibitory effects of FDP. High plasma levels of fibrinogen, induced by hypertransfusion of hemophiliacs with cryoprecipiate, can also inhibit platelet function and result in paradoxical bleeding (Hathaway et al, 1973; Edson, 1979). This phenomenon may be due, in part, to FDP (Edson, 1979).

Liver disease
The hemostatic problem in severe liver disease may also stem in part from the elevated FDP levels in the plasma of such patients. There appears to be a correlation between such levels and the bleeding time but not with the degree of abnormality of platelet aggregation (Ballard & Marcus, 1976). Although bleeding times and platelet counts were normal or nearly so in 16 patients with Wilson disease (hepatolenticular degeneration), 15 of them had some abnormality of platelet aggregation, most

frequently when collagen was used (Owen et al, 1976). Marked decreases of platelet membrane glycoprotein I were found in platelets of three cirrhotic patients (Ordinas et al, 1978). It was suggested that this acquired membrane protein abnormality, similar to that in congenital Bernard-Soulier disease, might be responsible for defective platelet adhesion to subendothelium and the observed prolongation of bleeding times.

Endocrine alterations

Patients with *hypothyroidism* may have prolonged bleeding times and decreased platelet retention in glass bead columns, in addition to mild decreases of certain plasmatic coagulation factors (Edson et al, 1975). Several of these patients had a bleeding tendency which improved with treatment of the hypothyroidism. *Pregnant* women, as well as those taking *oral contraceptives* (o/c), had increased rates of ADP-induced second-phase platelet aggregation (Yamazaki et al, 1979) and shortened plasma clotting times due to increased platelet procoagulant activity (Lecompte & Renaud, 1973). McGrath and Castaldi (1975) found increased platelet aggregation by collagen, and Leff et al (1979) found significantly increased platelet factor 3 activity and decreased serum antithrombin III activity in women taking o/c. Peters et al (1979) noted a change in the characteristics of platelet receptor sites for noradrenaline and serotonin between days 21 and 28 in healthy women taking o/c. Platelet aggregation induced by these agents varied accordingly, being greater at 21 days and less at 28 days in those on o/c than in controls. O/C users generated more platelet aggregating activity upon addition of arachidonic acid to their platelet microsomes than did age, sex, and family history matched controls (Schorer et al, 1978). Such alterations of platelet function may contribute to the increased risk of thrombosis associated with estrogen therapy.

The frequency of occlusive vascular complications in *diabetes mellitus* has prompted numerous investigations of the hemostatic mechanism in patients with this disorder. Platelet abnormalities observed include increased sensitivity to aggregation by ADP, epinephrine or arachidonic acid (Colwell et al, 1976; Dupuy et al, 1979), 'spontaneous' platelet aggregation and increased circulating platelet aggregates (Wu & Hoak, 1974), a paradoxical increase in lag time of collagen-induced aggregation and decreased membrane glucosyltransferase activity (Roux, 1977), and an activity in the plasma of diabetics not found in normal plasma which enhances ADP-induced platelet aggregation (Kwaan et al, 1972). The latter activity was not detected in another study (Lufkin et al, 1979). Increased plasma von Willebrand factor has been reported (Colwell et al, 1976; Lufkin et al, 1979), as has shortened platelet survival (Paton, 1979), which however was not correlated with the presence of vascular complications. No correlation was observed between platelet hyperaggregability and vascular complications (Dupuy et al, 1979). Kazmier et al (1979a), in contrast, found a greater shortening of platelet survival in diabetics with occlusive arterial disease than in those without. Kazmier et al (1979b) found plasma von Willebrand factor to increase with age and extent of peripheral arterial occlusive disease. Mean von Willebrand factor activity was normal in patients with uncomplicated diabetes. Increased plasma β-TG in diabetics was noted by two groups (Burrows et al, 1978; Preston et al, 1978) but not by another (Campbell et al, 1977). The discrepancy may stem in part from differences in sampling technique and from use by the first two groups of PGE_1 in the collection tubes to prevent in vitro release of β-TG from platelets. An increased production of malondialdehyde upon thrombin stimulation (Gensini et al, 1979) suggests that platelets of diabetics have increased activity of the prostaglandin metabolic pathway which leads to production of the platelet-aggregating endoperoxides and thromboxanes. Support for this concept comes from the observation (Butkus et al, 1979) that platelets from diabetic subjects produce more thromboxane B_2 from arachidonic acid than do platelets from non-diabetic subjects. The forearm veins of 10 type I diabetics generated significantly less PGI_2 than those of 10 sex- and age-matched controls (Silberbauer et al, 1979).

Lipid alterations

Modifications of plasma or platelet membrane lipid composition, either in vitro or in vivo, have frequently been found to have significant effects on platelet function, as tested in vitro. Accumulating evidence suggests that lipid-induced alterations of platelet function may contribute to the development of a hemorrhagic or thrombotic diathesis, and perhaps also to the pathogenesis of atherosclerotic vascular disease.

Enrichment of platelet membranes with *cholesterol*, by incubating platelets with cholesterol-rich liposomes in vitro, increases membrane microviscosity or rigidity, and renders platelets hyper-reactive to stimuli such as ADP, epinephrine, collagen or thrombin (Shattil et al, 1975; Colman, 1978; Insel et al, 1978; Shattil & Cooper, 1978; Stuart et al, 1980). The latter authors found increased thromboxane production in stimulated cholesterol-enriched platelets, suggesting that enhanced prostaglandin metabolism mediates the hyper-responsiveness of such platelets. Similar changes (increased thromboxane production) have also been found in platelets from hyper-cholesterolemic (type IIa) subjects (Bizios et al, 1977; Tremoli et al, 1979a, 1979b). These platelets have an increased cholesterol content in their membranes, relative to phospholipid (Shattil et al, 1977). Increased numbers of circulating platelet aggregates have also been observed in hypercholesterolemic subjects (Lowe et al, 1979b). Joist et al (1979) found significant shortening of template bleeding time and increased platelet factor 3 activity in hypercholesterolemic (type IIa) and in type IV hyperlipidemic subjects. These authors, and others (Freedman et al, 1979), could not demonstrate any consistent hypersensitivity of hypercholesterolemic platelets to various aggregating stimuli. Such variability points out the difficulty of interpreting platelet function tests in hyperlipidemic patients who may be nonhomogeneous with respect to: (1) the presence and extent of atherosclerotic vascular disease; (2) platelet survival and the pecentage of younger platelets in the circulation; or (3) other unknown metabolic variability producing altered platelet function.

Changes in the *fatty acid* content in the diet, in plasma or in platelet membranes have significant effects on platelet function, and may be related to bleeding, thrombosis or atherosclerosis. Acute increases in plasma triglycerides or in plasma free fatty acids (which normally are mostly albumin-bound) can be induced by eating, by intravenous infusion of lipids, by injection of heparin or by hormonal substances such as catecholamines or ACTH (Nordøy, 1974; Nordøy, 1976; O'Brien et al, 1976; Burstein et al, 1979; Nordøy, 1979; Nordøy & Svensson, 1979). While acute hypertriglyceridemia may predipose to activation of platelets and the coagulation mechanism, more marked potentiation of platelet excitability can be produced by acutely increased plasma free fatty acids, particularly saturated fatty acids. Healthy subjects who eat a saturated fat meal develop increased circulating platelet aggregates at 90 minutes; the value returns to baseline by 180 minutes (Lowe et al, 1979a).

Chronic or subacute alterations of the types of fatty acids in the diet are ultimately reflected in the fatty acid side chain composition of platelet membrane phospholipids (Nordøy, 1976), and indeed in the membrane phospholipids of other cells as well (Ahrens, 1979), including endothelial cells (Nordøy, 1979; Nordøy & Svensson, 1979). Of special interest are recent investigations correlating dietary fatty acid content with platelet function, suggesting that platelet (and endothelial cell) function may be significantly altered by dietary adjustments. Studies of an Eskimo population (Dyerberg & Bang, 1979) and a few Western Europeans (Siess et al, 1980) indicate that enrichment of the diet with the polyunsaturated fatty acid eicosapentaenoic acid (20:5) increases the plasma and platelet membrane phospholipid content of this fatty acid relative to arachidonic acid, resulting in decreased generation of TXA_2 by stimulated platelets, and ultimately resulting in a mild bleeding diathesis associated with prolongation of the bleeding time. Paradoxically, administration of aspirin to such Eskimos seems to shorten the bleeding time, suggesting either that actively inhibitory prostacyclins such as PGI_3 may be generated by endothelial cells from eicosapentaenoic acid (Dyerberg et al, 1978) or that platelets utilize eicosapentaenoic acid to produce triene prostaglandins (PGH_3 and TXA_3) which inhibit platelet activation (Needleman et al, 1979a). Further support for the importance of certain dietary fatty acids in platelet function comes from studies of other Western European populations (Renaud et al, 1978; Renaud et al, 1979) showing that the saturated fatty acid content of the diet correlates well with certain platelet functions (procoagulant activity; thrombin, collagen or ADP-induced aggregation), and perhaps with atherosclerotic complications, but does not correlate well with the type or extent of lipemia. Reduction of saturated fat ingestion, replaced to some extent by unsaturated fats, reversed some of the heightened platelet functions. It would therefore seem that dietary fats, in particular the content of certain saturated and unsaturated fatty acids, are importantly related to platelet functions and hemostatic balance, and moreover, that such altered platelet functions might be important mediators of the atherosclerotic process and its complications.

Further evidence supporting an important role for *platelets as mediators of atherosclerosis* comes from studies using animal models. Pigs with severe von Willebrand's disease have a severe bleeding disorder due mainly to defective adhesion of platelets to the vessel wall (Fuster et al, 1978). Such pigs are resistant to development of the advanced atherosclerosis often occurring in normal pigs, even if atherogenic diets are fed. Conversely, induction of platelet dysfunction by administration of aspirin and dipyridamole reduces atherosclerosis in normal pigs (Fuster et al, 1979). Thus, certain hypofunctional platelet disorders, either congenital or acquired, may protect against atherosclerosis.

Drugs which modify lipids can profoundly affect platelet functions. Clofibrate, administered in doses which did not significantly change lipemia, reversed platelet hypersensitivity in hypercholesterolemic (type IIa) patients (Carvalho et al, 1974). Studies with washed platelets in vitro indicate that clofibrate may directly affect platelet metabolism and function (Huzoor-Akbar & Ardlie, 1977a). Halofenate, another lipid-lowering agent has similar platelet inhibitory effects (Colman et al, 1976; Huzoor-Akbar & Ardlie, 1977b). Vitamin E (α-tocopherol), an antioxidant with known inhibitory action on lipid peroxidation, inhibits platelet aggregation and release, perhaps by interfering with platelet prostaglandin metabolism (Steiner & Anastasi, 1976; Wautier & Caen, 1979) or by affecting calcium flow across membranes. Ethanol, while it may elevate plasma lipids, seems also to be platelet inhibitory (Renaud et al, 1979).

Much uncertainty remains as to the in vivo mechanisms controlling platelet lipid composition, the mechanisms by which various membrane lipids modulate platelet function, and the relative importance of these phenomena in human disease processes. Particularly controversial at present is the effect of various dietary manipulations on human platelet function, or on many other processes ultimately dependent on cell membrane function.

Platelet abnormalities in various thromboembolic disorders

Shortened platelet survival and/or *accelerated platelet turnover* have been observed in patients with myocardial infarction, stroke, arterial and venous thromboembolism, postoperative state, febrile illness, disseminated intravascular coagulation, atherosclerosis, cardiovascular prostheses, neoplasia, hypertension, hypoxemia, vasculitis, thrombotic thrombocytopenic purpura, homocystinuria, rheumatic heart disease and occlusion of saphenous vein aorto-coronary bypass grafts (Harker & Slichter, 1974, Steele et al, 1976. Genton & Steele, 1977, Didisheim & Fuster, 1978). Shortened platelet survival in these conditions has not been observed by all investigators however and may depend upon the stage and severity of the disease, age, and other factors (Najean et al, 1979). The small degree of variability in platelet survival from patient to patient reported by Harker, Genton, and their associates was not experienced by Najean et al (1979).

Hyperaggregable platelets (which aggregate upon adding lower ADP, epinephrine, arachidonic acid or collagen concentrations than are required to aggregate normal platelets) have been observed in patients with angina pectoris after exercise (Yamazaki et al, 1970a), transient ischemic attacks (Dugdale et al, 1975; Andersen et al, 1976; Dougherty et al, 1977), acute stroke (Dougherty et al, 1977), and in hyperlipidemic subjects as reviewed above. *Circulating platelet aggregates* have been reported in the blood of 14 of 30 patients with recurrent deep venous thrombosis (Wu et al, 1976) (spontaneous platelet aggregation was seen in 13), and in patients with completed stroke or transient ischemic attacks when studied within 10 days of the acute event (Wu & Hoak, 1974; Dougherty et al, 1977), recent myocardial infarction or recent onset of peripheral vascular symptoms (Wu & Hoak, 1974), and coronary artery disease following exercise (Kumpuris et al, 1980). Others have not confirmed the presence of circulating platelet aggregates in several of these conditions (Prazich et al, 1977). Increased circulating platelet aggregates can be associated with certain plasma lipid alterations as reviewed in that section. Platelet hyperaggregability by the *screen filtration pressure* method was demonstrated in the blood of four young patients with stroke (Kalendovsky et al, 1975); two had classical migraine, and three had shortened platelet survival. Similar findings were reported in patients with essential hypertension, cerebral thrombosis or hemorrhage more than two months after onset (Kobayashi et al, 1976). Increased *platelet coagulant activities* were noted in patients with transient ischemic attacks (Walsh et al, 1976a), postoperative venous thrombosis (Walsh et al, 1976b), and primary retinal vein thrombosis (Walsh et al, 1977a).

Platelet adhesiveness was *reduced* following myocardial infarction or cerebral thrombosis (Yamazaki et al, 1970b) but was elevated in men or women who smoke cigarettes; the latter effect in women was not different whether or not they were taking o/c (Strolin-Benedetti et al, 1976). An activity in plasma which enhances ADP-induced platelet aggregation has been observed in patients with myocardial infarction and cerebrovascular disorders (Neri Serneri et al, 1976).

Elevated β-TG levels in the plasma have been reported in deep venous thrombosis (Ludlam et al, 1975, Smith et al, 1978, Cella et al, 1979) and arterial thrombosis (Ludlam & Anderson, 1977), preeclampsia (Redman et al, 1977), myocardial infarction with mural thrombosis (Denham et al, 1977), and peripheral vascular disease (Cella et al, 1979). β-TG was significantly correlated with PF4 and platelet survival in 62 patients with coronary artery disease (Doyle et al, 1980). Elevated β-TG levels have also been seen with charcoal hemoperfusion (Gimson et al, 1980) and in patients with DIC and TTP (examples of intravascular platelet destruction) but not ITP (platelet destruction considered to be extravascular) (Han et al, 1979). Plasma β-TG levels increase with age in normal subjects (Ludlam, 1979). Elevated levels in women taking o/c have been observed by two groups (Aranda et al, 1979, Duncan, 1979) but not by another (Ludlam & Anderson, 1977). The discrepancy may have been due to differences in techniques of sample collection: addition of theophylline (phosphodiesterase inhibitor) and PGE_1 (stimulator of adenylate cyclase) to the EDTA anticoagulant and keeping the blood sample on ice appear helpful in preventing spurious release of these factors from platelets following collection. Any difficulty in venipuncture may lead to release of these platelet components and thus render their determination in plasma questionable. Such variables in technique may also contribute to the varying normal values reported from different laboratories. *Elevated platelet factor 4* (PF4) levels in plasma have been reported in certain thrombotic states (O'Brien & Etherington, 1976). These include myocardial infarction (Handin et al, 1978), pulmonary emboli, prosthetic heart valves, severe cardiorespiratory failure (Handin et al, 1978), and coronary artery disease after exercise (Green et al, 1980). PF4 was significantly correlated with β-TG and platelet survival and turnover in 62 patients with coronary artery disease (Doyle et al, 1980).

Synthesis of *prostaglandin endoperoxides* (PGG_2, PGH_2) following platelet stimulation with collagen was elevated in some patients with arterial thrombosis, postoperative deep venous thrombosis, and recurrent venous thrombosis with shortened platelet survival (Lagarde & Dechavanne, 1977). Patients with Prinzmetal's angina reportedly have increased circulating levels of *thromboxane B_2* (TXB_2), a stable derivative of thromboxane A_2 (Lewy et al, 1979a). Elevated TXB_2 levels have also been observed in the plasma of some patients with angina, myocardial infarction, or stroke (Sakanishi et al, 1979). *PGD_2 activation of adenylate cyclase* in platelet membrane fractions was decreased in nine of 20 consecutive patients hospitalized with acute deep-vein thrombosis and/or plumonary embolism; the value returned toward normal after the acute thrombotic event in four of five patients who had follow-up studies. The authors speculated that since PGD_2 is synthesized in platelets in concentrations sufficient to inhibit aggregation and activate adenylate cyclase, diminished platelet sensitivity to this prostaglandin could contribute to thrombosis (Cooper, 1979).

While in many of these disorders the observed abnormalities of platelet function may simply represent responses of normal platelets to vascular disease, it is apparent that platelets play a major role in the propagation of many of these disorders. In some of them, the platelet dysfunction may be primordial.

Other disorders

It has been proposed that *migraine* is caused by an abnormality of platelet function (Hanington, 1978). Reduced platelet uptake of serotonin has been reported (Malmgren et al, 1978), and platelet monoamine oxidase concentration is lower than normal (Sandler, 1977). Some patients with *asthma* have an abnormal platelet aggregation response to epinephrine (Solinger et al, 1973). Three patients with severe *vitamin B_{12} deficiency* had absent second-wave platelet aggregation after ADP stimulation, total lack of aggregation in response to standard amounts of epinephrine or collagen, and in two patients, bleeding times of more than 20 minutes. Vitamin B_{12} therapy corrected these defects (Levine, 1973). Other nutritional factors reported to affect platelet function include *vitamin C deficiency* (scurvy) (Çetingil et al, 1958; McNicol & Douglas, 1967; Owen et al, 1975) and perhaps *deficiencies of iron or folate* (Edson, 1979). The possible influence of dietary lipid on platelet function has been outlined in the section on lipid alterations.

The dramatic clinical response of some patients with *thrombotic thrombocytopenic purpura* (TTP) to exchange transfusion with whole blood (Bukowski et al, 1976; Pisciotta et al, 1977), plasmapheresis (Bukowski et al, 1977), and transfusion of normal plasma (Byrnes & Khurana, 1977) has led to the hypothesis that a physiologic plasma-inhibitor of platelet aggregation is lacking in some patients with this disorder. Remuzzi et al (1978) reported that an inhibitor of platelet aggregation, having many of the characteristics of PGI_2, was lacking in venous tissue from their patient with TTP. In addition plasma from their patient, unlike normal plasma and the patient's own plasma after plasma infusion, was unable to stimulate synthesis of PGI_2-like activity in normal vascular tissues. Hensby et al (1979) found undetectable levels of the stable derivative of PGI_2, 6-oxo-$PGF_{1\alpha}$, in the plasma of their patient with TTP, a unique finding in their series. Infusion of synthetic PGI_2 raised the plasma level of 6-oxo-$PGF_{1\alpha}$ to normal but had no effect on the platelet count. This unresponsiveness could be due to the fact that the plasma of some patients with TTP contains a platelet aggregating factor (PAF) which can be neutralized by an inhibitor found in normal plasma, i.e. a platelet-aggregating-factor inhibitor (PAFI) (Lian et al, 1979; Brandt et al, 1979). In one patient who survived (Brandt et al, 1979), the PAF disappeared following recovery, and plasma from this patient at that time neutralized the PAF in the plasma of two patients with TTP during the thrombocytopenic phase. The plasma of several patients with acute thrombocytopenia from other causes also contained PAF. In summary, a current hypothesis of the pathogenesis of TTP is as follows: an initial event, perhaps endothelial damage, stimulates adherence and aggregation of platelets. PAF is released from platelets, and depletion of vascular PAFI also occurs. The rate and extent of these two processes determine whether a given patient with TTP will respond to plasma infusions (to replenish PAFI which then neutralizes PAF) or will require exchange transfusion (to remove PAF as well as replete PAFI) (Lian et al, 1979; Brandt et al, 1979).

Drugs
In addition to the potential of many drugs to produce thrombocytopenia by various mechanisms (not reviewed here), a long and growing list of drugs have been shown to alter platelet function. In fact medicaments are the commonest cause of platelet dysfunction. Such dysfunction is most often of the hypofunctional variety, sometimes resulting in or exacerbating a bleeding tendency, but some drugs may render platelets hyperfunctional, perhaps generating a thrombotic diathesis. A few drugs have been the subject of clinical trials for the prevention of various thrombotic disorders (reviewed by Didisheim & Fuster, 1978; by Wautier & Caen, 1979; and by Gent in this volume). The principal classes of platelet-active drugs and their probable mechanisms of action are listed in Table 2.7.

Aspirin and other nonsteroidal anti-inflammatory agents (NSAIA)
It has long been known that taking aspirin is associated with an increased risk of significant bleeding. The minimal prolongation of prothrombin time caused by therapeutic doses of aspirin seemed unlikely to explain the major bleeds that occasionally occur, and direct ulcerative action on gastric mucosa did not account for bleeding at other sites. Aspirin was noted in the fifties and sixties to prolong the bleeding time (Beaumont et al, 1956; Blatrix, 1963); the mechanism for this effect was clarified when aspirin was shown to inhibit collagen-induced platelet aggregation and the second wave of ADP-induced platelet aggregation, and to block release from platelets of ADP, a potent platelet-aggregating substance (Weiss & Aledort, 1967; Evans et al, 1968; O'Brien, 1968; Zucker & Peterson, 1968). More recently aspirin and other NSAIAs have been shown to intefere with platelet prostaglandin synthesis by inhibiting platelet fatty acid cyclo-oxygenase (Table 2.7). Inhibition of platelet cyclo-oxygenase reduces synthesis of the labile endoperoxides PGG_2 and PGH_2 from platelet membrane arachidonic acid, in turn decreasing production of TXA_2, the extremely potent mediator of platelet aggregation (see section on prostaglandin metabolism in Chapter 1). These two effects of aspirin and other NSAIA's — inhibition of ADP release and interference with prostaglandin synthesis — can now be understood by the observation that interference with endoperoxide production inhibits stimulus-induced ADP release. In the case of aspirin, the inhibition of platelet cyclo-oxygenase is seen following doses of 300–600 mg by mouth in humans, and results from irreversible acetylation of the enzyme (Burch et al, 1978a). Other NSAIA's have a reversible effect on this enzyme. This difference in action probably accounts for the different duration of effect, which in the case of aspirin is for the life of the platelet (7 to 10 days), whereas with other NSAIA's the effect only lasts for a few hours until the drug is cleared from the circulation (reviewed by Didisheim, 1980).

Aspirin inhibits synthesis of prostaglandin endoperoxides not only in platelets, but also in cultured endothelial cells (Jaffe & Weksler, 1979) and in microsomal preparations from arterial walls (Burch et al, 1978b). In endothelial cells and deeper in vessel walls, these endoperoxides are the precursors of PGI_2. Thus, aspirin can also block vessel wall production of PGI_2, the most potent endogenous inhibitor of platelet aggregation known at present. Cultured human endothelial cell cyclo-oxygenase is as sensitive to aspirin as platelet cyclo-oxygenase (Jaffe & Weksler, 1979). However, because endothelial cells can actively synthesize cyclo-oxygenase and platelets cannot,

Table 2.7 Drugs and agents reported to alter platelet function

Classes of drugs and agents	Actions
1. Platelet Cyclo-oxygenase Inhibitors Aspirin Nonsteroidal Anti-inflammatory Agents (NSAIA) Phenylbutazone, Indomethacin, Ibuprofen, Fenoprofen, Flurbiprofen, Naproxen, Sulfinpyrazone*	Inhibit production of endoperoxides, TXA_2, PGI_2
2. Platelet cAMP Phosphodiesterase Inhibitors Dipyridamole and related compounds: RA 233, RA 433, VK 744, VK 774 Methylxanthines: theophylline, caffeine, aminophylline, papaverine	Raise platelet cAMP
3. Prostaglandins Prostacyclin (PGI_2, PGX), PGE_1, PGD_2	Stimulate adenylate cyclase, raise cAMP Antagonize TXA_2
4. Thromboxane Synthetase Inhibitors benzydamine; imidazole and congeners 9,11-azo-13-oxa-15 hydroxyprostanoic acid 9–11 azoprosta-5-13 dienoic acid (U-51605) sodium-p-benzyl-4-[1-oxo-2-(4-chlorobenzyl)- 3-phenyl propyl] phenyl phosphonate (N-0164) 9,11 (epoxymethano) prostanoic acid 1(isopropyl-2-indolyl)-3-pyridyl-3-ketone (L-8027) onion; garlic	Inhibit production of TXA_2 from endoperoxides
5. Thromboxane Inhibitors Phtalazinol (EG-626)	Inhibit action of TXA_2
6. Membrane-Active Drugs† Antibiotics (Penicillins, Cephalosporins) Phenothiazines Tricyclic antidepressants Local anesthetics Propranolol	Alter platelet plasma membrane structure and/or function

7. Miscellaneous Agents† (Various or unknown actions)

Heparin	Vitamin E
Dextrans	Diuretics (Furosemide, ethacry-nic acid)
Microtubule inhibitors (colchicine, vinca alkaloids)	Adrenal corticosteroids
Lipid-altering agents	Estrogens
(clofibrate, halofenate, androgens)	Hydroxychloroquin
Nitroprusside, Nitrates	Glyceryl guaiacolate
Hydralazine	Ethanol
Sympathetic blocking agents	Ticlopidine
Monoamine oxidase inhibitors	Suloctidil
Serotonin antagonists	Tobacco smoking

* Listed here because structurally similar to phenylbutazone; sulfinpyrazone has little anti-inflammatory activity.
† Modified from Weiss (1972) and Packham & Mustard (1977).

the effect of a single dose of aspirin on endothelial cell prostacyclin production is of short duration (substantial recovery of PGI_2 production in 24 hours) in contrast to the effect on platelet TXA_2 synthesis, which persists for the lifetime of the platelet (Jaffe

& Weksler, 1979; Masotti et al, 1979). In addition, aspirin (acetylsalicylic acid) is rapidly hydrolyzed in plasma to salicylate which has a relatively long half-life, and which may inhibit the antiplatelet effects of subsequent doses of aspirin (Ali & McDonald, 1979). There is, therefore, some biochemical rationale for the use of low, infrequent doses of· aspirin (e.g. 300 mg every day or twice a day) to achieve an antiplatelet effect while maintaining significant capability of endothelial cells to produce PGI_2 (Kelton et al, 1978; O'Grady & Moncada, 1978). These theories have not yet been fully tested in vivo. Search continues for TXA_2 synthetase inhibitors which would be specific for inhibition of TXA_2 synthesis by platelets while totally sparing PGI_2 synthesis by the vessel wall.

Sulfinpyrazone (Anturane)

Sulfinpyrazone, devoid of anti-inflammatory activity, appears to act as a reversible inhibitor of cyclo-oxygenase (Ali & McDonald, 1977); hence, in contrast to aspirin, it is effective only as long as it is present in plasma. In vitro it appears to inhibit aspirin's effects on platelets (Ali & McDonald, 1979); thus the two agents might antagonize each other's effect on platelet function when administered together. In a randomized double blind study of the effect of sulfinpyrazone on myocardial reinfarction, patients taking sulfinpyrazone had a reduced platelet aggregation response to epinephrine as well as a milder potentiation of washed platelets to aggregation by thrombin compared with the placebo group (Latour et al, 1979). Sulfinpyrazone's reported effectiveness in reducing sudden cardiac death in patients who have had a myocardial infarct (Anturane Reinfarction Trial Research Group, 1978, 1980) may stem in part from an antiarrhythmic effect of this agent.

Dipyridamole and related agents

Dipyridamole (Persantin), other pyrimidopyrimidines and related compounds inhibit platelet cyclic AMP phosphodiesterase, resulting in maintenance of elevated platelet cAMP which inhibits platelet aggregation and the release reaction. Dipyridamole may potentiate the effect of PGI_2 in raising platelet cAMP and inhibiting platelet aggregation (Moncada & Korbut, 1978). The effect could explain the lack of demonstrable action of dipyridamole in in vitro tests of platelet function: PGI_2, because of its extremely short half-life, disappears from blood specimens before the platelet function tests can be performed. Harker and Slichter (1970, 1972) reported that combinations of dipyridamole and aspirin were as effective as four times the dosage of dipyridamole alone in normalizing the shortened platelet survival seen in patients with prosthetic heart valves; in contrast, when the low dose of dipyridamole or aspirin was given separately, no effect was observed. Buchanan et al (1979) found that both aspirin and sodium salicylate caused a significant (30 to 50 per cent) rise in the plasma concentration of simultaneously administered dipyridamole over that achieved with dipyridamole alone; this finding may explain the synergistic effect on platelet survival. There was also a prolongation of the suppression of collagen-induced platelet aggregation by dipyridamole when aspirin or sodium salicylate was given in addition. This effect appeared to be due to saturation of the glucuronide pathway which is the major route of clearance of dipyridamole from the circulation.

Penicillins and cephalosporins

A bleeding tendency, associated with prolongation of the bleeding time and impaired platelet aggregation, has been seen in patients receiving large doses of carbenicillin or penicillin G (McClure et al, 1970; Brown et al, 1974; Cazenave et al, 1977). In vitro in high concentrations, these substances can inhibit most platelet reactions such as shape change; adhesion to collagen-coated or subendothelial surfaces; platelet aggregation induced by ADP, epinephrine, collagen, thrombin or the ionophore A23187; platelet release of stored substances; generation of platelet factor 3; and clot retraction (Cazenave et al, 1977). Most other penicillins, including ampicillin, nafcillin, oxacillin and to a lesser extent, methicillin and ticarcillin, can exert similar, dose-dependent effects in vitro (Brown et al, 1976; Cazenave et al, 1977; Henry et al, 1979). Cephalosporins can also produce these effects (Cazenave et al, 1977), although clinically important bleeding has not been recognized. These antibiotics may intercalate into the lipid bilayer of the platelet plasma membrane and interfere with binding of various agonists to receptor sites (Cazenave et al, 1977; Henry et al, 1979; Shattil et al, 1979a). Such a mechanism would be consistent with the global effects of these drugs on platelet functions, and with the observed relationship between the lipid solubility of various congeners and their antiplatelet effects.

Other membrane-active drugs

A variety of other membrane-active drugs are known to inhibit various platelet functions in vitro. These include phenothiazines, tricyclic antidepressants, local anesthetics, antihistamines, cyproheptadine and propranolol. Clinical bleeding is unusual with use of these agents. These and other platelet-inhibitory drugs have been the subject of reviews (Weiss, 1972; Packham & Mustard, 1977; Weiss, 1978; Wautier & Caen, 1979).

Heparin

Heparin affects various platelet functions [reviewed by Gallus & Engel (1978)], but the mechanisms and clinical importance of heparin-induced platelet dysfunction are not yet clear. Heparin has been reported to enhance, inhibit, or have no effect on various platelet activation processes. In vitro, heparin often potentiates the activation of platelets by various stimuli (Bygdeman & Tangen, 1977; Eldor & Weksler, 1979; Michaelski et al, 1978; Chuang et al, 1979; Cofrancesco et al, 1979; Reches et al, 1979). Platelet counts performed on an automated counter are 30 per cent lower when heparin is used instead of EDTA as the anticoagulant (Didisheim et al, 1980), probably because heparin induces some platelets to form aggregates which are eliminated from counting. Conversely, intravenous administration of heparin in moderate or large doses (100 to 200 U/kg) prolongs the bleeding time and inhibits in vitro platelet aggregation and serotonin release induced by ADP, epinephrine and collagen in a significant proportion of human subjects (Heiden et al, 1977). It is not known whether heparin-induced alterations of plasma or platelet lipid compositions (due to heparin-induced release of lipoprotein lipases) might contribute to variable alterations of platelet function (Joist & Mustard, 1975). Heparin administration resulted in a signficant increase of plasma TXB_2 in 20 of 27 patients with angina pectoris (Lewy et al, 1979b); there was no correlation between TXB_2 and serum free fatty acid levels before or after heparin administration however. Heparin-induced thrombocytopenia has been recognized with increasing frequency in recent years (Bell et al, 1976b; Nelson et al, 1978; Cimo et al, 1979; Hussey et al, 1979; Kapsch et al, 1979). The relationship of this complication of heparin therapy to its actions listed above remains unclear.

Dextrans
Infusion of dextrans can prolong the bleeding time and impair platelet retention on glass bead columns, aggregation and generation of procoagulant activities (Bygdeman & Eliasson, 1967; Weiss, 1972). These effects are dose-related, more pronounced with dextrans of higher molecular weight, and may be delayed in onset. In vitro, dextrans potentiate platelet aggregation induced by certain stimuli, reminiscent of the sometimes paradoxical in vivo and in vitro effects of heparin on platelet function (Bygdeman & Tangen, 1977; Eldor & Weksler, 1979; Reches et al, 1979). While dextrans may interact with the platelet membrane, other more indirect mechanisms may be operative (Weiss, 1972). Åberg et al (1978) found dextran infusion to decrease factor VIII R:Ag and VIII R:WF activities while prolonging the bleeding time. These effects were more marked in patients with von Willebrand's disease, indicating that dextran infusion should be avoided in such patients and probably also in any patient with significant impairment of hemostasis.

Significance of acquired platelet dysfunction
The acquired qualitative platelet disorders are legion and are likely to be increasingly recognized in the future. In many instances these defects, by themselves, produce only in vitro abnormalities and little clinically significant bleeding or thrombosis. However, it is important to recognize that such acquired platelet dysfunction can aggravate a bleeding or thrombotic tendency in patients who have other hemostatic defects such as thrombocytopenia, congenital platelet dysfunction, abnormalities of the plasmatic coagulation mechanism, or certain systemic or vascular conditions which predispose to thrombohemorrhagic phenomena. In this regard, drug-induced platelet dysfunction deserves special consideration, not only for its role in iatrogenic hemostatic failure, but also for its potential therapeutic importance in thromboembolic disorders.

PERSPECTIVE

The varied and important roles of platelets in hemostasis and blood coagulation, both physiologic and pathologic, are becoming more clearly defined as the mechanisms of platelet function and interactions with blood vessels and plasmatic proteins become better understood. These unique cells are emerging not only as central elements in the hemostatic defense mechanism of the body, but also as important mediators of allied processes such as atherosclerosis and thrombosis, and certain immunologic, inflammatory and neoplastic phenomena. This decade can be expected to witness considerable crystallization of the essential roles and mechanisms of platelet participation in these processes. Improved recognition and the detailed study of congenital or acquired disorders of platelet function will further improve understanding of the mechanisms of normal platelet function.

ACKNOWLEDGMENTS

During the preparation of these reviews (Chapters 1 & 2), helpful discussions were provided by our colleagues, Doctors E. J. W. Bowie, Alexander Duncan, David N. Fass, Francis J. Kazmier, Kenneth G. Mann, Michael E. Nesheim, Lawrence A. Solberg, Jr., Paula B. Tracy, and James G. White. Additionally, the secretarial expertise of Kitty Johnson, Kathy Minten, and Dawn Stangler was indispensible.

BIBLIOGRAPHY

Åberg M, Hedner U, Bergentz S-E 1978 Effect of dextran 70 on factor VIII and platelet function in von Willebrand's disease. Thrombosis Research 12: 629–634

Ahrens E H 1979 Dietary fats and coronary heart disease: unfinished business. Lancet 2: 1345–1348

Ali M, McDonald J W D 1977 Effects of sulfinpyrazone on platelet prostaglandin synthesis and platelet release of serotonin. Journal of Laboratory and Clinical Medicine 89: 868–875

Ali M, McDonald J W D 1979 Interference by sulfinpyrazone and salicylate of aspirin inhibition of platelet cyclo-oxygenase activity. Prostaglandins and Medicine 3: 327–332

Andersen L A, Gormsen J 1976 Platelet aggregation and fibrinolytic activity in transient cerebral ischemia. Acta Neurologica Scandinavica 55: 76–82

Ando Y, Yamamoto M, Watanabe K, Ikeda Y, Toyama K, Yamada K 1979 Defective ^{125}I-factor VIII binding to platelets in patients with Bernard-Soulier syndrome and von Willebrand's disease. Thrombosis and Haemostasis 42: 374

Anturane Reinfarction Trial Research Group 1978 Sulfinpyrazone in the prevention of cardiac death after myocardial infarction. New England Journal of Medicine 298: 289–295

Anturane Reinfarction Trial Research Group 1980 Sulfinpyrazone in the prevention of sudden death after myocardial infarction. New England Journal of Medicine 302: 250–256

Aranda M, Saez M, Abril V, Cararach J, Castells E, Castellanos J M, 1979 B-thromboglobulin levels and oral contraceptives Lancet 2: 308–309

Ardlie N G, Coupland W, W, Schoefl G I 1976 Hereditary thrombocytopathy: a familial bleeding disorder due to impaired platelet coagulant activity. Australia New Zealand Journal of Medicine 6: 37–45

Ballard H S, Marcus J 1976 Platelet aggregation in portal cirrhosis. Archives of Internal Medicine 136: 316–319

Bang N U, Heidenreich R O, Trygstad C W 1972 Plasma protein requirements for human platelet aggregation. Annals of the New York Academy of Sciences 201: 280–299

Baumgartner H R, Tschopp T B, Weiss H J 1977 Platelet interaction with collagen fibrils in flowing blood: II. impaired adhesion-aggregation and bleeding disorders. Thrombosis and Haemostasis 37: 17–28

Beaumont J L, Caen J, Bernard J 1956 L' influence de l'acide salicylique dans les maladies hémorragiques. Sang 27: 243–248

Bell R L, Kennerly D A, Stanford N, Majerus P W 1979 Diglyceride lipase: a pathway for arachidonate release from platelets. Proceedings of the National Academy of Sciences, USA 76: 3238–3241

Bell T G, Meyers K M, Prieur D J, Fauci A. S, Wolff S M, Padgett G A 1976a Decreased nucleotide and serotonin storage associated with defective function in Chediak-Higashi syndrome cattle and human platelets. Blood 48: 175–184

Bell W R, Tomasulo P A, Alving E M, Duffy T P 1976b Thrombocytopenia occurring during the administration of heparin. Annals of Internal Medicine 85: 155–160

Berger S, Aledort L M, Gibert H S, Hanson J P, Wasserman L R 1973 Abnormalities of platelet function in patients with polycythemia vera. Cancer Research 33: 2683–2687

Beurling-Harbury C, Galvan C A 1978 Acquired decrease in platelet secretory ADP associated with increased postoperative bleeding in post-cardiopulmonary bypass patients and in patients with severe valvular heart disease. Blood 52: 13–23

Bithell T C, Parekh S J, Strong R R 1972 Platelet function studies in the Bernard-Soulier syndrome. Annals of the New York Academy of Sciences 201: 145–160

Bithell T C, Didisheim P, Cartwright G E, Wintrobe M M 1965 Thrombocytopenia inherited as an autosomal dominant trait. Blood 25: 231–240

Bizios R, Wong L K, Vaillancourt R, Lees R S, and Carvalho A C 1977 Platelet prostglandin endoperoxide formation in hyperlipidemias. Thrombosis and Haemostasis 38: 228

Blatrix C 1963 Allongement du temps de saignement sous l'influence de certains médicaments. Nouvelle Revue Française d'Hématologie 3: 346–350

Bolin R B, Ikumura T, Jamieson G A 1977 Changes in distribution of platelet membrane glycoproteins in patients with myeloproliferative disorders. American Journal of Hematology 3: 63–71

Boughton B J, Allington M J, King A 1978 Platelet and plasma β-thromboglobulin in myeloproliferative syndromes and secondary thrombocytosis. British Journal of Haematology 40: 125–132

Boughton B J, Corgett W E N, Ginsburg A D 1977 Myeloproliferative disorders: a paradox of in vivo and in vitro platelet function. Journal of Clinical Pathology 30: 228–234

Boxer G J, Holmsen H, Robkin L, Bang N U, Boxer O A, Baehner R L 1977 Abnormal platelet function in Chediak-Higashi syndrome. British Journal of Haematology 35: 521–533

Brandt J T, Kennedy M S, Senhauser D A 1979 Platelet aggregating factor in thrombocytopenic purpura. Lancet 1: 463–464

Brown C H III, Bradshaw M W, Natelson E A, Alfrey C P Jr, Williams T W Jr 1976 Defective platelet function following the administration of penicillin compounds. Blood 47: 949–956

Brown C H III, Natelson E A, Bradshaw M W, Williams T W, Alfrey C P 1974 The hemostatic defect produced by carbenicillin. New England Journal of Medicine 291: 265–270

Buchanan G R, Handin R I 1976 Platelet function in the Chediak-Higashi syndrome. Blood 47: 941–948

Buchanan M R, Rosenfeld, J, Gent M, Lawrence W, Hirsh J. 1979 increased dipyridamole plasma concentrations associated with salicylate administration. Relationship to effects on platelet aggregation in vivo. Thrombosis Research 15: 813–820

Bukowski R M, King J W, Hewlett J S 1977 Plasmapheresis in the treatment of thrombotic thrombocytopenic purpura. Blood 50: 413–417

Bukowski R M, Hewlett J S, Harris J W, Hoffman G C, Battle J D, Silverblatt E, Yang I Y 1976 Exchange transfusions in the treatment of thrombotic thrombocytopenic purpura. Seminars in Hematology 13: 219–232

Burch J W, Stanford N, Majerus P W 1978a Inhibition of platelet prostaglandin synthetase by oral aspirin. Journal of Clinical Investigation 61: 314–319

Burch J W, Baenziger N L, Stanford N, Majerus P W 1978b Sensitivity of fatty acid cyclo-oxygenase from human aorta to acetylation by aspirin. Proceedings of the National Academy of Sciences, USA 75: 5181–5184

Burrows A W, Chavin S I, Hockaday T D R 1978 Plasma-thromboglobulin concentrations in diabetes mellitus. Lancet 1: 235–237

Burstein Y, Berns L, Heldenberg D, Kahn Y, Werbin B Z, Tamir I 1979 Increase in platelet aggregation following a rise in plasma free fatty acids. American Journal of Hematology 4: 17–22

Butkus A, Skrinska V A, Schumacher O P 1979 Prostaglandin metabolism in platelets of patients with diabetes mellitus. Circulation 59–60 (Supplement 1) II. 219

Bygdeman S, Eliasson R 1967 Effect of dextrans on platelet adhesiveness and aggregation. Scandinavian Journal of Clinical and Laboratory Investigation 20: 17–23

Bygdeman S, Tangen O 1977 Studies on the mechanism of platelet aggregation and release reaction induced by collagen and adrenaline. Thrombosis Research 11: 141–148

Byrnes J J, Khurana M 1977 Treatment of thrombotic thrombocytopenic purpura with plasma. New England Journal of Medicine 297: 1386–1389

Caen J 1972 Glanzmann thrombasthenia. Clinics in Haematology 1: 383–392

Caen J P, Castaldi P A, Leclerc J C, Inceman S, Larrieu M J, Probst M, Bernard J 1966 Congenital bleeding disorders with long bleeding time and normal platelet count: I. Glanzmann's thrombasthenia (report of 15 patients). American Journal of Medicine 1: 4–26

Caen J P, Nurden A T, Jeannaeu C, Michel H, Tobelem G, Levy-Toledano S, Sultan Y, Valenci F, Bernard J 1976 Bernard-Soulier syndrome: a new platelet glycoprotein abnormality. Journal of Laboratory and Clinical Medicine 87: 586–596

Campbell I W, Davies J, Fraser D M, Pepper D S, Clarke B F, Duncan L J F, Cash J D, 1977 Plasma β-thromboglobulin in diabetes mellitus. Diabetes 26: 1175–1177

Cardamone J M, Edson J R, McArthur J R, Jacob H S 1972 Abnormalities of platelet function in the myeloproliferative disorders. Journal of the American Medical Association 221: 270–273

Carvalho A C A, Colman R W, Lees R S 1974 Platelet function in hyperlipoproteinemia. New England Journal of Medicine 290: 434–438

Castaldi P A, Rozenberg M C, Stewart J H 1966 The bleeding disorder of uraemia: a qualitative platelet defect. Lancet 2: 66–69

Cazenave J-P, Guccione M A, Packham M A, Mustard J F 1977 Effects of cephalothin and pencillin G on platelet function in vitro. British Journal of Haematology 35: 135–152

Cella G, Zahavi J, de Haas H A, Kakkar V V 1979 β-thromboglobulin, platelet production time and platelet function in vascular disease. British Journal of Haematology 43: 127–136

Çetingil A I, Ulutin O N, Karaca M 1958 A platelet defect in a case of scurvy. British Journal of Haematology 4: 350–354

Chediak J, Lambert E, Maxey B 1978 Correction of clot retraction in thrombasthenia by ATP and reistocetin. Thrombosis Research 12: 875–882

Chediak J, Telfer M C, Vander Laan B, Maxey B, Cohen I 1979 Cycles of agglutination-disagglutination induced by ristocetin in thrombasthenic platelets. British Journal of Haematology 43: 113–126

Chesney C, Colman R S, Pichet L 1974 A syndrome of platelet-release abnormality and mild hemophilia. Blood 43: 821–830

Chesney C M, Baker A S, Carvalho A D, Ozer A, Meissner G F, Colman R W 1977 Adenylate cyclase and phosphodiesterase activity in the platelet release abnormality. Thrombosis and Haemostasis 38: 971–983

Chuang J Y K, Mohammad S F, Mason R G 1979 Effect of heparin on aggregation, release reaction and thromboxane A₂ synthesis in human platelets. Thrombosis and Haemostasis 42: 83

Cimo P L, Moake J L, Weinger R S, Ben-Menachem Y, Khalil K G 1979 Heparin-induced thrombocytopenia: association with a platelet aggregating factor and arterial thromboses. American Journal of Hematology 6: 125–133

Clancy R, Jenkins E, Firkin B 1972 Qualitative platelet abnormalities in idiopathic thrombocytopenic purpura. New England Journal of Medicine 286: 622–626

Clare N M, Montiel M M, Lifschitz M D, Bannayan G A 1979 Alport's syndrome associated with macrothrombopathic thrombocytopenia. American Journal of Clinical Pathology 72: 111–117

Cofrancesco E, Radaelli F, Pogliani E, Amici N, Torri G G, Casu B 1979 Correlation of sulfate content and degree of carboxylation of heparin and related glycosaminoglycans with anticomplement activity: relationships to the anticoagulant and platelet-aggregating activities. Thrombosis Research 14: 179–187

Colman R W 1978 Platelet function in hyperbetalipoproteinemia. Thrombosis and Haemostasis 39: 284–293

Colman R W, Bennett J S, Sheridan J F, Cooper R A, Shattil S J 1976 Halofenate: a potent inhibitor of normal and hypersensitive platelets. Journal of Laboratory and Clinical Medicine 88: 282–291

Colwell J A, Halushka P V, Sarji K, Levine J, Sagel J, Nair R M G 1976 Altered platelet function in diabetes mellitus. Diabetes 25 (Supplement 2): 826–831

Cooper B 1979 Diminished platelet adenylate cyclase activation by prostaglandin D₂ in acute thrombosis. Blood 54: 684–693

Cooper B, Ahern D 1979 Characterization of the platelet prostaglandin D₂ receptor. Journal of Clinical Investigation 64: 586–590

Cooper B, Schafter A I, Puchalsky D, Handin R I 1978 Platelet resistance to prostaglandin D₂ in patients with myeloproliferative disorders. Blood 52: 618–626

Cooper H A, Clemetson K J, Lüscher E F 1979 Human platelet membrane receptor for bovine von Willebrand factor (platelet aggregating factor): an integral membrane glycoprotein. Proceedings of the National Academy of Sciences, USA 76: 1069–1073

Cowan D H, Graham R C Jr, Baunach D 1975 The platelet defect in leukemia: platelet ultrastructure, adenine nucleotide metabolism, and the release reaction. Journal of Clinical Investigation 56: 188–200

Cronberg S, Nilsson I N, Zetterqvist E 1967 Investigation of a family with members with both severe and mild degree of thrombasthenia. Acta Paediatrica Scandinavica 56: 189–197

Czapek E E, Deykin D, Salzman E, Lian E C, Hellerstein L J, Rosoff C V 1978 Intermediate syndrome of platelet dysfunction. Blood 52: 103–113

Dameshek W 1969 Foreword and a proposal for considering paroxysmal nocturnal hemoglobinuria as a candidate myeloproliferative disorder. Blood 33: 263–264

Davis J W, McField J R, Phillips P S, Graham B A 1972 Effects of exogenous urea, creatinine and guanidinosuccinic acid on human platelet aggregation in vitro. Blood 39: 388–397

Day H J, Holmsen H 1972 Platelet adenine nucleotide 'storage pool deficiency' in thrombocytopenic absent radii syndrome. Journal of the American Medical Association 221: 1053–1054

Denham M J, Fisher M, James G, Hassan M 1977 β-thromboglobulin and heparin-neutralizing activity test in clinical conditions. Lancet 1: 1154

Didisheim P 1980 Analgesic and anti-inflammatory drugs: their effects on hemostasis. In: U Seligsohn (ed) Hemophilia-key issues, Castle House, London (in press)

Didisheim P, Bunting D 1966 Abnormal platelet function in myelofibrosis. American Journal of Clinical Pathology 45: 566–573

Didisheim P, Fuster V 1978 Actions and clinical status of platelet-suppressive agents. Seminars in Hematology 15: 55–72

Didisheim P, Stropp J Q, Defily M, Borowick J H 1980 Effect of prostacyclin (PGI₂) and PGE₁ on platelet-surface interactions. Proceedings of 18th Congress, International Society of Hematology, Montreal, Quebec, Canada

Dixon R H, Rosse W F 1977 Mechanism of complement-mediated activation of human blood platelets in vitro. Journal of Clinical Investigation 59: 360–368

Dougherty J H Jr, Levy De E. Weskler B B 1977 Platelet activation in acute cerebral ischemia. Serial measurements of platelet function in cerebrovascular disease. Lancet 1: 821–824

Dowling S V, Muntz R H, D'Souza S, Ekert H 1976 Platelet release abnormality associated with a variant of von Willebrand's disease. Blood 47: 265–274

Doyle D J, Chesterman C N, Cade J F, McGready J R, Rennie G C, Morgan F J 1980 Plasma concentrations of platelet-specific proteins correlated with platelet survival. Blood 55: 82–84

Dugdale M, Salky N, Robinson H, Robertson J T 1975 Platelets and transient ischemic attacks (TIAs). Stroke 6: 229

Duncan A 1979 Beta-thromboglobulin and oral contraception. Lancet 2: 631

Dupuy E, Guillausseau P J, Gaudeul P, Kartalis G, Wild A M, Pastureau A, Soria C, Malbec D, Duprey J, Luhetzki J, Caen J P 1979 Fonctions plaquettaires des diabétiques ayant une angiopathie. Nouvelle Presse Médicale 8: 3123–3125

Dyerberg J, Bang H O 1979 Lipid metabolism, atherogenesis, and haemostasis in Eskimos: the role of the prostaglandin-3 family. Haemostasis 8: 227–233

Dyerberg J, Bang H O, Stoffersen E, Moncada S, Vane J R 1978 Eiocosapentaenoic acid and prevention of thrombosis and atherosclerosis? Lancet 2: 117–119

Edson J R 1979 Acquired qualitative abnormalities of platelet function. In: Schmidt R M (ed) CRC Handbook Series in Clinical Laboratory Science. Section I: Hematology Volume I. CRC Press, Boca Raton, Florida, p. 463–469

Edson J R, Fecher D R, Doe R P 1975 Low platelet adhesiveness and other hemostatic abnormalities in hypothyroidism. Annals of Internal Medicine 82: 342–346

Ekert H, Sheers M 1974 Preoperative and postoperative platelet function in cyanotic congenital heart disease. Journal of Thoracic and Cardiovascular Surgery 67: 184–190

Eknoyan G, Wacksman S J, Glueck H I, Will J J 1969 Platelet function in renal failure. New England Journal of Medicine 280: 677–681

Eldor A, Weksler B B 1979 Heparin and dextran sulfate antagonise PGI_2 inhibition of platelet aggregation. Thrombosis Research 16: 617–628

Epstein C J, Sahud M A, Piel D F, Gookman J R, Bernfield M R, Cushner J H, Ablin A R 1972 Hereditary macrothrombocytopathia, nephritis and deafness. American Journal of Medicine 52: 299–310

Evans G, Packham M A, Nishizawa E E, Mustard J F, Murphy E A 1968 The effect of acetylsalicylic acid on platelet function. Journal of Experimental Medicine 128: 877–894

Freedman D, Mielke C H, Rodvien R, Kalal K, Tun P, Malloy M J, Kane J 1979 Abnormal platelet function in dysbetalipoproteinemia. Circulation 59 and 60 (Supplement II): II–270

Friedman L L, Bowie E J W, Thompson J H, Brown A L, Owen C A 1964 Familial Glanzmann's thrombasthenia. Mayo Clinic Proceedings 39: 908–918

Fujimura K, Taketomi Y, Kuramoto A 1979 Analysis of platelet membrane glycoproteins in myeloproliferative disorders. Thrombosis and Haemostasis 42: 46

Fuster V, Fass D N, Bowie E J W 1979 Resistance to atherosclerosis in pigs with genetic and therapeutic inhibition of platelet function. Thrombosis and Haemostasis 42: 270

Fuster V, Bowie E J W, Lewis J C, Fass D N, Owen C A, Brown A L 1978 Reistance to arteriosclerosis in pigs with von Willebrand's disease. Journal of Clinical Investigation 61: 722–730

Gallus A, Engel G 1979 Heparin. The Society of Hospital Pharmacists of Australia, Woden, Australia, 1–126

Ganguly P, Sutherland S B, Bradford H R 1978 Defective binding of thrombin to platelets in myeloid leukemia. British Journal of Haematology 39: 599–605

Garay S M, Gardella J E, Fazzini E P, Goldring R M 1979 Hermansky-Pudlak syndrome: pulmonary manifestations of a ceroid storage disorder. American Journal of Medicine 66: 737–747

Gartner T K, Phillips, D R, Gerrard J M, White J G 1979 Platelet functional defect causing Glanzmann's thrombasthenia. Thrombosis and Haemostasis 42: 195

Gartner T K, Williams D C, Minion F C, Phillips D R 1978 Thrombin-induced platelet aggregation is mediated by a platelet plasma membrane-bound lectin. Science 200: 1281–1283

Gausis N, Fortune D, W, Whiteside M-G 1969 The May-Hegglin anomaly: a case report and chromosome study. British Journal of Haematology 16: 619–620

Gensini G F, Abbate R, Favilla S, Neri-Serneri G G 1979 Changes of platelet function and blood clotting in diabetes mellitus. Thrombosis and Haemostasis 42: 983–993

Genton E, Steele P 1977 Platelet survival: value for the diagnosis of thromboembolism and evaluation of antithrombotic drugs. In: Mills D C B, Pareti F I (eds) Platelets and Thrombosis, Proceedings of the Serono Symposia, Academic Press, New York, Volume 10, 157–166

Gerrard J M, Schollmeyer J V, Phillips D R, White J G 1979a Alpha-actinin deficiency in thrombasthenia: possible identity of a-actinin and glycoprotein III. American Journal of Pathology 94: 509–528

Gerrard J M, White J G, Rao G H R, Krivit W, Witkop C J 1975 Labile aggregation stimulating substance (LASS): the factor from storage pool deficient platelets correcting defective aggregation and release of aspirin treated normal platelets. British Journal of Haematology 29: 657–665

Gerrard J M, Phillips D R, Rao G H R, Plow E F, Walz D W, Ross R, Harker L A, White J G 1979b The role of α-granules and their contents in platelet function: studies of the gray platelet syndrome, a selective deficiency of these organelles. Blood 54 (Supplement 1): 241a

Gerrard J M, Stoddard S. F, Shapiro R S, Coccia P F, Ramoay N K C, Nesbit M E, Rao G H R, Krivit W, White J G 1978 Platelet storage pool deficiency and prostaglandin synthesis in chronic granulocytic leukemia. British Journal of Haematology 40: 597–607

Gerritsen S M, Akkerman J W N, Sixma J J 1978 Correction of the bleeding time in patients with storage pool deficiency by infusion of cryoprecipitate. British Journal of Haematology 40: 153–160

Gerritsen S M, Akkerman J W N, Nijmeijer B, Sixma J J, Witkop C J, White J 1977 The

Hermanski-Pudlak syndrome: evidence for a lowered 5-hydroxytryptamine content in platelets of heterozygotes. Scandinavian Journal of Haematology 18: 249–256

Gimson A E S, Langley P G, Hughes R D, Canalese J, Mellon P J, Williams R, Woods H F, Weston M J 1980 Prostacyclin to prevent platelet activation during charcoal haemoperfusion in fulminant hepatic failure. Lancet 1: 173–175

Ginsburg A D 1975 Platelet function in patients with high platelet counts. Annals of Internal Medicine 82: 506–511

Godwin H A, Ginsburg A D 1974 May-Hegglin anomaly: a defect in megakaryocytic fragmentation? British Journal of Haematology 26: 117–128

Goudemand M, Parquet-Gernez A 1973 L'anomalie de May-Hegglin. Nouvelle Revue Française d'Hématologie 13: 568–573

Green L H, Seroppian E, Handin R I 1980 Platelet activation during excercise-induced myocardial ischemia. New England Journal of Medicine 302: 193–197

Gröttum K A, Solum N O 1969 Congenital thrombocytopenia with giant platelets: a defect in the platelet membrane. British Journal of Haematology 16: 277–290

Gröttum K A, Hovig T, Holmsen H, Abrahamsen A F, Jeremic M, Seip M 1969 Wiskott-Aldrich syndrome: qualitative platelet defects and short platelet survival. British Journal of Haematology 17: 373–388

Hagedorn A B, Bowie E J W, Owen C A 1979 Hemostatic disorders and platelet nucleotide release in myeloproliferative disease. Thrombosis and Haemostasis 42: 45

Ham J M, Lawrence J C 1977 Heparin, heparin-activated enzymes and platelets. Haemostasis 6: 26–34

Han P, Turpie A G G, Genton E 1979 Plasma β-thromboglobulin: differentiation between intravascular and extravascular platelet destruction. Blood 54: 1192–1196

Handin R I, McDonough M, Lesch M 1978 Elevation of platelet factor four in acute myocardial infarction: measurement by radioimmunoassay. Journal of Laboratory and Clinical Medicine 91: 340–349

Hanington E 1978 Migraine: a blood disorder? Lancet 2: 501–502

Hardisty R M, Hutton R A 1967 Bleeding tendency associated with 'new' abnormality of platelet behaviour. Lancet 1: 983–985

Hardisty R M, Wolff H II 1955 Haemorrhagic thrombocythaemia: a clinical and laboratory study. British Journal of Haematology 1: 390–405

Hardisty R M, Mills D C B, Ketsa-ard K 1972 The platelet defect associated with albinism. British Journal of Haematology 23: 697–692

Harker L A, Slichter S J 1970 Studies of platelet and fibrinogen kinetics in patients with prosthetic heart valves. New England Journal of Medicine 283: 1302–1305

Harker L A, Slichter S J 1972 Platelet and fibrinogen consumption in man. New England Journal of Medicine 287: 999–1005

Harker L A, Slichter S J 1974 Arterial and venous thrombo-embolism: kinetic characterization and evaluation of therapy. Thrombosis et Diathesis Haemorrhagica 31: 188–202

Hathaway W E, Mahasanduna C, Clarke J, Humbert J R 1973 Paradoxical bleeding in intensively transfused hemophiliacs: alteration of platelet function. Transfusion 13: 6–12

Heiden D, Mielke C H Jr, Rodvien R 1977 Impairment by heparin of primary haemostasis and platelet (^{14}C) 5-hydroxytryptamine release. British Journal of Haematology 36: 427–436

Henry D, Audet P, Shattil S J 1979 Relationships between the structure of penicillins and their anti-platelet activity. Blood 54 (Supplement 1): 243a

Hensby C N, Lewis P J, Hilgard P, Mufti G J, Hows J, Webster J 1979 Prostacyclin deficiency in thrombotic thrombocytopenic purpura. Lancet 2: 748

Hermansky F, Cieslar P 1976 Thrombopathies héréditaires par trouble de libération. Nouvelle Revue Française d'Hématologie 16: 413–420

Hermansky F, Pudlak P 1959 Albinism associated with hemorrhagic diathesis and unusual pigmented reticular cells in the bone marrow: report of two cases with histochemical studies. Blood 14: 162–169

Hoagland H C, Silverstein M N 1978 Primary thrombocythemia in the young patient. Mayo Clinic Proceedings 53: 578–580

Holcomb G R, Strand J C, Kaye M P 1979 The protective effect of prostacyclin on platelet function following cardiopulmonary bypass. Blood 54 (Supplement 1): 244a

Horowitz H I, Stein I M, Cohen B D, White J G 1970 Further studies on the platelet-inhibitory effect of guanidinosuccinic acid and its role in uremic bleeding. American Journal of Medicine 49: 336–345

Horowitz H I, Cohen B D, Martinez P, Papayoanou M F 1967 Defective ADP-induced platelet factor 3 activation in uremia. Blood 30: 331–340

Howard M A, Hutton R A, Hardisty R A 1973 Hereditary giant platelet syndrome: a disorder of a new aspect of platelet function. British Medical Journal 4: 586–588

Hussain S, Schwartz J M, Friedman S A, Chua S N 1978 Arterial thrombosis in essential thrombocythemia. American Heart Journal 96: 31–36

Hussey C V, Bernhard V M, McLean M R, Fobian J E 1979 Heparin induced platelet aggregation: in vitro confirmation of thrombotic complications. Annals of Clinical and Laboratory Science 9: 487–493

Hutton R A, O'Shea M J 1968 Haemostatic mechanism in uraemia. Journal of Clinical Pathology 21: 406–411

Huzoor-Akbar, Ardlie N H 1977a Effects of clofibrate on platelets and evidence of the involvement of platelet lipids in platelet function. Thrombosis Research 10: 95–105

Huzoor-Akbar, Ardlie N G 1977b The effect of halofenate-free acid on aggregation, the release reaction, coagulant activity, and lipid metabolism of human platelets. Thrombosis and Haemostasis 38: 612–619

Inceman S, Tangün Y 1972 Platelet defects in the myeloproliferative disorders. Annals of New York Academy of Sciences 201: 251–261

Ingerman C M, Smith J B, Shapiro S, Sedar A, Silver M J 1978 Hereditary abnormality of platelet aggregation attributable to nucleotide storage pool deficiency. Blood 52: 332–344

Insel P A, Nirenberg P, Turnbull J, Shattil S J 1978 Relationships between membrane cholesterol, α-adrenergic receptors, and platelet function. Biochemistry 17: 5269–5274

Jaffe E A, Weksler B B 1979 Recovery of endothelial cell prostacyclin production after inhibition by low doses of aspirin. Journal of Clinical Investigation 63: 532–535

Jamieson G A, Okumura T, Fishback B, Johnson M M, Egan J J, Weiss H J 1979 Platelet membrane glycoproteins in thrombasthenia, Bernard-Soulier syndrome, and storage pool disease. Journal of Laboratory and Clinical Medicine 93: 652–660

Jenkins C S P, Phillips D R, Clemetson K J, Meyer D, Larrieu M J, Lüscher E F 1976 Platelet membrane glycoproteins implicated in ristocetin-induced aggregation: studies on the proteins of platelets from patients with Bernard-Soulier syndrome and von Willebrand's disease. Journal of Clinical Investigation 57: 112–124

Jerushalmy Z, Zucker M B 1966 Some effects of fibrinogen degradation products (FDP) on blood platelets. Thrombosis et Diathesis Haemorrhagica 15: 413–419

Joist J H, Mustard J F 1975 Heparin, lysolecithin and platelet function. In: Bradshaw R A, Wessler S (eds) Heparin (Structure, Function, and Clinical implications). Plenum Press, New York, p 255–261

Joist J H, Baker R K, Schonfeld G 1979 Increased in vivo and in vitro platelet function in type II hyperlipoproteinemia. Thrombosis Research 15: 95–108

Kalendovsky Z, Austin J, Steele P 1975 Increased platelet aggregability in young patients with stroke; diagnosis and therapy. Acta Neurologica 32: 13–20

Kapsch D N, Adelstein E H, Rhodes G R, Silver D 1979 Heparin-induced thrombocytopenia, thrombosis, and hemorrhage. Surgery 86: 148–155

Kasturi J, Saraya A K 1978 Platelet functions in dysproteinaemia. Acta Haematologica 59: 104–113

Kaywin P, McDonough M, Insel P A, Shattil S J 1978 Platelet function in essential thrombocythemia: decreased epinephrine responsiveness associated with a deficiency of platelet α-adrenergic receptors. New England Journal of Medicine 299: 505–509

Kazmier F J, Fuster V, Chesebro J H, O'Fallon W M, Palumbo P J 1979a Platelet survival half-life (PS) in atheroscelerosis and diabetes mellitus. Circulation 59 and 60 (Supplement II): 270

Kazmier F J, Owen C A Jr, O'Fallon W M, Palumbo P J, Bowie E J W 1979b Willebrand antigen (VIII R:AG) and ristocetin co-factor (VIIR:RWF) in atherosclerosis and diabetes mellitus. Circulation 59 and 60 (Supplement II): 271

Keenan J, P, Wharton J, Shepherd A J N, Bellingham A J 1977 Defective platelet lipid peroxidation in myeloproliferative disorders: a possible defect of prostaglandin synthesis. British Journal of Haematology 35: 275–283

Kelton J G, Hirsh J, Carter C J, Buchanan M R 1978 Thrombogenic effect of high dose aspirin in rabbits. Relationship to inhibition of vessel wall synthesis of prostaglandin I_2-like activity. Journal of Clinical Investigation 62: 892–895

Kinlough-Rathbone R L, Chahil A, Perry D W, Packham M A, Mustard J F 1979 Effect of amino sugars that block platelet lectin activity on fibrinogen binding to washed rabbit or human platelets. Thrombosis and Haemostasis 42: 249a

Kobayashi I, Fujita T, Yamazaki H 1976 Platelet aggregability measured by screen filtration pressure method in cerebrovascular disease. Stroke 7: 406–409

Kubisz P 1973 Thrombocytopathia with abnormalities in platelet release reaction. Acta Haematologica 49: 349–360

Kumpuris A G, Luchi R J, Waddel C C, Miller R R 1980 Production of circulating platelet aggregates by exercise in coronary patients. Circulation 61: 62–65

Kunicki T J, Aster R H 1978 Deletion of the platelet-specific alloantigen Pl^{A1} from platelets in Glanzmann's thrombasthenia. Journal of Clinical Investigation 61: 1225–1231

Kunicki T J, Johnson M M, Aster R H 1978 Absence of the platelet receptor for drug-dependent antibodies in the Bernard-Soulier syndrome. Journal of Clinical Investigation 62: 716–719

Kurstjens R, Bolt C, Vossen M, Haznen C 1968 Familial thrombopathic thrombocytopenia. British Journal of Haematology 15: 305–317

Kwaan H C, Colwell J A, Cruz S, Suwanwela N, Dobbie C 1972 Increased platelet aggregation in diabetes mellitus. Journal of Laboratory and Clinical Medicine 80: 236–246

Lackner H, Karpatkin S 1975 On the 'easy bruising' syndrome with normal platelet count: a study of 75 patients. Annals of Internal Medicine 83: 190–196

Lagarde M, Dechavanne M 1977 Increase of platelet prostaglandin cyclic endoperoxides in thrombosis. Lancet 1: 88

Lagarde M, Byron P A, Vargaftig B B, Dechavanne M 1978 Impairment of platelet thromboxane A_2 generation and of the platelet release reaction in two patients with congenital deficiency of platelet cyclo-oxygenase. British Journal of Haematology 38: 251–266

Latour J-G, Théroux P, Bourassa M G 1979 Platelet aggregation follow-up of a controlled sulfinpyrazone reinfarction trial. Circulation 59 and 60 (Supplement II): 271

Lecompte F, Renaud S 1973 Influence of pregnancy and oral contraceptives on platelets in relation to coagulation and aggregation. Thrombosis et Diathesis Haemorrhagica 29: 510–517

Leff B, Henriksen R A, Owen W G 1979 Effect of oral contraceptive use on platelet prothrombin converting (platelet factor 3) activity. Thrombosis Research 15: 631–638

Levine P H 1973 A qualitative platelet defect in severe vitamin B_{12} deficiency: response, hyperresponse, and thrombosis after vitamin B_{12} therapy. Annals of Internal Medicine 78: 533–539

Lewis J H, Zucker M B, Ferguson J H 1956 Bleeding tendency in uremia. Blood 11: 1073–1076

Lewy R I, Smith, J B, Silver M J, Saia J, Walinsky P, Wiener L 1979a Detection of thromboxane B_2 (TXB_2) in peripheral blood of patients with Prinzmetal's angina. Clinical Research 27: 462a

Lewy R I, Wiener L, Smith J B, Walinsky P, Silver M J 1979b Intravenous heparin initiates in-vivo synthesis and release of thromboxane in angina pectoris. Lancet 2: 97

Lian EC-Y, Harkness D R, Byrnes J J, Wallach H, Ninez R 1979 Presence of a platelet aggregating factor in the plasma of patients with thrombotic thrombocytopenic purpura (TTP) and its inhibition by normal plasma. Blood 53: 333–338

Logan L J, Rapaport S I, Maher I 1971 Albinism and abnormal platelet function. New England Journal of Medicine 284: 1340–1345

Lorez H P, Richards J G, Da Prada M, Picotti G B, Paretti F I, Capitanio A, Mannucci P 1979 Storage pool disease: comparative fluorescence microscopical, cytochemical and biochemical studies on amine-storing organelles of human blood platelets. British Journal of Haematology 43: 293–305

Lowe G D O, Johnston R V, Drummond M M, Forbes C D, Prentice C R M 1979a Induction of circulating platelet-aggregates in healthy subjects by a saturated fat meal. Thrombosis Research 16: 565–568

Lowe G D O, Reavey M M, Third JLHC, Bremmer W F, Forbes C D, Prentice C R M, Lawrie T D V 1979b Increased plasma fibrinogen and circulating platelet-aggregates in type II hyperlipoproteinaemia. Clinical Science 56: 21p

Ludlam C A 1979 Evidence for the platelet specificity of β-thromboglobulin and study of its plasma concentrations in healthy individuals. British Journal of Haematology 41: 271–278

Ludlam C A and Anderson J L 1977 The significance of platelet function tests in the evaluation of hemostatic and thrombotic tendencies. In: H J Day, H Holmsen, M B Zucker (eds) Proceedings of a workshop on platelets, Philadelphia, U.S. Government Press

Ludlam C A, Bolton A E, Moore S, Cash J D 1975 New rapid method for the diagnosis of deep venous thrombosis. Lancet 2: 259–260

Lufkin E G, Fass D N, O'Fallon W M, Bowie E J W 1979 Increased von Willebrand factor in diabetes mellitus. Metabolism 28: 63–66

Lusher J M, Schneider J, Mizukami I, Evans R K 1968 The May-Hegglin anomaly: platelet function, ultrastructure and chromosome studies. Blood 32: 950–961

Maldonado J 1974a 'Swiss-cheese' platelets. Annals of Internal Medicine 81: 860–861

Maldonado J E 1974b Dysplastic platelets and circulating megakaryocytes in chronic myeloproliferative disease: II. ultrastructure of circulating megakaryocytes. Blood 43: 811–820

Maldonado J E, Pierre R V 1975 The platelets in preleukemia and myelomonocytic leukemia: ultrastructural cytochemistry and cytogenetics. Mayo Clinic Proceedings 50: 573–587

Maldonado J E, Pintado T, Pierre R V 1974 Dysplastic platelets and circulating megakaryocytes in chronic myeloproliferative disease. I. The platelets: ultrastructure and peroxidase reaction. Blood 43: 797–809

Malmgren R, Olsson P, Tornleng G, Unge G 1978 Acetylsalicylic asthma and migraine: a defect in serotonin (5 HT) uptake in platelets. Thrombosis Research 13: 1137–1139

Malmsten C, Hamberg M, Svensson J, Samuelsson B 1975 Physiological role of an endoperoxide in human platelets: hemostatic defect due to platelet cyclo-oxgenase deficiency. Proceedings of the National Academy of Sciences, USA 72: 1446–1450

Malmsten C, Kindahl H, Samuelsson B, Levy-Toledano S, Tobelem G, Caen J P 1977 Thromboxane synthesis and the platelet release reaction in Bernard-Soulier syndrome, thrombasthenia Glanzmann and Hermansky-Pudlak syndrome. British Journal of Haematology 35: 511–520

Masotti G, Piggesi L, Galanti G, Abbate R 1979 Differential inhibition of prostacyclin production and platelet aggregation by aspirin. Lancet 2: 1213–1216

Maurer H M, Wolff J A, Buckingham S, Spielvogel A R 1972 'Impotent' platelets in albinos with prolonged bleeding times. Blood 39: 490–499

Maurer H M, Still W J S, Caul J, Valdes O S, Laupus W E 1971 Familial bleeding tendency associated with microcytic platelets and impaired release of platelet adenosine diphosphate. Journal of Pediatrics 78: 86–94

McClure P D, Casserly J G, Monsier C, Crozier D 1970 Carbenicillin-induced bleeding disorder. Lancet 2: 1307–1308

McClure P D, Ingram G I C, Stacey R S, Glass U H, Matchett M O 1966 Platelet function tests in thrombocythaemia and thrombocytosis. British Journal of Haematology 12: 478–498

McCoy E E, Enns L 1978 Sodium transport, ouabain binding, and (Na^+/K^+) — ATPase activity in Down's syndrome platelets. Pediatric Research 12: 685–689

McGrath K M, Castaldi P A 1975 Changes in coagulation factors and platelet function in response to progestational agents. Haemostasis 4: 65–72

McKenna R, Bachmann F, Whittaker B, Gilson J R, Weinberg M 1975 The hemostatic mechanism after open-heart surgery II. Frequency of abnormal platelet functions during and after extracorporeal circulation. Journal of Thoracic and Cardiovascular Surgery 70: 298–308

McNicol G P, Douglas A S 1967 Platelet abnormality in human scurvy. Lancet 1: 975–978

Meyers K M, Seachord C I, Prieur D, Holmsen H 1979b A serotonin induced biphasic aggregation by platelets from cats with the Chediak-Higashi syndrome. Thrombosis and Haemostasis 42: 195

Meyers K M, Holmsen H, Seachord C I, Gorham J, Prieur D 1979a Characterization of platelets from mink and cats with the Chediak-Higashi syndrome. Thrombosis and Haemostasis 42: 218

Michaelski R, Lam D A, Pepper D S, Kakkar V V 1978 Neutralization of heparin in plasma by platelet factor 4 and protamine sulfate. British Journal of Haematology 38: 561–571

Milton J G, Frojmovic M M 1979 Invaginated plasma membrane of human platelets: evagination and measurement in normal and 'giant platelets'. Journal of Laboratory and Clinical Medicine 93: 162–170

Minkes M S, Joist J H, Needleman P 1979 Arachidonic acid-induced platelet aggregation independent of ADP-release in a patient with a bleeding disorder due to platelet storage pool disease. Thrombosis Research 15: 169–179

Moake J, Olson J, Troll J, Peterson D, Cimo P, Weinger R 1979 Defective binding of ^{125}I-von Willebrand factor (vWF) to Bernard-Soulier platelets. Blood 54 (Supplement 1): 253a

Moncada S, Korbut R 1978 Dipyridamole and other phosphodiesterase inhibitors act as antithrombotic agents by potentiating endogenous prostacyclin. Lancet 1: 1286–1289

Murphy S 1972 Hereditary thrombocytopenias. Clinics in Haematology 1: 359–368

Najean Y, Dassin E, Renner C, Wacquet M 1979 Cinétique plaquettaire au cours des maladies artérielles. Artérites, prothéses valvulaire et vasculaire: 73 observations. Nouvelle Presse Médicale 8: 3813–3816

Needleman P, Wyche A, Raz A 1979b Platelet and blood vessel arachidonate metabolism and interactions. Journal of Clinical Investigation 63: 345–349

Needleman P, Raz A, Minkes M S, Ferrendelli J A, Sprecher H 1979a Triene prostaglandins: prostacyclin and thromboxane biosynthesis and unique biological properties. Proceedings of the National Academy of Sciences, USA 76: 944–948

Neemeh J A, Bowie E J W, Thompson J H Jr, Didisheim P, Owen C A Jr 1972 Quantitation of platelet aggregation in myeloproliferative disorders. American Journal of Clinical Pathology 57: 336–347

Nelson J C, Lerner R, G, Goldstein R, Cagin N A 1978 Heparin-induced thrombocytopenia. Archives of Internal Medicine 138: 548–552

Neri Serneri G G, Abbate R, Gensini G F, Mugnaini C, Laggi A 1976 Occurrence of a plasmatic aggregating activity in some patients with increased platelet aggregation. European Symposium on Platelet Aggregation, Coagulation, Fibrinolysis and Atherosclerosis, Palermo

Nishimura J, Okamoto S, Ibayashi H 1979 Abnormalities of platelet adenine nucleotides in patients with myeloproliferative disorders. Thrombosis and Haemostasis 41: 787–795

Nordøy A 1974 Plasma and platelet lipids in man. Haemostasis 2: 103–117

Nordøy A 1976 Lipids as triggering factors in thrombosis. Thrombosis and Haemostasis 35: 32–48

Nordøy A 1979 Albumin-bound fatty acids, platelets and endothelial cells in thrombogenesis. Haemostasis 8: 193–202

Nordøy A, Svensson B 1979 The simultaneous effect of albumin-bound fatty acids on platelets and endothelial cells. Thrombosis Research 15: 215–226

Nurden A T, Caen J P 1974 An abnormal platelet glycoprotein pattern in three cases of Glanzmann's thrombasthenia. British Journal of Haematology 28: 253–260

Nurden A T, Caen J P 1975 Specific roles for platelet surface glycoproteins in platelet function. Nature 255: 720–722

Nurden A T, Rendu F, Kunicki T, Caen J P 1979 Characterization of the molecular defects of the platelets of two patients with the gray platelet syndrome. Blood 54 (Supplement 1): 254a

Nyman D, Eriksson A W, Lehmann W, Blombäck M 1979 Inherited defective platelet aggregation with arachidonate as the main expression of a defective metabolism of arachidonic acid. Thrombosis Research 14: 739–746

O'Brien J R 1967 Platelets: a Portsmouth syndrome? Lancet 2: 258

O'Brien J R 1968 Effects of salicylates on human platelets. Lancet 1: 779–783
O'Brien J R, Etherington M D 1976 An inverse relation between platelet factor 4 in the platelet and in the plasma. Thrombosis and Haemostasis 36: 649–651
O'Brien J R, Etherington M D, Jamieson S 1976 Acute platelet changes after large meals of saturated and unsaturated fats. Lancet 1: 878–880
O'Grady J, Moncada S 1978 Aspirin: a paradoxical effect on bleeding time. Lancet 2: 780
Okuma M, Uchino H 1979 Altered arachidonate metabolism by platelets in patients with myeloproliferative disorders. Blood 54: 1258–1271
Ordinas A, Maragall S, Castillo R, Nurden A T 1978 A glycoprotein I defect in the platelets of three patients with severe cirrhosis of the liver. Thrombosis Research 13: 297–302
Owen C A Jr, Bowie E J W, Thompson J H Jr 1975 The diagnosis of bleeding disorders 2d ed. Little, Brown & Co., Boston
Owen C A, Goldstein N P, Bowie E J W 1976 Platelet function and coagulation in patients with Wilson disease. Archives of Internal Medicine 136: 148–152
Packham M A, Mustard J F 1977 Clinical pharmacology of platelets. Blood 50: 555–573
Pareti F I, Capitanio A, Mannucci P M 1976 Acquired storage pool disease in platelets during disseminated intravascular coagulation. Blood 48: 511–515
Pareti F I, Day H J, Mills D C B 1974 Nucleotide and serotonin metabolism in platelets with defective secondary aggregation. Blood 44: 789–800
Pareti F I, Smith J B, D'Angelo A, Mannucci P M 1979b The congenital deficiency of platelet thromboxane and vessel wall prostacyclin results in a mild bleeding disorder which no thrombotic tendency. Blood 54 (Supplement 1): 255a
Pareti F I, Dawes J, Franchi F, Mannucci P, Pepper D S 1979a Content and release of β-thromboglobulin and platelet factor 4 in patients with qualitative platelet defects. Thrombosis Research 16: 537–542
Pareti F I, Mannucci P M, Asti D, Guarani A, Gugliotta L, Tura S 1979c Acquired storage pool disease in myeloproliferative disorders. Thrombosis and Haemostasis 42: 44
Parmley R T, Poon M C, Crist W M, Malluh A 1979 Giant platelet granules in a child with the Chediak-Higashi syndrome. American Journal of Hematology 6: 51–60
Paton R C 1979 Platelet survival in diabetes mellitus using an aspirin-labelling technique. Thrombosis Research 15: 793–802
Peters J R, Elliott J M, Grahame-Smith D G 1979 Effect of oral contraceptives on platelet noradrenaline and 5-hydroxytryptamine receptors and aggregation. Lancet 2: 933–936
Pisciotta A V, Garthwaite T, Darin J, Aster R H 1977 Treatment of thrombotic thrombocytopenic purpura by exchange transfusion. American Journal of Hematology 3: 73–82
Pittman M A, Graham J B 1964 Glanzmann's thrombopathy: an autosomal recessive trait in one family. American Journal of Medical Sciences 247: 293–303
Prazich J A, Rapaport S A, Samples J R, Engler R 1977 Platelet aggregate ratios-standardization of technique and test results in patients with myocardial ischemia and patients with cerebrovascular disease. Thrombosis Haemostasis 38: 597–605
Preston F E, Ward J D, Marcola B, Porter N R, Timperley W R, O'Malley B C 1978 Elevated β-thromboglobulin levels and circulating platelet aggregates in diabetic microangiopathy. Lancet 1: 238–240
Quick A J 1965 Hereditary thrombopathic thrombocytopenia: sex-linked inheritance pattern. American Journal of the Medical Sciences 250: 527–530
Quick A J 1966 Salicylates and bleeding: the aspirin tolerance test. American Journal of the Medical Sciences 252: 265–269
Rabiner S F 1972 Uremic bleeding. In: Spaet T H (ed) Progress in Hemostasis and Thrombosis, Grune & Stratton, New York, Volume 1, p 233–250
Rabiner S F, Molinas F 1970 The role of phenol and phenolic acids on the thrombocytopathy and defective platelet aggregation of patients with renal failure. American Journal of Medicine 49: 346–351
Raccuglia G 1971 Gray platelet syndrome: a variety of qualitative platelet disorder. American Journal of Medicine 51: 818–828
Reches A, Eldor A, Salomon Y 1979 Heparin inhibits PGE$_1$-sensitive adenylate cyclase and antagonizes PGE$_1$ antiaggregating effect in human platelets. Journal of Laboratory and Clinical Medicine 93: 638–644
Redman C W G, Allington M J, Bolton F G, Stirrat G M 1977 Plasma-β-thromboglobulin in pre-eclampsia. Lancet 2: 248
Regan M G, Lackner H, Karpatkin S 1974 Platelet function and coagulation profile in lupus erythematosus. Annals of Internal Medicine 81: 462–468
Remuzzi G, Mecca G, Cavenaghi A E, Donati M B, de Gaetano G 1977 Prostacyclin-like activity and bleeding in renal failure. Lancet 2: 1195–1197
Remuzzi G, Misiani R, Mecca G, de Gaetano G, Donati M B, Riuniti O 1978 Thrombotic thrombocytopenic purpura-a deficiency of plasma factors regulating platelet-vessel-wall interaction? New England Journal Of Medicine 299: 311

Remuzzi G, Mecca G, Marchesi D, Livio M, de Gaetano G, Donati M B, Silver M J 1979 Platelet hyperaggregability and the nephrotic syndrome. Thrombosis Research 16: 345–354

Renaud S, Morazain R, McGregor L, Baudier F 1979 Dietary fats and platelet functions in relation to atherosclerosis and coronary heart disease. Haemostatis 8: 234–251

Renaud S, Dumont E, Godsey F, Suplisson A, Thevenon C 1978 Platelet functions in relation to dietary fats in farmers from two regions of France. Thrombosis and Haemostasis 40: 518–531

Rendu F, Lebret M, Nurden A, Caen J P 1979 Detection of an acquired platelet storage pool disease in three patients with a myeloproliferative disorder. Thrombosis and Haemostasis 42: 794–795

Rendu F, Breton-Gorius J, Trugnan G, Castro-Malaspina H, Andrieu J-M, Bereziat G, Lebret M, Caen J P 1978 Studies on a new variant of the Hermansky-Pudlak syndrome: qualitative, ultrastructural, and functional abnormalities of the platelet dense bodies associated with phospholipase A defect. American Journal of Haematology 4: 387–399

Rosse W F 1977 Paroxysmal nocturnal hemoglobinuria In: Williams W J, Beutler E, Erslev A J, Rundles R W (eds) Hematology, 2d ed, McGraw-Hill, New York, p 560–570

Roth G J, Stanford N, Majerus P W 1975 Acetylation of prostaglandin synthetase by aspirin. Proceedings of the National Academy of Sciences, USA 72: 3073–3076

Roux E, Cherbit G, Reganault F 1977 Collagen-induced platelet aggregation and collagen glycosyl-transferase activity in diabetic patients. Thrombosis Research 11: 847–858

Russell N H, Keenan J P, Bellingham A J 1979 Thrombocytopathy in preleukaemia: association with a defect of thromboxane A_2 activity. British Journal of Haematology 41: 417–425

Sahud M A, Aggeler P M 1969 Platelet dysfunction — differentiation of a newly recognized primary type from that produced by aspirin. New England Journal of Medicine 280: 453–459

Sakanishi N, Koh H, Kishi Y, Omori K, Yajima M, Numano F, Nishiyama K, Numano F, Maezawa H 1979 Plasma thromboxane B_2 concentration in healthy Japanese and in patients with atherosclerosis. Circulation 59 & 60 (Supplement II): 246

Sandler M 1977 Transitory platelet mono-amine oxidase deficit in migraine: some reflections. Headache 17: 153–158

Schorer A E, Gerrard J M, White J G, Krivit W 1978 Oral contraceptive use alters the balance of platelet prostaglandin and thromboxane synthesis. Prostaglandins and Medicine 1: 5–11

Semeraro N, Cortellazzo S, Colucci M, Barbui T 1979 A hitherto underscribed defect of platelet coagulant activity in polycythaemia vera and essential thrombocythaemia. Thrombosis Research 16: 795–802

Sharp A A 1977 Diagnosis and management of disseminated intravascular coagulation. British Medical Bulletin 33: 265–272

Shattil S J, Cooper R A 1978 Role of membrane lipid composition, organization, and fluidity in human platelet function. In: Spaet T H (ed) Progress in Hemostasis and Thrombosis, Grune & Stratton, New York, Volume 4, p 59–86

Shattil S J, Bennett J S, Colman R W, Cooper R A 1977 Abnormalities of cholesterol-phospholipid composition in platelets and low-density lipoproteins of human hyperbetalipoproteinemia. Journal of Laboratory and Clinical Medicine 89: 341–353

Shattil S J, Anaya-Galindo R, Bennet J, Colman R W, Cooper R A 1975 Platelet hypersensitivity induced by cholesterol incorporation. Journal of Clinical Investigation 55: 636–643

Shattil S J, Bennett J, McDonough M, Turnbull J, Vilaire G 1979a Carbenicillin and penicillin G impair platelet function by inhibiting the binding of agonists to the platelet surface. Thrombosis Haemostasis 42: 76

Siess W, Scherer B, Böhlig B, Roth P, Kurzmann I, Weber P C 1980 Platelet-membrane fatty acids, platelet aggregation, and thromboxane formation during a mackerel diet. Lancet 1: 441–444

Silberbauer K, Schernthaner G, Sinzinger H, Winter M, Piza-Katzer H 1979 Iuveniler Diabetes mellitus: verminderte Prostacyclin (PGI$_2$) synthesis in der Gefässwand. Vasa 8: 213–216

Silverstein M N 1975 Agnogenic Myeloid Metaplasia. Publishing Sciences Group, Acton, Massachusetts

Smith R C, Duncanson J, Ruckley C V, Webber R G, Allan N C, Dawes J, Bolton A E, Hunter W M, Pepper D S, Cash J D 1978 β-thromboglobulin and deep vein thrombosis. Thrombosis and Haemostasis 39: 338–345

Smith T P, Dodds W J, Tartaglia A P 1973 Thrombasthenic-thrombopathic thrombocytopenia with giant 'Swiss-cheese' platelets: a case report. Annals of Internal Medicine 79: 828–834

Solinger A, Bernstein I L, Glueck H I 1973 The effect of epinephrine on platelet aggregation in normal and atopic subjects. Journal of Allergy and Clinical Immunology 51: 29–34

Spaet T H, Lejnieks F, Gaynor E, Goldstein M L 1969 Defective platelets in essential thrombocythemia. Archives of Internal Medicine 124: 135–142

Stachurska J, Lopacink S, Gerdin B, Saldecu T, Koroscik A, Kopec M 1979 Effects of proteolytic degradation products of human fibrinogen and of human factor VIII on platelet aggregation and vascular permeability. Thrombosis Research 15: 663–672

Steele P, Battock, D, Pappas G, Genton E 1976 Correlation of platelet survival time with occlusion of saphenous vein aorto-coronary bypass grafts. Circulation 53: 685–687

Steiner M, Anastasi J 1976 Vitamin E: an inhibitor of the platelet release reaction. Journal of Clinical
Investigation 57: 732–737
Stewart J H, Castaldi P A 1967 Uraemic bleeding: a reversible platelet defect corrected by dialysis.
Quarterly Journal of Medicine 36: 409–423
Strolin-Benedetti M, Gutty D, Strolin P 1976 A comparative study of the effect of oral contraceptives and
cigarette smoking on platelet adhesiveness. Haemostasis 5: 14–20
Stuart M J, Gerrard J M, White J G 1980 Effect of cholesterol on production of thomboxane B₂ by platelets
in vitro. New England Journal of Medicine 302: 6–10
Stuart M J, Miller M L, Davey F R, Wolk J A 1979 The post-aspirin bleeding time: a screening test for
evaluating haemostatic disorders. British Journal of Haematology 43: 649–659
Sultan Y, Jeanneau C 1971 Myeloproliferative disorders and platelet aggregation In: Caen J (ed) Platelet
Aggregation, Masson & Cie, Paris, p 193–197
Sultan Y, Bernal-Hoyos J, Levy-Toledano S, Jeanneau C, Caen J P 1974 Dominant inherited familial factor
VIII deficiency (von Willebrand disease) associated with thrombocytopathic thrombobyctopenia.
Pathologie Biologie 22: 27–36
Tremoli E, Folco G, Agradi E, Galli C 1979a Platelet thromboxanes and serum cholesterol. Lancet 1:
107–108
Tremoli E, Maderna P, Sirtori M, Sirtori C R 1979b Platelet aggregation and malondialdehyde formation in
type IIa hypercholesterolemic patients. Haemostasis 8: 47–53
Ulutin O N 1976 The platelets: fundamentals and clinical applications. Kagit ve Basin Isleri A. S., Istanbul
Vainer P H, Bussel A 1976 Etudes sur les glycoprotéines membranaires et la glycosylation des protéines des
plaquettes dans la leucémie myéloïde chronique. Nouvelle Revue Française d'Hématologie 16: 447–454
Vainer P H, Bussel A 1977 Glycoprotéines de surface altérées des plaquettes de leucémie myéloïde
chronique (altered platelet surface glycoproteins in chronic myeloid leukemia). International Journal of
Cancer 19: 143–149
Vainer H, Bussel A 1979 Defective platelet surface markers in chronic myeloid leukemia (CML).
Thrombosis and Haemostasis 42: 45
Vigliano E M, Horowitz H I 1967 Bleeding syndrome with IgA myeloma: interaction of protein and
connective tissue. Blood 29: 823–836
Vossen M E M H, Stadjouders A M, Kurstjens R, Haanen C 1968 Observations on platelet ultrastructure
in familial thrombocytopathic thrombocytopenia. American Journal of Pathology 53: 1021–1031
Walsh P N, Murphy S, Barry W E 1977b The role of platelets in the pathogenesis of thrombosis and
hemorrhage in patients with thrombocytosis. Thrombosis and Haemostasis 38: 1085–1096
Walsh P N, Pareti F I, Corbett J J 1976a Platelet coagulant activities and serum lipids in transient cerebral
ischemia. New England Journal of Medicine 295: 854–858
Walsh P N, Goldberg R E, Tax R L, Margargal L E 1977a Platelet coagulant activities and retinal vein
thrombosis. Thrombosis and Haemostasis 38: 399–406
Walsh P N, Rogers P H, Marder V J, Gagnatelli G, Escovitz E S, Sherry S 1976b The relationship of
platelet coagulant activities to venous thrombosis following hip surgery. British Journal of Haematology
32: 421–437
Wautier J L, Caen J P 1979 Pharmacology of platelet-suppressive agents. Seminars in Thrombosis and
Hemostasis 5: 293–315
Weinfeld A, Branchög I, Kutti J 1975 Platelets in the myeloproliferative syndromes. Clinics in
Haematology 4: 373–392
Weiss H J 1967 Platelet aggregation, adhesion and adenosine diphosphate release in thrombopathia
(platelet factor 3 deficiency). American Journal of Medicine 43: 570–578
Weiss H J 1972 The pharmacology of platelet inhibition. In: Spaet T H (ed) Progress in hemostasis and
thrombosis, Grune & Stratton, New York, Volume 1, p 199–231
Weiss H J 1978 Antiplatelet therapy. New England Journal of Medicine 298: 1344–1347; 1403–1406
Weiss H J, Aledort L M 1967 Impaired platelet-connective tissue reaction in man after aspirin ingestion.
Lancet 2: 495–497
Weiss H J, Lages B A 1977 Possible congenital defect in platelet thromboxane synthetase. Lancet 1:
760–761
Weiss H J, Rogers J 1972 Thrombocytopathia due to abnormalities in platelet release reaction — studies on
six unrelated patients. Blood 39: 187–196
Weiss H J, Tschopp T B, Baumgartner II R 1975 Impaired interaction (adhesion-aggregation) of platelets
with the subendothelium in storage-pool disease and after aspirin ingestion. New England Journal of
Medicine 293: 619–623
Weiss H J, Chervenick P A, Zalusky R, Factor A 1969 A familial defect in platelet function associated with
impaired release of adenosine diphosphate. New England Journal of Medicine 281: 1264–1270
Weiss H J, Willis A L, Kuhn D, Brand H 1976 Prostaglandin E₂ potentiation of platelet aggregation
induced by LASS endoperoxide: absent in storage pool disease, normal after aspirin ingestion. British
Journal of Haematology 32: 257–272

Weiss H J, Tschopp T B, Baumgartner H R, Sussman II, Johnson M M, Egan J J 1974 Decreased adhesion of giant (Bernard-Soulier) platelets to subendothelium. American Journal of Medicine 57: 920–925

Weiss H J, Witte L D, Kaplan K L, Lages B A, Chernoff A, Nossel H L, Goodman D S, Baumgartner H R 1979b Heterogeneity in storage pool deficiency: studies on granule-bound substances in 18 patients including variants deficient in α-granules, platelet factor 4, β-thromboglobulin and platelet derived growth factor. Blood 54: 1296–1319

White J G 1979 Ultrastructural studies of the gray platelet syndrome. American Jounral of Pathology 95: 445–462

White J G, Witkop C J 1972 Effects of normal and aspirin platelets on defective secondary aggregation in the Hermansky-Pudlak syndrome: a test for storage pool deficient platelets. American Journal of Pathology 68: 57–66

White J G, Edson J R, Desnick S J, Witkop Jr C J 1971 Studies of platelets in variant of the Hermansky-Pudlak syndrome. American Journal of Pathology 63: 329–332

Wu K K 1978 Platelet hyperaggregability and thrombosis in patients with thrombocythemia. Annals of Internal Medicine 88: 7–11

Wu K K, Hoak J C 1974 A new method for the quantitative detection of platelet aggregates in patients with arterial insufficiency. Lancet 2: 924–926

Wu K K, Barnes R W, Hoak J C 1976 Platelet hyperaggregability in idiopathic recurrent deep vein thrombosis. Circulation 53: 687–691

Wu K K, Chen Y C, Walasek J, Smith C 1979 Hereditary bleeding disorder due to primary defects in platelet release mechanism. Thrombosis and Haemostasis 42: 194

Yamazaki H, Kobayashi I, Shimamoto Y 1970a Enhancement of ADP-induced platelet aggregation by exercise test in coronary patients and its prevention by pyridinolcarbamate. Thrombosis et Diathesis Haemorrhagica 24: 438–449

Yamazaki H, Odakura T, Takeuchi K, Sano T 1970b Adhesive platelet count and blood coagulability in myocardial infarction and cerebral thrombosis. Thrombosis et Diathesis Haemorrhagica 24: 450–460

Yamazaki H, Motomiya T, Kikutani N, Sakakibara C, Watanabe S, Numata M, Noguchi K 1979 Platelet aggregation during menstrual cycle and pregnancy. Thrombosis Research 14: 333–340

Zahavi J, Marder V J 1974 Acquired storage pool disase of platelets associated with circulating antiplatelet antibodies. American Journal of Medicine 56: 883–890

Zucker M B, Peterson J 1968 The effect of salicylates on the hemostatic properties of platelets in man. Journal of Clinical Investigation 47: 2169–2180

Zucker S, Mielke C H 1972 Classification of thrombocytosis based on platelet function tests: correlation with hemorrhagic and thrombotic manifestations. Journal of Laboratory and Clinical Medicine 80: 385–394

Zucker S, Mielke C H, Durocher J R, Crosby W H 1972 Oozing and bruising due to abnormal platelet function (thrombocytopathia): a family study of the syndrome. Annals of Internal Medicine 76: 725–731

Zuzel M, Cawley J C, Paton R C, Burns G F, McNicol G P 1979 Platelet function in hairy-cell leukemia. Journal of Clinical Pathology 32: 814–821

3. Structure and function in blood coagulation

Robert F. Baugh and Cecil Hougie

It has been a relatively short time since the last edition of this volume, and although the advances of the past four years do not seem as significant as the preceding years', our comprehension of the in vivo processes of blood coagulation have increased. The scope of research in blood coagulation is now much too broad to be covered adequately in one chapter. If a more complete view is desired, several recent reviews are available (Baugh & Hougie, 1977, 1979; Hougie & Baugh, 1980; Davie et al, 1979; Ratnoff, 1979). It is hoped that this review will be complimentary to those cited and concentrate on areas which have not previously been covered.

RECENT DEVELOPMENTS

It is the nature of research that the more difficult problems are usually the last to be solved. Thus factor VIII is still an enigma in clotting although recent results suggest it may finally be lending itself to experiments which can be critically evaluated. The unequivocal understanding of how a biochemical entity functions at the molecular level requires that the purified component possess recognizable biologic activity and be available in quantities great enough to undergo the series of experiments which reveals its molecular architecture. With factor VIII this has been a problem. Purity has never been convincingly demonstrated, the amounts available have been small and the biological activity has been extremely labile. It has always been a problem in biochemical research that the exciting and enlightening experiments are dependent on purification procedures which are often time-consuming and tedious. The effort expended on purification does not seem to justify the rewards of modern day research. Thus experiments are performed with reagents which have not been well characterized, leading to results which are difficult to interpret. Eventually, the problem may resolve itself due to the enormous effort expended on researching it. Factor VIII, and possibly factor V, will have a major effect on our understanding of the clotting mechanism once their structure and function are fully known. In our present vision of the clotting mechanism as a cascade sequence (Fig. 3.1), factors VIII and V participate as structural co-factors. Some of the more recent evidence on factors VIII and V would suggest roles other than purely as structural co-factors. Hopefully sufficiently large purified amounts of these two clotting factors will become available so their functions can be firmly established.

Table 3.1 presents an updated list of the known coagulation factors. The amino acid sequence of fibrinogen has essentially been completed (Hessel et al, 1979; York & Blomback, 1979; Cotrell et al, 1979; Watt et al, 1979; Strong et al, 1979) and future studies should concentrate on how the sequence is expressed in the quaternary structure of the molecule as it undergoes the transition from fibrinogen in solution to a

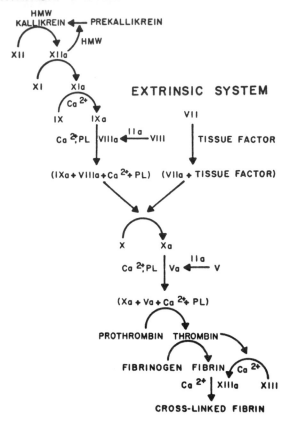

Fig. 3.1   Cascade mechanism of blood coagulation. PL: phospholipid; Ca^{2+}: calcium ion; HMW: high molecular weight kininogen.

fibrin gel. Sequence data are also being completed, possibly within the next two years, for all of the vitamin K-dependent clotting factors. Protein S is still a vitamin K-dependent plasma protein in search of a function (DiScipio & Davie, 1979) and the structure and function of tissue factor has received little attention during the past few years. With the introduction of synthetic peptides which function as substrates for the vitamin K-dependent carboxylation of glutamic acid residues, the system responsible for carboxylating the vitamin K-dependent clotting factors should also be deciphered soon (Decottignies-Le Marechal et al, 1979).

Factor V
There have been four recent reports on the purification of bovine factor V in more or less homogeneous form (Saraswathi et al, 1978; Esmon, 1979; Nesheim et al, 1979; Bartlett et al, 1980). The preparation isolated in the laboratory of Mann was a single chain glycoprotein which had a molecular weight of 330 000. The single chain nature of the molecule was established by sedimentation equilibrium studies of the native molecule and on the molecule in 6M guanidinium chloride with and without disulfide

Table 3.1 Blood clotting factors

Factor	Common name	Molecular weight[a]	≃ Concentration in 1 ml plasma
I	Fibrinogen	340 000 (330 000)	3 mg
II	Prothrombin	72 000 (38 000)	200 μg
III	Tissue factor	220 000–320 000	0
IV	Calcium ions	—	—
V	Proaccelerin	290 000–400 000, 1 000 000	≃50 μg
VI	Activated V	—	
VII	Proconvertin	63 000 (63 000)	2 μg
VIII	Antihemophilic factor	85 000, 89 000, 93 000	≃0.2 μg
IX	Christmas factor	55 400 (46 500)	3–4 μg
X	Stuart factor	55 000 (40 000)	6–8 μg
XI	Plasma thromboplastin antecedent	160 000 (160 000)	7 μg
XII	Hageman factor	90 000 (90 000)	40 μg
XIII	Fibrin stabilizing factor	320 000 (320 000)	
—	Prekallikrein	88 000 (88 000)	25–40 μg
—	High molecular weight kininogen	180 000	80 μg
—	Protein C	62 000 (60 000)	5 μg
—	Protein S	69 000	?
—	von Willebrand factor	1.2–5 million	7 μg

[a]Molecular weight of activated form given in parentheses.

bond reduction. The sedimentation coefficient was unusually low (9–19S), suggesting that the molecule is not globular.

In contrast to the finding of Mann and his co-workers (Nesheim et al, 1979), the preparation of Esmon appeared as a tightly spaced doublet on SDS-gel acrylamide electrophoresis. The molecular weight before disulfide bond reduction was 320 000, corresponding closely with the value obtained by Mann and co-workers, but was 280 000 following reduction. Thrombin at 4°C completely cleaved both bands of the doublet seen on the reduced and unreduced SDS-acrylamide gels with the formation of two new species with molecular weights corresponding to 210 000 and 115 000; there was a concomitant 3- to 4-fold increase in specific activity. These changes, which were attributed to the formation of an intermediate, were not inhibited by 1 mM benzamidine/HCl and remained constant until the temperature was increased to 37°C when there was an additional 3-fold increase in factor V activity with disappearance of the higher molecular weight band of 210 000 and the formation of a new species with a molecular weight of 73 000, while the 115 000 molecular weight band of the intermediate remained unchanged. The SDS polyacrylamide gel pattern corresponded to that of thrombin activated factor V, which was obtained by activating factor V with thrombin and then isolating the factor V activity by ion exchange chromatography. The heavy (115 000) and light chains (73 000) could be separated into two peaks by chromatography of the thrombin-activated factor V (Va) in the presence of EDTA and neither of these peaks alone had any factor V activity, even on the addition of Mg^{2+} or Ca^{2+}. However, when combined the activity slowly regenerated on the addition of Ca^{2+} or Mg^{2+}; if the mixture was then rechromatographed in the presence of Ca^{2+}, a single and biologically active protein peak was obtained with the disappearance of the light chain of the intermediate from its usual elution position. Protein C degraded the slower-migrating band of the factor V doublet, but did not inactivate the protein; it degraded both light and heavy chains of Va with loss of factor V activity.

The preparation of factor V obtained in the laboratory of Colman (Saraswathi et al, 1978) by venipuncture when subjected to SDS polyacrylamide gel electrophoresis under non-reducing conditions gave two major bands with molecular weights of 430 000 and 290 000; in the presence of dithiothreitol the lighter subunit remained unchanged, but the disulfide bridges of the heavier subunit were reduced to produce two chains each of 200 000 daltons (Saraswathi et al, 1978). They believe factor V to be composed of two subunits, a light (1) chain linked in a dimer (1_2) by disulfide bridges and a heavy (h) chain, noncovalently linked to the light chain. They postulate the heavy chain of their preparation to be the same as the single chain molecule of both Esmon's and Mann's preparations (Ittyerah et al, 1980a). Disc electrophoresis of purified native factor V in gels of 3 to 6 per cent acrylamide concentration all gave three protein bands, all of which were associated with factor V activity, and these results were interpreted as indicating that the three protein bands represent charge isomers of factor V. In contrast to factor V prepared from venepuncture blood, factor V prepared from slaughterhouse blood by postmortem exsanguination could be activated by thrombin only 6-fold, compared to 18-fold. Factor V from venipuncture blood had an apparent molecular weight of 1–2 million based on the elution pattern on Sepharose 4B compared to the 560 000 of slaughterhouse blood, but in each case only one peak was obtained. Their data indicate that progressive reductions in the molecular weight of factor V are brought about by proteolysis during blood collection at the slaughterhouse; they postulate that both chains of the factor V molecule are fragmented but in both cases the fragments are apparently attached to the factor V molecule by disulfide linkages and are revealed as multiple bands upon SDS-electrophoresis under reducing conditions.

The detrimental effect of proteases, which are present in abundance and almost impossible to exclude from slaughterhouse blood on factor V structure were confirmed by Hanahan and his co-workers (Bartlett et al, 1980). Factor V purified from either human or bovine blood collected by venipuncture always had an apparent molecular weight in the range of 800 000 to 1 000 000, as determined by gel filtration. If blood from the slaughterhouse was collected in 2 mM DFP, the apparent high molecular weight form of factor V was preserved but lower concentrations of DFP (about 0.1 mM) or the usual protease inhibitors were ineffective, and the molecular weight of factor V prepared from such plasma was less than 500 000. They also observed that if there was a large amount of tissue involvement during the collection of the blood, low molecular weight forms were present even in the presence of high concentrations of DFP. It was considered unlikely that the very high molecular weight factor V represented an aggregated form of the lower molecular weight species since DFP preserved the high molecular weight form, and the high molecular weight factor V maintained its apparent size when rechromatographed in low or high salt media; in addition, changes in pH from 6 to 7.5 during the preparation did not alter the apparent size.

The activity of native factor V may increase as much as 80-fold following thrombin activation giving rise to spuriously high purification values, it is therefore difficult to compare the specific activities of preparations from different laboratories. Unlike other workers in the field who report in terms of Va activity, Mann's group report the activity in terms of total factor V or that activity observed after activation by thrombin. They compared the specific activities of the preparations of other workers with theirs by multiplying activation quotients (the ratio of the activity observed after thrombin treatment to the activity observed before thrombin treatment) by reported factor Va specific activities. Using this criteria, the specific activity of their preparation is 1250 units/mg, representing a purification of 2500 which is greatly in excess of those of the other groups.

The differences in the molecular characteristics of the factor V preparations of different laboratories all well versed in protein isolation are difficult to explain. This is particularly so since all four methods gave highly reproducible results. The preparations of Nesheim et al and Esmon had identical molecular weights, but the preparation of Esmon gave a doublet on SDS gel electrophoresis in contrast to the single band obtained by Nesheim et al. One explanation of this discrepancy could be that the preparation of Esmon contained a degradation product of factor V removed by one of the steps in the Nesheim et al procedure. The apparent greater homogeneity and specific activity of the latter procedure may be explained on the basis that the method involved more steps and included hydrophobic chromatography on octyl Sepharose and also phenyl Sepharose chromatography. Some of the differences might be attributed to the method of collection for Saraswathi et al and Bartlett et al both used venipuncture blood while Nesheim et al and Esmon used slaughterhouse blood. However, Nesheim et al found it made no difference to their preparation whether it was drawn by venipuncture or obtained from the slaughterhouse. The preparation of Nesheim et al could be activated 80-fold by thrombin which is considerably higher than those of other workers; this suggests that the preparation had no previous exposure to thrombin and was in the native state despite the fact that slaughterhouse blood was used. It may be that the degraded forms of factor V observed by both Bartlett et al and Saraswathi et al in slaughterhouse blood are removed completely in the Nesheim et al procedure and partially in the Esmon procedure. Variations in reported molecular weight may, in part, be explained by the different techniques used; thus if factor V is a rod-like molecule as Nesheim et al propose, the use of gel filtration to estimate molecular weights will lead to erroneous molecular weight estimates, especially when using globular proteins as standards. Sedimentation velocity experiments used alone for determining the molecular weight of factor V would also be of limited value because of the rod-like shape of the factor V molecule.

Using double diffusion analysis in agar an antibody produced against the preparation of Nesheim gave a single precipitin band against both purified bovine plasma factor V as well as bovine plasma (Tracy et al, 1979). The same workers also found that immunoelectrophoresis of the antibody against whole bovine plasma also produced a single precipitin arc, another indication that the antibody was specific for bovine plasma factor V. On the other hand, an antibody against factor V prepared in Colman's laboratory gave two precipitin arcs on the immunoelectrophoresis of bovine plasma, one close to the origin and the other migrating towards the anode, the two components exhibited a reaction of non-identity, it was postulated that these represented l_2 and h subunits of factor V (Ittyerah et al, 1980b). However, immunoelectrophoresis would not be expected to separate multimeric subunits of a protein non-covalently associated (Mann, 1980). Bartlett et al state that an antibody raised against the high molecular weight (1 000 000) bovine factor V did not cross-react with the lower molecular weight species: these experiments were attributable to a worker in their laboratory and the results are unpublished. Despite their differences all the preparations shortened the clotting time of aged plasma in the presence of tissue extract and this activity increased on incubation of the preparation with thrombin; in the case of the factor V prepared by Nesheim et al it also accelerated the factor Xa-catalyzed activation of human prethrombin 1. The possibility that more than one factor may be involved in the shortening of the prothrombin time of aged plasma does not appear to have been seriously considered and in none of the recent reports is it specifically stated whether the preparations corrected the defect of plasma from a patient with a congenital deficiency of factor V.

Factor VIII

Factor VIII is the coagulant protein which is inactive, decreased or absent in individuals with hemophilia A. It is also usually decreased in von Willebrand's disease, but the characteristic feature of this condition is a decrease or apparent structural abnormality in von Willebrand's factor, a plasma protein required for plate-let adhesion. Factor VIII:C and von Willebrand factor are difficult to separate from one another and there is clearly a close association between the two proteins; for example, both proteins increase proportionately following strenuous exercise (Brown et al, 1979). Accordingly, protein preparations containing coagulant as well as platelet-aggregation activity have been referred to as factor VIII/vWf. Preparations containing both activities have been purified 5000- to 10 000-fold. These prepara-tions, referred to as factor VIII/vWf, show a single sharp precipitin line upon immunoelectrophoresis and have a molecular weight greater than one million (Schmer et al, 1972; Legaz et al, 1973). Upon reduction, they form subunits with an apparent molecular weight of about 200 000 as measured by SDS polyacrylamide gel elec-trophoresis (Schmer et al, 1972; Legaz et al, 1973). Although many workers report that they have obtained homogeneous preparations of factor VIII/vWf, such claims are based on the finding of a single band after reduction on SDS polyacrylamide gels and this is clearly a function of the amount of protein applied to the gel. Thus, when 100 μg of one preparation of factor VIII-vWf was electrophoresed on a 5 per cent SDS-polyacrylamide disc gel, no protein appeared to enter the gel and on reduction a single band was observed with a molecular weight of approximately 230 000. When 400 μg protein/gel was applied, some protein entered the gels and a minor band corresponding to a molecular weight of 180 000 was seen; following reduction eight bands could be clearly visualized corresponding to molecular weights ranging from 230 000 to 30 000 with 65 per cent of the protein in the 182 000 to 230 000 band (Lane et al, 1979).

All the most recent data indicate that the coagulant moeity (VIII:C) is a trace protein, and for this reason difficult to visualize on gels. It has been known for some time that it can be dissociated from the von Willebrand factor by a number of techniques, including gel filtration in the presence of high salt or calcium chloride, ion exchange chromatography and by antigen-antibody chromatography (Rick & Hoyer, 1973; Wagner et al, 1973; Weiss & Hoyer, 1973; Austen, 1974; Baugh et al, 1974; Brown et al, 1974). Accordingly, it is now generally believed that factor VIII/vWf is a molecular complex comprising a high molecular weight protein (von Willebrand factor) and a low molecular weight subunit (VIII:C), although a few investigators maintain that factor VIII/vWf is a covalently linked subunit structure which has both coagulant and platelet aggregating activities (Switzer & McKee, 1976; Switzer et al, 1979).

The biochemical characterization of factor VIII has been thwarted by low yields in the purification process, often less than 2 per cent, and the inherent instability of the molecule. Some of the problems have been partially overcome by use of large amounts of bovine plasma (Vehar & Davie, 1980). The steps in their isolation procedure included glycine precipitation, DEAE Sephadex column chromatography, Sephadex G-200 gel filtration and factor X-Sepharose column chromatography; chromatography and gel filtration were carried out in the presence of a reducing agent (0.5 mM dithiothreitol). The final preparation migrated as a triplet on sodium dodecyl sulfate/urea-polyacrylamide gel electrophoresis with apparent molecular weights of 93 000, 88 000 and 85 000. The overall purification was 320 000 with a yield of little more than 1 per cent. An antibody raised in rabbits against the purified factor VIII did not react with von Willebrand factor and neutralized factor VIII coagulant activity. The final preparation could be activated 30-fold by thrombin; both thrombin and Xa activation converted the gel triplet to a doublet with cleavage of all three of the original bands, suggesting that these are closely related forms. As the SDS/urea-polyacrylamide gel electrophoretic pattern for the activated form differed completely from that of the precursor, this suggests that their preparation is free of activated factor VIII. The presence of the latter species as in the case of factor V gives spuriously high purification figures. Dithiothreitol, which was present in their final preparation, enhances the VIII:C activity as measured by the one-stage test so that accurate specific activities could not be determined. The yields were very low and as the authors point out improvements are necessary. However, the isolation of highly purified VIII:C which appears to be free of von Willebrand factor in amounts sufficient to characterize represents a major accomplishment.

Protein C

Protein C is a vitamin K-dependent protein which was discovered by Stenflo in 1976. He applied an ammonium sulfate cut of a barium citrate eluate of bovine plasma to a DEAE Sephadex column and obtained four peaks which were labeled sequentially A, B, C and D. The third peak (C) contained the new protein which was arbitrarily labeled protein C. Stenflo found that while the new protein had an amino acid composition similar to that of the other vitamin K dependent clotting proteins, it did not share with them any main antigenic determinants. It was composed of a light and heavy chain linked by interchain disulfide bridges. The NH_2-terminal amino acid sequence was determined and a γ-carboxyglutamic acid residue was found in positions 6 and 7 which established that protein C was a vitamin K-dependent protein; the sequence was very homologous to that of prothrombin, factor VII, IX and X. Unlike the other vitamin K-dependent clotting factors, Stenflo found that bovine protein C disappears completely during dicoumarol administration and no immunoreactive form was present. It appeared to have no action in the blood coagulation system and Stenflo postulated that since it was vitamin K-dependent it was likely to exert its function on the surface of biological membranes.

The findings of Stenflo were almost immediately confirmed by Kisiel et al (1976; 1977b). They estimated the molecular weight of the protein to be 58 000 by sodium dodecyl sulfate gel electrophoresis which was in close agreement with the value obtained by Stenflo. However, sedimentation equilibrium experiments indicated a minimal molecular weight of 62 000: this figure corresponded exactly with the sum of the molecular weights of the light and heavy chains obtained by SDS gel electrophoresis which were 21 000 and 41 000, respectively (Kisiel et al, 1976). The amino acid composition of bovine protein C and the heavy and light chains have been determined (Stenflo, 1976; Kisiel et al, 1976); the native protein contains approximately 18 per cent carbohydrate by weight and this includes hexose, glucosamine and neuraminic acid. Protein C, like the other vitamin K-dependent clotting factors, is inactive in its native zymogen form, but following activation exhibits serine esterase activity. It differs from them in that when activated it has only anticoagulant properties. It may be activated by thrombin, trypsin and the factor X activating protein present in Russell's viper venom (Kisiel et al, 1976; 1977b; 1979; Walker et al, 1979). Activation by thrombin and the factor X activator of Russell's viper venom appear identical and are accompanied by a reduction in the molecular weight of the heavy chain with no detectable change in the light chains. Amino-terminal analysis of the heavy chains of the protein C zymogen and activated protein C show that the terminal amino acid of the latter coincide exactly with that observed in residues 15 through 28 in the heavy chain of the precursor molecule; it was concluded from this and other data that the latter is cleaved at an Arg-Ile peptide bond in positions 14 and 15 of the heavy chain (Fig. 3.2). The molecular weight of the released tetradecapeptide is in good agreement with the difference observed by SDS gel electrophoresis between the heavy chain of protein C and the heavy chain of the activated protein C. Activation by trypsin is accompanied by a similar reduction in the heavy chain, but in contrast to activation by Russell's viper venom-X additional proteolysis of the light chain was observed (Kisiel et al, 1976).

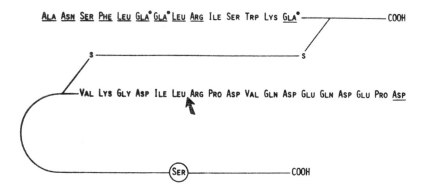

Fig. 3.2 Partial structure of human protein C. The residues underlined are identical to those found in bovine protein C. Gla★ (γ-carboxyglutamic acid) shown in positions 6, 7, and 14 of the light chain is tentative. The arrow indicates the probable site of cleavage in the heavy chain of protein C by thrombin. Reprinted from Kisiel (1979) with permission from the author and the American Society of Clinical Investigation.

Activated protein C has amidase activity against the chromogenic substrate Bz-Phe-Val-Arg-p-nitroanilide (S-2160) and also against S-2302, S-2238 and S-2266. There was no hydrolysis with S-2227 and S-2251, while only weak amidase activity was observed with the factor Xa specific substrate S-2222. The data indicate that it has a substrate specificity more similar to that of thrombin than Xa or plasmin. Prior treatment of activated protein C to remove endogenous Ca^{2+} results in a virtual loss of amidase activity which may be restored by addition of Ca^{2+} (Kisiel et al, 1977b). The active form of protein C like the other serine esterases is inhibited by diisopropyl fluorophosphate (DFP). Bovine protein C isolated from serum appears to behave indistinguishably from that of plasma on SDS gel electrophoresis, while the yield from serum is essentially the same as that from plasma (Kisiel et al, 1976). While their experiments did not rule out the possibility that a small amount of protein C may have undergone some molecular change, they believe that no major change occurs as a result of either intrinsic or extrinsic coagulation. This conclusion is consistent with the subsequent findings of these workers (Kisiel et al, 1977b) that only about 10 per cent of protein C is activated by either a complex of Xa-phospholipid calcium or factor VII-tissue factor calcium ions as determined by SDS gel electrophoresis.

Human protein C has now been characterized (Kisiel, 1979). It has the same molecular weight as the bovine molecule and is composed of heavy and light chains which are of the same molecular weight as their bovine counterparts. The amino acid and carbohydrate compositions of the two proteins are remarkably similar with the notable exceptions of their histidine, valine and N-acetyl glucosamine contents. Each contains ten residues of γ-carboxyglutamic acid per mol of protein (DiScipio & Davie, 1979). The amino-terminal sequence of the light chain of the human molecule is identical to that of the bovine protein, but the terminal sequences of the heavy chains are different (Kisiel, 1979). The amino acid sequence in the active site of activated protein C is homologous with that found in the active site regions of the four vitamin K-dependent clotting factors (Fig. 3.3).

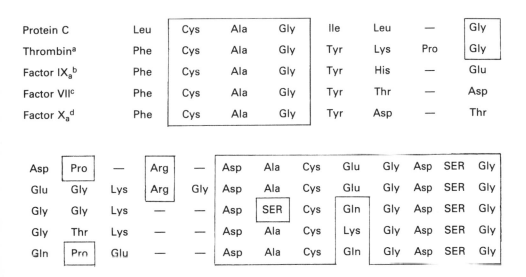

Fig. 3.3 Active-site sequence of activated protein C and the four vitamin K-dependent coagulation proteins. Amino acid residues in protein C that are identical with the coagulant proteins are shown in blocks. Dashes refer to spaces that have been inserted to bring the five proteins into alignment for better homology. The active-site serine analogous to serine-195 in chymotrypsin is shown in capital letters. Reprinted with permission of the authors (Kisiel et al, 1977a) and the American Chemical Society.

Anticoagulant activity

In their first study, Kisiel et al (1976) noted significant inhibition of clotting in the presence of activated protein C. Bovine activated protein C markedly prolonged the activated partial thromboplastin time (APTT) of bovine plasma, with relatively little effect on the APTT of human plasma, while human activated protein C markedly prolonged the APTT of human plasma with significantly less effect on bovine plasma (Kisiel et al, 1977b; Kisiel, 1979). Activated protein C has no detectable effect on the coagulant activities of factors XII, XI or X or on the activated forms of these factors; it also has no effect on factor VII, prothrombin or plasminogen (Kisiel et al, 1977b). On the other hand, it inactivates factor VIII (Vehar & Davie, 1980) and the thrombin activated form of factor V (Kisiel et al, 1977b; Kisiel, 1979; Walker et al, 1979). The inactivation of Va by activated protein C is dependent on calcium ions; there may also be an absolute requirement for phospholipid (Kisiel et al, 1977b); and phospholipid markedly enhances the reaction (Kisiel et al, 1977b; Walker et al, 1979). Unlike prothrombin, which appears to bind to negatively charged phospholipid only in the presence of Ca^{2+} ions, protein C binds to phospholipid both in the presence and absence of calcium (Walker et al, 1979). However, the molecule appears to contain endogenous calcium ions, since prior treatment of activated protein C with EDTA inactivates it and the activity is restored by incubation with calcium ions (Kisiel et al, 1977). Factor V purified by the method of Esmon (1979) gives a doublet on SDS gels; following treatment with activated protein C the slower-migrating band of the factor V was degraded; factor Va underwent more extensive degradation and both heavy and light chains were cleaved (Walker et al, 1979).

Activated protein C causes rapid loss of the coagulant activity of highly purified factor VIII which contains no detectable von Willebrand's factor; this inactivation requires both the presence of Ca^{2+} and phospholipid; the rate of inactivation of the thrombin-activated form of factor VIII is significantly faster than that of the unactivated form (Vehar & Davie, 1980). The coagulant activity of factor VIII/vWf is also readily inactivated by protein C, but this effect is not dependent on the addition of phospholipid. The inactivation is only observed when factor VIII/vWf is preincubated with calcium chloride for several hours prior to the addition of activated protein C, and addition of EDTA before adding the protein C prevents most of the inactivation. The loss of coagulant activity of purified factor VIII by activated protein C is associated with the disappearance of the 93 000 molecular weight band of the highly purified factor VIII, the two faster-moving bands of the triplet are not affected (Vehar & Davie, 1980).

Platelets contain activated factor V-like activity which can be expressed by freeze thawing platelets (Østerud, et al, 1977) or by the thrombin treatment of platelets (Miletich et al, 1978a). A complex of thrombin treated platelets, Xa and calcium has potent prothrombin conversion activity (Tracy et al, 1979) and it has been proposed that the platelet factor Va constitutes the receptor site on the platelet for Xa (Kane et al, 1980). Comp and Esmon (1979) found that the prior incubation of thrombin-activated platelets with activated protein C inhibits the binding of Xa to the platelets. There was a decrease of prothrombin converting activity and this was not increased by raising the concentration of factor Xa, suggesting that the inhibition by activated protein C was not competitive with respect to factor Xa concentration. When Xa was added first to the thrombin activated platelets, the rate of inhibition was significantly slowed; this finding was interpreted as indicating that binding of the Xa occurs at a site at or near the activated factor V platelet receptor sites and the Xa protects the latter from degradation or cleavage from the platelet by protein C. DFP-treated activated protein C had no effect on factor Xa binding (Comp & Esmon, 1979).

The role of protein C in hemostasis

The physiological role of protein C is unknown. Its concentration in human plasma appears to be four to five times less than that in bovine plasma, but this estimate is based on the amounts of the protein that can be isolated from equivalent amounts of plasma and such differences may be due to other factors such as differences in stability of the two proteins (Kisiel, 1979). So far no specific quantitative assay for protein C is available, but since the purified protein and antibody are both available, immunological methods should soon become available.

The concentration of protein C in serum appears to be similar to that of plasma, but Kisiel et al (1977a) calculated that it would take the activation of as little as 1 per cent of the protein C to result in a sufficient concentration of activated protein C to rapidly inactivate factor V at physiological concentrations. To have any significant action on clotting, protein C has to act fairly rapidly and its activation might occur in concert with the activation of factor VIII and factor V. Of its known actions, its effect on factor VIII is likely to be more important than that on factor V.

An isolated increase of protein C would be expected to result in a hypocoagulable state and a decrease in hypercoagulability. Unless there is adequate depression of the prothrombin time, the reduction of Protein C would counter-balance the coumarin-induced defect and make the treatment ineffective. These and other questions regarding the significance of protein C should become elucidated in the coming years when quantitation of this protein becomes widespread.

ALTERNATE PATHWAYS

The concept of two independent pathways, the intrinsic and extrinsic, both leading to the formation of prothrombinase, has been and remains an invaluable one for the study of blood coagulation. Since a deficiency of a clotting factor involved in only one pathway results in clinical bleeding, even at the time the theory was first enunciated by Biggs et al in 1953, it was understood that the two pathways did not act in isolation, but were in some way interrelated. The findings that trace amounts of thrombin enhanced the activity of factors VIII and V many fold was the first recognized link.

The first traces of thrombin formed would be expected to be derived through the more rapid extrinsic system and therefore a defect in this system, as in factor VII deficiency, results in a concomitant impairment of the intrinsic system through a delay in the conversion of factors VIII and V to their more reactive states. It has recently been shown by Østerud and Rapaport (1978) that the reaction product of tissue factor, factor VII and calcium activates factor IX. They found that an incubation mixture of tissue factor, factor VII, factor IX and Ca^{2+} generated factor IXa clotting activity and that on sodium dodecyl sulfate polyacrylamide gel electrophoresis of such a mixture the single band of native factor IX was replaced by the heavy and light chain bands of factor IXa. Indeed, the tissue factor-factor VII-Ca^{2+} complex activated factor IX at the same rate as factor XIa (Østerud & Rapaport, 1977).

The contact phase not only initiates the intrinsic system, but also plays a role in the extrinsic system. The generation of kallikrein is associated with the activation of factor VII in plasma stored in the cold (Gjonnaess, 1972) and in plasma incubated with kaolin (Saito & Ratnoff, 1975), however purified kallikrein does not directly activate purified factor VII (Saito & Ratnoff, 1975; Seligsohn et al, 1979) unless factor IXa is added to the reaction mixture (Laake & Østerud, 1974; Seligsohn et al, 1979). Activated forms of factor XII directly activate bovine factor VII (Radcliffe et al, 1977; Kisiel et al, 1977a) and also human factor VII (Seligsohn et al, 1979). The reaction of IXa on factor VII occurs in the absence of added phospholipid and in the absence of Ca^{2+}; it occurs at 37°C as well as 4°C (Seligsohn et al, 1979) so that the potential importance of this pathway of factor VII activation is not necessarily limited to the phenomenon of cold-activation of plasma factor VII (Seligsohn et al, 1978a). Factor VII activity was found to increase when kallikrein was added to either factor XII-deficient plasma or to factor IX-deficient plasma and it appears that kallikrein can indirectly activate factor VII in plasma through the generation of at least two materials, factor XIIa and factor IXa (Seligsohn et al, 1979) (See Fig. 3.4). Factor VII may also be activated by factor Xa and thrombin (Radcliffe & Nemerson, 1975).

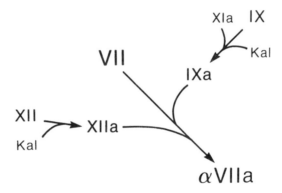

Fig. 3.4 Pathways described by Seligsohn et al, 1979 for activating factor VII. VIIa is the activated two chain form of factor VII. Kal: plasma kallikrein. Reprinted with permission of the authors (Seligsohn et al, 1979) and the American Society for Clinical Investigation, Inc.

The activation of factor VII referred to above involves cleavage of an internal peptide bond of the native single chain molecule with the formation of a two-chain molecule held together by disulfide bond(s) (Radcliffe & Nemerson, 1975; Kisiel et al, 1977a). Factor VII can be measured by a coupled amidolytic assay using as the substrate a mixture of purified factor X, tissue factor and calcium; the amount of factor X formed at the end of three minutes is measured with a chromogenic substrate and is a function of the amount of factor VII; this assay when used together with the conventional type of one-stage clotting assay gives a measure of the degree of factor VII activation (Seligsohn et al, 1978b). Thus, when plasma factor VII is activated by kaolin, clotting or cold, the one-stage assay values are strikingly increased, but no increase is observed with the amidolytic assay. After interaction of factor VII with tissue factor, a factor VII phospholipid complex thought to contain no tissue factor can be isolated; unlike the two chain activated VII discussed above, which can only activate factor X in the presence of tissue factor, the factor VII-phospholipid complex can directly activate factor X (Østerud et al, 1972).

INTERACTIONS OF PLATELETS WITH COAGULATION FACTORS

The in vitro techniques used in assaying blood coagulation factors frequently lead to a diminished appreciation of the role platelets play in the clotting mechanism. Platelets have long been thought to be the principal in vivo source of the phospholipid required by the clotting mechanism, but in vitro this requirement is more easily satisfied by a purified or semi-purified extraneous source of phospholipid such as cephalin. The phospholipid activity of platelets, referred to as platelet factor 3, is not apparent unless platelets have been damaged or aggregated by an external agent such as collagen or ADP. It is only in the past few years that it has become apparent that platelet factor 3 activity is more involved than simply providing a phospholipid source for coagulation reactions (Weiss, 1975; Gordon, 1976). Platelets play a major role in the cessation of bleeding. Platelets first adhere to the site of vascular damage, and through a series of complex reactions not fully understood, a platelet mass forms at the site of the wound. This mass, referred to as a platelet plug, consists of platelets which have aggregated and released the contents of the various storage organelles present in platelets. It is thought that at some time during the formation of the platelet plug the coagulation system comes into play and a fibrin:platelet mass is formed through the interaction of platelets and clotting factors (Weiss, 1975; Gordon, 1976).

Thrombin
Thrombin is one of the more important physiological activators of human blood platelets. Thrombin activation of platelets leads to shape changes, secretion of stored granule materials and aggregation. Accompanying these changes are the exposure of platelet factor 3 activity (Rittenhouse-Simmons & Deykin, 1977), increased prostaglandin synthesis (Smith & Silver, 1976), and membrane fluidity changes (Nathan et al, 1979). These actions are probably part of the mechanism for expanding and consolidating the platelet:fibrin mass at the site of a vascular lesion. The binding of thrombin to a platelet membrane is a complex process and as a result some controversy exists over the exact mechanism by which thrombin activates platelets. In terms of the structure of thrombin, the binding and resultant activation of platelets are due to different parts of the thrombin molecule. The experiments of Tollefsen & Majerus (1976) show that DFP-thrombin binds to the platelet membrane in the same manner as does native thrombin (Tollefsen et al, 1974). DFP-treated thrombin has no protease activity due to the reaction of DFP with the active site serine. DFP-treated thrombin bound to platelets did not lead to activation and aggregation of platelets. Thus the active site of thrombin was required for platelet activation. Two types of bindings were initially observed, high and low affinity binding, with approximately 500 high affinity sites per platelet, while there was some question as to the number of low affinity sites. The relationship between the two sites was not clear. Tollefsen & Majerus (1976) later suggested only one class of binding site existed based on the dissociation rates of labeled thrombin from platelet membranes and the isolation of a single type of gluteraldehyde-linked platelet protein:thrombin complex. The two

classes of binding sites were postulated to arise out of negative cooperativity where the binding of thrombin to a high affinity site converted other unoccupied high affinity sites to low affinity sites. Workman et al (1977) suggested that two distinct binding sites existed based on the behavior of a chemically modified thrombin. In particular, N-bromosuccinimide and 2-hydroxy-5-nitrobenzyl bromide treatment of thrombin, which modified a single tryptophan residue near the fibrinogen binding region in thrombin, abolished thrombin binding to high affinity sites, yet some activity was retained in activating the platelets. The interpretation of these results was that the thrombin molecule possessed two regions which bound to platelets, both of which were distinct from thrombin's catalytic site. One region, that involved in thrombin binding to fibrinogen, was also involved in binding to the high affinity sites on the platelet, while the other bound to the low affinity site. It has generally been conceded that platelet activation by thrombin requires binding to the high affinity sites, but as platelet activation was still present either the high affinity sites still bound the modified thrombin, or the high affinity sites were not required for the platelet activation.

Tam et al (1979) used hirudin to measure the dissociation of thrombin from platelets. They found that hirudin, which forms a complex with thrombin, abolished binding to the high affinity sites, but not the low affinity sites. Hirudin also caused the thrombin to be released from the high affinity sites in two different modes. If hirudin was added after a short preincubation of thrombin with the platelets, bound thrombin was released rapidly. However, as the length of the preincubation period was increased, thrombin was released more slowly. This phenomenon was dependent on catalytically active thrombin. The results suggested that once binding of thrombin occurred, a modification of the binding site took place which depended on the catalytic activity of thrombin. However the conversion of the rapidly dissociating thrombin to the more slowly dissociating form was too slow to account for platelet activation unless only a small fraction of the slowly dissociating form was required for platelet activation.

Another approach to studying thrombin interactions with platelets has been to concentrate on isolating and characterizing the platelet membrane receptor for thrombin. Okumura et al (1978) have isolated a platelet membrane protein which seems to fulfil many of the requirements of a thrombin receptor (Okumura et al, 1976; Okumura & Jamieson, 1976). The protein has been termed glycocalicin, which is a reference to the fact it is found in the platelet glycocalyx, the layer of loosely bound proteins which adhere to the platelet membrane. It apparently is closely related to another platelet membrane protein, termed glycoprotein I, which is found in the platelet membrane. Both proteins share common antigenic determinants. The identity of these glycoproteins as the thrombin receptor was based on the competitive inhibition of thrombin binding to both high and low affinity sites by purified glycocalicin. Glycocalicin (molecular weight 150 000) could be fragmented by treatment with proteases to yield a peptide of 45 000 molecular weight and a macroglycopeptide with a molecular weight of 120 000. The macroglycopeptide was devoid of any activity, while the peptide fragment was actually a more effective inhibitor of thrombin binding to platelets than was intact glycocalicin. Based on these and other findings it was concluded that glycocalicin and glycoprotein I were functionally identical and acted together as the platelet receptor for thrombin.

Factor X and factor V

The availability of purified preparations of factor X and factor V has allowed binding studies to be carried out with both of these clotting factors. These are the two clotting factors which form a complex with Ca^{2+} and phospholipid and in their activated forms convert prothrombin to thrombin. Miletich et al (1977; 1978a) have shown that factor Xa binds to the platelet surface after the platelet release reaction occurs. The binding had the property of being a receptor-ligand interaction as it was specific, saturable, reversible and correlated with the generation of thrombin. The affinity of the binding site for Xa was quite high as less than 1 per cent of the potential physiological concentration of Xa saturated the binding sites. The Xa receptor was distinct from the thrombin receptor as 1) calcium was required, 2) binding only occurred after the release reaction, and 3) thrombin did not compete for the Xa binding site. One of the more interesting observations was that the catalytic activity of Xa was approximately 50 000-fold greater when bound to the platelet membrane. In contrast substituting phospholipid for platelets only resulted in a 50-fold increase in catalytic activity. The binding capacity of the receptor was destroyed by thrombin treatment. Thus, the receptor had characteristics which distinguished it from being only platelet phospholipid.

It is possible the platelet receptor for factor Xa is factor Va. It has been known for some time that platelets contain factor V activity. It has never been clear whether this was an intrinsic activity of platelets or represented platelet bound plasma factor V. Using an antibody raised against purified bovine factor V, Tracy et al (1979) were able to show that approximately 600 factor V molecules were present per bovine platelet. The platelet factor V appeared to be similar to plasma factor V in that it had the same antigenic determinants, similar clotting activities and plasma V could exchange with platelet factor V. Further studies on the binding of factor V to platelets indicated that both factor V and factor Va bound to the platelet membrane. Factor Va binding showed two classes of binding sites with approximately 900 high affinity sites ($K_d = 3 \times 10^{-10}$ M) and as many as 3500 lower affinity sites ($K_d = 3 \times 10^{-9}$ M). In contrast factor V showed only 800 to 900 binding sites with a dissociation constant of 3×10^{-9} M. Thus the conversion of factor V to Va resulted in significantly better binding to the platelet membrane. Unlike factor Xa, platelet activation had no measurable effect on the amount of factor V or Va bound to the platelet membrane. Several investigators have reported that factor V does not bind either factor Xa or prothrombin unless it has been converted to factor Va (Suttie & Jackson, 1977; Freeman et al, 1977). Thus, if factor Va is the platelet receptor for Xa, the number of high affinity Va sites on platelets exceeds the number of Xa binding sites of high affinity by a factor of 3. Several other lines of evidence suggest Va may be the binding site for Xa, however; Miletich et al (1978b) found that patients with hereditary factor V deficiency had decreased factor Xa binding sites on their platelets. The deficiency could be corrected by incubating the platelets with the supernatant obtained from thrombin-treated normal platelets which contained factor V activity. Furthermore, factor Xa binding to thrombin-activated platelets could be inhibited by incubating the platelets with a naturally occurring human antibody to factor V. Comp and Esmon have shown that protein C, which inactivates factor V, destroys the factor Xa binding sites in platelets if incubated with platelets before Xa is added. Xa bound to platelets protects the binding site from attack by protein C.

Although much of the data is still tentative, the studies on factor V and X binding to platelets provide the basis for visualizing some of the complementary roles of platelets and clotting factors in normal hemostasis. Factor V, found on the platelet membrane, may possibly be activated to factor Va by platelet activation reactions which occur at the site of a vascular lesion. A platelet activator of factor V has been suggested by Østerud et al (1977) who found that platelets would express factor Va activity after treatment with collagen. Factor Xa would then bind to Va on the platelet surface and thrombin production would be ensured at the site where a fibrin network is required to solidify the platelet plug. Several questions remain about such a hypothesis. One is that prothrombin binding to platelets has not yet been demonstrated (Tollefsen et al, 1975; Dahlbäck & Stenflo, 1978), although to some extent this must occur if Xa on the platelet surface converts prothrombin to thrombin. This may be a problem in translating in vitro experiments into in vivo reality. Prothrombin has been shown to bind to phospholipid micelles, a property which resides in the N-terminal propiece which is cleaved off by factor Xa (Nelsestuen & Lim, 1977; Nelsestuen & Broderius, 1977; Lim et al, 1977). Perhaps this is a property which is not significant for prothrombin in vivo. Another question is what is the role of factor V. It has been suggested that factor V binds via Ca^{2+} bridges to prothrombin, making prothrombin more accessible to proteolysis by factor Xa (Vogel et al, 1976). However, if Xa protects Va from inactivation by protein C, as has been proposed by Comp & Esmon (1979), and platelets do not bind prothrombin, it is difficult to see how factor V could be interacting directly with prothrombin. A final question is what does factor V interact with on the platelet surface. Platelet activation, which both releases and exposes platelet factor 3 activity (phospholipid), does not have any effect on the binding of factor V. Thus phospholipid may not be the binding site for factor V. Future experiments with these purified clotting factors should help resolve some of these questions.

Other clotting factors
It has been suggested that other clotting factors interact with platelets, but the evidence is controversial and no definitive proof exists. Walsh (1972) observed that platelets could activate both factors XII and XI to initiate the contact phase of intrinsic coagulation. The activation of XII by platelets was reported to be dependent upon platelet activation. Factor XI activation by platelets required the presence of collagen. Both mechanisms of activation were believed to represent activities of platelets independent of platelet factor 3 activity. Several other investigators have tried to verify these findings but have been unable to show the platelet dependent activation of either factor XII or XI (Vicic et al, 1979; Vecchione & Zucker, 1975; Østerud et al, 1979). Platelets do contain a number of hydrolytic enzymes, many of which are released upon platelet activation, but none of the enzymes has been characterized with respect to specificity (Phillips & Jakabova, 1977; Lipscomb & Walsh, 1979). The interaction of platelets with the contact phase clotting factors at present is an enigma. Since platelets do contain proteases, it is quite possible they may have a role in contact phase activation, but evidence for this is not very firm.

Another possible point of interaction of platelets with clotting factors is the factor VIII-factor IX complex of the intrinsic system. In many ways this step is similar to the factor X-factor V step, as both phospholipid and calcium ions are required for maximum catalytic activity (Hougie et al, 1967). Platelets have not been shown to have any significant activity in binding either factor VIII or factor IX, even though extensive efforts have been directed to this area. Although platelets have been shown to possess significant factor V activity, both by clotting and antigenic determinations, platelets do not contain either factor VIII clotting activity or any significant amount of factor VIII antigen as measured by a human antibody to factor VIII (Peake, 1979). Platelets do contain the von Willebrand factor (factor VIII related antigen) (Slot et al, 1978; Bouma et al, 1975), release the von Willebrand factor under certain types of stimulation (Koutts et al, 1978; Zucker et al, 1979) and also possess a platelet membrane binding site for the von Willebrand factor (Green & Muller, 1978; Kao et al, 1979; Schreider-Trip et al, 1979; Zucker et al, 1977). However the von Willebrand factor found in platelets does not have any detectable coagulant activity. Plasma von Willebrand factor is thought to be involved in the process of platelet adhesion to vascular subendothelium, one of the first steps in forming a platelet plug at the site of a vascular lesion (Hovig & Stormorken, 1974; Sakaricssen et al, 1979). It appears that the same platelet membrane site which binds thrombin may also be the site for the von Willebrand factor (Okumura et al, 1978). The von Willebrand factor is one of three large plasma proteins which have been demonstrated to either bind to or be present on the platelet membrane. Fibrinogen and cold insoluble globulin have also been shown to interact with the platelet membrane. Fibrinogen binding to platelet membranes has been thought to be necessary for certain types of platelet aggregation, especially ADP-induced platelet aggregation (Niewiarowski et al, 1972; Soria et al, 1978; Marguerie et al, 1980). Cold insoluble globulin, also known as fibronectin (Mosesson, 1977; Ruoslahti & Vaheri, 1975), has been postulated to be the collagen-binding site on the platelet membrane (Bensusan et al, 1978). Each of these large proteins appears to be involved in the formation of a platelet plug and eventual consolidation of the plug at the site of a vascular lesion. The exact mechanisms and structural features of each in mediating various platelet functions in this process is only just beginning to be understood.

Platelet-derived coagulation factors

It has been extremely difficult to ascertain whether platelets contain any of the plasma coagulation factors as endogenous constituents. Four factors have contributed to this difficulty: (1) the morphology of the platelet with its sponge-like system of canals (canaliculi) which are in contact with the external environment, (2) the loosely adherent layer of proteins referred to as the glycocalyx, (3) the sensitivity of platelets to various antagonists which stimulate the release reactions in apparently uncoupled fashions, and (4) the ability of platelets to phagocytize external products. Of the plasma coagulation factors only three, fibrinogen, the von Willebrand factor and factor XIII have been identified internally in platelets. The data for the von Willebrand factor is probably the strongest as it has been shown that megakaryocytes, the parent cell-type of platelets, synthesize the von Willebrand factor (Nachman et al, 1977). Platelets contain a factor XIII which is distinct from plasma factor XIII in that it does not have the formulation a_2b_2 in peptide chain arrangement, but instead has the formulation of a_2, possessing no b chains. The a chains in both plasma and platelet factor XIII appear to be indistinguishable (Schwartz et al, 1971; Schwartz et al, 1973). There has been some controversy over the nature of platelet fibrinogen. Ganguly has suggested that platelet fibrinogen may be different from plasma fibrinogen based on differences in molecular weight, clottability, subunit structure, and plasmin degradation patterns (James & Ganguly, 1975; James et al, 1977). Others have suggested that these differences may be due to artifacts of the isolation procedures (Doolittle et al, 1974). The role of platelet fibrinogen is unclear. It is released upon platelet activation, yet it does not bind to platelet membranes, nor will it support platelet aggregation, as does plasma fibrinogen.

Platelet factor 3 and factor 4 are two coagulant activities directly associated with platelets. Platelet factor 4 is a platelet-released low molecular weight protein (minimum molecular weight of 7000) which can neutralize the anticoagulant activity of heparin (Levine & Wohl, 1976; Handin & Cohen, 1976). Platelet factor 4 is released from the α storage granules of platelets complexed with a high molecular weight glycoprotein which is rich in chondroitan sulfate. The role of platelet factor 4 is speculative at this time, although in addition to its heparin-neutralizing ability it has been noted to inhibit collagenase (Hiti-Harper et al, 1978). Platelet factor 3, usually thought of as the phospholipid component of platelet membranes, even though recognized for many years, may be the poorest understood of the coagulant activities of platelets. Although our knowledge of the interactions of purified coagulation factors with platelets and platelet membranes is increasing, it is still difficult to explain platelet factor 3 activity simply in terms of the phospholipid composition of platelet membranes.

BLOOD COAGULATION AND THE KININ, COMPLEMENT AND FIBRI-NOLYTIC SYSTEMS

The coagulation, kinin, complement and fibrinolytic systems are all part of the body's intricate defense mechanism against mechanical or biological intrusion. As each of these systems becomes more clearly understood, it is becoming apparent they should not be conceived of as separate systems, but rather as interacting components of the overall defense mechanism. Several reviews are available if a more detailed treatment of each system is desired (Kondo & Takemura, 1979; Mills, 1979; Movat, 1978; Murano, 1978; Ryan et al, 1979; Stormorken, 1979). Only interactions which bear on the coagulation mechanism will be examined.

The systems are detailed in Figures 3.5, 3.6 and 3.7 and Tables 3.2 and 3.3. Each is found in plasma, is multi-component, involves the action of proteases which must be activated from an inactive circulating precursor, involve cascade sequences in which a small stimulus is amplified, and each system is partially controlled by a series of inhibitors which act either by destroying the activity of a component or by neutralizing one of the proteases. Each of these attributes has for years suggested close links to the coagulation mechanism. The central point in examining these interrelationships appears to revolve around the contact phase of blood coagulation, i.e. factor XII, prekallikrein, high molecular weight kininogen and factor XI. This cyclic pathway, in which XIIa converts prekallikrein to kallikrein and kallikrein in turn converts XII to XIIa, is an interesting enigma in coagulation. It is still not certain as to how this cycle is activated. Three possibilities are frequently mentioned: (1) XII binds to a surface (membrane) producing a conformationally altered single chain XIIa* which has limited proteolytic activity. The XIIa* then cleaves XII to XIIa or

Table 3.2   Complement factors

Component	Molecular weight	Serum concentration[a]
	Classical pathway	
C1q	400 000	180
C1r	168–198 000	101
C1s	85 000	110
C2	117 000	25
C3	190–220 000	1600
C4	206 000	640
C5	190–220 000	80
C6	95 000	75
C7	110 000	55
C8	163 000	80
C9	79 000	230
	Alternate pathway	
Initiating factor	170 000	—
Factor B	80–93 000	100–200 μg
Factor D	22–25 000	—
C3	180 000	1600
C3b	171 000	—
Properdin	184–220 000	10–20

[a] μg/ml plasma

Table 3.3   Kinin and fibrinolytic factors

Component	Molecular weight	Plasma concentration (μg/ml)
	Kinin	
Prekallikrein	88 000	25–40
Hageman factor (Factor XII)	90 000	40
High molecular weight kininogen	180 000	80
Low molecular weight kininogen	80 000	400
	Fibrinolytic	
Hageman factor (Factor XII)	90 000	40
Prekallikrein	88 000	25–40
Plasminogen	92 000 (88 000)	$\approx$ 100
Factor XI or other plasma factor	—	—
Tissue derived activators	—	—

prekallikrein to kallikrein and thus the cycle is initiated, (2) XII bound to a surface does not have catalytic activity, but due to a conformational change upon binding is more susceptible to proteolysis by traces of active proteases always present in plasma (Revak et al, 1977). (3) As yet undetected factors are responsible for triggering the contact phase. High molecular weight kininogen is involved in the cycle as it has been shown to acelerate both the conversion of XII to XIIa and prekallikrein to kallikrein (Griffin & Cochrane, 1976; Meier et al, 1977).

Kinin system

The kinin system in plasma is intimately involved with the coagulation system. Two forms of kininogens circulate in the plasma referred to as low molecular weight kininogen (LMWK) and high molecular weight kininogen (HMWK). With the exception of LMWK, each component of the plasma kinin system is a recognized

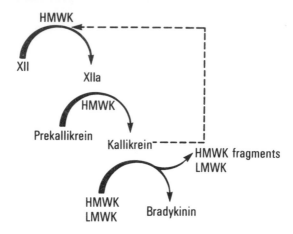

Fig. 3.5   Plasma kallikrein system. HMWK: high molecular weight kininogen; LMWK: low molecular weight kininogen.

component of the coagulation system. HMWK is cleaved by kallikrein to produce the vasoactive peptide bradykinin and several other fragments (Nakayasy & Nagasawa, 1979; Kerbiriou & Griffin, 1979; Kaplan, 1979). With bovine HMWK (molecular weight 76 000 vs. 180 000 for human) one of these fragments inhibits the kaolin-mediated activation of factor XII (Han et al, 1978). Several investigators have shown that HMWK following treatment with kallikrein to remove the vasoactive and inhibitory peptides, no longer functions in accelerating the conversion of prekallikrein to kallikrein or factor XII to XIIa (Chan et al, 1979; Thompson et al, 1978). Thus, the production of the vasoactive bradykinin inhibits contact activation in two manners, by the generation of inhibitory peptides and by the removal of the active co-factor. HMWK has been reported to circulate in plasma complexed with both factor XI and prekallikrein (Thompson et al, 1979). Whether HMWK is susceptible to proteolysis by kallikrein when it is complexed is not yet known. It will be interesting to see how the contact phase factors kinetically form both activated factor XI and vasoactive peptides.

Fibrinolytic system

The contact phase clotting factors again play a significant role in the activation of the fibrinolytic system which essentially involves the conversion of plasminogen to plasmin. Those components which convert plasminogen to plasmin are collectively referred to as plasminogen activators and are found both in plasma and various tissues. A potent antiplasmin, which forms a 1:1 stoichiometric complex with plasmin, is also found in plasma (Wiman & Collen, 1977). Several different plasminogen converting activities have been described in plasma. Factor XIIa appears capable of converting plasminogen to plasmin, but this may be a minor pathway (Kluft et al, 1979). More important seem to be XIIa-mediated activation pathways. Kallikrein and XIa have both been suggested to convert plasminogen to plasmin (Mandle & Kaplan, 1979). Plasmin is a broad specificity serine esterase and it has several possible roles in regulating the clotting cascade. Plasmin can inhibit clotting by inactivating factors V, VIII and HMWK, and it has been demonstrated to convert

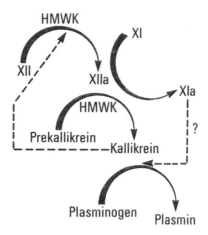

Fig. 3.6 Plasma fibrinolytic system. HMWK: high molecular weight kininogen.

prekallikrein to kallikrein, activate and degrade factor XII as well as degrade factor IX. Whether these activities have a significant role in vivo is still to be established.

Complement system

The complement system is far more complex than either the fibrinolytic or kinin system in terms of both number of components and actions. As such, interactions with the coagulation system are more difficult to assess. A factor XII dependent pathway has been described which converts C1 to its active esterase (Donaldson, 1968). The pathway has not been described yet, but both plasmin and kallikrein have been shown capable of converting the C1s component of C1 to its active form (Lepow et al, 1958; Sumi et al, 1973). C1 esterase inhibitor, on the other hand, has been postulated to be the principle plasma inhibitor of kallikrein (Trump et al, 1978). Zimmerman et al (1971) described abnormal prothrombin consumption in rabbits deficient in C6, which could be corrected by the addition of C6. A study of a patient deficient in C6 showed that thrombin-induced platelet aggregation was reduced in the patient and could be restored by adding C6 (Wautier et al, 1979). Polly and Nachman (1979) have shown that the C5–C9 complex is taken up by platelets during thrombin activation and, though not a prerequisite for thrombin-induced platelet aggregation, greatly enhances the response. These and other observations lead to the proposal of a third pathway for the activation of complement independent of either the classical or alternative pathways. Thrombin associated with the platelet membrane was assumed to form a C3 convertase which entered the complement sequence at the level of the C3 stage and activated the terminal components through C9 (Polley & Nachman, 1978). On the reverse side, the C3b fragment from C3 has been shown to induce monocytes to expose tissue factor activity initiating the extrinsic system of blood coagulation (Prydz et al, 1977). The same phenomenon has been shown for the C5 chemotactic fragment and leukocytes (Muhfelder et al, 1979). The complexities of both the complement system and coagulation system are such that additional links between the two systems will probably be established during the coming years.

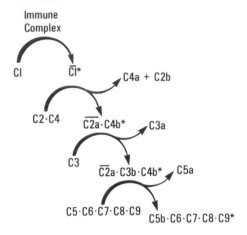

Fig. 3.7   Classical complement activation as a cascade mechanism. The bar over a component indicates it possesses esterolytic activity. The * indicates the complex is membrane bound. C3a and C5a are activation peptides released having chemotactic activity. C4a and C2b have no such activity. The alternate pathway for the activation of complement enters the sequence at the level of C3. Adapted from Müller-Eberhard (1975).

SUMMARY

Progress over the past decade in understanding the molecular mechanisms of blood coagulation has been impressive. The problems associated with basic research in this area are many and intuitive and clever approaches have yielded results which can be translated into better medical care. It was not too long ago when biochemists looked upon the components of blood as the garbage dump of the body, a discouraging outlook which for years prevented rigorous attempts at examining the clotting mechanism and its components. That has changed and the next decade promises refinements and significant advances in our understanding of the intricacies of blood clotting.

REFERENCES

Austen D E G 1974 Factor VIII of small molecular weight and its aggregation. Brit. J. Haematol. 27: 89–100

Bartlett S, Latson P, Hanahan D 1980 High molecular weight factor V of bovine and human plasma. Biochemistry 19: 273–77

Baugh R, Hougie C 1977 Biochemistry of blood coagulation. In: Poller L (ed) Recent Advances in Blood Coagulation, 2nd edn. Churchill Livingstone, New York. p 1–34

Baugh R, Hougie C 1979 The chemistry of blood coagulation. Clin. Haematol. 8: 3–30

Baugh R F, Brown J, Sargeant R, Hougie C 1974 Separation of human factor VIII activity from the von Willebrand's antigen and ristocetin platelet aggregating activity. Biochim. Biophys. Acta 371: 360–67

Bensusan H B, Koh T L, Henry K G, Murray B A, Culp L A 1978 Evidence that fibronectin is the collagen receptor on platelet membranes. Proc. Nat. Acad. Sci. (U.S.) 75: 5864–68

Biggs R, Douglas A S, Macfarlane R G 1953 The formation of thromboplastin in human blood. J. Physiol. 119: 89–101

Bouma B N, Hordijk-Hos J M, de Graaf S, Sixma J J, van Mourik J A 1975 Presence of factor VIII-related antigen in blood platelets of patients with von Willebrand's disease. Nature 257: 510

Brown J, Baugh R, Hougie C 1979 Effect of exercise on the factor VIII complex: A correlation of the von Willebrand antigen and factor VIII coagulant antigen increase. Thromb. Res. 15: 15: 61–67

Brown J E, Baugh R F, Sargeant R B, Hougie C 1974 Separation of bovine factor VIII-related antigen (platelet aggregating factor) from bovine antihemophilic factor. Proc. Soc. Exp. Biol. Med. 147: 608–11

Chan J, Movat H, Burrowes C 1979 High molecular weight kinonogen: Its inability to correct the clotting of kininogen-deficient plasma after cleavage of bradykinin by plasma kallikrein, plasmin or trypsin. Thromb. Res. 14: 817–24

Comp P C, Esmon C T 1979 Activated protein C inhibits platelet prothrombin-converting activity. Blood 54: 1272–81

Cotrell B A, Strong D D, Watt K W K, Doolittle R F 1979 Amino acid sequence studies on the α chain of human fibrinogen. Exact location of cross-linking receptor sites. Biochemistry 18: 5405–9

Dahlbäck B, Stenflo J 1978 Binding of bovine coagulation factor Xa to platelets. Biochemistry 17: 4938–45

Davie E, Fujikawa K, Kurachi K, Kisiel W 1979 The role of serine proteases in the blood coagulation cascade. Adv. Enzymol. 48: 277–318

Decottignies-LeMarechal P, Rikong-adie H, Azerad R, Guadry M 1979 Vitamin K-dependent carboxylation of synthetic substrates. Nature of the products. Biochem. Biophys. Res. Commun. 90: 700–707

DiScipio R, Davie E 1979 Characterization of protein S, a γ-carboxyglutamic acid containing protein from bovine and human plasma Biochemistry 18: 899–904

Donaldson V 1968 Mechanism of activation of C′1 esterase in hereditary angioneurotic edema plasma in vitro: the role of Hageman factor, a clot-promoting agent. J. Exp. Med. 127: 411–29

Doolittle R F, Takagi T, Cottrell B A 1974 Platelet and plasma fibrinogens are identical gene products. Science 185: 368–70

Esmon C T 1979 The subunit structure of thrombin-activated factor V. Isolation of activated factor V, separation of subunits, and reconstitution of biological activity. J. Biol. Chem. 254: 964–73

Freeman J P, Guillan M C, Begeand A, Jackson C M 1977 Activation of bovine blood coagulation factor V, a prerequisite for it to bind both prothrombin and factor Xa. Fed. Proc. 36: 675 Abstract

Gjønnaess H 1972 Cold promoted activation of factor VII activity during the spontaneous coagulation of blood. Thromb. Diath. Haemorrh. 28: 155–68

Gordon J L (ed) 1976 Platelets in Biology and Pathology. Elsevier/North-Holland Inc., New York

Green D, Muller H P 1978 Platelet-binding of the von Willebrand factor. Thromb. Haemos. 39: 684–94

Griffin J H, Cochrane C 1976 Mechanisms for the involvement of high molecular weight kininogen in surface-dependent reactions of Hageman factor. Proc. Nat. Acad. Sci. (U.S.) 73: 2554–58, 1976

Han Y N, Kato H, Iwanaga S, Oh-ishi S, Katori M 1978 Primary structure of bovine high molecular-weight kininogen. Characterization of carbohydrate-free fragment 1·2 (fragment X) released by the action of plasma. J. Biochem. 83: 213–23

Handin R, Cohen H 1976 Purification and binding properties of human platelet factor four. J. Biol. Chem. 251: 4273–81

Hessel B, Mabino M, Iwanaga S, Blomback B 1979 Primary structure of human fibrinogen and fibrin. Structural studies on NH_2-terminal part of Bβ chain. Eur. J. Biochem. 98: 521–62

Hiti-Harper J, Wohl H, Harper E 1978 Platelet factor 4: An inhibitor of collagenase. Science 199: 991–92

Hougie C, Baugh R 1980 Current views on blood coagulation and hemostatic mechanism. In: Thomson J (ed) Blood Coagulation and Haemostasis: A Practical Guide. Churchill Livingstone, New York

Hougie C, Denson K W E, Biggs R 1967 A study of the reaction product of factor VIII and factor IX by gel filtration. Thrombos. Diathes. haemorrh. 18: 211–22

Hogiv T, Stormorken H 1974 Ultrastructural studies on the platelet plug formation in bleeding time wounds from normal individuals and patients with von Willebrand's disease. Acta Path. Microbiol. Scand. 248/S2: 105–23

Ittycrah T R, Rawala R, Colman R W 1980a Studies on the structure of bovine factor V. Fed. Proc. 39: 544

Ittyerah T R, Rawala R, Colman R W 1980b Function of the subunits of factor V. In: Mann K G, Taylor F B Jr (eds) Regulation of Coagulation. Elsevier North Holland, New York

James H L, Ganguly P 1975 Identity of human platelet fibrinogen. Biochem. Biophys. Res. Commun. 63: 659

James H L, Ganguly P, Jackson C W 1977 Characterization and origin of fibrinogen in blood platelets. A review with recent data. Thrombos. Haemost. 38: 439–55

Kane W H, Lindhout M J, Jackson C M, Majerus P 1980 Factor V_a-dependent binding of factor Xa to human platelets. J. Biol. Chem. 255: 1170–74

Kaplan A P 1979 Structure-function correlation of human kininogen. Monogr. Allergy 14: 212–17

Kao K J, Pizzo S V, McKee P A 1979 Platelet receptors for human factor VIII-von Willebrand protein — functional correlation of receptor occupancy and ristocetin-induced platelet aggregation. Proc. Nat. Acad. Sci. (U.S.) 76: 5317–20

Kerbiriou D, Griffin J 1979 Human high molecular weight kininogen. Studies of the structure-function relationships and of proteolysis of the molecule occurring during contact activation. J. Biol. Chem. 254: 12020–27

Kisiel W 1979 Human plasma protein C: Isolation, characterization, and mechanism of activation by

alpha-thrombin. J. Clin. Invest. 64: 761–69
Kisiel W, Ericsson L H, Davie E W 1976 Proteolytic activation of protein C from bovine plasma. Biochemistry 15: 4893–4900
Kisiel W, Fujikawa K, Davie E 1977a Activation of bovine factor VII (proconvertin) by factor XIIa (activated Hageman factor). Biochemistry 16: 4189–94
Kisiel W, Canfield W M, Ericsson L H, Davie E W 1977b Anticoagulant properties of bovine plasma protein C following activation by thrombin. Biochemistry 16: 5824–31
Kluft C, Trumpi-Kalshoven M, Jie A, Veldhuyzen-Stolk E 1979 Factor XII-dependent fibrinolysis: A double function of plasma kallikrein and the occurrence of a previously undescribed factor XII- and kallikrein-dependent plasminogen activity. Thromb. Haemost. 41: 756–73
Kondo M, Takemura S 1979 Biological effects and the mechanism of complement activation-interaction among complement, coagulation, fibrinolysis and kinin generation system. Nippon Rinsho 37: 1038–43
Koutts J, Walsh P N, Plow E F, Fenton J W, Bouma B N, Zimmerman T S 1978 Active release of human platelet factor-VIII related antigen by adenosine diphosphate, collagen, and thrombin. J. Clin. Invest. 62: 1255–63
Laake K, Østerud B 1974 Activation of purified plasma factor VII by human plasmin, plasma kallikrein and activated components of the human intrinsic blood coagulation system. Thromb. Res. 5: 759–79
Lane J, Ekert H, Vafiadis A 1979 Affinity chromatography of human factor VIII using human and rabbit antibodies to factor VIII. Thrombos. Haemostas. 42: 1306–15
Legaz M E, Schmer G, Counts R B, Davie E W 1973 Isolation and characterization of human factor VIII (antihemophilic factor) J. Biol. Chem. 248: 3946–55
Lepow I, Ratnoff O, Levy L 1958 Studies on the activation of a proesterase associated with partially purified first component of human complement. J. Exp. Med. 107: 451–74
Levine S, Wohl H 1976 Human platelet factor 4: Purification and characterization by affinity chromatography. J. Biol. Chem. 251: 324–28, 1976.
Lim, T K, Bloomfield V A, Nelsestuen G L 1977 Structure of the prothrombin- and blood clotting factor X-membrane complexes. Biochemistry 16: 4177–71
Lipscomb M S, Walsh P N 1979 Human platelets and factor XI localization in platelet membranes of factor XI-like activity and its functional distinction from plasma factor XI. J. Clin. Invest. 63: 1006–14
Mandle R, Kaplan A 1979 Hageman factor-dependent fibrinolysis: generation of fibrinolytic activity by the interaction of human activated factor XI and plasminogen. Blood 54: 850–62
Marguerie G A, Edgington T S, Plow E F 1980 Interaction of fibrinogen with its platelet receptor as part of a multi-step reaction with ADP-induced platelet aggregation. J. Biol. Chem. 255: 154–161
Meier H, Pierce J, Colman R, Kaplan A 1977 Activation and function of human Hageman factor. The role of high molecular weight kininogen and prekallikrein. J. Clin. Invest. 60: 18–31, 1977
Miletich J, Jackson C, Majerus P 1977 Interaction of coagulation factor Xa with human platelets. Proc. Nat. Acad. Sci. (U.S.) 74: 4033–36
Miletich J, Jackson C, Majerus P 1978a Properties of the factor Xa binding site on human platelets. J. Biol. Chem. 235: 6908–16
Miletich J, Majerus D, Majerus P 1978b Patients with congenital factor V deficiency have decreased factor Xa binding sites on their platelets. J. Clin. Invest. 62: 824–31
Mills I H 1979 Kallikrein, kininogen and kinins in control of blood pressure. Nephron 23: 61–71
Mosesson M W 1977 Cold-insoluble globulin (CIg), a circulating cell surface protein. Thrombosis Haemostas. 38: 742–51
Movat H Z 1978 The kinin system: its relation to blood coagulation, fibrinolysis and the formed elements of the blood. Rev. Physiol. Biochem. Pharmacol. 84: 143, 1978
Muhfelder T, Niemetz J, Kreutzer D, Beebe D, Ward P, Rosenfeld S 1979 C5 chemotactic fragment induces leukocyte production of tissue factor activity: a link between complement and coagulation. J. Clin. Invest. 63: 147–50, 1979
Müller-Eberhard H 1975 Complement. Ann. Rev. Biochem. 44: 697–724
Murano G 1978 The 'Hageman' connection: interrelationships of blood coagulation, fibrino(geno)lysis, kinin generation, and complement activation. Am. J. Hematol. 4: 409–17
Nachman R, Levine R, Jaffe E 1977 Synthesis of factor VIII antigen by cultured guinea pig megakaryocytes. J. Clin. Invest. 60: 914–21
Nakayasu T, Nagasawa S 1979 Studies on human kininogens. I. Isolation, characterization and cleavage by plasma kallikrein of high molecular weight (HMW)-kininogen. J. Biochem. (Tokyo) 85: 249–58
Nathan I, Fleischer G, Livne A, Dvilansky A, Parola A 1979 Membrane microenvironmental changes during activation of human blood platelets by thrombin. J. Biol. Chem. 254: 9822–28
Nelsestuen G L, Broderius M 1977 Interaction of prothrombin and blood-clotting factor X with membranes of varying composition. Biochemistry 16: 4172–77
Nelsestuen G L, Lim T K 1977 Equilibria involved in prothrombin and blood clotting factor X-membrane binding. Biochemistry 16: 4164–71

Nesheim M, Myamel K, Hibbard L, Mann K 1979 Isolation and characterization of single chain bovine factor V. J. Biol. Chem. 254: 508–17

Niewiarowski S, Regoeczi E, Mustard J F 1972 Platelet interaction with fibrinogen and fibrin. Comparison of the interaction of platelets with that of fibroblasts, leukocytes and erythrocytes. Ann. N.Y. Acad. Sci. 201: 72–83

Okumura T, Jamieson G 1976 Platelet glycocalicin: 1. Orientation of glycoprotein of the human platelet surface. J. Biol. Chem. 251: 5944–49

Okumura T, Lombart C, Jamieson G 1976 Platelet glycocalicin. 2. Purification and characterization. J. Biol. Chem. 251: 5950–5955

Okumura T, Hasitz M, Jamieson G 1978 Platelet glycocalicin. Interaction with thrombin and role as thrombin receptor of the platelet surface. J. Biol. Chem. 253: 3535–43

Østerud B, Rapaport S 1977 Activation of factor IX by the reaction product of tissue factor and factor VII: Additional pathway for initiating blood coagulation. Proc. Nat. Acad. Sci. (U.S.) 74: 5260–64

Østerud B, Rapaport S, Lavine K 1977 Factor V activity of platelets: Evidence for an activated factor V molecule and for a platelet activator. Blood 49: 819–34, 1977

Østerud B, Harper E, Rapaport S, Lavine K 1979 Evidence against collagen activation of platelet associated factor XI as a mechanism for initiating intrinsic clotting. Scand. J. Haemat. 22: 205–13

Østerud B, Berre A, Otnaess A, Bjørklid E, Prydz H 1972 Activation of the coagulation factor VII by tissue thromboplastin and calcium. Biochemistry 11: 2853–57

Peake I R 1979 Factor VIII clotting antigens studied by immunoradiometric assay. Thromb. Haem. 42: 343–

Phillips D R, Jakábová M 1977 Ca^{2+}-dependent protease in human platelets. Specific cleavage of platelet polypeptides in the presence of added Ca^{2+}. J. Biol. Chem. 252: 5602–5

Polley M. Nachman R 1978 The human complement system in thrombin-mediated platelet function. J. Exp. Med. 147: 1713–26

Polley M, Nachman R 1979 Human complement in thrombin-mediated platelet function: uptake of the C5–C–9 complex. J. Exp. Med. 149: 633–45

Prydz H, Allison A, Schlorlemmer H 1977 Further link between complement activation and blood coagulation. Nature 270. 173–74

Radcliffe R, Nemerson Y 1975 The activation and control of factor VII by activated factor X and thrombin. Isolation and characterization of a single chain form of factor VII. J. Biol. Chem. 250: 388–95

Radcliffe R, Bagdasarian A, Colman R, Nemerson Y 1977 Activation of blood factor VII by Hageman factor fragments. Blood 50: 611–17

Ratnoff O D 1979 The physiology of blood coagulation. Behring Inst. Mitt. 63: 135–55

Revak S, Cochrane C, Griffin J 1977 The binding and cleavage characteristics of human Hageman factor during contact activation. J. Clin. Invest. 59: 1167–75

Rick M E, Hoyer L W 1973 Immunological studies of antihemophilic factor (AHF) (factor VIII). V. Immunologic properties of AHF subunits produced by salt dissociation. Blood 42: 737–47

Rittenhouse-Simmons S, Deykin D 1977 The mobilization of arachidonic acid in platelets exposed to thrombin or ionophore A23187. Effect of adenosine triphosphate deprivation. J. Clin. Invest. 60: 495–98

Ruoslahti E, Vaheri A 1975 Interaction of soluble fibroblast surface antigen with fibrinogen and fibrin. Identity with cold insoluble globulin of human plasma. J. Exp. Med. 141: 497–500

Ryan J W, Oza N B, Martin L C, Pena G A 1979 Components of the kallikrein kinin system in urine. Adv. Exp. Med. Biol. 120A: 313–23

Saito H, Ratnoff O 1975 Alteration of factor VII activity by activated Fletcher factor (a plasma kallikrein): A potential link between the intrinsic and extrinsic blood clotting systems. J. Lab. Clin. Med. 85: 405–15

Sakariassen K, Bolhuis P, Sixma J 1979 Human blood platelet adhesion to artery subendothelium is mediated by factor VIII-von Willebrand factor bound to the subendothelium. Nature 279: 636–38

Saraswathi S, Rawala R, Colman R W 1978 Subunit structure of bovine factor V. Influence of proteolysis during blood collection. J. Biol. Chem. 253: 1024–29

Schmer G, Kirby E P, Teller D C, Davie E W 1972 The isolation and characterization of bovine factor VIII (antihemophilic factor) J. Biol. Chem. 247: 2512–21

Schreider-Trip M D, Jenkins, C S P, Kahlé H, Sturle A, Ten Cate J W 1979 Studies on the mechanism of ristocetin-induced platelet aggregation: binding of factor VIII to platelets. Brit. J. Haematol. 43: 99–112

Schwartz M L, Pizzo S V, Hill R, McKee P A 1971 The subunit structures of human plasma and platelet factor XIII (fibrin-stabilizing factor). J. Biol. Chem. 246: 5851–54

Schwartz M L, Pizzo S V, Hill R, McKee P 1973 Human factor XIII from plasma and platelets. Molecular weights, subunit structure, proteolytic activation, and cross linking of fibrinogen and fibrin. J. Biol. Chem. 248: 1395–1407

Seligsohn U, Østerud B, Rapaport S 1978a A coupled amidolytic assay for factor VII: Its use with a clotting assay to determine the activity of factor VII. Blood 52: 978–88

Seligsohn U, Østerud B, Griffin J, Rapaport S 1978b Evidence for the participation of both activated XII and activated IX in cold-promoted activation of factor VII. Thromb. Res. 13: 1049–57

Seligsohn U, Østerud B, Brown S, Griffin J, Rapaport S 1979 Activation of human factor VII in plasma and in purified systems. J. Clin. Invest. 64: 1056–65

Slot J W, Bouma B N, Montgomery R, Zimmerman T S 1978 Platelet factor VIII-related antigen-immunofluorescent localization. Thromb. Res. 13: 871–82

Smith J, Silver M J 1976 Prostaglandin synthesis by platelets and its biological significance. In: Gordon J (ed) Platelets in Biology and Pathology. North-Holland Publishing, New York, p 331–52

Soria J, Soria C, Betrand O, Samama M 1978 Fibrinogen and platelet aggregation. Role of the Glycopeptidic part and of the fibrinopeptide B. Description of a new technique of fibrinoglycopeptide isolation. Biochem. Biophys. Res. Comm. 82: 442–50

Stenflo J 1976 A new vitamin K-dependent protein. Purification from bovine plasma and preliminary characterization. J. Biol. Chem. 71: 2730–33

Stormorken H 1979 Interrelations between the coagulation-, the fibrinolytic and the kallikrein-kinin system. Scand. J. Haematol. 34: 24–7

Strong D D, Watt W K, Cottrell B A, Doolittle R F 1979 Amino acid sequence studies on the α chain of human fibrinogen. Complete sequence of the largest cyanogen bromide fragment. Biochemistry 18: 5399–5404

Sumi H, Muramatu M, Fujii S 1973 The relation of C1sa, a subunit of the activated first component of complement, to other plasma enzymes. Biochim. Biophys. Acta 327: 207–12

Suttie J W, Jackson C M 1977 Prothrombin structure, activation, and biosynthesis. Physiol. Rev. 57: 1–70

Switzer M, McKee P 1976 Studies on human antihemophilic factor: Evidence for a covalently linked subunit structure. J. Clin. Invest. 57: 925–37

Switzer M, Pizzo S, McKee P 1979 Is there a precursive, relatively procoagulant-inactive form of normal antihemophilic factor (factor VIII)? Blood 54: 916–27

Tam S, Fenton J, Detwiler T 1979 Dissociation of thrombin from platelets by hirudin. J. Biol. Chem. 254: 8723–25

Thompson R E, Mandle R, Kaplan A 1978 Characterization of human high molecular weight kininogen. Procoagulant activity associated with the light chain of kinin free high molecular weight kininogen. J. Exp. Med. 147: 488–99

Thompson R, Mandle R, Kaplan A 1979 Studies of the binding of pre-kallikrein and factor XI to high molecular weight kininogen and its light chain. Proc. Nat. Acad. Sci. (U.S.) 76: 4862–66

Tollefsen D, Majerus P 1976 Evidence for a single class of thrombin-binding sites on human platelets. Biochemistry 15: 2144–49

Tollefsen D, Feagler J, Majerus P 1974 the Binding of thrombin to the surface of human platelets. J. Biol. Chem. 249: 2646–51

Tollefsen D, Jackson C, Majerus P 1975 Binding of the products of prothrombin activation to human platelets. J. Clin. Invest. 56: 241–45

Tracy P, Peterson J, Nesheim M, McDuffie F, Mann K 1979 Interaction of coagulation factor V and Va with platelets. J. Biol. Chem. 254: 10354–61

Trumpi-Kalshoven M, Kluft C 1978 C1 inhibitor: the main inhibitor of human plasma kallikrein. Adv. Biosci. 22: 93–101

Vecchione J, Zucker M 1975 Procoagulant activity of platelets in recalcified plasma. Brit. J. Haematol. 31: 423–28

Vehar G, Davie E 1980 Preparation and properties of bovine factor VIII (antihemophilic factor). Biochemistry 19: 401–10

Vicic W, Ratnoff O, Saito H, Goldsmith G 1979 Platelets and surface-mediated clotting activity. Brit. J. Haematol. 43: 91–98

Vogel C N, Butkowski R J, Mawn K G, Lundlbad R 1976 Effect of polylysine on the activation of prothrombin. Polylysine substitutes for calcium ions and factor V in the factor Va catalyzed activation of prothrombin. Biochemistry 15: 3265–69

Wagner R H, Cooper H A, Owen W G 1973 Dissociation of antihemophilic factor and separation of a small active fragment. Thromb. Diathes. Haemorrh. 54: 185–90

Walker F, Sexton P, Esmon C 1979 The inhibition of blood coagulation by activated protein C through the selective inactivation of activated factor V. Biochim. Biophys. Acta 571: 333–42

Walsh P 1972 The role of platelets in the contact phase of blood coagulation. Brit. J. Haematol. 22: 237–54

Watt K W K, Cottrell B A, Strong D D, Doolittle R F 1979 Amino acid sequence studies on the α chain of human fibrinogen. Overlapping sequences providing the complete sequence. Biochemistry 18: 5410–15

Wautier J, Peltier A, Caen J 1979 Complement (C6) and platelet activation by thrombin in humans. Thromb. Res. 15: 589–91

Weiss H 1975 Platelet physiology and abnormalities of platelet function. New Engl. J. Med. 293: 580–88

Weiss H J, Hoyer L W 1973 von Willebrand factor. Dissociation from antihemophilic factor procoagulant activity. Science 182: 1149–51

Wiman B, Collen D 1977 Purification and characterization of human antiplasmin, the fast-acting plasmin inhibitor in plasma. Eur. J. Biochem. 78: 19–26

Workman E, White G, Lundblad 1977 Structure-function relationships in the interaction of α-thrombin with blood platelets. J. Biol. Chem. 252: 7118–23

York J, Blombäck B 1979 The sites of the lactoperoxidase-catalyzed iodination of human fibrinogen. J. Biol. Chem. 254: 8766–95

Zimmerman T, Arroyave C, Müller-Eberhard H 1971 A blood coagulation abnormality in rabbits deficient in the sixth component of complement (C6) and its correction by purified C6. J. Exp. Med. 134: 1491–1600

Zucker M B, Brockman M J, Kaplan K L 1979 Factor-VIII-related antigen in human blood platelets — localization and release by thrombin and collagen. J. Lab. Clin. Med. 94: 675–82

Zucker M B, Kim S, McPherson J, Grant R A 1977 Binding of factor VIII to platelets in the presence of ristocetin. Brit. J. Haemat. 35: 535–49

4. Contact activation of coagulation

Derek Ogston

The sequences of reactions culminating in the formation of thrombin are traditionally termed the intrinsic and extrinsic pathways of coagulation. The initiation of the intrinsic pathway involves the participation of a number of agents and, physiologically, the contact with a surface. In our present state of knowledge contact activation of the coagulation system involves the interaction of factor XII (Hageman factor), factor XI (plasma thromboplastin antecedent; PTA) and components of the kallikrein-kinin system — prekallikrein and high molecular weight kininogen (HMW kininogen). Knowledge of the requirement for these agents in the coagulation sequence has been initiated by the discoveries of patients with hereditary deficiency of individual factors.

Hereditary deficiency of components of the contact activation system

Hageman trait is an uncommon hereditary disorder of blood coagulation resulting from a functional deficiency of factor XII (Ratnoff & Colopy, 1955). In spite of a greatly prolonged clotting time in glass tubes there is no bleeding tendency. The deficiency of factor XII is usually inherited as an autosomal recessive characteristic; in an exceptional family there appeared to be autosomal dominant inheritance (Bennett et al, 1972). The great majority of individuals with Hageman trait lack factor XII-antigen (Saito et al, 1976), but the plasma of a small number with deficient clotting activity have been found to contain an agent immunologically indistinguishable from normal factor XII (Saito et al, 1979b).

Factor XI deficiency, transmitted as an autosomal recessive trait, is usually associated with a mild bleeding tendency, but patients may be asymptomatic. No evidence has been obtained for the presence of factor XI antigen significantly in excess of factor XI activity, indicating that hereditary factor XI deficiency results from absence of the factor XI molecule (Forbes & Ratnoff, 1972; Rimon et al, 1976).

A further coagulation defect characterized by an abnormality of the intrinsic coagulation mechanism with a greatly prolonged whole blood clotting time and partial thromboplastin time was described by Hathaway (1965), and ascribed to deficiency of an agent termed Fletcher factor. The individuals with this deficiency had no haemorrhagic tendency. Subsequently this factor was identified as plasma kallikrein (Wuepper, 1973). The deficiency occurs through an autosomal recessive mode of inheritance (Abildgaard & Harrison, 1974).

More recently a number of families have been identified with a different abnormality of their intrinsic coagulation system. This defect has been recognised as due to a deficiency of the high molecular weight form of kininogen and the disorders have been variously referred to as Fitzgerald trait (Saito et al, 1975); Williams trait (Colman et al, 1975); Flaujeac trait (Wuepper et al, 1975) and Reid trait (Lutcher, 1976). The defect is again inherited as an autosomal recessive.

Fitzgerald trait plasma contains a normal concentration of the lower molecular weight form of kininogen (LMW kininogen) whereas both HMW and LMW kininogen are deficient in Williams and Flaujeac trait plasma. The level of prekallikrein associated with deficiency of HMW kininogen is also variable: prekallikrein is considerably reduced in Fitzgerald plasma, but normal in Flaujeac plasma. Williams plasma has a partial deficiency. All the individuals described with deficiency of HMW kininogen have been asymptomatic.

BIOCHEMISTRY OF COMPONENTS OF THE CONTACT ACTIVATION SYSTEM

Factor XII

Human factor XII is a single polypeptide chain with a molecular weight of 80 000 (Revak et al, 1974; Chan & Movat, 1976). Bovine factor XII has also been found to consist of a single-chain glycoprotein of molecular weight 74 000 to 78 000 (Fujikawa et al, 1977b; Claeys & Collen, 1978).

The mean concentration of factor XII in human plasma determined by radial immunodiffusion was found to be 29 µg/ml by Revak et al (1974).

The site of synthesis of factor XII is unknown; the liver is suggested by the decreased plasma concentration in patients with hepatic cirrhosis (Saito et al, 1976).

Activation of factor XII takes place on contact of normal plasma with a large variety of negatively charged surfaces such as glass or kaolin (Ratnoff & Rosenblum, 1958). Physiological materials with this property include collagen (Wilner et al, 1968; Harpel, 1972) and platelet membranes (Walsh, 1972b), and recently homogenates of cultured rabbit endothelial cells have been shown to be capable of activating rabbit factor XII (Wiggins et al, 1980). It has been proposed that binding of factor XII to a negatively charged surface results in a conformational change in the molecule with exposure of active sites and accompanying exposure of hydrophobic sites; evidence to support this view has been provided by data obtained with circular dichroism spectroscopy (McMillin et al, 1974) and fluorescence spectroscopy (Fair et al, 1977).

Human activated factor XII has esterase and proteolytic activity with the ability to hydrolyse N-α-acetylglycyl-lysine methyl ester (AGLMe) and to cleave prekallikrein (Ulevitch et al, 1974). AGLMe acts as a competitive inhibitor of prekallikrein activation suggesting that both esterase and protease activities share a common site on factor XIIa. Both activities are inhibited by diisopropylfluorophosphate (DFP) pointing to the conclusion that factor XIIa is a serine protease. Activated bovine factor XII is also inhibited by DFP (Fujikawa et al, 1977a).

Surface binding of factor XII has been shown by Revak and colleagues (1977) to result in cleavage of the molecule into two fragments of 52 000 and 28 000 molecular weight; cleavage took place at two closely spaced sites, one of which was within a disulphide loop. Cleavage at the site external to the disulphide bond released the 28 000 molecular weight fragment from the surface, whereas this fragment remained surface bound if the split took place at the site within the disulphide loop so that it was disulphide-linked to the 52 000 molecular weight fragment. In this way a two-chain enzyme was formed (Fig. 4.1). The sites in the molecule responsible for the binding of factor XII to the surface are located in the 52 000 molecular weight fragment (Revak et al, 1976), while the enzymatically active site is located in the 28 000 molecular

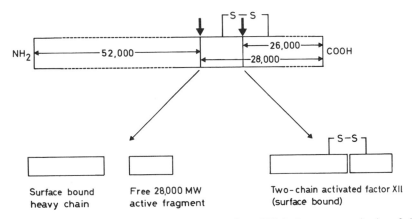

Fig. 4.1. Schematic representation of cleavage of human factor XII during contact activation of plasma.
↑ = Sites of cleavage.

weight fragment. Bovine factor XIIa is also composed of a heavy and light chain linked by one or more disulphide bonds (Fujikawa et al, 1977a); evidence from amino acid sequence studies suggests that factor XII is converted to its activated form by cleavage of a specific arginyl-valine bond.

Apart from solid-phase activation of factor XII on contact with negatively charged surfaces, fluid phase activation takes place on the incubation of factor XII with proteases such as kallikrein or plasmin. The fragments of factor XII produced have the property of converting prekallikrein to kallikrein (Kaplan & Austen, 1971; Cochrane & Wuepper, 1971). Revak and her colleagues (1974) demonstrated that treatment of purified factor XII with plasmin, kallikrein or trypsin results in cleavage at two primary sites yielding fragments of molecular weights 52 000, 40 000 and 28 000; the prekallikrein-activating ability was associated with the 28 000 moiety. The clot-promoting activity of this active fragment is, however, much less than that of the parent molecule.

In more recent studies the surface bound two-chain active factor XII molecule and the free 28 000 molecular weight fraction have been compared in respect of their ability to cleave radiolabelled prekallikrein and factor XI (Revak et al, 1978). Both were capable of cleaving, and thereby activating, prekallikrein, but only the two-chain enzyme cleaved factor XI and then only when it was surface bound. It was concluded, therefore, that the initiation of intrinsic coagulation through the activation of factor XI is a localised event occurring at the site of contact activation.

Debate exists on the requirement for cleavage of factor XII into a two-chain molecule to achieve activation and the acquisition of clot-promoting properties. One view is that the conformational changes induced by negatively charged agents expose enzymatically active groups on the factor XII molecule. In support of this view Ratnoff and Saito (1979b) have shown that purified factor XII, activated by exposure to ellagic acid adsorbed to Sephadex gels, had amidolytic properties when studied in the fluid phase after separation from the gels; no cleavage of the factor XII could be demonstrated by SDS-polyacrylamide gel electrophoresis. The alternative view is that activation of factor XII requires it to be cleaved within a disulphide loop to form a two-chain molecule. Consistent with this view are experimental results demonstrating that surface binding of the single chain form of factor XII does not increase the incorporation of the active site titrant [³H] — DFP (Griffin, 1977a; Meier et al, 1977).

Factor XI

Human factor XI is a glycoprotein composed of two identical polypeptide chains held together by disulphide bond(s). The molecular weight estimated by SDS-polyacrylamide gel electrophoresis has varied from 140 000 (Kurachi & Davie, 1977) to 160 000 (Bouma & Griffin, 1977), but these have been considered to be falsely high: a value closer to the 124 000 found by sedimentation equilibrium studies for bovine factor XI (Koide et al, 1977) is believed to be more accurate (Kurachi & Davie, 1977). The concentration of factor XI in normal plasma has been estimated to be 4 µg/ml (Bouma & Griffin, 1977). Using a radioimmunoassay Saito & Goldsmith (1977) obtained a value of 6 µg/ml.

The activation of factor XI by factor XIIa involves the cleavage of a peptide bond in each of the two chains. Activated factor XI is composed, therefore, of four polypeptide chains linked by disulphide bonds. The estimated molecular weights of the heavy and light chains are 35 000 and 25 000 respectively, and the active site serines are located in each of the light chains (Kurachi & Davie, 1977).

Plasma prekallikrein and kallikrein

Kallikrein is an enzyme which releases the pharmacologically active polypeptide kinins from their precursors termed kininogen or prokinin. The kallikreins are basically of two types, plasma and glandular, which differ in their reaction to kininogens and other substrates, in their behaviour towards inhibitors, in their physicochemical properties, and in their immunochemistry. There are two forms of kininogen in plasma, a high molecular weight type (HMW kininogen) and a lower molecular weight form (LMW kininogen). While glandular kallikrein preferentially cleaves LMW kininogen with the release of lysyl-bradykinin (kallidin), plasma kallikrein has HMW kininogen as its preferred substrate and the kinin released is bradykinin.

Plasma kallikrein circulates in an inactive precursor form (prekallikrein). The plasma prekallikrein level, assayed by radial immunodiffusion, has been found to have a mean value of close to 100 µg/ml (Bagdasarian et al, 1974; Gallimore et al, 1978; Heber et al, 1978). The molecular weight of human plasma kallikrein is approximately 100 000 (Wuepper & Cochrane, 1972; Gallimore et al, 1978). Micro-heterogeneity has been described by Laake & Venneröd (1974) with five to six peaks on isoelectric focusing between pH 7.7 and 9.4.

The only established plasma activators of prekallikrein are factor XII (Margolis, 1958) and its fragments (Kaplan & Austen, 1970). Claims have been made that plasmin can activate prekallikrein directly (Vogt, 1964; Andreenko & Suvorov, 1976), but this is disputed (Burrowes et al, 1971). It is likely that plasmin influences prekallikrein indirectly through the formation of prekallikrein-activating factor XII fragments.

Activation of prekallikrein involves limited proteolysis with the formation of a two-chain molecule linked by one or more disulphide bonds, but without change in molecular weight. The active centre of kallikrein appears to reside in the light chain (Mandle & Kaplan, 1977).

High molecular weight kininogen

The existence of two forms of kinogen in human plasma was first reported by Jacobsen (1966): these are now designated HMW and LMW kininogen. Human HMW kininogen isolated by Thompson and associates (1978) was a single chain protein of about 120 000 daltons. Cleavage by kallikrein resulted in a size reduction of 15 000 daltons and the release of bradykinin. The kinin-free kininogen consisted of a heavy chain of 66 000 daltons and a light chain of 37 000 daltons linked by disulphide bonds. The light chain was responsible for the coagulant activity of HMW kininogen while the heavy chain was found to share antigenic determinants with LMW kininogen and had no coagulant activity. The decrease in the plasma level in patients with cirrhosis suggests that kininogen is synthesized by the liver (Saito et al, 1976).

Bovine HMW kininogen has been more extensively studied. It is a glycoprotein with an estimated molecular weight of about 76 000 (Komiya et al, 1974). When incubated with bovine plasma kallikrein equimolar amounts of bradykinin, kinin-free kininogen and a peptide termed fragment 1.2 are released (Han et al, 1975b). On further incubation fragment 1.2 is further cleaved into fragment 1, a glycoprotein with a molecular weight of 8000 (Han et al, 1976), and fragment 2, a histidine-rich peptide of molecular weight 4584 (Han et al, 1975a). The kinin-free kininogen is composed of a heavy chain of molecular weight 48 000 and a light chain of molecular weight 16 000 held together by a disulphide bond (Kato et al, 1976). Fragment 1.2, fragment 2 and fragment X, a carbohydrate-free fragment 1.2, all suppress kinin formation in plasma by contact activation and inhibit the activation of factor XII by kaolin (Oh-ishi et al, 1977; Han et al, 1978). Matheson and associates (1976) found, however, that fragment 1.2 increased vascular permeability.

Opinion differs on whether kinin-free kininogen can still function as a coagulation factor. Chan and colleagues (1976, 1979) found that kallikrein digestion of human HMW kininogen diminished its coagulant activity whereas other investigators have reported that kinin-free kininogen retains full coagulant activity (Colman et al, 1975; Matheson et al, 1976; Schiffman et al, 1977; Saito, 1977).

HMW kininogen complexes with prekallikrein and factor XI

The existence of prekallikrein-HMW kininogen complexes in plasma has been demonstrated (Mandle et al, 1976; Donaldson et al, 1977), and Scott and Colman (1980) have provided evidence to support the concept that free prekallikrein exists in equilibrium with such complexes. They also suggest that when HMW kininogen binds to kallikrein it retards the destruction of the kallikrein activity by competing for binding sites which would otherwise be available to C1 inactivator.

Complex formation between HMW kininogen and factor XI has also been found (Thompson et al, 1977). This complex was separable from the prekallikrein-HMW kininogen complex indicating that prekallikrein and factor XI bind to different molecules of HMW kininogen.

ROLES OF HMW KININOGEN AND PREKALLIKREIN IN CONTACT-ACTIVATED COAGULATION

Activation of the intrinsic coagulation mechanism takes place on contact of normal plasma with a surface, but a mixture of highly purified factor XII and factor XI incubated with kaolin does not result in the generation of clot-promoting activity (Schiffman & Lee, 1974). It is now recognised that both prekallikrein and HMW kininogen are also required although their precise roles in the intrinsic pathway are not finally established.

Maximal rates of activation of the procoagulant activity of factor XI were found by Griffin and Cochrane (1976) to require factor XII, HMW kininogen and a surface. HMW kininogen accelerated the activation of factor XI by factor XIIa, the activation of prekallikrein by factor XIIa, and activation of factor XII by kallikrein. Surface binding of factor XII in the presence of HMW kininogen rendered the molecule much more susceptible to cleavage into its two-chain activated form by kallikrein (Griffin, 1978). On the basis of these findings a hypothesis was formulated for the mechanism of contact activation of factor XII: factor XII and HMW kininogen form a complex on a negatively charged surface which induces a conformational change in the factor XII molecule and thereby renders it susceptible to proteolytic cleavage. The surface-bound factor XIIa activates prekallikrein and factor XI and the generated kallikrein reciprocally activates more factor XII and thereby augments the quantity of factor XIIa (Fig. 4.2). In partial agreement with this hypothesis Meier and associates (1977)

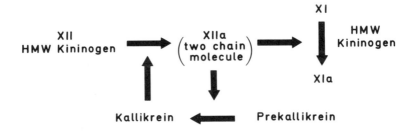

Fig. 4.2 Diagrammatic representation of the hypothesis of reciprocal activation of factor XII and prekallikrein.

also concluded from their experiments that kallikrein functions as an activator of factor XII by a positive feedback mechanism: HMW kininogen did not affect the binding of factor XII to a surface, but enhanced its ability to activate prekallikrein and factor XI. They suggested that HMW kininogen, circulating as a complex with prekallikrein, places the proenzyme in an optimal position for its reciprocal interaction with factor XII. An enhancement of the prekallikrein- and factor XI-activating function of factor XII fragments by HMW kininogen was observed by Liu et al (1977). Contrary to these findings and conclusions, Ratnoff and Saito (1979a) found that the acquisition of clot-promoting properties of factor XII, activated by ellagic acid adsorbed to Sephadex gels, did not require prekallikrein whereas HMW kininogen was required for the interaction of activated factor XII and factor XI in the fluid phase. They concluded that HMW kininogen is not required for conversion of factor XII to its active form, but that it is needed for the expression of its coagulant properties. Factor XII fragments, however, did not required HMW kininogen to activate factor XI (Saito, 1977), suggesting two ways of activating factor XI.

A further role for HMW kininogen was revealed by Wiggins and colleagues (1977):

using ^{125}I-labelled factor XI and prekallikrein they found that HMW kininogen links both molecules to a surface where they could be cleaved by surface-bound factor XIIa.

Recent findings suggest that kallikrein itself may influence the role of HMW kininogen in contact activation: the accelerating effect of HMW kininogen on kaolin-mediated activation of factor XII was found to be markedly increased by brief treatment with kallikrein, suggesting that a 'nicked' form of kininogen is produced (Kato et al, 1979): the complex with prekallikrein was formed through the light chain and interaction with kaolin through the fragment 1.2 region.

The possibility of an alternative pathway for the activation of factor XII, independent of HMW kininogen, has been raised by experiments reported by Fujikawa and colleagues (1979). The conversion of bovine factor XII to its two-chain form could be achieved by kallikrein in the presence of HMW kininogen and a surface. Factor XII, however, was also readily activated by kallikrein in the presence of dextran sulphate of molecular weight 500 000 even in the absence of a surface such as kaolin.

If the activation of factor XII does take place by reciprocal interaction between surface-bound factor XII and prekallikrein it is pertinent to consider how the initiation of the cycle is achieved. One explanation, in accord with the findings of Ratnoff and Saito (1979a, b), is that binding of factor XII to a surface alone can induce some activation. Further support for such a view is provided by the finding that surface-bound single-chain factor XII does react very slowly with DFP, indicating inherent activity of single-chain forms which might trigger surface-dependent coagulation (Griffin, 1977b). Recently, Wiggins and Cochrane (1979) have demonstrated that single-chain factor XII, incubated with kaolin, can cleave other factor XII molecules in the absence of prekallikrein.

The mechanism for the activation of factor XII may be yet more complex. Chan and his colleagues (1977) have reported studies suggesting the presence in plasma of an agent, separable from factors XII and XI, prekallikrein/kallikrein, HMW kininogen, and plasminogen/plasmin, which enhanced the activation of factor XII. Of possible physiological relevance is the finding that a cationic protein derived from the granules of human eosinophils has a stimulating effect on factor XII-dependent reactions (Venge et al, 1979).

Influence of factor XIIa on factor VII

There is now abundant evidence that the intrinsic and extrinsic coagulation systems are linked, at least in vitro, through the enhancement of the coagulant activity of factor VII by components of the contact system. Gjonnaess (1972) found that cold-promoted activation of factor VII depended on the presence of factor XII and kallikrein: they postulated that factor XIIa activated prekallikrein and the kallikrein increased factor VII activity. Favouring a role for kallikrein was the observation that the increase in activity of factor VII on exposure to surfaces did not take place in Fletcher factor plasma (Stormorken & Abildgaard, 1974; Saito & Ratnoff, 1975). Purified kallikrein did not increase the activity of purified factor VII suggesting that an additional agent as required. HMW kininogen was incriminated as this agent on the finding that the activity of factor VII in the plasma of a patient with Fitzgerald trait was not augmented by kaolin (Saito et al, 1975). However, the requirement for kallikrein and kininogen in the activation of factor VII by factor XIIa has been questioned by more recent observations. Using purified bovine reagents Kisiel and associates (1977) found that conversion of factor VII to its two-chain active form could be readily achieved by factor XIIa alone, while Radcliffe and colleagues (1977) demonstrated that factor XII fragments were capable of catalysing a 55-fold increase in factor VII activity. In vivo the role of kallikrein may be to produce active factor XII fragments.

INTERACTION OF COMPONENTS OF CONTACT ACTIVATION SYSTEM WITH PLATELETS

A variety of observations have suggested that platelets may play a significant role in the contact activation system. Factor XI appears to be firmly bound to the platelet membrane being retained after successive washes (Horowitz & Fujimoto, 1965; Walsh, 1972a), and to be bound to isolated platelet membranes (Karpatkin & Karpatkin, 1969). More recently, Tuszynski and Walsh (1979), using an antibody raised in rabbits against human factor XI, have detected factor XI antigen on the platelet surface by fluorescein-labelled goat anti-rabbit IgG. In contrast, factor XII is readily removed from platelets by washing and is, therefore, unlikely to be significantly adsorbed onto the membrane (Horowitz & Fujimoto, 1965; Walsh, 1972a).

Walsh (1972b) has described experiments to demonstrate that the addition of adenosine diphosphate (ADP) to normal or factor XII-deficient platelets results in the formation of an agent which is capable of activating plasma factor XII and thereby promoting the clotting of platelet-poor plasma. Further studies on washed ADP- or collagen-treated human platelets incubated with purified factor XII were reported by Walsh & Griffin (1979): enhancement of coagulant activity and factor XII cleavage were shown, both required kallikrein and were enhanced by HMW kininogen. These experiments provide further evidence that platelets promote the proteolytic activation of factor XII.

Studies by Walsh (1972c) raised the possibility of an alternative pathway for the activation of factor XI, and thereby the intrinsic coagulation pathway, which by-passes factor XII: he showed that collagen could induce coagulant activity in platelets washed to free them of loosely adsorbed coagulation factors. The platelet coagulant activity was independent of factor XII, but required the presence of factor XI.

Tuszynski and Walsh (1979) have reported that platelets from patients without detectable plasma factor XI contained factor XI antigen and activity. Such patients had minimal bleeding manifestations and their platelets behaved normally in contact activation when incubated with collagen. These patients contrasted with a patient with the hereditary giant platelet syndrome who experienced severe bleeding: this patient's platelets lacked factor XI and failed to initiate intrinsic coagulation in response to collagen. It was concluded that the platelet membrane factor XI can substitute for plasma factor XI in the coagulation mechanism and may be required for haemostasis even when plasma XI is present.

INHIBITORS OF THE CONTACT ACTIVATION SYSTEM

Control of the contact activation system may be achieved by prevention of the initial activation or by the inhibition of one of the activated components of the system — factor XII, factor XI or kallikrein.

There is evidence that substances in normal plasma inhibit the activation of factor XII by surface contact through interference with the adsorption of factor XII to a surface, although this inhibition is not detectable when factor XII and kallikrein are present. Separation of the inhibitory agents from factor XII has been achieved using SP-Sephadex C-50 column chromatography (Saito et al, 1974).

Inhibitors of factor XIIa

A number of the plasma protease inhibitors have been shown to be capable of neutralising the biological actions of activated factor XII. Inhibition of factor XIIa by C1 inactivator was shown by Forbes and colleagues (1970) and later inhibition of factor XII fragments was also demonstrated (Schreiber et al, 1973). Antithrombin III was shown to inhibit activated factor XII and its fragment in a progressive and time-dependent reaction with the formation of a 1:1 stoichiometric complex (Stead et al, 1976); the interaction was markedly accelerated by heparin. The effect of various protease inhibitors on factor XIIa was examined by Chan and associates (1977a); only C1 inactivator and antithrombin III had inhibitory activity. In contrast to the finding of Stead et al (1976), heparin had only a moderate enhancing effect on the antithrombin III inhibitory activity. Alpha$_2$-macroglobulin and α_1-antitrypsin had no effect on factor XIIa. Recently the fast-acting plasmin inhibitor, α_2-antiplasmin, has been shown to be capable of inhibiting the clot-promoting and prekallikrein-activating activity of factor XII fragments when tested at physiological concentrations (Saito et al, 1979a). Hedner (1979) has reported that a protein, previously described as an inhibitor of plasminogen activation, functions as an immediate inhibitor of factor XIIa, but its characterisation is not complete.

Inhibitors of factor XIa

Activated factor XIa is also susceptible to inhibition by a variety of the plasma protease inhibitors. C1 inactivator (Forbes et al, 1970), α_1-antitrypsin (Heck & Kaplan, 1974) and antithrombin III (Damus et al, 1973) have each been shown to possess such inhibitory properties. A further factor XIa inhibitor has been described (Nossel & Niemetz, 1965; Ratnoff et al, 1972), but its nature and distinction from other protease inhibitors is not yet established. The clot-promoting activity of factor XIa is also inhibited by α_2-antiplasmin (Saito et al, 1979a).

Inhibitors of plasma kallikrein

The neutralisation of plasma kallikrein can be achieved by a variety of the plasma protease inhibitors. The principle inhibitor is probably C1 inactivator (Ratnoff et al, 1969; Gigli et al, 1970; Gallimore et al, 1979). Alpha$_2$-macroglobulin also forms complexes with kallikrein (Harpel, 1973); in such a complex it retains a proportion of its kininogenase activity, and in plasma the complex protects the free kallikrein from neutralisation by other inhibitors so that slow cleavage of kinin from kininogen proceeds (Vogt & Dugal, 1976).

In studies by McConnell (1972) α_1-antitrypsin was claimed to have kallikrein-inhibiting activity in addition to α_2-macroglobulin and C1 inactivator. Habel and colleagues (1976) found, however, that α_1-antitrypsin did not inhibit plasma kallikrein and it is likely that the α_1-antitrypsin fractions in McConnell's experiments were contaminated with antithrombin III which does inhibit kallikrein, particularly in the presence of heparin (Burrowes et al, 1975). Complex formation between antithrombin III and kallikrein has been demonstrated (Venneröd et al, 1976). The studies of Saito and associates (1979a) have demonstrated that α_2-antiplasmin is also capable of inhibiting the amidolytic, kininogenase and clot-promoting activities of plasma kallikrein. In contrast to these reports Gallimore and colleagues (1979), using a chromogenic peptide substrate assay, found little or no inhibition of plasma kallikrein by α_1-antitrypsin, antithrombin III or α_2-antiplasmin, but they found a further inhibitor, distinct from C1 inactivator and α_2-macroglobulin.

PHYSIOLOGICAL ROLE OF THE CONTACT ACTIVATION SYSTEM

The lack of clinical effects from deficiencies of components of the contact activation system leading to the activation of factor XI in the intrinsic coagulation sequence makes it difficult to ascribe a basic physiological function to these components. The absence of an essential role for the system in fibrin formation is further shown by the clear evidence now available that deficiency of factor XII does not protect from thrombosis (Pizzuto et al, 1979), including venous thrombosis with its predominant fibrin component as illustrated by John Hageman's fatal pulmonary embolism (Ratnoff et al, 1968). A number of patients with factor XII deficiency have suffered a myocardial infarction (Glueck & Roehill, 1966; Hoak et al, 1966), although the significance of this in relation to the contact activation system is open to doubt in view of the platelet composition of arterial thrombi and the lack of equation of myocardial infarction with coronary thrombosis. Myocardial infarction has also been recorded in Fletcher factor deficiency (Currimbhoy et al, 1976).

The absence of a bleeding tendency and the liability to venous thrombosis in individuals with factor XII deficiency suggests that alternative pathways are available for the activation of factor XI or later components of the intrinsic pathway in order to achieve the generation of thrombin and consequent fibrin formation. One possibility, considered above, is that the factor XI activation may be achieved by platelets on interaction with collagen (Walsh, 1972c). A further possibility is that small quantities of thrombin or activated factor X, generated through the extrinsic pathway, may stimulate the intrinsic system by enhancing the functional activity of factor VIII or activating factor IX.

Surface activation of the coagulation system can be readily demonstrated in the test-tube, and in experimental animals the infusion of surface-activated plasma induces intravascular clotting providing the vessel is clamped (Swedenborg et al, 1979). Evidence is available to indicate that activation of the contact system can occur in vivo, albeit in pathological states. For example, a case of disseminated intravascular coagulation with hypofibrinogenaemia followed intravenous injection of a kaolin-containing medication has been reported (Beresford, 1971). More recent evidence has come from studies of patients with polycythaemia vera who had reductions in the levels of factor XII, prekallikrein and kallikrein inhibitors in the presence of intravascular coagulation demonstrated by an increase in soluble fibrin complexes (Carvalho & Ellman, 1976). Activation of factor XII is also implicated in the disseminated intravascular coagulation of gram negative sepsis (Mason & Colman,

1971) with reductions in the factor XII level (Mason et al, 1970) and a decrease in plasma prekallikrein (O'Donnell et al, 1976) and plasma kininogen (Hirsch et al, 1974).

While this chapter has concentrated on the interactions of factor XII, prekallikrein and kininogen in the activation of the coagulation system it must be appreciated that the same components participate in reactions leading to plasmin and kinin function. The mechanisms by which the contact activation system is directed down a single pathway is unknown. Indeed, it must be concluded that our understanding of the precise role of the contact activation system in normal haemostasis or in pathological thrombosis lags behind knowledge of the biochemistry of the constituent proteins and their interactions.

REFERENCES

Abildgaard C F, Harrison J 1974 Fletcher factor deficiency. Blood 43: 641–644
Andreenko G V, Suvorov A V 1976 Effect of plasmin on kallikreinogen. Biochemistry (Biokhimiya) 41: 460–463
Bagdasarian A, Lahiri B, Talamo R G, Wong P, Colman R W 1974 Immunochemical studies of plasma kallikrein. Journal of Clinical Investigation 54: 1444–1454
Bennett B, Ratnoff O D, Holt J B, Roberts H R 1972 Hageman trait (Factor XII deficiency): a probable second genotype inherited as an autosomal dominant characteristic. Blood 40: 412–415
Beresford H R 1971 Coagulation defects after I. V. kaolin. New England Journal of Medicine 285: 522
Burrowes C E, Habal F M, Movat H Z 1975 The inhibition of human plasma kallikrein by antithrombin III. Thrombosis Research 7: 175–183
Burrowes C E, Movat H Z, Soltay M J 1971 The kinin system of human plasma VI. The action of plasmin. Proceedings of the Society for Experimental Biology and Medicine 138: 959–966
Bouma B N, Griffin J H 1977 Human blood coagulation Factor XI. Prufication, properties, and mechanism of activation by activated Factor XII. Journal of Biological Chemistry 252: 6432–6437
Carvalho A, Ellman L 1976 Activation of the coagulation system in polycythemia vera. Blood 47: 669–677
Chan J Y C, Movat H Z 1976 Purification of factor XII (Hageman factor) from human plasma. Thrombosis Research 8: 337–349
Chan J Y C, Burrowes C E, Habal F M, Movat H Z 1977a The inhibition of activated factor XII (Hageman factor) by antithrombin III: the effect of other plasma proteinase inhibitors. Biochemical and Biophysical Research Communications 74: 150–158
Chan J Y C, Burrowes C E, Movat H Z 1977b Activation of factor XII (Hageman factor): enhancing effect of a potentiator. Thrombosis Research 10: 309–313
Chan J Y C, Habal F M, Burrowes C E, Movat H Z 1976 Interaction between factor XII (Hageman factor), high molecular weight kininogen and prekallikrein. Thrombosis Research 9: 423–433
Chan J Y C, Movat H Z, Burrowes C E 1979 High molecular weight kininogen: its inability to correct the clotting of kininogen-deficient plasma after cleavage of bradykinin by plasma kallikrein, plasmin or trypsin. Thrombosis Research 14: 817–824
Claeys H, Collen D 1978 Purification and characterization of bovine caogulation factor XII (Hageman factor). European Journal of Biochemistry 87: 69–74
Cochrane C G, Weupper K D 1971 The first component of the kinin-forming system in human and rabbit plasma. Its relationship to clotting factor XI (Hageman factor). Journal of Experimental Medicine 134: 986–1004
Colman R W, Bagdasarian A, Talamo R C, Scott C F, Seavey M, Guimaràes J A, Pierce J V, Kaplan A P 1975 Williams trait. Human kininogen deficiency with diminished levels of plasminogen proactivator and prekallikrein associated with abnormalities of the Hageman factor-dependent pathways. Journal of Clinical Investigation 56: 1650–1662
Currimbhoy Z, Vinciguerra V, Palakavongs P, Kuslanksy P, Degnan T J 1976 Fletcher factor deficiency and myocardial infarction. American Journal of Clinical Pathology 65: 970–974
Damus P S, Hicks M, Rosenberg R D 1973 Anticoagulant action of heparin. Nature 246: 355–357
Donaldson V H, Kleniewski J, Saito H, Sayed J K 1977 Prekallikrein deficiency in a kindred with kininogen deficiency and Fitzgerald trait clotting defect. Evidence that high molecular weight kininogen and prekallikrein exist as a complex in normal human plasma. Journal of Clinical Investigation 60: 571–583

Fair B D, Saito H, Ratnoff O D, Rippon W B 1977 Detection by fluorescence of structural changes accompanying the activation of Hageman factor (factor XII). Proceedings of the Society for Experimental Biology and Medicine 155: 199–202

Forbes C D, Tatnoff O D 1972 Studies on plasma thromboplastin antecedent (factor XI), PTA deficiency and inhibition of PTA by plasma, pharmacologic inhibitors and specific antiserum. Journal of Laboratory and Clinical Medicine 79: 113–127

Forbes C D, Pensky, J, Ratnoff O D 1970 Inhibition of activated Hageman factor and activated plasma thromboplastin antecedent by purified C͞I inactivator. Journal of Laboratory and Clinical Medicine 76: 809–815

Fujikawa K, Heimark R L, Kurachi K, Davie E W 1979 Activation of bovine factor XII (Hageman factor). Thrombosis and Haemostasis 42: 35

Fujikawa K, Kurachi K, Davie E W 1977a Characterization of bovine factor XIIa (activated Hageman factor). Biochemistry 16: 4182–4188

Fujikawa K, Walsh K A, Davie E W 1977b Isolation and characterization of bovine factor XII (Hageman factor). Biochemistry 16: 2270–2278

Gallimore M J, Amundsen E, Larsbraaten M, Lyngaas K, Fareid E 1979 Studies on plasma inhibitors of plasma kallikrein using chromogenic peptide substrate assays. Thrombosis Research 16: 695–703

Gallimore M J, Fareid E, Stormorken H 1978 The purification of a human plasma kallikrein with weak plasminogen activator activity. Thrombosis Research 12: 409–420

Gigli I, Mason J W, Colman R W, Austen K F 1970 Interaction of plasma kallikrein with C͞I-inactivator. Journal of Immunology 104: 574–581

Gjonnaess H 1972 Cold promoted activation of factor VII. III. Relation to the kallikrein system. Thrombosis et Diathesis Haemorhagica 28: 182–193

Glueck H I, Roehill W 1966 Myocardial infarction in a patient with Hageman (factor XII) defect. Annals of Internal Medicine 64: 390–396

Griffin J H 1977a New hypothesis for the molecular mechanism of surface-dependent activation of Hageman factor (factor XII). Thrombosis and Haemostasis 38: 50

Griffin J H 1977b Molecular mechanisms of surface-dependent activation of Hageman factor (HF) (coagulation factor XII). Federation Proceedings 36: 314

Griffin J H 1978 Role of surface in surface-dependent activation of Hageman factor (blood coagulation Factor XII). Proceedings of the National Academy of Sciences 75: 1998–2002

Griffin J H, Cochrane C G 1976 Mechanisms for the involvement of high molecular weight kininogen in surface-dependent reactions of Hageman factor. Proceedings of the National Academy of Sciences 73: 2554–2558

Habel F M, Burrowes C E, Movat H Z 1976 Generation of kinin by plasma kallikrein and plasmin and the effect of α^1-antitrypsin and antithrombin III on the kininogenases. In: Sicuteri F, Back N, Haberland G L (eds) Kinins, pharmacodynamics and biological role. Plenum Press, New York, p 23

Han Y N, Kato H, Iwanaga S, Oh-ishi S, Katori M 1978 Primary structure of bovine plasma high-molecular weight kininogen. Characterization of carbohydrate-free fragment 1.2 (fragment X) released by the action of plasma kallikrein and its biological activity. Journal of Biochemistry 83: 213–221

Han Y N, Kato H, Iwanaga S, Suzuki T 1976 Bovine plasma high molecular weight kininogen: the amino acid sequence of fragment 1 (glycopeptide) released by the action of plasma kallikrein and its location in the precursor protein. FEBS Letters 63: 197–200

Han Y N, Komiya M, Iwanaga S, Suzuki T 1975a Studies on the primary structure of bovine high-molecular weight kininogen. Amino acid sequence of a fragment ('Histidine-rich peptide') released by plasma kallikrein. Journal of Biochemistry 77: 55–68

Han Y N, Komiya M, Kato H, Iwanaga S, Suzuki T 1975b Primary structure of bovine high molecular weight kininogen: chemical compositions of kinin-free kininogen and peptide fragments released by plasma kallikrein. FEBS Letters 57: 254–258

Harpel P C 1972 Studies on the interaction between collagen and a plasma kallikrein-like activity. Evidence for a surface-active enzyme system. Journal of Clinical Investigation 51: 1813–1822

Harpel P C 1973 Studies on human plasma α_2-macroglobulin-enzyme interactions. Evidence for proteolytic modification of the subunit chain structure. Journal of Experimental Medicine 138: 508–521

Hathaway W E, Belhasen L P, Hathaway H S Evidence for a new thromboplastin factor: Case report, coagulation studies and physicochemical studies. Blood 26: 521–532

Heber H, Geiger R, Heimburger N 1978 Human plasma kallikrein: purification, enzyme characterization and quantitative determination in plasma. Hoppe-Seyler's Zeitschrift für Physiologische Chemie 359: 659–669

Heck L W, Kaplan A P 1974 Substrates of Hageman factor I. Isolation and characterization of human factor XI (PTA) and inhibition of the activated enzyme by α_1-antitrypsin. Journal of Experimental Medicine 140: 1615–1630

Hedner U 1979 Inhibition of Hageman factor by a fibrinolytic inhibitor. Thrombosis and Haemostasis 42: 262

Hirsche E F, Nagajima T, Oshima G, Erdös E G, Herman C M 1974 Kinin system responses in sepsis after trauma in man. Journal of Surgical Research 17: 147–153

Hoak J C, Swanson L W, Warner E D 1966 Myocardial infarction associated with severe factor XII deficiency. Lancet 2: 884–886

Horowitz H I, Fujimoto M M 1965 Association of factors XI and XII with blood platelets. Proceedings of the Society for Experimental Biology and Medicine 119: 487–492

Jacobsen S 1966 Substrates for plasma kinin-forming enzymes in human, dog and rabbit plasma. British Journal of Pharmacology 26: 403–411

Kaplan A P, Austen K F 1970 A prealbumin activator of prekallikrein. Journal of Immunology 105: 802–811

Kaplan A P, Austen K F 1971 A prealbumin activator of prekallikrein II. Derivation of activators of prekallikrein from active Hageman factor by digestion with plasmin. Journal of Experimental Medicine 133: 696–712

Kato H, Han Y N, Iwanga S, Suzuki T, Komiya M 1976 Bovine plasma HMW and LMW kininogens. Structural differences between heavy and light chains derived from kinin-free proteins. Journal of Biochemistry 80: 1299–1311

Kato H, Sugo T, Ikari N, Hashimoto N, Iwanaga S, Fujii S 1979 Role of bovine HMW kininogen in contact-mediated activation of factor XII: Demonstration of a nicked form, 'active kininogen', with maximal cofactor activity by limited proteolysis. Thrombosis and Haemostasis 42: 262

Kisiel W, Fujikawa K, Davie E W 1977 Activation of bovine factor VII (proconvertin) by factor XIIa (activated Hageman factor). Biochemistry 16: 4189–4194

Koide T, Kato H, Davie E W 1977 Isolation and characterization of bovine factor XI (plasma thromboplastin antecedent). Biochemistry 16: 2279–2286

Komiya M, Kato H, Suzuki T 1974 Bovine plasma kininogens I. Further purification of high molecular weight kininogen and its physicochemical properties. Journal of Biochemistry 76: 811–822

Kurachi K, Davie E W 1977 Activation of human factor XI (plasma thromboplastin antecedent) by factor XIIa (activated Hageman factor). Biochemistry 16: 5831–5839

Laake K, Österud B 1974 Activation of purified plasma factor VII by human plasmin, plasma kallikrein, and activated components of the human intrinsic blood coagulation system. Thrombosis Research 5: 759–772

Laake K, Venneröd A M 1974 Factor XII induced fibrinolysis: studies on the separation of prekallikrein, plasminogen proactivator, and factor XI in human plasma. Thrombosis Research 4: 285–302

Liu C Y, Scott C F, Bagdasarian A, Pierce J V, Kaplan A P, Colman R W 1977 Potentiation of the function of Hageman factor fragments by high molecular weight kininogen. Journal of Clinical Investigation 60: 7–17

Lutcher C L. 1976 Reid trait: A new expression of high molecular weight kininogen (HMW-kininogen) deficiency. Clinical Research 24: 47

McConnell D J 1972 Inhibitors of kallikrein in human plasma. Journal of Clinical Investigation 51: 1611–1623

McMillin C R, Saito H, Ratnoff O D, Walton A G 1974 The secondary structure of human Hageman factor (factor XII) and its alteration by activating agents. Journal of Clinical Investigation 54: 1312–1322

Mandle R Jr, Kaplan A P 1977 Hageman factor substrates. Human plasma prekallikrein: mechanism of activation by Hageman factor and participation in Hageman factor-dependent fibrinolysis. Journal of Biological Chemistry 252: 6097–6104

Mandle Jr R, Colman R W, Kaplan A P 1976 Identification of prekallikrein and HMW kininogen as a circulating complex in human plasma. Proceedings of the National Academy of Sciences 73: 4179–4183

Margolis J 1958 Activation of plasma by contact with glass:evidence for a common reaction which releases plasma kinin and initiates coagulation. Journal of Physiology 144: 1–22

Mason J W, Colman R W 1971 The role of Hageman factor in disseminated intravascular coagulation induced by sepsis neoplasia or liver disease. Thrombosis et Diathesis Haemorrhagica 26: 325–331

Mason J W, Kleeberg U R, Dolan P, Colman R W 1970 Plasma kallikrein and Hageman factor in gram negative bacteremia. Annals of Internal Medicine 73: 545–551

Matheson R T, Miller D R, Lacombe M-J, Han Y N, Iwanaga S, Kato H, Wuepper K D 1976 Flaujeac factor deficiency. Reconstitution with highly purified bovine high molecular weight kininogen and delineation of a new permeability enhancing peptide released by plasma kallikrein from bovine high molecular weight kininogen. Journal of Clinical Investigation 58: 1395–1406

Meier H L, Pierce J V, Colman R W, Kaplan A P 1977 Activation and function of human Hageman factor. The role of high molecular weight kininogen and prekallikrein. Journal of Clinical Investigation 60: 18–31

Nossel H L, Niemetz J 1965 A normal inhibitor of the blood coagulation contact reaction product. Blood 25: 712–723

O'Donnell T F, Clowes G H Jr, Talamo R C, Colman R W 1976 Kinin activation in the blood of patients with sepsis. Surgery, Gynecology and Obstetrics 143: 539–545

Oh-ishi S, Katori M, Han Y N, Iwanaga S, Kato H, Suzuki T 1977 Possible physiological role of new peptide fragments released from bovine high molecular weight kininogen by plasma kallikrein. Biochemical Pharmacology 26: 115–120

Pizzuto J, Garcia N, Reyna M P, Conte G, Ambriz R 1979 Factor XII deficiency and thrombosis. Thrombosis and Haemostasis 42: 236

Radcliffe R, Bagdasarian A, Colman R, Nemerson Y 1977 Activation of bovine factor VII by Hageman factor fragments. Blood 50: 611–617

Ratnoff O D, Colopy J E 1955 A familial hemorrhagic trait associated with a deficiency of a clot-promoting fraction of plasma. Journal of Clinical Invetigation 34: 602–613

Ratnoff O D, Rosenblum J M 1958 Role of Hageman factor in the initiation of clotting by glass: evidence that glass frees Hageman factor from inhibition. American Journal of Medicine 25: 160–168

Ratnoff O D, Saito H 1979a Interactions among Hageman factor, plasma kallikrein, high molecular weight kininogen, and plasma thromboplastin antecedent. Proceedings of the National Academy of Sciences 76: 958–961

Ratnoff O D, Saito H 1979b Amidolytic properties of single-chain activated Hageman factor. Proceedings of the National Academy of Sciences 76: 1461–1463

Ratnoff O D, Busse R J, Sheon R P 1968 The demise of John Hageman. New England Journal of Medicine 279: 760–761

Ratnoff O D, Pensky J, Donaldson V H, Amir J 1972 The inhibitory properties of plasma against activated plasma thromboplastin antecedent (factor XIa) in hereditary angioneurotic edema, Journal of Laboratory and Clinical Medicine 80: 803–809

Ratnoff O D, Pensky J, Ogston D, Naff G B 1969 The inhibition of plasmin, plasma kallikrein, plasma permeability factor and the C'lr subcomponent of the first component of complement by serum C'1 esterase inhibitor. Journal of Experimental Medicine 129: 315–331

Revak S D, Cochrane C G 1976 The relationship of structure and function in human Hageman factor. The association of enzymatic and binding activities with separate regions of the molecule. Journal of Clinical Investigation 57: 852–860

Revak S D, Cochrane C G, Bouma B N, Griffin J H 1978 Surface and fluid phase activities of two forms of activated Hageman factor produced during contact activation of plasma. Journal of Experimental Medicine 147: 719–729

Revak S D, Cochrane C G, Griffin J H 1977 The binding and cleavage characteristics of human Hageman factor during contact activation. Comparison normal plasma with plasma deficient in factor XI, prekallikrein, or high molecular weight kininogen. Journal of Clinical Investigation 59: 1167–1175

Revak S D, Cochrane C G, Johnston A R, Hugli T E 1974 Structural changes accompanying enzymatic activation of human Hageman factor. Journal of Clinical Investigation 54: 619–627

Rimon A, Schiffman S, Feinstein D I, Rapaport S I 1976 Factor XI activity and factor XI antigen in homozygous and heterozygous factor XI deficiency. Blood 48: 165–174

Saito H 1977 Purification of high molecular weight kininogen and the role of this agent in blood coagulation. Journal of Clinical Investigation 60: 584–594

Saito H, Goldsmith G H 1977 Plasma thromboplastin antecedent (PTA, factor XI): a specific and sensitive radioimmunoassay. Blood 50: 377–385

Saito H, Ratnoff O D 1975 Alteration of factor VII activity by activated Fletcher factor (a plasma kallikrein): a potential link between the intrinsic and extrinsic blood-clotting systems. Journal of Laboratory and Clinical Medicine 85: 405–415

Saito H, Goldsmith G H, Moroi M, Aoki N 1979a Inhibitory spectrum of α_2-plasmin inhibitor. Proceedings of the National Academy of Sciences 76: 2013–2017

Saito H, Goldsmith G, Waldmann R 1976a Fitzgerald factor (high molecular weight kininogen) clotting activity in human plasma in health and disease in various animal plasmas. Blood 48: 941–947

Saito H, Ratnoff O D, Donaldson V H, Haney G, Pensky J 1974 Inhibition of the adsorption of Hageman factor (Factor XII) to glass by normal human plasma. Journal of Laboratory and Clinical Medicine 84: 62–73

Saito H, Ratnoff O D, Pensky J 1976b Radio-immunoassay of human Hageman factor (factor XII). Journal of Laboratory and Clinical Medicine 88: 506–514

Saito H, Ratnoff O D, Waldmann R, Abraham J P 1975 Fitzgerald trait. Deficiency of a hitherto unrecognised agent, Fitzgerald factor, participating in surface-mediated reactions of clotting, fibrinolysis, generation of kinins, and the property of diluted plasma enhancing vascular permeability (PF/Dil). Journal of Clinical Investigation 55: 1082–1089

Saito H, Scott J G, Movat H Z, Scialla S J 1979b Molecular heterogeneity of Hageman trait (factor XII deficiency). Evidence that two of 49 subjects are cross-reacting material positive (CRM+). Journal of Laboratory and Clinical Medicine 94: 256–265

Schiffman S, Lee P 1974 Preparation, characterization, and activation of a highly prufied factor XI: evidence that a hitherto unrecognized plasma activity participates in the interaction of factors XI and XII. British Journal of Haematology 27: 101–114

Schiffman S, Lee P, Feinstein D I, Pecci R 1977 Relationship of contact activation factor (CAC) procoagulant activity to kininogen. Blood 49: 935–945

Schreiber A D, Kaplan A P, Austen K F 1973 Inhibition by CĪINA of Hageman factor fragment activation of coagulation, fibrinolysis and kinin generation. Journal of Clinical Investigation 52: 1402–1409

Scott C F, Colman R W 1980 Function and immunochemistry of prekallikrein-high molecular weight kininogen complex in plasma. Journal of Clinical Investigation 65: 413–421

Stead N, Kaplan A P, Rosenberg R D 1976 Inhibition of activated factor XII by antithrombin-heparin cofactor. Journal of Biological Chemistry 251: 6481–6488

Stormorken H, Abildgaard C F 1974 The Fletcher factor-prekallikrein deficiency: a diagnostic test which identifies heterozygotes. Thrombosis Research 5: 373–378

Swedenborg J, Kourias E, Olsson P 1979 Coagulation activity of surface activated plasma in vivo. Thrombosis Research 16: 231–237

Thompson R E, Mandle R Jr, Kaplan A P 1977 Association of factor XI and high molecular weight kininogen in human plasma. Journal of Clinical Investigation 60: 1376–1380

Thompson R E, Mandle R Jr, Kaplan A P 1978 Characterization of human high molecular weight kininogen. Journal of Experimental Medicine 147: 488–499

Tuszynski G P, Walsh P N 1979 Platelet membrane factor XI substitutes for plasma factor XI. Thrombosis and Haemostasis 42: 36

Ulevitch R J, Letchford D, Cochrane C G 1974 A direct enzymatic assay for the esterolytic activity of activated Hageman factor. Thrombosis et Diathesis Haemorrhagica 31: 30–39

Venge P, Dahl R, Hällgren R 1979 Enhancement of factor XII dependent reactions by eosinophil cationic protein. Thombosis Research 14: 641–649

Venneröd A M, Laake K, Solberg A K, Strömland S 1976 Inactivation and binding of human plasma kallikrein by antithrombin III and heparin. Thrombosis Research 9: 457–466

Vogt W 1964 Kinin formation by plasmin: an indirect process mediated by activation of kallikrein. Journal of Physiology 170: 153–166

Vogt W, Dugal B 1976 Generation of an esterolytic and kinin-forming kallikrein-α_2-macroglobulin complex in human serum by treatment with acetone. Naunyn-Schmiedebergs Archives of Pharmacology 294: 75–84

Walsh P N 1972a Albumin density gradient separation and washing of platelets and the study of platelet coagulant activities. British Journal of Haematology 22: 205–217

Walsh P N 1972b The role of platelets in the contact phase of blood coagulation. British Journal of Haematology 22: 237–254

Walsh P N 1972c The effects of collagen and kaolin on the intrinsic coagulant activity of platelets. Evidence for an alternative pathway in intrinsic coagulation not requiring factor XII. British Journal of Haematology 22: 393–405

Walsh P N, Griffin J H 1979 Human platelets promote the proteolytic activation of factor XII. Thrombosis and Haemostasis 42: 36

Wiggins R C, Cochrane C G 1979 The autoactivation of rabbit Hageman factor. Journal of Experimental Medicine 150: 1122–1133

Wiggins R C, Bouma B N, Cochrane C G, Griffin J Γ¯ 1977 Role of high-molecular weight kininogen in surface-binding and activation of coagulation factor XI and prekallikrein. Proceedings of the National Academy of Sciences 74: 4636–4640

Wiggins R C, Cochrane C G, Griffin J H 1979 Rabbit blood coagulation factor XI. Purification and properties. Thrombosis Research 15: 475–486

Wiggins R C, Loskutoff D J, Cochrane C G, Griffin J H 1980 Activation of rabbit Hageman factor by homogenates of cultured rabbit endothelial cells. Journal of Clinical Investigation 65: 197–206

Wilner G D, Nossel H L, Leroy E C 1968 Activation of Hageman factor by collagen. Journal of Clinical Investigation 47: 2608–2615

Wuepper K D 1973 Prekallikrein deficiency in man. Journal of Experimental Medicine 138: 1345–1355

Wuepper K D, Cochrane C G 1972 Plasma prekallikrein: isolation, characterisation, and mechanism of action. Journal of Experimental Medicine 135: 1–20

Wuepper K D, Miller D R, Lacombe M J 1975 Flaujeac trait: deficiency of human plasma kininogen. Journal of Clinical Investigation 56: 1663–1672

5. Progress in fibrinolysis

*E. J. P. Brommer   P. Brakman   F. Haverkate   C. Kluft
D. Traas   G. Wijngaards*

INTRODUCTION

As soon as fibrin is deposited in a ruptured vessel or in a wound, its eventual breakdown is prepared for: plasminogen, the zymogen of plasmin, is adsorbed onto the surface of the fibrin polymers, together with activators that are present locally or in the circulating blood.

Activation of plasminogen to plasmin will take place upon the surface of fibrin, and plasmin, tempered by specific inhibitors, will break down fibrin to split products that are carried away and removed elsewhere from the circulating blood.

This view of plasmin-mediated, 'classical' fibrinolysis, which encompasses the specificity of plasmin for fibrin and the latest ideas on the role of the main plasmin inhibitor, α_2-antiplasmin, has emerged slowly and is based on several lines of evidence. The course of events depicted above can for the purpose of clarity be divided into four parts, which will be dealt with successively:

1. Plasminogen and plasmin.
2. Plasminogen activators.
3. Inhibitors of fibrinolysis.
4. Breakdown of fibrin to degradation products.

This will be followed by a brief review of recent advances in the knowledge of alternative, non-plasmic fibrinolysis.

Plasminogen and plasmin

In normal physiology, the plasminogen-plasmin enzyme system is still regarded as the main fibrinolytic system in the blood. Plasminogen is present in plasma and serum at a fairly constant level of 10–20 mg/100 ml or ~1–2 μmol/l. It is probably synthesized in the liver. Definite proof is still lacking but this is suggested by low levels of plasminogen in liver disease, and by the change of the genetic type of plasminogen to that of the donor after hepatic homotransplantation (Raum et al, 1980).

Plasminogen can be assayed immunologically (radial diffusion plates are available commercially), or functionally. Functional assay, formerly performed in a caseinolytic test system or on plasminogen-free fibrin plates, is substantially simplified by the commercial availability of the synthetic substrates such as S-2251, or Chromozym PL, and non-commercial variants suitable for specific purposes. In the functional assay methods plasminogen is activated to plasmin by urokinase (UK) or streptokinase (SK): the amount of substrate hydrolyzed during a fixed period of time or the rate of hydrolysis is a measure of the concentration of plasminogen.

The structure of plasminogen has been unravelled further in the last few years. The complete amino-acid sequence of its single polypeptide chain, consisting of 791

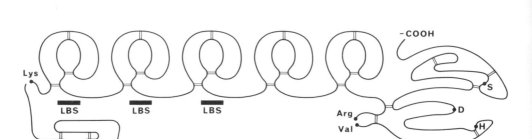

Fig. 5.1   Model of plasmin(ogen) molecule. Three lysine-binding sites (LBS) are tentatively indicated near kringle structures of heavy chain. Native plasminogen has NH₂-terminal amino glutamic acid (Glu), partially degraded Lys-plasminogen ends with lysine 78 (Lys). Active centre in light chain is composed of serine (S), histidine (H) and arginine (D) residues. Activation occurs by cleavage of peptide bond between arginine 561 (Arg) and valine 562 (Val). Disulphide bridges are indicated.

residues, MW 92 000, is now known. For detailed information the reader is referred to review articles by Wiman (1978) and by Wallén (1978) and to the contribution of Sottrup-Jensen et al (1978).

Essentially, the plasmin(ogen) molecule appears to consist of two parts, one harbouring the active site and highly homologous to pancreatic serine esterases and to the corresponding chains of prothrombin and factor Xa, the other bearing the binding regions, rendering it an affinity for fibrin. The latter part contains five almost identical triple loop structures, named kringles after Scandinavian biscuits of this form. Comparable kringle structures have been found to be constituents of prothrombin and factor X molecules, indicating a descent of these related serine esterases from a common ancestor molecule.

The activation of plasminogen to plasmin by urokinase and presumably by other activators occurs by the cleavage of a peptide bond between the two above-mentioned parts of the molecule, splitting the single polypeptide chain into two smaller ones, a heavy chain with the binding region and a light chain with the active centre. Although these chains remain linked to each other by disulphide bridges, this cleavage is enough to elicit the proteolytic ability of the enzyme: plasmin.

The activation of plasminogen to plasmin is susceptible to modulation not only for therapeutic purposes but also under normal conditions. Most data collected up to now are compatible with the hypothesis that the binding of the (pro)enzyme to its substrate is of utmost importance for the regulation of fibrinolysis (Collen & Wiman, 1979b). Breakdown of fibrin by plasmin in vitro is counteracted by relatively high concentration of ε-aminocaproic acid (EACA) or analogous substances like tranexamic acid etc., used for this purpose also in clinical medicine. This inhibiting action has been related to the binding of EACA to plasmin(ogen) and is used as the principle of the isolation of plasminogen from blood. Lysine, if bound with its α-amino group to Sepharose, resembles EACA and binds plasminogen. When plasma is passed through a column made up of this Lysine-Sepharose, the plasma can be cleared almost completely of plasminogen. The adsorbed plasminogen can be recovered from the column by elution with EACA (Deutsch & Mertz, 1970).

The effect has been attributed to the presence of so-called 'lysine-binding sites' of the plasminogen molecule. Presumably, complementary structures, resembling EACA are exposed on the surface of fibrin molecules and display an affinity for the lysine-binding sites of plasminogen and plasmin (Wiman & Wallén, 1977).

Lysine-binding sites have been located in at least three of the kringles of the plasminogen molecule. Kinetic studies have provided evidence for the existence of two or three more lysine-binding sites of the molecule, the exact location of which is not yet known. At least one of the lysine-binding sites supposedly has a function in the conformation of the plasminogen molecule (Wiman & Wallén, 1975), which impedes the conversion of plasminogen to plasmin.

In purified systems, low concentrations of EACA enhance the activation of plasminogen by UK, presumably by the induction of a conformational change in the plasminogen molecule. This might be brought about by the release of a 'lysine-binding site', occupied by a complementary group of the same molecule. This conformational change is reversible, and enables the plasminogen molecule to attach itself faster to fibrin; it also facilitates the activation by UK.

In vivo this conformational change of plasminogen, rendering the molecule susceptible for activation appears to be obtained by complexing with α_2-antiplasmin (Wiman et al, 1979). This explains perhaps why no adverse effects in the sense of paradoxical hyperfibrinolysis or fibrinogenolysis are seen during oral therapy with EACA or tranexamic acid, while very low concentrations will exist in the blood regularly.

For some time it has been known that the activation of plasminogen to the functioning enzyme plasmin involves two enzymatic cleavages (Wiman & Wallén, 1973). A small peptide chain, MW $\sim$ 8000, is split off from the NH_2-terminal part of the plasminogen molecule. The new molecule is named Lys-plasminogen after its new NH_2-terminal amino acid, a lysine residue; the native plasminogen, with glutamine as its NH_2-terminus, is called Glu-plasminogen. This partial degradation has an enhancing effect upon the activation of the enzyme by UK and it increases the affinity for fibrin (Thorsen, 1975) and for α_2-antiplasmin (Wiman et al, 1979) probably by the exposure of lysine-binding sites. This is also manifested by the greater adsorption to plasma clots (Soria et al, 1978; Juhan et al, 1979). The cleavage can be achieved in vitro by plasmin. In vivo presumably traces of plasmin in the clot are enough to convert Glu-plasminogen to Lys-plasminogen. This conversion occurs easily during isolation procedures and only rigorous precautions have enabled it to be proved that in normal blood only Glu-plasminogen exists.

Actual activation to plasminogen occurs by cleavage of the peptide bond between Arg_{561} and Val_{562} converting the zymogen to the enzyme plasmin.

In vitro, plasmin is a potent proteolytic enzyme, capable of attacking many proteins, among which are several clotting factors. In vivo its action is largely restricted to the breakdown of fibrin. This specificity is brought about by at least three factors.

1. plasminogen (especially Lys-plasminogen) attaches itself preferentially to fibrin,
2. plasminogen activators also have an affinity for fibrin; their activity is greatly enhanced by contact with fibrin; so plasminogen is converted to plasmin primarily at the surface of fibrin,

3. free plasmin is immediately bound and neutralized by α_2-antiplasmin or α_2-macroglobulin.

Unrestrained action of plasmin in the body, even if only directed towards fibrin would be detrimental and would lead to precocious removal of fibrin deposits and hence to bleeding. The action of plasmin is therefore controlled by a number of factors (apart from the synthesis of fibrinolytic (pro)enzymes):

1. the availability of plasminogen activator might be a limiting factor;
2. inhibitors curtail the proteolytic activity of plasmin by competing for lysine-binding sites of plasminogen and plasmin, or by blocking the active site of free enzyme.

These factors will be dealt with separately.

Plasminogen activators

The active enzyme plasmin is formed by partial proteolysis of plasminogen. This is brought about by specific enzymes, called plasminogen activators. Urokinase is the most extensively studied plasminogen activator of human origin. It is found in great quantities in the urine and is secreted by cultured human embryonic kidney cells, in amounts large enough to produce it on a commercial scale. Until recently, knowledge of plasminogen activation was largely derived from studies with urokinase (reviewed by Duckert, 1978).

Plasminogen activator in the blood

Despite great progress in technical facilities the presence of urokinase in the blood is still a matter of dispute. The plasminogen activator found in the blood is supposed to be released by the vascular endothelium. As early as 1959, Todd demonstrated with a histological technique that plasminogen activator was present in the endothelial lining of blood vessels. Recently, the synthesis of activator by endothelial cells has been confirmed in cell cultures (Loskutoff & Edgington, 1977). Plasminogen activator can be extracted from various animal and human tissues or can be harvested from tissue cultures (Bernik et al, 1979). Rijken et al (1979) succeeded in the purification and characterization of an activator from human uterine tissue. It appeared to have a molecular weight of 69 000 dalton and to consist of two chains with molecular weights of 31 000 and 38 000, held together by disulphide bridges. The serine residue of the active site was located on the lighter chain. The plasminogen activator showed a strong tendency to adsorb onto surfaces. In a later study Rijken (1980) was able to produce an antibody against this plasminogen activator, with which he demonstrated the identity of the tissue-derived plasminogen activator and the vascular activator. The tissue activator appeared to differ both immunologically and functionally from urokinase.

Functional differences between urokinase and tissue activator of animal origin had been found earlier. In contrast to urokinase, tissue activator is adsorbed onto fibrin clots (Thorsen et al, 1972) and in a purified system plasmin formation by tissue activator is greatly enhanced by the presence of fibrin (Camiolo et al, 1971; Wallen, 1978), but not by urokinase. These properties of tissue activator can now confidently be ascribed to the circulating plasminogen activator. Thus, since both plasminogen and its activator are adsorbed onto the surface of fibrin, it is reasonable to assume that in the living organism activation of plasminogen to plasmin will occur preferentially, if not solely, at this locus. Therefore, plasmin will be generated only when fibrin is present.

Extrinsic and intrinsic plasminogen activation system
Normal blood or plasma, taken from a resting individual exerts practically no fibrinolytic action in a clot lysis test or on plasminogen-rich fibrin plates. Fibrinolytic activity can only be detected after reduction of the influence of inhibitors by dilution or by euglobulin fractionation. The fibrinolytic activity of the blood, measured in this way, reflects predominantly the level of circulating plasminogen activator and changes in fibrinolytic activity, observed in these tests should be attributed mainly to differences in the level of vascular endothelial activator.

In the fibrin plate method, the greater part of the fibrinolytic activity of euglobulin fractions can be inhibited by C1 inactivator, a naturally occurring inhibitor of a component of the complement system (Trumpi-Kalshoven, 1978). The small fibrinolytic fraction, resistant to C1 inactivator was shown by Rijken (1980) to correspond with the activity, extinguished by antibody against tissue-derived plasminogen activator. It is referred to as 'extrinsic' plasminogen activator, to distinguish it from the remaining lytic activity in the euglobulin fractions, attributed to an 'intrinsic' activation system. The fibrinolytic activity of euglobulin fractions increases dramatically during physical or mental straining. 'Venous occlusion' of the forearm by maintaining the pressure in a circular cuff for 5 to 25 minutes above diastolic blood pressure also is a potent stimulus for the fibrinolytic activity of the blood.

In the fibrin plate method this gain of activity is resistant to inhibition by C1 inactivator (Kluft, 1978). Therefore, it can be attributed to a rise in extrinsic, i.e., vascular plasminogen activator.

Physiological and pharmacological regulation of fibrinolysis
It is generally accepted that the vascular plasminogen activator is released by the vascular endothelium under the influence of specific stimuli. The factors transmitting the stimulus to the vessel wall are not yet fully understood.

Adrenalin has a stimulating effect. Yet, the conclusion that the release is under adrenergic control is premature. The stimulating effect of exogenous adrenalin can be blocked only partially by β-receptor blocking drugs (Cash & Woodfield, 1969; Ingram & Vaughan Jones, 1969; Gader et al, 1974; Mannucci, 1974). During exercise a high level of adrenalin occurs and fibrinolytic activity rises not withstanding β-blockade (Britton et al, 1976). α-blockade seems not to influence the fibrinolytic effect induced by adrenalin (Tanser & Smellie, 1964; Cash et al, 1970; Rosing et al, 1978). Obviously, adrenalin can induce a rise in plasminogen activator via other, still unknown ways.

Intravenous injection of vasopressin, a vasoactive drug related to antidiuretic hormone, raises the level of plasminogen activator in the blood (Mannucci, 1974). Some of its analogues, e.g., DDAVP (1-desamino-8-D-arginine vasopressin), though practically devoid of vasoactive effect, are among the most potent drugs with respect to the heightening of the activator level in the blood (Gader et al, 1974; Cash et al, 1978; Åberg et al, 1979).

This substance also raises the concentration of clotting factor VIII (Mannucci et al, 1975; Prowse et al, 1979; Åberg et al, 1979), which is released by vascular endothelium by the same stimuli as plasminogen activator.

The mode of action of DDAVP is unknown. DDAVP has no effect upon the release of plasminogen activator in isolated pig ears (Markwardt & Klöcking, 1976, 1978) or in rat hindquarters (Emeis et al, 1981). A complex interaction between vessel wall and central nervous influences was surmised by Markwardt & Klöcking (1976). Cash et al (1978) found no change in activator level in venous blood of a volunteer after intra-arterial administration of DDAVP in the same arm. Cash put forward the hypothesis that a hypothalamic hormone might mediate the stimulus. Indeed, Cort and Dodds (1979) found a substance, released by the brains of dogs and capable of inducing a rise in factor VIII in peripheral vessels. The humoral transmitter was released by the brain in response to DDVAP or an analogue into the internal carotid artery.

Relevance of systemic plasminogen activator level

What is the significance of the concentration of plasminogen activator as measured in blood? The rise of activator level during stress suggests that it has a physiological role in circumstances of 'fight and flight'. It is conceivable, but not proven, that the higher the plasminogen activator level, the faster the removal of fibrin from the bloodstream. Possibly, the rise is intended to keep pace with the increase in factor VIII under the same circumstances.

The rate of fibrin formation, occurring even during normal life as a result of wear and tear, might be elevated during stress. A concomitant plasmin generation may be expected. Collen et al (1977) tried to answer the question whether the changes in clotting and fibrinolytic parameters during exercise are accompanied by actual prothrombin and/or plasminogen activation followed by fibrinogen to fibrin conversion and fibrino(geno)lysis. They measured the turnover of fibrinogen, plasminogen and prothrombin in untrained healthy volunteers during strenuous exercise. A temporary, significant increase in the catabolism of fibrinogen and plasminogen was observed. The appearance of plasmin-antiplasmin complexes indicated plasmin generation during the experiment, and the partial degradation of fibrinogen noted in blood samples taken two hours after exercise, indicated the action of plasmin. From the fact that prothrombin turnover did not change measurably, the authors concluded that fibrinogenolysis occurred without (increased) fibrin formation. It seems justifiable to conclude from the above-mentioned study, that increased plasmin generation takes place during strenuous exercise. However, the formation of small amounts of fibrin is not excluded. At present, most investigators including Collen (1979), favour the view that plasmin is formed in blood only in the presence of fibrin.

Since we know that excessive fibrinolysis — as in congenital α_2-antiplasmin deficiency (see below) — can cause spontaneous haemorrhage, one might expect bleeding if high plasminogen activator levels result in plasmin generation.

To our knowledge bleeding has never been reported in healthy individuals in situations where high fibrinolytic activity can be anticipated or measured. Only in patients with compromised coagulation, as in severe haemophilia, has the conjecture been made (Astrup et al, 1961).

Owing to its effect on the release of factor VIII, DDAVP is used in the treatment of haemorrhage in moderate haemophilia and Von Willebrand's disease (Mannucci et al, 1977; Lowe et al, 1977; Boulton & Smith, 1978; Kobayashi, 1979). To avoid possible bleeding complications by the concomitant rise of the plasminogen activator level, clinicians give tranexamic acid simultaneously. In the treatment of haemorrhage from oesophageal varices with vasopressin, however, this is not common practice. Yet vasopressin proves to be effective in the control of bleeding due to the vasoconstrictive action (see Conn et al, 1975). Does the fibrinolytic activity measured in venous blood represent adequately the ability of the body to get rid of fibrin formed during everyday life? This important question cannot yet be answered conclusively. It is the more relevant and important since low levels of plasminogen activator are incriminated as the cause of thromboembolism and since oral fibrinolytic therapy is aimed at the elevation of basal activator concentrations.

Local factors enhancing fibrinolysis
Can local fibrin formation exert an additional stimulus to the vessel wall in order to create a higher activator level locally? Markwardt and Klöcking (1976, 1978) and Emeis et al (1980) demonstrated in experimental animals that bradykinin, formed during contact activation, is a potent stimulator of activator release. Possibly this plays a part locally at the site of fibrin deposition or formation. Can the plasminogen activator concentration close to a clot be raised by circulating proenzymes, for instance, via the contact activation system?

The concept of an intrinsic pathway leading to the activation of plasminogen as opposed to an extrinsic system is attractive, not least, because of the parallel with the coagulation cascade. Several groups of investigators have presented evidence for an activator system in plasma, capable of activating plasminogen. Probably, many different proteins are engaged and various sequences of enzymatic reactions may induce an increase in fibrinolytic activity in vitro.

The involvement of factor XII in contact activation of fibrinolysis was suggested by the observation by Niewiarowski and Prou-Wartelle in 1959, that kaolin-induced euglobulin clot lysis was slower in Hageman trait plasma than in normal plasma. Other factors involved in surface-mediated initiation of blood coagulation, such as high molecular kininogen and prekallikrein (see Ogston's contribution to this volume), also influence the results of fibrinolytic assays (Kluft, 1979). Apart from activated Hageman factor (Goldsmith et al, 1978), kallikrein and factor XIa, both dependent upon the presence of surface-mediated Hageman factor, are capable of activating plasminogen directly (Mandle & Kaplan, 1979). In a purified system, however, they are weak activators. Kluft (1980) estimated the activity of kallikrein to be in the order of 10^4 less than the activity of urokinase and tissue activator. The requirement for fibrinolysis of a proactivator, distinct from the factors known to be associated with contact activation, is still in dispute.

In 1974, Astrup and Rosa showed that fibrinolytic activity could be generated by dextran sulphate even in the absence of Hageman factor. They postulated a factor XII-independent proactivator system in human blood. The measurement of the fibrinolytic activity upon fibrin plates using dextran sulphate proves to be a useful supplement to the existing test methods (Kluft, 1979).

Venous occlusion or addition of tissue activator causes an increase in the fibrinolytic activity of euglobulin fractions prepared in the presence of dextran sulphate. This increment appeared to be resistant to C1 inactivator but could be neutralized by an antibody against tissue activator (Rijken, 1980). On the contrary, the fibrinolytic activity of euglobulin fractions from plasma taken without previous stimulation and prepared with dextran sulphate and flufenamate (a synthetic fibrinolytic agent that suppresses inhibitors) was not influenced by anti-tissue activator antibody, but could be blocked by C1 inactivator, indicating the intrinsic generation of activity. Thus, in vitro, an inventory can be made of the extrinsic and intrinsic pathways of plasminogen activation, and in clinical material their functional integrity can be tested. A new adjuvant in the distinction of the various pathways was found in an inhibitor derived from the blood fluke Schistosoma mansoni. A substance extracted from this parasite appears to counteract specifically the factor XII-independent plasminogen activation in the dextran sulphate-triggered assay (Kluft, et al, 1978).

Significance of intrinsic activation system
The physiological relevance of the extrinsic fibrinolytic system is beyond doubt. On the contrary, the role of the intrinsic system in the removal of fibrin in vivo is uncertain. In plasma samples of normal resting individuals, the amount of extrinsic activator is very low. On account of the almost total suppression of fibrinolytic action by C1 inactivator in this case, euglobulin clot lysis is assumed to be caused mainly by the intrinsic fibrinolytic system. Yet an antibody directed against the extrinsic tissue activator abolishes clot lysis completely (Rijken, 1980). This suggests that the intrinsic activation of fibrinolysis, observed in regular euglobulin fractions, is not an independent system, but is contingently tied to the action of tissue activator. Since the dextran sulphate-induced lysis is only partially suppressed by anti-tissue activator, as was discussed before, it may be concluded that some polyanions can generate fibrinolytic activity independently of the extrinsic system. It is intriguing to know whether fibrinolysis can be enhanced within the body in a comparable way, for instance, by polyanionic substances like chondroitin sulphate (Coccheri et al, 1978).

Clinical support for the contribution of an intrinsic fibrinolytic system to the removal of fibrin is meagre. An unimpaired contact activation system does not seem to be important for normal physiology: factor XII-deficiency (Hageman trait), lack of prekallikrein (Fletcher trait) or of high molecular kininogen (Fitzgerald trait) are all symptomless conditions, detected only accidentally. The thromboembolic events in the terminal disease of Mr Hageman (Ratnoff et al, 1968) does not contradict this. Hedner (1973) found a high level of an inhibitor of fibrinolysis in patients with a thrombotic tendency. This inhibitor appeared to inactivate factor XIIa in a clotting assay (Hedner & Martinsson, 1978). She also described a number of patients with thrombosis, who had an IgG antibody against factor XIIa (Hedner & Nilsson, 1976). If a causal relationship exists between the inactivation of factor XIIa in vitro and thrombosis, and if thrombosis in these patients was a consequence of impaired fibrinolysis, it might be suggested that factor XII is important for fibrinolysis, perhaps more than for coagulation.

Clinical evidence for impaired fibrinolysis, caused by a deficient factor XII-independent pathway has not yet been presented.

Inhibitors of fibrinolysis
The last few years have witnessed a revolution in the concept of the physiological

function of fibrinolytic inhibitors. Several plasma proteins and low molecular weight substances in blood and urine have been isolated, which evidently reduce fibrinolysis in vitro, or can even bind plasmin. However, the discovery of the fast-acting α_2-plasmin inhibitor (α_2-antiplasmin) has pushed into the background the other inhibiting substances except α_2-macroglobulin.

α_2-antiplasmin is a single-chain polypeptide, MW 65-70 000, migrating on electrophoresis as an α_2-globulin, and synthesized by liver parenchymal cells (Aoki & Yamanaka, 1978). It binds plasmin very effectively, forming a 1:1 stoichiometric complex, devoid of protease activity (Muellertz & Clemmensen, 1976; Moroi & Aoki, 1976; Wiman & Collen, 1977). It prevents the occurrence of free plasmin in blood even to the extent that infusion of purified plasmin (up to a certain amount of course) is harmless (Hedner et al, 1978; Collen & Verstraete, 1979). Generalized plasmin action, as is aimed at in thrombolytic therapy, is obtained only after binding of all available α_2-antiplasmin by plasmin. In purified systems, α_2-antiplasmin reacts slowly with urokinase, kallikrein, factor Xa and thrombin (Moroi & Aoki, 1976, 1977). In plasma α_2-antiplasmin does not bind thrombin or chymotrypsin (Edy & Collen, 1977) nor leucocyte proteases like elastase and chymotrypsin-like enzyme (Ohlssen & Collen, 1977). α_2-antiplasmin inhibits plasmin, and in addition it decreases the binding of Lys-plasminogen to fibrin 30 times more effectively than EACA (Aoki et al, 1978b).

During clotting of blood, approximately 22 per cent of α_2-antiplasmin is covalently bound to fibrin. This binding is dependent upon the presence of factor XIII (fibrin-stabilizing factor, FSF) and calcium ions (Sakata & Aoki, 1980). This explains why serum levels of α_2-antiplasmin are lower than plasma levels. Sakata & Aoki demonstrated that the adsorption of α_2-antiplasmin on to fibrin was an effective mechanism for the inhibition of fibrinolysis by plasmin. Since thrombin is necessary for the activation of FSF, α_2-antiplasmin was not bound to fibrin during clotting initiated by batroxobin, a snake venom. This may help to understand why defibrination in vivo by snake venoms does not give rise to thromboembolic phenomena.

α_2-antiplasmin can be measured immunologically and functionally. The functional assay determines α_2-antiplasmin indirectly by its immediate inhibiting action on the proteolytic activity of plasmin on a synthetic substrate (Naito & Aoki, 1978; Edy et al, 1978; Gallimore et al, 1979). The plasma level of α_2-antiplasmin is about 60 mg/l or 0.9 μM (Aoki & Yamanaka, 1978). The normal plasminogen concentration in plasma is about 1.5 μM. It can be calculated from these molar concentrations that enough α_2-antiplasmin is present to bind about 70 per cent of plasmin, if all plasminogen was to be converted and provided that the plasmin formed is within reach of α_2-antiplasmin. However, about one-third of the α_2-antiplasmin present in normal blood does not appear to bind plasmin as effectively as the rest (Clemmensen, 1979). The equilibrium between these two forms of α_2-antiplasmin may be important for the physiological regulation of fibrinolysis (Clemmensen et al 1979). In any case the effective level will be lower than the level actually measured, and sufficient to bind approximately 50 per cent of total plasmin. The calculation is still more complicated by the fact that the level of free plasminogen is reduced by a factor of two by complex formation with another natural inhibitor of fibrinolysis, histidine-rich protein (Lijnen et al, 1980).

The bleeding tendency of two cases of congenital α_2-antiplasmin deficiency (Koie et al, 1978; Kluft et al, 1979) denotes the relevance of this inhibitor for haemostasis. The study of these cases helped enormously in the comprehension of the function of this inhibitor and at the same time threw doubt upon the physiological importance of other inhibitors with regard to fibrinolysis. This is strengthened by the fact that familial α_2-macroglobulin deficiency is an asymptomatic condition (Bergquist & Nilsson, 1979).

Since both plasminogen concentration and plasminogen activator level in plasma are normal in congenital α_2-antiplasmin deficiency (Aoki, 1979), one might expect signs of plasmin action, for example manifesting itself in the breakdown of fibrinogen. Nevertheless, no fibrinogenolysis could be detected, while the bleeding tendency in this condition points to a too rapid removal of fibrin by unrestrained plasmin action. This is obviously not controlled by normal or even elevated levels of α_2-macroglobulin, α_1-antitrypsin, C1-esterase inhibitor and other inhibiting substances. Lipinski and Gurewich (1979) regarded this observation as an argument for their hypothesis of the existence of an anti-activator. The circulating anti-activator-activator complex would dissociate only in the presence of fibrin, thus protecting other proteins like fibrinogen. Rational deductions are, however, the following (Collen, 1979): (1) plasmin is only formed from plasminogen within the clot or upon the surface of fibrin, (2) the activity of plasmin is mitigated by α_2-antiplasmin and (3) other inhibitors have little influence upon the fibrin splitting action of plasmin. Acquired α_2-antiplasmin deficiency may occur in liver disease (Aoki & Yamanka, 1978; Teger-Nilsson, 1978). When the plasminogen level does not drop to the same extent, the occurrence of free plasmin in the blood can be anticipated in an earlier stage during plasminogen activation. Apart from calamities like DIC, excessive fibrinolysis as a consequence of α_2-antiplasmin deficiency is to be expected only when level are the very low, or when it is absent. This is the case in homozygous congenital α_2-antiplasmin deficiency.

The presence of plasmin-α_2-antiplasmin complexes in plasma signifies plasmin formation, hence fibrinolysis. Collen et al (1977) developed a rapid latex agglutination test to measure plasmin-α_2-antiplasmin complexes in human plasma. Due to the rather long survival time of these complexes ($T\frac{1}{2} = \sim12$ hrs), the detection of the complex may provide information on the involvement of fibrinolysis in complicated haemorrhagic and thrombotic disorders. In case of considerable fibrinolysis α_2-antiplasmin levels will fall and changes in fibrinogen and plasminogen will also be seen. The monitoring of these values in plasma has been proposed as a useful parameter during thrombolytic therapy (Collen & Verstraete, 1979).

Recently, Lijnen et al (1980) discovered a new natural inhibitor of fibrinolysis. The so-called 'histidine-rich glycoprotein', described in 1972 by Haupt and Heimburger, appears to interfere with the binding of plasminogen to fibrin by the interaction with one or more of the lysine-binding sites of plasminogen, comparable to EACA.

Apart from circulating inhibitors, inhibitors present in tissues, e.g., in the arterial wall (Noordhoek Hegt & Brakman, 1977) and in blood platelets (Mui et al, 1975; Joist et al, 1976) should receive attention, because they might have an essential, though local function in regulating fibrinolysis in the body. Recently, a fast-acting plasmin inhibitor has been isolated from platelets and purified by Sandbjerg Hansen and Clemmensen (1980). It differs from the known plasma proteinase inhibitors. Functionally it shows similarities to α_2-antiplasmin, it has an equally high reaction rate with purified plasmin. This supports the idea that the platelet inhibitor is primarily an inhibitor of plasmin. From various human tissues, inhibitors can be extracted in water with physiological salt concentration, isolated and purified.

Placenta has been studied most extensively. The placental inhibitor, however, could not be demonstrated in the blood of pregnant women. Nevertheless, it is not excluded that the fall in fibrinolytic activity of the blood during pregnancy is caused by the production of this inhibitor (Holmberg & Åstedt, 1979). Concerning the specificity of this inhibitor, Wijngaards (1979) found that placental preparations inhibited urokinase, both in a fibrinolytic test system and on synthetic substrates. This inhibitor behaved slightly differently towards tissue activator; the activity on a synthetic substrate was unaffected, whereas considerable inhibition was found in fibrinolytic assays. Similar methods are being applied in the search for inhibitors derived from tumour tissue and for pathological fibrinolytic inhibitors in plasma of patients with thrombotic tendency (see below).

Fibrin degradation

Some interesting developments in the research of fibrin degradation are noteworthy. Though tests for assay of FDP are commercially available and in general use in hospital laboratories, much has still to be learned about the processes determining the type of degradation products appearing in the blood, about the discrimination between fibrinolysis and fibrinogenolysis in vivo and about the properties and physiological functions of the different degradation products.

The first small fragment split off from fibrin by plasmin, the carboxy-terminal of the Aα-chain, has been isolated by Harfenist and Canfield (1975) and determined by radioimmunoassay (Harfenist et al, 1975). A radioimmunoassay has also been developed for a (MW 28 000) fragment obtained by chemical cleavage with cyanogenbromide, and partially identical with the early plasmic product (Blombäck et al, 1976). Gollwitzer et al (1977) employed a radioimmunoassay for the demonstration of a similar fragment (MW 30 000) in order to detect early plasmin action in patients. The values found in healthy donors were very low and indicated that less than 0.1 per cent of fibrinogen Aα-chain is degraded under normal conditions. This estimation differs considerably from that obtained by the authors referred to above and from the results obtained with a different method used by Semeraro et al (1977). These investigators found approximately 13 per cent degraded Aα-chains in purified normal fibrinogen, but had to leave open the question of whether the degradation occurred in vivo or — at least partially — during the isolation procedure in vitro.

Gollwitzer et al found an increase in Aα-chain fragments in patient sera correlating with an increased level of soluble monomer complexes. Clinical application of a radioimmunoassay raised against isolated and purified fragment A, a comparable early plasmin degradation product, was reported by Takagi and Kawai (1978). They found a significant increase of this fragment A above normal levels in a variety of diseases, but unfortunately they did not mention correlation with other data which could confirm actual breakdown of fibrin. Despite the obvious difficulties of this approach to the demonstration of plasmin action in disease, the theoretical advantages warrant further evaluation.

According to Nossel (1979), a modified fibrinopeptide B assay can be used to detect plasmin action; Bβ-chain fragments are cleaved from the amino-terminal of the

Bβ-chain of fibrin(ogen) to form fragment X. Levels of this Bβ-chain fragment (Bβ 1–42) rose in association with pulmonary embolism and with resolution of thrombosis.

Some progress has been achieved in the discrimination between fibrinolysis and fibrinogenolysis in patient plasma by determination of cross-linked fibrin degradation products and of neo-antigens expressed on fibrin fragments after cleavage. Lane et al (1977) could not conclusively demonstrate D-dimer fragments in serum of patients during thrombolytic therapy, by means of polyacrylamide gel electrophoresis of a solid phase immunoprecipitate (immunoabsorption by shaking diluted serum with anti-fibrinogen-coated sepharose, Lane et al, 1976). With the same technique, however, they obtained strong evidence for the presence of D-dimer fragments in serum of patients with disseminated intravascular coagulation (Lane et al, 1978).

Immunological techniques depend on the availability of suitable antisera. Plow and Edgington (1971; 1973a, 1973b) were fortunate to produce an antibody discerning neo-antigenic determinants of D-fragments of fibrinogen, distinct from antigen or fibrin derived D-fragments. With this antibody they were able to demonstrate both fibrin and fibrinogen breakdown in various diseases: dependent upon the patient examined, the percentage of fibrin-derived FDP ranged from 0–100 per cent. Remarkably, in a case of fatal haemorrhage during abruptio placentae, studied by these authors, fibrinogen degradation products were found exclusively. This observation needs confirmation before definite conclusions may be drawn.

Later in other centres, studies could be performed with antibodies which allowed fibrinolysis and fibrinogenolysis to be distinguished. Budzynski et al (1979) produced an antibody directed against antigenic markers which distinguished D-dimer fragments from plasmic derivatives of non-cross-linked fibrin and fibrinogen. But they had not then developed a method that could be applied to clinical material. Lee-Own et al (1979) also managed to raise an antibody against D-dimer and D'Alisa et al (1979) and Lahiri et al (1979) reported on their successful production of an antibody against chemically reduced cross-linked γ-chain fragments and the development of a radioimmunoassay capable of detecting minute amounts of the cross-linked γ-peptides. It is to be hoped that these previously unattainable developments will eventually lead to widely applicable methods for clinical use. The future production of monoclonal antibodies by mouse myeloma and spleen cell hybridomas is promising in this respect.

Analysis of fibrin(ogen) degradation products and their properties has been performed principally by means of breakdown of fibrinogen in vitro. The discovery by Haverkate and Timan (1977) that the presence of calcium ions in physiological concentrations is essential for obtaining late fragments, comparable to those expected to originate in vivo, explained many controversies in the literature. Furthermore, it allowed the localization of the structural abnormality of fibrinogen Pontoise, obtained from a case of dysfibrinogenemia, in the β-chain of the D-moiety (Haverkate et al, 1978).

Leucocyte proteases
Other proteolytic enzymes may attack fibrin independently of the classical fibrinolytic system described above. Proteases derived from leucocytes have received much attention during recent years. Their place in human pathology is, however, far from established. They might be less fastidious than plasmin and not degrade fibrin

preferentially. They may also attack other plasma proteins, including fibrinogen, resulting in a condition designated 'primary fibrinogenolysis'. A number of leucocyte proteases capable of cleaving fibrinogen and fibrin at physiological pH have been described. They include elastase (Ohlsson & Olsson, 1974) and a chymotrypsin-like protease (Schmidt & Havemann, 1974). Both enzymes could be demonstrated immunologically in the plasma of patients with acute leukaemia and septicaemia, whereas in normal plasma and in some other diseases they were undetectable (Egbring et al, 1977). The enzymes appeared to form a complex with antiproteases (α_1-antitrypsin and α_2-macroglobulin) rapidly after their release from leucocytes, but this did not abolish their amidolytic activity on synthetic substrates. The complexes are, however, inactive towards larger natural substrates (Reilly & Travis, 1980). The degradation products resulting from the cleavage of fibrinogen or fibrin by these enzymes in vitro are different from those produced by plasmin (Plow & Edgington, 1975, 1978; Hafter et al, 1980). They can be distinguished by laborious gel filtration and electrophoretic techniques but an elegant method has been devised by Bilezikian and Nossel (1977), based on the presence of fibrinopeptides A and B upon slightly larger dialysable fragments split off by leucocyte proteases. It should be feasible to apply this method to clinical material. Indeed (Gramse et al, 1979) reported her experience with this method in patients and demonstrated FPA-like peptides in blood samples of patients with acute myeloblastic leukaemia and septicaemia. Furthermore, she found high molecular weight fragments, specific for fibrinogen degradation by elastase, by means of an antibody against neo-antigenic determinants upon these fragments (Gramse et al, 1978). Ohlsson (1979) succeeded in elaborating a radioimmunoassay for human granulocyte elastase and found with this method an increase above normal in 6 out of 22 patients with acute myeloblastic leukaemia. Gel filtration experiments confirmed that essentially all elastase in the plasma was bound by α_1-antitrypsin.

These developments herald a new era in the diagnosis of defibrination syndromes, primary or secondary fibrinolysis and fibrinogenolysis. Distinction between plasmic and non-plasmic digestion of fibrinogen or fibrin is of obvious clinical importance, both for diagnosis and for treatment.

FIBRINOLYSIS IN DISEASE AND DISEASES OF FIBRINOLYSIS

If not a continuous process taking place upon the endothelial lining of normal blood vessels, as proposed by Nolf in 1908, fibrin deposition and removal probably occur on many places in the body in answer to microtrauma, by daily wear and tear.

It is conceivable that the speed of clotting on the one hand and the speed of clot lysis on the other are critical, and that considerable changes in this 'haemostatic balance' produce clinical symptoms, either haemorrhage or thromboembolism.

Spontaneous bleeding can be a consequence of impairment of coagulation but also of unrestricted fibrinolysis, as we have learned from the few cases of congenital α_2-antiplasmin deficiency.

A *thrombotic tendency* likewise may be the result of one of two disturbances of the haemostatic balance: either too prompt fibrin formation or too slow removal of fibrin deposited in a blood vessel, may cause thrombosis, at least theoretically.

In liver disease the blood level of several fibrinolytic factors, either produced or cleared by the liver, may be abnormal. The possible consequences have been reviewed recently by Ratnoff (1977).

Recurrent thrombosis

Virtually all factors of the fibrinolytic system have been incriminated as potentially capable of causing a thrombotic tendency. Often, however, the claim is based on the concurrence of the deviation of a single laboratory test and an ill-defined clinical condition, or rather while other possible causal factors are not assessed, e.g. a high fibrinogen level, increased platelet stickiness, spontaneous aggregation, circulating activated clotting factors, etc. Moreover, it is extremely difficult to obtain reliable data from fibrinolytic assays: the fibrinolytic activity falls during storage of the samples and apparently arises from contact with foreign surfaces like metal (puncture needle) glass and proteins adherent to platelets may influence results.

Low or abnormal plasminogen

Low *plasminogen* levels represent a bad prognosis in liver disease (Biland et al, 1978). In several liver diseases, however, synthesis of other proteins may be impaired likewise and low plasminogen levels cannot be regarded as causing thrombosis if, for instance, antithrombin III levels are not determined, not to mention levels of fibrinogen and other clotting factors including factor XIII and, in the case of cirrhosis, clearance of plasminogen activator, i.e. level of circulating extrinsic (tissue) activator.

Aoki et al (1978a) studied a patient with recurrent thrombosis who appeared to have an inherited abnormality of the structure and function of the plasminogen molecule. The enzymatic activity of plasminogen in a caseinolytic assay was abnormally low, but a normal level of immunoreactive plasminogen was found. Other members of this family, too, were regarded as heterozygotes because they had half-normal levels of activity. One member, apparently homozygote, had practically no plasminogen activity. Nevertheless, the proband was the only one who suffered from thrombosis. The authors suggest that this condition predisposes to a thrombotic tendency once the initial thrombotic event has occurred. Similar plasminogen abnormalities may not be too rare. Robbins et al (1979) reported on five cases of abnormal plasminogen, that were not normally able to be activated by urokinase or streptokinase. Once formed, plasmin seemed to behave perfectly normally.

In our opinion, the thrombotic tendency described in congenital dysfibrinogenemia should be studied from the same fibrinolytic point of view: the affinity for plasmin might be altered adversely by a molecular deviation of fibrin, analogous to the defective binding of thrombin in some cases of dysfibrinogenemia (Liu et al, 1979).

Impaired activation of plasminogen

Nilsson and her group added further cases to the published list of patients with thrombosis, who appeared not to respond to venous occlusion and/or infusion of DDAVP (Johansson et al, 1978). A causal relationship was suggested. Steele et al (1978) also found impaired response to venous occlusion associated with recurrent thrombosis. However, they did not find decreased lytic activity as an isolated abnormality. Furthermore, normalization of blood lytic activity did not reduce the occurrence of venous thrombosis. Widespread endothelial damage causes deficiency of blood and tissue fibrinolytic activity, as Browse et al (1977) reported in patients with vascular disorders, accompanied by recurrent superficial thrombophebitis or venous liposclerosis. Angles-Cano et al (1979) observed the absence of a rise in plasminogen activator after venous occlusion in patients with systemic lupus erythematosus which might predispose to the thromboembolic events known to occur in this disease.

Fibrinolytic shut-down after surgical operations might be responsible for deep-vein thrombosis (DVT) (Comp et al, 1979). Little is known about the relative importance of the many factors involved. The surgical procedure itself or the anaesthesia obviously are not the only factors, as the eventual development of DVT after surgery can be predicted preoperatively by assessment of the fibrinolytic activity in a euglobulin clot lysis test (Clayton et al, 1976; Rakoczi et al, 1978). This statement, which is in disagreement with earlier observations (Becker, 1972), is remarkable since resting levels of fibrinolytic activity are seldom regarded as indicative of the fibrinolytic potential of the blood. Response to stimulation or diurnal rhythm presumably are better parameters. In the case of the preoperative forecast of postoperative DVT, Vermylen and Chamone (1979) postulated that thrombosis could already be developing before the operation. This problem might be solved by the recently introduced technique of Nossel et al (1979), who found elevated fibrinopeptide A levels, signalling thrombin action, several days preceding postoperative thrombosis, whereas the level of $B\beta$ 1–42, indicating plasmin action, rose only after pulmonary embolism or DVT had become manifest.

Taberner et al (1979) observed — contrary to expectation — that in patients in whom DVT eventually developed, α_2-antiplasmin concentration did not rise as soon after operation as in patients without DVT. In their opinion this delay in recovery is secondary to an impairment of fibrinolysis.

In some other conditions low fibrinolytic activity has been found in plasma without any artificial stimulus. In Behçet's syndrome, a puzzling disease characterized by oral and genital lesions, uveitis, skin eruptions and thrombophlebitis, low fibrinolytic activity has been observed by Chajek et al (1973). In this disease the matter is complicated by the presence of substances which interfere with euglobulin precipitation, while a true impairment of fibrinolysis in this disease may be caused by inhibitors (Kluft et al, 1980).

Likewise, a correlation between a prolonged euglobulin clot lysis time and thrombosis has been reported in malignancy (Samuels, 1979). Here also inhibitors should be determined before a judgement can be passed.

Excessive inhibition of fibrinolysis

Abnormally high inhibition of several different fibrinolytic factors, detected in widely varying test systems, have been described in connection with thrombosis. As early as 1961, Nilsson et al described pathological inhibition of fibrinolysis in a lysis test as a cause of thrombosis. In 1966 Brakman et al observed different inhibitory activities in plasma using a fibrin plate assay. Dependent upon the enzyme used they could define inhibiting activity against plasmin, urokinase or tissue activator. They attributed the thrombotic tendency of a number of patients to the presence of an inhibitor against tissue activator (Brakman & Astrup, 1970). High levels of urokinase inhibition have been described in malignancy (Hisazumi et al, 1974).

Recently, Yuen et al (1979) reported the finding of increased inhibitory activity against fibrinolysis in malignant solid tumour tissue using a histochemical fibrin slide technique. Isolation and characterization of tumour-derived inhibitors, as well as their assessment in blood and comparison with other inhibitors is awaited with interest.

In blood of patients with the microembolism syndrome as a consequence of traumatic insufficiency, a substance inhibiting fibrinolysis was detected by Bagge et al (1978) in a clot lysis method. Isolation and purification of the inhibitor yielded a protein immunologically identical to α_2-antiplasmin (Bagge et al, 1979).

Based on the premise that an intact intrinsic activator system is essential for fibrinolysis, disturbance of contact activation may be expected to lead to persistence of fibrin deposits and thrombi. The terminal thromboembolism of Mr Hageman has been mentioned already. Hedner and Nilsson (1976) described an IgG-antibody directed against factor XIIa in patients with a history of thrombosis and in their judgement, a causal relationship is plausible. In a family with severe thrombotic tendency they discovered a new inhibitor, which inactivated bovine factor XIIa in a clotting assay. The inhibitor was characterized as an α_2-globulin, MW 75 000 (Hedner, 1973). Recently it appeared to be immunologically and functionally distinct from α_2-anti-plasmin (Hedner & Collen, 1976).

Obviously, fibrinolysis can be impeded by many different substances, each only detectable by a particular method. The impairment may reach such a degree as to promote thrombosis. Simple screening techniques for the detection of impairment of fibrinolysis are clearly needed for adequate diagnosis in a larger number of patients and for the tracing of pathological inhibitors in various disease states.

During recent years it has been appreciated that not only quantitative changes in blood levels of (pro)enzymes and substrates can cause impairment of fibrinolysis, but also qualitative alterations of molecular structure of these proteins. Congenital abnormalities of structure and functional behaviour of plasminogen and fibrinogen have already been found. One should be prepared to detect functionally abnormal molecules of other fibrinolytic factors, too.

Haemorrhage

There is little doubt that premature removal of fibrin from the tear of a damaged blood vessel will promote bleeding.

'Hyperfibrinolysis' has long been listed as a cause of haemorrhage but this concept was based mainly on the bleeding tendency in disseminated intravascular coagulation. Apart from the fact that the short euglobulin clot lysis time and comparable parameters in this condition are largely due to the low fibrinogen level, it is doubtful whether bleeding in this syndrome is caused by 'hyperfibrinolysis' in the sense of pathologically increased fibrinolytic activity, surpassing the demand. Rather, bleeding should be attributed to imperfect fibrin clot formation due to the presence of large amounts of fibrin split products, interfering with fibrin polymerization.

Likewise, the term 'activated fibrinolysis', often used in biochemical papers, is a misnomer, when used to designate clinical conditions where signs of plasmin action, like FDP's or plasmin-α_2-antiplasmin complexes, are detectable.

For the clinician, terms like 'hyperfibrinolysis' and 'activated fibrinolysis' are associated with inappropriate stimulation of processes that are to be counteracted. In most clinical situations this counteraction will be unhelpful, if not detrimental. Is haemorrhage ever a consequence of a disturbance of the regulation of fibrinolysis? The only fibrinolytic factor known to be regulated in a physiological sense by neuro-hormonal control, is the level of extrinsic plasminogen activator, revealed for instance by euglobulin lysis tests. Evidence for bleeding due to inappropriately high levels of activator is lacking, with the possible exception of stress-induced bleeding in severe coagulation disorders. The only clinical condition in which bleeding is attributed irrefutably to a too rapid fibrinolysis is congenital α_2-antiplasmin deficiency. As discussed previously, the precocious lysis of fibrin in this disorder is ascribed to the action of plasmin, unrestrained by the inhibitor. This condition is exceedingly rare: despite a large-scale search for it in many centres only two cases have been described to date.

NEW TRENDS IN FIBRINOLYTIC THERAPY

Excellent review articles cover the present day status of therapeutic potential (Vogel, 1978; Duckert, 1978; Verstraete, 1978; Samama, 1979; etc.). Discussion of this subject will be confined to a few remarks about interesting, though not yet fully explored, new ways in fibrinolytic treatment.

With regard to thrombolytic therapy, some authors claim that the efficacy of treatment with urokinase or streptokinase can be improved by modulations of the usual regimen. Verstraete et al (1978) re-evaluated the intermittent administration of streptokinase and drew attention to the good therapeutic results without bleeding complications. Brochier et al (1977) and Kakkar (1978) reported successful treatment of pulmonary emboli and deep vein thrombosis with intermittent infusions of plasminogen and streptokinase. Combination of streptokinase (Kakkar, 1978) or urokinase (Juhan et al, 1979) with heparin in order to prevent ongoing fibrin deposition was not satisfactory. In view of the many relations between thrombin action and fibrinolysis, this experience raises intriguing questions about the cause of this failure. In experimental animals the efficacy of urokinase, inferred from the results of euglobulin lysis assays, could be improved by the simultaneous administration of low molecular weight dextran sulphate (Matsuo et al, 1978).

Fundamental questions about the action of thrombolytics in whole blood or plasma have been answered recently. High doses of urokinase are required to induce fibrinolysis in plasma or in the patient. Analyzing the changes in α_2-antiplasmin level during thrombolytic therapy with urokinase and streptokinase, Collen and Verstraete (1979) observed that depletion of α_2-antiplasmin was accompanied by extensive systemic fibrinolysis, whereas only moderate fibrinolysis occurred when α_2-antiplasmin level fell to 50 per cent of normal. Studies with infusions of human plasmin confirmed the hypothesis that plasminaemia only occurred after depletion of α_2-antiplasmin. Hayashi and Yamada (1979) also found a correlation between fibrinolysis and low α_2-antiplasmin levels after urokinase treatment. Remarkably, immunoreactive α_2-antiplasmin sometimes remained as high as 30 to 60 per cent of preinfusion values despite definitive thrombolytic effect (Samama, 1978; Hedner et al, 1978; Aoki, 1979; Hayashi & Yamada, 1979). Part of the α_2-antiplasmin appears to remain in the circulation in an altered, inactive form (Collen & Wiman, 1979b). Attempts to induce thrombolysis by the inhibition of α_2-antiplasmin with synthetic fibrinolytic agents have not been very successful. In the case of ortho-thymotic acid, the failure has been attributed to the narrow range of its effective concentration (Prandini et al, 1978). Yet, the exploitation of the principle of inducing thrombolysis by capturing α_2-antiplasmin seems to be warranted.

The combination of an anabolic steroid, stanazolol, with a biguanide, phenformin or metformin, still appears to be the most effective mode of long-term oral fibrinolytic therapy (Samama, 1979; Burnand et al, 1980). The practical application of this therapy has been curtailed by the withdrawal of biguanides from the market in some countries. In at least one study, therapy with anabolic steroids alone was able to maintain previously diminished euglobulin lysis within a normal range for a long time (Walker & Davidson, 1979). However, Steele et al (1978) question whether normalization of lytic activity will reduce the occurrence of thrombosis. Unfortunately, methods to check the biological effect of the fibrinolytic activity measured, are still lacking. Again, the need for suitable test methods is evident.

CONCLUSION

A survey of the last few years' contributions to the knowledge of fibrinolysis reveals stimulating advances in many respects. On the other hand some elementary questions are still open and progress in therapeutic possibilities is disappointing.

The application and perfection of affinity chromatography has advanced biochemical research in this field enormously. Notable accomplishments have been made in unravelling structures, improving isolation procedures, and in determining kinetic aspects of the main factors involved in fibrinolysis. Interestingly, former diverging theories on the mechanism by which the action of plasmin in the blood is restricted to fibrin are united in the latest views on fibrinolysis. Above all, the appreciation of the role of lysine-binding sites in the attachment of plasmin on to fibrin, and the discovery of the functions of the main natural inhibitor, α_2-antiplasmin, have augmented our knowledge of the complex process resulting in removal of fibrin from the body. A positive acquisition — from the clinicians' point of view — is the insight gained into the function of fibrinolysis in the maintenance of the haemostatic balance.

Involvement of fibrinolysis in many critical and life-threatening disorders, often accompanied by bleeding, was known for a long time, but convincing evidence that an unimpaired fibrinolytic system is fundamental to normal physiology emerged only during the last few years. Especially the discovery that α_2-antiplasmin deficiency gives rise to a serious haemorrhagic diathesis has aided in the understanding not only of the importance of fibrinolysis but also of some of its basal mechanisms. It has to be stressed that some of the major advances were due largely to the alertness of the clinician in notifying unusual cases of bleeding or thrombosis and referring them to specialized centres.

The successful production of specific antibodies has enabled major advances to be made in the assay of plasminogen activators, leucocyte proteases and fibrin(ogen) degradation products. Enzyme studies have been greatly facilitated by sensitive and specific synthetic substrates. Simple screening techniques are, however, badly needed to be employed in the clinical laboratory for the detection and control of abnormal fibrinolysis. This will help to close the gap between clinic and laboratory.

Supported by Praeventiefonds, project number 28–443.

BIBLIOGRAPHY

Åberg M, Nilsson I M, Vilhardt H 1979 The release of fibrinolytic activator and factor VIII after injection of DDAVP. In: Davidson J F, Čepelák V, Samama M M, Desnoyers P C (eds) Progress in Chemical Fibrinolysis and Thrombolysis, Raven Press, New York, Vol 4, p 92–97

d'Alisa R M, Lahiri B, Birkens S, Yang C C, Canfield R E, Nossel H L, Butler V P 1979 Antibodies to carboxy-terminal fibrin γ-γ-cross-linked peptide. Federation Proceedings 38: 996

Angles-Cano E, Sultan Y, Clauvel J P 1979 Predisposing factors to thrombosis in systemic lupus erythematosus. Possible relation to endothelial cell damage. Journal of Laboratory and Clinical Medicine 94: 312–323

Aoki N, Moroi M, Matsuda K, Tachiya K 1977 The behaviour of α_2-plasmin inhibitor in fibrinolytic states. Journal of Clinical Investigation 60: 361–369

Aoki N, Moroi M, Sakada Y, Yoshida N, Matsuda M 1978 An abnormal plasminogen. A hereditary molecular abnormality found in a patient with recurrent thrombosis. Journal of Clinical Investigation 61: 1186–1195

Aoki N, Moroi M, Tachiya K 1978b Effects of α_2-plasmin inhibitor on fibrin clot lysis. Its comparison with α_2-macroglobulin. Thrombosis and Haemostasis 39: 22–31

Aoki N, Yamanaka T 1978 The α_2-plasmin inhibitor levels in liver disease. Clinica Chimica Acta 84: 99–105

Aoki N, Saito H, Kamiya T, Koie K, Sakata Y, Kobakura M 1979 Congenital deficiency of α_2-plasmin inhibitor associated with severe hemorrhagic tendency. Journal of Clinical Investigation 63: 877–884

Astrup T, Brakman P, Ollendorff P, Rasmussen J 1961 Haemostasis in haemophilia in relation to the haemostatic balance in the normal organism and the effect of peanuts. Thrombosis et Diathesis Haemorrhagica 5: 329–340

Astrup T, Rosa A T 1974 A plasminogen proactivator-activator system in human blood effective in absence of Hageman factor. Thrombosis Research 4: 609–613

Bagge L, Björk I, Saldeen T, Wallin R 1978 Purification of a fibrinolysis inhibitor in serum from post-traumatic patients. Thrombosis and Haemostasis 39: 97–108

Bagge L, Saldeen T 1978 The primary fibrinolysis inhibitor and trauma. Thrombosis Research 13: 1131–1136

Becker J 1972 Fibrinolytic activity of the blood and its relation to postoperative venous thrombosis of the lower limbs. Acta Chirurgica Scandinavica 138: 787–792

Bergquist D, Nilsson I M 1979 A family with α_2-macroglobulin deficiency. Thrombosis and Haemostasis 42: 219 (Abstract)

Bernik M B, Rijken D C, Wijngaards G 1979 Production of two immunologically distinct plasminogen activators by human tissue in culture. Thrombosis and Haemostasis 42: 414

Biland L, Duckert F, Prisender S, Nijman D 1978 Quantitative estimation of coagulation factors in liver disease. The diagnostic and prognostic value of factor XIII, factor V and plasminogen. Thrombosis and Haemostasis 39: 646–656

Bilezikian S B, Nossel H L 1977 Unique pattern of fibrinogen cleavage by human leukocyte proteases. Blood 50: 21–28

Blombäck M, Blombäck B, Holmqvist H 1976 Immunological characterization of early fibrinogen degradation products. Thrombosis Research 8: 567–577

Boulton F E, Smith A 1979 DDAVP and cryoprecipitate in mild haemophilia. Lancet ii: 535

Brakman P, Mohler E R, Astrup T 1966 A group of patients with impaired plasma fibrinolytic system and selective inhibition of tissue activator-induced fibrinolysis. Scandinavian Journal of Haematology 3: 389–398

Brakman P, Astrup T 1970 Selective inhibition of tissue plasminogen activator in thrombotic disease. XIIIth International Congress on Hematology, Munich, Abstract Volume p 173

Britton B J, Wood W C, Smith M, Hawkey C, Irving M H 1976 The effect of beta adrenergic blockade upon exercise-induced changes in blood coagulation and fibrinolysis. Thrombosis and Haemostasis 35: 396–402

Brochier M, Planiol T, Griguer P, Raynaud P, Fauchier J P, Charbonnier B, Latour F, Pellois A 1977 Intérêt du traitement séquentiel lysyl-plasminogène-urokinase en thérapeutique thrombolytique. Coeur et Médecine Interne 16: 513–521

Browse N L, Gray L, Jarrett P E M, Morland M 1977 Blood and vein-wall fibrinolytic activity in health and vascular disease. British Medical Journal 1: 478–481

Budzinski A Z, Marder V J, Parker M E, Shames P, Brizuela B S, Olexa S A 1979 Antigenic markers on fragment DD, a unique plasmic derivative of human crosslinked fibrin. Blood 54: 794–804

Burnand K, Clemenson G, Morland M, Jarrett P E M, Browse N L 1980 Venous lipodermatosclerosis: treatment by fibrinolytic enhancement and elastic compression. British Medical Journal 1: 7–11

Camiolo S M, Thorsen S, Astrup T 1971 Fibrinogenolysis and fibrinolysis with tissue plasminogen activator, urokinase, streptokinase-activated human globulin and plasmin. Proceedings of the Society for Experimental Biology and Medicine 138: 277–280

Cash J D, Woodfield D G 1969 Alterations of fibrinolysis and blood coagulation. Lancet i: 54

Cash J D, Woodfield D G, Allan A G E 1970 Adrenergic mechanisms in the systemic plasminogen activator response to adrenaline in man. British Journal of Haematology 18: 487–494

Cash J D 1978 Control mechanism of activator release. In: Davidson J F, Rowan R M, Samama M M, Desnoyers P C (eds) Progress in Chemical Fibrinolysis and Thrombolysis, Raven Press, New York, Vol 3, p 65–75

Cash J D, Gader A M A, Mulder J L, Cort J H 1978 Structure-activity relations of the fibrinolytic response to vasopressins in man. Clinical Science and Molecular Medicine 54: 403–409

Chajek T, Aronowski E, Izak G 1973 Decreased fibrinolysis in Behçet's disease. Thrombosis et Diathesis Haemorrhagica 29: 610–618

Clayton J K, Anderson J A, McNicol G P 1976 Preoperative prediction of postoperative deep vein thrombosis. British Medical Journal 2: 910–912

Clemmensen I 1979 Different molecular forms of α_2-antiplasmin. In: Collen D, Wiman B, Verstraete M (eds) Physiological Inhibitors of Coagulation and Fibrinolysis, p 131–136

Clemmensen I, Thorsen S, Müllertz S 1979 Functional properties of two different molecular forms of α_2-plasmin inhibitor. Thrombosis and Haemostasis 42: 103 (Abstract)

Coccheri S, De Rosa V, Cavallaroni K, Poggi M 1978 Activation of fibrinolysis by means of sulfated polysaccharides: present status and perspectives. In: Davidson J F, Rowan R M, Samama M M, Desnoyers P C (eds) Progress in Chemical Fibrinolysis and Thrombolysis, Raven Press, New York, Vol 3, p 461–475

Collen D, de Cock F, Cambiaso C, Masson P 1977 A latex agglutination test for rapid quantitative estimation of the plasmin-antiplasmin complex in human plasma. European Journal of Clinical Investigation 7: 21–26

Collen D, Semeraro N, Tricot J P, Vermylen J 1977 Turnover of fibrinogen, plasminogen, and prothrombin during exercise in man. Journal of Applied Physiology 42: 865–873

Collen D 1979 α_2-antiplasmin inhibitor deficiency. Lancet i: 1039–1040

Collen D, Verstraete M 1979 α_2-antiplasmin consumption and fibrinogen breakdown during thrombolytic therapy. Thrombosis Research 14: 631–639

Collen D, Wiman B 1979a Physiological inhibitors of fibrinolysis with special reference to antiplasmin, the fast-acting plasmin inhibitor. In: Neri Serneri G G, Prentice C R M (eds) Haemostasis and Thrombosis, Academic Press, New York, p 187–194

Collen D, Wiman B 1979b Turnover of antiplasmin, the fast-acting plasmin inhibitor of plasma. Blood 53: 313–324

Collen D, Wiman B 1979c The fast-acting plasmin inhibitor of human plasma. In: Davidson J F, Čepelák V, Samama M M, Desnoyers P C (eds) Progress in Chemical Fibrinolysis and Thrombolysis, Churchill Livingstone, Vol 4, p 11–19

Comp P C, Jacocks R M, Taylor F B 1979 The dilute whole blood clot lysis assay: a screening method for identifying postoperative patients with a high incidence of deep venous thrombosis. Journal of Laboratory and Clinical Medicine 93: 120–127

Conn H O, Ramsby G R, Storer E H, Mutchnick M G, Joshi P H, Phillips M M, Cohen G A, Fields G N, Petrosky D 1975 Intra-arterial vasopressin in treatment of upper gastrointestinal haemorrhage: prospective, controlled clinical trial. Gastroenterology 68: 211–221

Cort J H, Dodds W J 1979 Evidence for the existence of a factor VIII releasing factor from the brain released by the action of vasopressin-like cyclic nonapeptides. Blood 54, Suppl 1: p 274a

Duckert F 1978 Urokinase. In: Markwardt F (ed) Fibrinolytics and Antifibrinolytics, Springer, Berlin, p 209–237

Deutsch D G, Mertz E T 1970 Plasminogen: purification from human plasma by affinity chromatography. Science 170: 1095–1096

Edy J, Collen D 1977 The interaction in human plasma of antiplasmin, the fast-reacting plasmin inhibitor, with plasmin, thrombin, trypsin and chymotrypsin. Biochimica et Biophysica Acta 484: 423–432

Edy J, Collen D, Verstraete M 1978 Quantitation of the plasma protease inhibitor antiplasmin with the chromogenic substrate S-2251. In: Davidson J F, Rowan R M, Samama M M, Desnoyers P C (eds) Progress in Chemical Fibrinolysis and Thrombolysis, Raven Press, New York, Vol 3, p 315–322

Egbring R, Schmidt W, Fuchs G, Havemann K 1977 Demonstration of granulocytic protease in plasma of patients with acute leukemia and septicemia with coagulation defects. Blood 49: 219–231

Emeis J J Plasminogen activator in perfusates from isolated perfused rat hindquarter. In preparation

Gader A M A, Da Costa J, Cash J D 1974a The effect of propranolol, alprenolol and practolol on the fibrinolytic and factor VIII responses to adrenaline and salbutamol in man. Thrombosis Research 4: 25–33

Gader A M A, Da Costa J, Cash J D 1974b 1-desamino-8-D-arginine vasopressin and fibrinolysis in man. Scottish Medical Journal 19: 56–57

Gallimore M J, Amundsen E, Aasen A O, Larsbraaten M, Lyngaas K, Svendsen L 1979 Studies on plasma antiplasmin activity using a new plasmin specific chromogenic tripeptide substrate. Thrombosis Research 14: 51–50

Goldsmith G, Saito H, Ratnoff O D 1978 The activation of plasminogen by Hageman factor (factor XII) and Hageman factor fragments. Journal of Clinical Investigation 62: 54–60

Gollwitzer R, Hafter R, Timpl R, Graeff H 1977 Immunological assay for a carboxyterminal peptide of the fibrinogen Aα-chain in normal and pathological human sera. Thrombosis Research 11: 859–868

Gramse M, Bingenheimer C, Havemann K 1978 Granulocyte elastase and its interference with fibrinogen. In: Havemann K, Janoff A (eds) Neutral proteases of human polymorphonuclear leukocytes, Urban and Schwarzenberg, Baltimore-München, p 347–355

Gramse M, Plow E F, Bilezikian S, Havemann K 1979 Two radioimmunoassays for the detection of elastase-like protease-specific fibrinogen degradation products in patients with leukemia and septicemia. Abstract Vth Meeting of the International Society of Haematology, European/African Division, Hamburg, p 27

Hafter R, Petri K, Schiessler H, Graeff H 1980 Vergleich der Spaltungsspezifität von PMN-Leukozytenelastase (LE) und Plasmin gegenüber Fibrinogen, Fibrin und quervernetztem Fibrin. Blut 40: 37

Harfenist E J, Canfield R E 1975 Degradation of fibrinogen by plasmin. Isolation of an early cleavage product. Biochemistry 14: 4110–4117

Harfenist E J, Lauer R C, Canfield R E, Nossel H L 1975 Isolation, characterization and radioimmunoassay of a peptide resulting from limited proteolysis of human fibrinogen by plasmin. Abstract Vth Congress of the International Society of Thrombosis and Haemostasis, Paris, p 408

Haupt H, Heimburger N 1972 Hoppe Seyler's Zeitschrift fuer Physiologische Chemie 353: 1125–1132 and 1133–1140

Haverkate F, Timan G 1977 Protective effect of calcium in the plasmin degradation of fibrinogen and fibrin fragments D. Thrombosis Research 10: 803–812

Haverkate F, Timan G, Soria J, Soria C, Samama M M 1978 Studies on the structure of the fragment D moiety of abnormal fibrinogens: influence of calcium ions. Thrombosis Research 13: 689–692

Hayashi S, Yamada K 1979 Role of α_2-plasmin inhibitor in the appearance of fibrinolytic activity during urokinase administration, and an evaluation of the optimal urokinase dosage. Thrombosis Research 16: 393–400

Hedner U 1973 Studies on an inhibitor of plasminogen activation in human serum. Thrombosis et Diathesis Haemorrhagica 30: 414–424

Hedner U, Collen D 1976 Immunochemical distinction between the inhibitors of plasminogen activation and antiplasmin in human plasma. Thrombosis Research 8: 875–879

Hedner U, Nilsson I-M 1976 Acquired anticoagulants against factors XI and XII in patients with severe thrombotic disease. XVI International Congress of Hematology, Kyoto, Abstract 8–88, p 341

Hedner U, Johansson L, Nilsson I M 1978 Effects of porcine plasmin on the coagulation and fibrinolytic systems in humans. Blood 51: 157–164

Hedner U, Martinsson G 1978 Inhibition of activated Hageman factor by an inhibitor of the plasminogen activation. Thrombosis Research 12: 1015–1023

Holmberg L, Åstedt B 1979 Characterization of placental inhibitor of fibrinolysis. In: Davidson J F, Čepelák V, Samama M M, Desnoyers P C (eds) Progress in Chemical Fibrinolysis and Thrombolysis, Churchill Livingstone, Edinburgh-London, Vol 4, p 402–405

Hornebeck W, Starkey P M, Gordo J L, Legrand Y, Pignaud G, Robert L, Caen J P, Ehrlich H P, Barrett A J 1980 The elastase-like enzyme of platelets. Thrombosis and Haemostasis 42: 1681–1683

Ingram G I C, Vaughan Jones R 1969 Alterations of fibrinolysis and blood coagulation. Lancet i: 310

Isacson S 1970 Effect of prednisone on the coagulation and fibrinolytic system. Scandinavian Journal of Haematology 7: 212–216

Johansson L, Hedner U, Nilsson I M 1978 A family with thromboembolic disease associated with deficient fibrinolytic activity in vessel wall. Acta Medica Scandinavica 203: 477–480

Joist J H, Niewiarowski S, Nath N, Mustard J F 1976 Platelet antiplasmin: its extrusion during the release reaction, subcellular localization, characterization, and relationship to antiheparin in pig platelets. Journal of Laboratory and Clinical Medicine 87: 659–669

Juhan I 1979 Modifications in coagulation parameters induced by treatment associating urokinase (2000 U CTA/kg/h) with heparin. Thrombosis and Haemostasis 42: 945–954

Juhan I, Roux F, Calas M F, Durand F, de la Forte C, Buonocuore M, Juhan C 1979 Binding of ^{99m}Tc-Lys- and ^{99m}Tc-Glu-plasminogen to fibrin. Thrombosis and Haemostasis 42: 390 (Abstract)

Kluft C 1978a Blood fibrinolysis. Thesis, Leiden

Kluft C 1978b Levels of plasminogen activators in human plasma: new methods to study the intrinsic and extrinsic activators. In: Davidson J F, Rowan R M, Samama M M, Desnoyers P C (eds) Progress in Chemical Fibrinolysis and Thrombolysis, Raven Press, New York, Vol 3, p 141–154

Kluft C 1979 Studies on the fibrinolytic system in human plasma: Quantitative determination of plasminogen activators and proactivators. Thrombosis and Haemostasis 41: 365–383

Kluft C, Trumpi-Kalshoven M M, Deelder A M 1979 Factor XII-independent activator generation in human plasma. In: Davidson J F, Čepelák V, Samama M M, Desnoyers P C (eds) Progress in Chemical Fibrinolysis and Thrombolysis, Churchill Livingstone, Edinburgh–London–New York, p 362–367

Kluft C, Vellenga E, Brommer E J P 1979 Homozygous α_2-antiplasmin deficiency. Lancet ii: 206

Kluft C, Wijngaards G, Michiels J J 1980 Factual or artificial inhibition of fibrinolysis and the occurrence of venous thrombosis in Behçet's disease. Scand J Haemat 143: 80–124

Kluft C 1980 Plasminogen activators in human plasms, factor XII-dependent fibrinolysis. In: Peters H (ed) Proteides of the biological fluids. Pergamon Press, Oxford, Vol 28: 372–8

Kobayashi I 1979 Treatment of hemophilia A and von Willebrand's disease patients with an intranasal dripping of DDAVP. Thrombosis Research 16: 775–779

Koie K, Ogata K, Kamiya T, Takamatsu J, Kohakura M 1978 α_2-plasmin inhibitor deficiency (Miyasato disease). Lancet ii: 1334–1336

Lahiri B, Birkens S, Canfield R 1979 Isolation of a crosslinked peptide from human fibrin and development of a radioimmunoassay. Federation Proceedings 38: 996

Lane D A, Scully M F, Kakkar V V 1976 A method for characterizing serum fibrinogen and fibrin degradation products. Thrombosis Research 9: 191–200

Lane D A, Robbins P A, Rampling M W, Kakkar V V 1977 SDS polyacrylamide gel characterization of serum FDP produced in response to ancrod and streptokinase/plasminogen infusion in man. British Journal of Haematology 36: 137–148

Lane D A, Preston F E, Van Ross M E, Kakkar V V 1978 Characterization of serum fibrinogen and fibrin fragments produced during disseminated intravascular coagulation. British Journal of Haematology 40: 609–615

Lee-Own V, Gordon Y B, Chard T 1979 The detection of neo-antigenic sites on the D-dimer peptide isolated from plasmin digested crosslinked fibrin. Thrombosis Research 14: 77–84

Levin E G, Loskutoff D J 1979 Serum-induced suppression of plasminogen activator production in endothelial cells. Blood Suppl 1: 288a

Lipinski B, Nowak A, Gurewich V 1974 Fibrinolysis versus fibrinogenolysis in man: resistance of fibrinogen to breakdown by fibrinolytic activity induced by venous occlusion. Experientia 30: 84–85

Liu C Y, Nossel H L, Kaplan K L 1979 Defective thrombin binding by abnormal fibrin associated with recurrent thrombosis. Thrombosis and Haemostasis 42: 181 (Abstract)

Loskutoff D J, Edgington T S 1977 Synthesis of a fibrinolytic activator and inhibitor by endothelial cells. Proceedings of the National Academy of Sciences of the United States of America 74: 3903–3907

Lowe G, Pettigrew A, Middleton S, Forbes C D, Prentice C R M 1977 DDAVP in haemophilia. Lancet ii: 614–615

Lijnen H R, Hoylaerts M, Collen D 1980 Isolation and characterization of a human plasma protein with affinity for the lysine binding sites in plasminogen. J Biol Chem 255:10214–22

Mandle R J, Kaplan A P 1979 Hageman-factor-dependent fibrinolysis: Generation of fibrinolytic activity by the interaction of human activated factor XI and plasminogen. Blood 54: 850–862.

Mannucci P M, Ruggeri Z M, Pareti F I, Capitanio A 1977 1-Deamino-8-D-arginine vasopressin: A new AMP? Thrombosis Research 4: 539–549

Mannucci P M, Åberg M, Nilsson I M, Robertson B 1975 Mechanism of plasminogen activator and factor VIII increase after vasoactive drugs. British Journal of Haematology 30: 81–93

Mannucci P M, Ruggeri Z M, Pareti F I, Capitanio A 1977 1-Deamino-8-D arginine vasopressin: A new pharmacological approach to the management of haemophilia and von Willebrand's disease. Lancet i: 869–872

Markwardt F, Klöcking H P 1976 Studies on the release of plasminogen activator. Thrombosis Research 8: 217–223

Markwardt F, Klöcking H P 1978 Einfluss von Mediatoren auf die Freisetzung von Plasminogenaktivatoren. Acta Biologica et Medica Germanica 37: 1603–1610

Matsuo O, Kawaguchi T, Kosugi T, Mihara H 1978 Sustained fibrinolytic activity in the euglobulin fraction induced by concomitant administration of urokinase and dextran sulphate. Thrombosis Research 13: 1125–1130

Moroi M, Aoki N 1976 Isolation and characterization of α_2-plasmin inhibitor from human plasma. Journal of Biological Chemistry 251: 5956–5965

Moroi M, Aoki N 1977 Inhibition of proteases in coagulation, kinin-forming and complement systems by α_2-plasmin inhibitor. Journal of Biochemistry 82: 969–972

Mui P T K, James H L, Ganguly P 1975 Isolation and properties of a low molecular weight antiplasmin from human blood platelets and serum. British Journal of Haematology 29: 627–637

Müllertz S, Clemmensen I 1976 The primary inhibitor of plasmin in human plasma. Biochemical Journal 159: 545–553

Naito K, Aoki N 1978 Assay of α_2-plasmin inhibitor activity by means of a plasmin specific tripeptide substrate. Thrombosis Research 12: 1147–1156

Niewiarowski S, Prou-Wartelle O 1959 Rôle du facteur contact (Facteur Hageman) dans la fibrinolyse. Thrombosis et Diathesis Haemorrhagica 3: 593–603

Nilsson I M, Krook H, Sternby N H, Söderberg E, Söderström N 1961 Severe thrombotic disease in a young man with bone marrow and skeletal changes and with a high content of an inhibitor in the fibrinolytic system. Acta Medica Scandinavica 169: 323–337

Nossel H L 1979 Fibrinogen proteolysis and deep vein thrombosis. Thrombosis and Haemostasis 42: 823 (Abstract)

Nossel H L, Canfield R, Kaplan K, Kernoff P, Lagama K, Owen J, Wasser J, Yudelman I 1979 Fibrinogen Bβ-chain proteolysis by thrombin and plasmin — a regulatory mechanism in hemostasis and thrombosis. Thrombosis and Haemostasis 42: 427 (Abstract)

Ohlsson K, Olsson I 1974 The neutral proteases of human granulocytes. Isolation and partial characterization of granulocyte elastase. European Journal of Biochemistry 42: 519–527

Ohlsson K, Collen D 1977 Comparison of the reaction of neutral granulocyte proteases with the major plasma protease inhibitors and with antiplasmin. Scandinavian Journal of Clinical and Laboratory Investigation 37: 345–350

Ohlsson K 1979 Immunoreactive granulocyte elastase in human serum. Abstract Vth Meeting of the International Society of Haematology, European/African Division, Hamburg, p 25

Plow E F, Hougie C, Edgington T S 1971 Neoantigenic expressions engendered by plasmin cleavage of fibrinogen. Journal of Immunology 107: 1496–1500

Plow E F, Edgington T S 1973a Immunobiology of fibrinogen. Emergence of neoantigenic expressions during physiological cleavage in vitro and in vivo. Journal of Clinical Investigation 52: 273–282

Plow E F, Edgington T S 1973b Discriminating neoantigenic differences between fibrinogen and fibrin derivatives. Proceedings of the National Academy of Sciences USA 70: 1169–1173

Plow E F, Edgington T S 1975 An alternative pathway of fibrinolysis. I. The cleavage of fibrinogen by leukocyte proteases at physiological pH. Journal of Clinical Investigation 56: 30–38

Plow E F, Edgington T S 1978 The fibrinolytic pathway of leukocytes. In: Havemann K, Janoff A (eds) Neutral proteases of human polymorphonuclear leukocytes, Urban and Schwarzenberg, Baltimore-München, p 330–345

Prandini M H, Wiman B, Samama M M, Collen D 1978 Effects of the synthetic fibrinolytic agents ortho-thymotic acid and S-1623 on the reaction between human plasmin and antiplasmin. Thrombosis Research 13: 165–173

Prowse C V, Sas G, Gader A M A, Cort J H, Cash J D 1979 Specificity in the factor VIII response to vasopressin infusion in man. British Journal of Haematology 41: 437–447

Rakoczi I, Chamone D, Collen D, Verstraete M 1978 Prediction of postoperative leg-vein thrombosis in gynaecological patients. Lancet i: 509–510

Ratnoff O D, Busse R J, Sheon R P 1968 The demise of John Hageman. New England Journal of Medicine 279: 760–761

Ratnoff O D 1977 The surface-mediated initiation of blood coagulation and related phenomena. In: Ogston D, Bennett B (eds) Haemostasis: Biochemistry, Physiology, and Pathology, J. Wiley & Sons, London–New York–Sydney–Toronto, p 25–55

Ratnoff O D 1977 The haemostatic defects of liver disease. In: Ogston D, Bennett B (eds) Haemostasis: Biochemistry, Physiology, and Pathology, J. Wiley & Sons, London–New York–Sydney–Toronto, p 446–466

Raum D, Marcus D, Alper C A, Levey R, Taylor P D, Starzl T 1980 Synthesis of human plasminogen by the liver. Science 288: 1036–1037

Reilly C R, Travis J 1980 The degradation of human elastin by neutrophil proteinases. Biochimica et Biophysica Acta 621: 147–157

Robbins K C, Wohl R C, Summaria L 1979 Variant plasminogens in patients with a history of venous thrombosis. Thrombosis and Haemostasis 42: 190 (Abstract)

Rosing D R, Redwood D R, Brakman P, Astrup T, Epstein S E 1978 The fibrinolytic response of man to vasoactive drugs measured in arterial blood. Thrombosis Research 13: 419–428

Rijken D C, Wijngaards G, Zaal-de Jong M, Welbergen J 1979 Purification and partial characterization of plasminogen activator from human uterine tissue. Biochimica et Biophysica Acta 580: 140–153

Rijken D C 1980 Plasminogen activator from human tissue. Thesis Leiden

Sakata Y, Aoki N 1980 Cross-linking of α_2-plasmin inhibitor to fibrin by fibrin-stabilizing factor. Journal of Clinical Investigation 65: 290–297

Samama M M 1979 Oral fibrinolytic therapy. In: Neri Serneri C G, Prentice C R M (eds) Haemostasis and Thrombosis, Academic Press, New York, p 271–278

Samama M M, Conard J, Cazenave B, Derlon A, Gaudric A, Coscas G 1979 Modifications of α_2-plasmin inhibitor during treatments by a defibrinating agent. Thrombosis and Haemostasis 42: 277 (Abstract)

Samuels A J 1979 Prolonged euglobulin clot lysis time as an index of fibrinolytic impairment in human subjects. Blood 54 Suppl 1: 301a

Sandberg Hansen M, Clemmensen I 1980 Partial purification and characterization of a new fast-acting plasmin inhibitor from human platelets. Biochemical Journal 187: 173–180

Schmidt W, Havemann K 1974 Isolation of elastase-like and chymotrypsin-like neutral proteases of human granulocytes. Hoppe-Seyler's Zeitschrift fur Physiologische Chemie 355; 1077–1082

Semeraro N, Collen D, Verstraete M 1977 On the origin of the Aα-chain heterogeneity of human fibrinogen. Biochimica et Biophysica Acta 492: 204–214

Soria J, Soria C, Samama M M 1978 A plasminogen assay using a chromogenic synthetic substrate: results from clinical work and from studies of thrombolysis. In: Davidson J F, Rowan R M, Samama M M, Desnoyers P C (eds) Progress in Chemical Fibrinolysis and Thrombolysis, Raven Press, New York, Vol 3, p 337–346

Sottrup-Jensen L, Claeys H, Zajdel M, Petersen T E, Magnusson S 1978 The primary structure of human plasminogen: isolation of two lysine-binding fragments and one 'mini'-plasminogen (MW 38 000) by esterase-catalyzed-specific limited proteolysis. In: Davidson J F, Rowan R M, Samama M M, Desnoyers P C (eds) Progress in Chemical Fibrinolysis and Thrombolysis, Raven Press, New York, Vol 3, p 191–209

Steele P, Ellis J, Genton E 1978 Effects of platelet suppressant, anticoagulant and fibrinolytic therapy in patients with recurrent venous thrombosis. American Journal of Medicine 64: 441–445

Taberner D A, Poller L, Burslem R W 1979 Antiplasmin levels after surgery: the failure of α_2-antiplasmin rise in patient with venous thrombosis. British Journal of Haematology 43: 493

Takagi K, Kawai T 1978 Radioimmunoassay of an early plasmin degradation product of human fibrinogen, 'fragment A', and its clinical application. Thrombosis and Haemostasis 39: 1–11

Tanser A R, Smellie H 1964 Observations on adrenalin-induced fibrinolysis in man. Clinical Science 26: 375–380

Thorsen S, Glas-Greenwalt P, Astrup T 1972 Differences in the binding to fibrin of urokinase and tissue plasminogen activator. Thrombosis et Diathesis Haemorrhagica 28: 65–74

Thorsen S 1975 Differences in the binding to fibrin of native plasminogen and plasminogen modified by proteolytic degradation. Biochimica et Biophysica Acta 393: 55–65

Thorsen S 1978 Influence of fibrin on the effect of 6-amino-hexanoic acid on fibrinolysis caused by tissue plasminogen activator or urokinase. In: Davidson J F, Rowan R M, Samama M M, Desnoyers P C (eds) Progress in Chemical Fibrinolysis and Thrombolysis, Raven Press New York, Vol 3, p 269–283

Todd A S 1959 The histological localization of plasminogen activator. Journal of Pathology and Bacteriology 78: 281–283

Trumpi-Kalshoven M M 1978 The relevance of C̄1-inhibitor in the inhibition of the fibrinolytic activity of plasmin. In: Davidson J F, Rowan R M, Samama M M, Desnoyers P C (eds) Progress in Chemical Fibrinolysis and Thrombolysis, Raven Press, New York, Vol 3, p 257–267

Vermylen J G, Chamone D A F 1979 The role of the fibrinolytic system in thromboembolism. Progress in Cardiovascular Diseases 21: 255–266

Verstraete M, Vermylen J, Schetz J 1978 Biochemical changes noted during intermittent administration of streptokinase. Thrombosis and Haemostasis 39: 61–68

Walker I D, Davidson J F 1978 Long-term fibrinolytic enhancement with anabolic steroid therapy: a five-year study. In: Davidson J F, Rowan R M, Samama M M, Desnoyers P C (eds) Progress in Chemical Fibrinolysis and Thrombolysis, Vol 3, Raven Press, New York, p 491–499

Wallén P 1978 Chemistry of plasminogen and plasminogen activation. In: Davidson J F, Rowan R M, Samama M M, Desnoyers P C (eds) Progress in Chemical Fibrinolysis and Thrombolysis, Raven Press, New York, Vol 3, p 167–181

Whitaker A N, Rowe E A, Masci P P, Gaffney P J 1979 Identification of D-dimer-E complex in disseminated intravascular coagulation. Thrombosis and Haemostasis 42: 274 (Abstract)

Wiman B, Collen D 1977 Purification and characterization of human antiplasmin, the fast-acting plasmin inhibitor in plasma. European Journal of Biochemistry 78: 19–26

Wiman B, Wallén P 1973 Activation of human plasminogen by an insoluble derivative of urokinase. Structural changes of plasminogen in the course of activation to plasmin and demonstration of a possible intermediate compound. European Journal of Biochemistry 36: 25–31

Wiman B, Wallén P 1975 Structural relationship between 'glutamic acid' and 'lysine' forms of human plasminogen and their interaction with the NH_2-terminal activation peptide as studied by affinity chromatography. European Journal of Biochemistry 50: 489–494

Wiman B, Wallén P 1977 The specific interaction between plasminogen and fibrin. A physiological role of the lysine-binding site in plasminogen. Thrombosis Research 10: 213–222

Wiman B 1978 Biochemistry of the plasminogen to plasmin conversion. In: Gaffney P J, Balkuv-Ulutin S (eds) Fibrinolysis: Current Fundamental and Clinical Concepts, Academic Press, London–New York–San Francisco, p 47–60

Wiman B, Lijnen H R, Collen D 1979 On the specific interaction between the lysine-binding sites in plasmin and complementary sites in α_2-antiplasmin and in fibrinogen. Biochimica et Biophysica Acta 579: 142–154

Wijngaards G 1979 Determination of plasminogen activator inhibiting activity of an extract of human placenta. In: Davidson J F, Čepelák V, Samama M M, Desnoyers P C (eds) Progress in Chemical Fibrinolysis and Thrombolysis, Churchill Livingstone, Edinburgh–London–New York, Vol 4, p 368–373

Yuen P, Kwaan H C, Ho F 1979 Fibrinolysis in solid tumors. Thrombosis and Haemostasis 42: 340 (Abstract)

6. Antithrombin and related inhibitors of coagulation

Ulrich Abildgaard

THE HAEMOSTATIC BALANCE

Blood platelets and clotting factors interact to arrest bleeding, but may also cause thrombosis. Excess fibrin may be removed by fibrinolysis which counteracts thrombosis, but is unable to control the initial stages of thrombus formation. The existence of control mechanisms within the coagulation and platelet aggregation systems have long been anticipated, but are less well understood than are the activation mechanisms. The activation sequence in coagulation involves negative feedback effects which tend to limit thrombin formation.

Activated coagulation factors present in the blood stream are also rapidly taken up by the normal liver. Although such mechanisms diminish the effects of activation of the coagulation, their antithrombotic effect is uncertain.

ANTITHROMBIN

The background
Following the demonstration of the enzymatic action of thrombin on fibrinogen, the results of simple experiments showed that the blood possessed the ability to inactivate thrombin (Schmidt, 1892). The substance responsible for this effect was termed antithrombin (Morawitz, 1905), and it was early assumed that antithrombin and thrombin formed an inactive complex (Weymouth, 1913). But progress in antithrombin research was slow and most of the present knowledge of the mechanism of antithrombin action and the clinical consequences of antithrombin deficiency has been obtained during the last 15 years.

Nomenclature
Antithrombin is one of the proteinase inhibitors of the blood. It inactivates all the clotting enzymes except factor VIIa. The role of the other proteinase inhibitors in blood coagulation is at present uncertain, but α_2-macroglobulin may account for a minor part of the inactivation of thrombin by normal plasma. The hypothesis that heparin accelerates the reaction between antithrombin and thrombin (Quick, 1938) was confirmed 30 years later. Claims that 'heparin cofactor' can be separated from antithrombin (Ganrot, 1969; Porter et al, 1967) are no longer tenable. The Roman numeral classification system (Fell et al, 1954) distinguished between antithrombin II (heparin cofactor) and antithrombin III (slow inactivation of thrombin). As a single plasma protein exerts both antithrombin II and III activities, and the other 'antithrombins' are not enzyme inhibitors, this nomenclature is no longer in use. It was recommended that the suffix 'III' should be kept for antithrombin to emphasise

that it was not an antibody, but this is not really needed now. In the present review, the term antithrombin (abbreviation AT) will be used, in agreement with recent publications (Abildgaard, 1979; Nordenman et al, 1980; Rosenberg & Lam, 1979; Thunberg et al, 1979). The review will refer to some earlier key observations, but will focus on developments that have appeared since the previous review by Lane and Biggs (1977) in the second volume in this series.

Biochemical aspects

Chemical structure

AT is an α_2-globulin with ellipsoid form and semiaxes 1.9, 3.7, and 5.2 nm (Furugren et al, 1977). The single polypeptide chain contains about 425 amino acids, to which are attached four glycosamine-based oligosaccharide units and glycolipid (Danishefsky et al, 1978). The molecular weight is about 58 000 (Nordenman et al, 1977), rather than the original estimate of 63 700 (Abildgaard, 1967a). The pI of the intact molecule is 5.1 (Fagerhol & Abildgaard, 1970). Upon unfolding, acidic residues are exposed in the AT molecule, resulting in a pI of 4.8 (Einarsson et al, 1977). About 10 per cent of the polypeptide chain has an α-helix structure, and about 40 per cent β-structure (Nordenman et al, 1977).

Comparison of the amino acid sequence reveals a relatively high degree of homology with α_1-antitrypsin, suggesting that the two inhibitors have evolved from a common ancestor (Petersen et al, 1979).

Interaction with clotting enzymes and glycosaminoglycans

Heparin accelerates the reaction between AT and clotting enzymes, by which equimolar, inactive complexes are formed. Heparin belongs to the glycosaminoglycans (GAGs), which are sulphated carbohydrates widely distributed in human and animal tissues. Heparin, prepared from bovine lung or porcine intestinal mucosa, is used as an anticoagulant drug. Endogenous heparin has not been demonstrated convincingly in human blood. The physiological implications of in vitro studies with heparin are therefore uncertain. Two other GAGs, heparan sulphate and dermatan sulphate, have a weak heparin-like activity, and due to their distribution in vascular tissues, may act as stationary anticoagulants. The situation is rendered even more complex by the demonstration that heparin can be separated into high and low activity fractions. It seems logical first to review this last finding, and then discuss the binding between heparin and AT, and finally the inactivation of the clotting enzymes.

Heparin fractions

The heterogeneity of heparin has long been recognized, and it was known that the anticoagulant activity tended to increase with increasing molecular weight and apparently also with the degree of sulphation. A breakthrough in the fractionation of heparin was the application of the Sepharose-AT column. Three groups independently separated commercial heparin by affinity chromatography on such columns. The heparin which did not bind to the Sepharose-AT, or which was eluted at low salt concentrations, is termed low affinity or low activity (LA) heparin (Lam et al, 1976; Höök, et al, 1976; Andersson et al, 1976). At most one third of the molecules in commercial heparin preparations carry more than 90 per cent of the activity.

Consequently, the specific activity of the high affinity or high activity (HA) is at least three times that of commercial heparin. HA heparin fractions are invaluable for the study of the molecular reactions between heparin, AT and the enzymes. It is not definitely established which sequence in heparin is responsible for the high activity; the results of Rosenberg and Lam (1979) suggest that a tetrasaccharide is essential, whereas the result of Lindahl et al (1979) indicates that a sequence of 12 to 14 sugar units is required for the high biological activity. A heparin fragment containing 10 to 16 sugar units has recently been shown to greatly potentiate the inhibition of factor Xa by AT, but to have little effect on thrombin inactivation and platelet aggregation and also to be relatively little influenced by heparin neutralizing components in plasma (Holmer et al, 1980).

Binding between heparin and AT
The binding of heparin to AT is dependent on the ionic strength and pH. Thus, the acceleration of AT activity virtually disappears when ionic strength exceeds 0.3 or pH 9.0 (Abildgaard, 1969a). At physiological ionic strength and pH the binding constant of HA heparin to AT is about $10^7 M^{-1}$ (Jordan et al, 1979), while that of the LA heparin is about $5 \times 10^4 M^{-1}$ (Nordenman & Björk, 1978). It has been suggested that there is only one binding site (Danielsson & Björk, 1978) or two binding sites on the AT molecule (Piepkorn et al, 1978). The structure of the binding site is not known. Rosenberg & Damus (1973) suggested that lysine was required for heparin binding. Tryptophan is probably involved in the binding, as fluorescence studies have demonstrated an increase in tryptophan fluorescence when heparin is bound to AT (Einarsson & Andersson, 1977). It is doubtful if these changes represent conformational changes of the AT molecule (Björk & Larsson, 1980).

Fluorescence studies suggest that both low and high activity heparin bind to antithrombin in molar ratios of 1:1 (Nordenman & Björk, 1978), but high molecular weight heparin (20 000 daltons) appears to have two binding sites for AT (Rosenberg et al, 1979).

Heparin has also been fractionated on DEAE-Sephadex (Piepkorn et al, 1978) and on α-thrombin-agarose (Griffith et al, 1978). Even these procedures can be used to prepare high activity heparin fractions.

Inactivation of clotting enzymes by AT
Thrombin and AT form an inactive complex in a 1:1 molar ratio (Abildgaard 1969b. Rosenberg & Damus, 1973), but unless the inhibitor is in molar excess, the complex undergoes degradation. Modified AT, in the form of a two chain molecule, may be released from the complex (Jesty, 1979; Fish & Björk, 1979) and appears to be identical to a modified AT which can be produced by thrombin action under special conditions (Jörnvall et al, 1979) and which has been visualized in SDS gels (Rosenberg & Damus, 1973; Shandra & Bang, 1977). The significance of this thrombin modified AT is uncertain. The observation fits, however, well in with the general idea that AT is a 'pseudo-substrate' for thrombin. Fish and Björk (1979) suggest that thrombin and AT form an enzyme-substrate complex and a specific bond in AT is cleaved. Thereafter, the complex becomes highly unstable, and the modified AT molecule might either dissociate as free modified AT, or form a final tight, inactive AT-thrombin complex. The tightening of the complex may involve a covalent acyl

ester bond (Owen et al, 1976), or merely a conformational change in the three dimensional structure of the modified AT. Jesty (1979) suggests that even if the formation of the complex is reversed, the released enzyme is inactive. Studies on the spectral changes show that AT undergoes conformational changes upon binding to thrombin (Villanueva & Danishefsky, 1979).

During activation of prothrombin to thrombin, two enzymatically inactive fragments are released. Walker and Esmon (1979) have demonstrated that prothrombin fragment 2 inhibits the inactivation of thrombin by AT. This finding seems to imply that at the site of thrombin formation, where fragment 2 concentration will be relatively high, inactivation by AT is impeded, while thrombin which diffuses away will not be protected against AT. This mechanism is another example of the regulatory role of the peptides formed by prothrombin activation, and which seems to modulate the appearance of coagulant activity.

Rosenberg and Damus (1973) showed that intact serine at the active site of thrombin was essential for reaction with AT. By limited proteolysis, thrombin capable of converting fibrinogen to fibrin (α-thrombin) can be converted to γ-thrombin which acts on some low molecular substrates, but has minimal clotting ability. Chang and coworkers (1979) showed that AT reacts in an essentially identical manner with α-thrombin and with γ-thrombin. In addition, they showed that fibrinogen did not affect the reaction between γ-thrombin with AT, in accordance with earlier kinetic data (Abildgaard, 1967b).

The inactivation of the other clotting enzymes proceeds in a similar fashion to that of the thrombin-AT reaction and leads to the formation of stable enzyme-inhibitor complexes. In purified systems containing physiological AT-concentration, half-lives of about 37 seconds for thrombin, and 90 seconds for Xa were found (Ødegård et al, 1977). AT inactivates factor IXa, XIa and XIIa at slow rates, the thrombin half-lives are probably in the 10 to 25 minutes' range (Østerud et al, 1976; Kurachi et al, 1976; Stead et al, 1976). Factor VIIa, in contrast, is not inhibited by AT (Godal et al, 1974; Jesty, 1978).

Factor Xa may be protected from AT when bound to phospholipids (Marciniak, 1973). Newer data indicate that factor Xa binds to platelets (Miletich et al, 1977; Dahlbäck & Stenflo, 1978), and is thereby protected against AT (Miletich et al, 1978). Such mechanisms might act to prolong thrombin and fibrin formation at the site of a haemostatic plug, but also probably in a thrombus, whereas the inactivation by AT of thrombin and Xa will proceed relatively more rapidly in the circulating blood.

In each of the reactions between AT and clotting enzymes, the inactivation rate is dependent on the AT concentration. With excess AT, pseudo first order reaction kinetics are found. As fibrin formation by activation of the intrinsic pathway involves the successive activation of at least four of these enzymes, it is more easy to realize that a relatively modest decrease of the AT concentration may result in a considerably greater clotting response (Dombrose et al, 1971; Reeves, 1980). It seems rational that the early enzymes, which only appear at relatively low concentrations, are more slowly inactivated than thrombin, which when present in excessive concentrations, rapidly coagulates the blood.

Influence of heparin on thrombin inactivation by AT
N-terminal analysis (reflecting fibrin formation) showed that moderate concentrations

of heparin increased the inactivation rate twentyfold (Abildgaard, 1968b). Stopflow technique combined with recording of the displacement of proflavin from thrombin as AT is bound, showed that heparin accelerated the inactivation by a factor of 200 to 400 (Li et al, 1976). By radioesterolytic methods (Jordan et al, 1979), or by amidolytic methods (Abildgaard, 1979), it was found that heparin increased the inactivation rate 2000 to 2300 fold. Translating these results to normal human plasma which has an antithrombin concentration of about 3 µmol/1, thrombin half-life in the absence of heparin is probably about 30 to 40 seconds. At heparin concentrations usually found during heparin treatment, the thrombin half-life is reduced to about 0.5 seconds, whereas it may be reduced to about 20 mseconds at very high heparin concentrations (Abildgaard, 1979).

These effects of heparin may be demonstrated both with HA heparin and crude heparin. On a weight basis, the activity of LA heparin is about 10 to 15 per cent of that of HA heparin (Nordenman et al, 1980; Jordan et al, 1979).

Influence of heparin on the inactivation of factor Xa by AT
As activation of factor X precedes that of prothrombin, its inhibition could have a stronger anticoagulant effect than the inhibition of thrombin. Studies with conventional clotting methods in fact suggested that heparin exerted its main anticoagulant effect via factor Xa (Yin, 1974). Further studies have confirmed the existence of species differences in inactivation rates, and shown the importance of assessing directly the enzymatic activity of factor Xa. With chromogenic substrates, it has been shown that human Xa is inactivated more slowly than thrombin, both in the absence and presence of heparin (Ødegård et al, 1977; Stürzebecher, 1977). Furthermore, LA heparin is even less efficient in factor Xa than in thrombin inactivation (Nordenman et al, 1980). In contrast, low molecular HA heparin is more efficient in factor Xa than in thrombin inactivation (Thunberg et al, 1979; Holmer et al, 1980). Plasma contains a component which particularly inhibits the effect of high molecular weight heparin on the Xa-AT reaction (Macgregor et al, 1979).

The mechanism of heparin action
The precise way in which heparin exerts its catalytic role on the inactivation of clotting enzymes has not been established. Three different models have been proposed for the reaction sequence: (1) Heparin binds to AT, thereby inducing conformational changes which facilitate the binding of thrombin. Upon the formation of a stable thrombin-AT complex, heparin is released and joins another AT molecule (Rosenberg & Damus, 1973; Li et al, 1976). (2) Heparin binds to thrombin, thereby facilitating its reaction with antithrombin (Machovic et al, 1975). (3) Heparin binds to AT, inducing a conformational change. Secondly, thrombin binds simultaneously to antithrombin and heparin, whereupon heparin is released (Holmer et al, 1979).

According to hypothesis (1) and (3), heparin binds primarily to AT. This is supported by several findings, such as the high anticoagulant activity of heparin with high affinity to AT, and by results of mixing experiments with stopflow technique (Li et al, 1976). Finally there is evidence to suggest that the binding of heparin to thrombin actually reduces the speed of thrombin neutralization (Jordan et al, 1979; Feinman, 1979). On the other hand, AT appears to have a higher affinity to thrombin-heparin complex than to thrombin or heparin alone (Hatton & Regoeczi,

1977). Further, active site blocked thrombin inhibits the heparin enhanced AT-thrombin reaction (Griffith et al, 1979), and the inactivation of a β-thrombin is not accelerated by heparin (Borsody & Machovic, 1979). Finally, kinetic studies may be interpreted to suggest that heparin acts by increasing the affinity of thrombin towards AT (Stürzebecher, 1977).

At present, it is not possible to decide which of the three models describes the actual molecular mechanism. It is evident, however, that in vivo, the concentration of AT will always by far exceed that of thrombin, and any heparin present in the blood will be bound to AT. Factor Xa has less affinity for heparin than has thrombin, and the reaction sequence probably follows model (1) above.

Inactivation of clotting enzymes by AT and haparan sulphate/dermatan sulphate
Of the various glycosaminoglycans (GAGs) found in human tissue, heparin sulphate (HS) and dermatan sulphate (DS) prolong APTT clotting times. Concentrations of HS and DS, about 70 times that of heparin, were required to obtain similar anticoagulant effects (Teien et al, 1976). HS apparently exerts its effect in a heparin like manner, i.e. by accelerating the inactivation of clotting enzymes by AT (Teien et al, 1976; Hatton et al, 1978). With esterolytic methods, Hatton et al (1978) found that even DS accelerated AT activity. Using chromogenic substrates, Teien et al (1976) obtained results which suggested that DS exerted its anticoagulant effect by some other mechanism, possibly by the inhibition of factor IXa. In view of the presence of HS and DS in the vascular wall, these findings suggest their importance as stationary anticoagulants, promoting the inactivation of clotting enzymes by AT at the endothelial surface.

Clinical aspects

Assay at AT
The clotting assays for determining AT activity tend to be complicated and only show moderate precision and accuracy. A contributing factor is the defibrination of plasma which is done to avoid (varying) adsorption of thrombin to fibrin during the initial inactivation stage. In a second stage, the remaining thrombin (or Xa) activity is measured. As thrombin activity is relatively low, fibrin is formed slowly, and the individual error in observation of gelation time tends to be great. Assay of AT in serum (Gerendas, 1960; von Kaulla & von Kaulla, 1967) eliminates defibrination, but serum AT is dependent both on the plasma AT concentration and on the (varying) consumption during in vitro coagulation. Nevertheless, these methods may be used to detect very low AT levels, such as are found in liver cirrhosis and in congenital deficiency (Conard & Samama, 1978). The gel method of Lane et al (1975) seems particularly well suited for the screening of large series (Lane & Biggs, 1977).

The method of Hensen and Loeliger (1963) is the first really quantitative plasma method, and it enabled Egeberg to detect the first family with AT deficiency (Egeberg, 1965). The method was later simplified and improved (Abildgaard et al, 1970; Howie et al, 1973). An elegant clotting assay using factor Xa was reported by Gitel & Wessler (1975). With the advent of immunoassays and, particularly with the chromogenic methods these clotting methods are now mainly regarded as reference methods.

Following immunization with homogeneous AT (Heimburger, 1967; Abildgaard, 1968a) *immunoassays* could be performed on large series of plasma samples. The radial immunodiffusion method requires at least 20 hours, but presents fewer methodological problems with AT than immunoelectrophoresis (Grimmer & Fagerhol, 1977). As in activity assays, serum AT is usually about 70 per cent of plasma AT in immunoassays (Fagerhol & Abildgaard, 1970), depending on to what extent the thrombin-AT complex has been antigenic in the immunized animal (McKay, 1980). Thus, with some antisera, similar plasma and serum AT values have been found. Such a result may also be obtained if EDTA or citrate is omitted in a gel buffer. In this case, thrombin is apparently formed during diffusion, and even if citrated/EDTA plasma is applied, the assay measures serum AT. This point is apparently neglected in some immunoassay studies. It is also possible to quantitate AT by nephelometry (Egbring et al, 1980) and by radioimmunoassay (Chan et al, 1979).

Synthetic chromogenic substrates, modelled after the activation site in prothrombin and factor X, have proved invaluable for the assay of coagulation inhibitor activities. In the first amidolytic AT method, plasma was defibrinated (Blombäck et al, 1974), but by selecting appropriate physiochemical conditions, fibrin formation could be avoided and the plasma samples assayed directly (Ødegård et al, 1975). Chromogenic methods recording the inactivation of thrombin and of Xa, both in the absence and presence of heparin, have been described. As judged by comparison with immunoassays in clinical materials, the results of all these methods seem to reflect mainly the AT concentration in the test plasma (Ødegård & Lie, 1978). It is particularly true for the methods with heparin. But even without heparin, the rate of thrombin inactivation is mainly determined by the AT concentration, whereas additional Xa inhibitors also influence Xa inactivation without heparin (Ødegård et al, 1976).

The chromogenic substrates H-D-Phe-Pip-Arg-pNA (S-2238 from Kabi) and Tos-Gly-Pro-arg-pNA (Chromozyme TH from Pentapharm/Bothringer) are well suited for AT assays (Abildgaard et al, 1977). Assay kits with these substrates have come into widespread use. The same substrates are also well fitted for assay of heparin in plasma (Lie et al, 1978). AT assays with these substrates have been automated (Kahlé et al, 1978b; Scully & Kakkar, 1977) as have methods using factor Xa and the chromogenic substrate Bz-Ile-Glu-Gly-Arg-pNA (S-2222 from Kabi) (Ødegård et al, 1978).

Regarding the choice of assay method for routine work, most immunoassays are simple, cheap and require about 20 hours, but do not detect all congenital AT deficiencies (Sas et al, 1974). The clotting assays are cheap, but their low accuracy and precision explain why they are now used less. The amidolytic assays measure AT activity and their precision and accuracy are as good or even better than the immunoassays (Bounameaux et al, 1978). The relatively high cost of the substrates limits their use but with newer methods, using more dilute solutions, costs will be reduced.

EXPRESSION OF RESULTS

The many different ways of expressing the results of AT assays cause confusion. With semiquantitative clotting assays (Gerendas, 1960; von Kaulla & von Kaulla, 1967), there is no alternative to expressing the results in seconds.

With quantitative AT assays, whether dependent on activity or immunological, it seems rational to express the results in g/l (formerly mg/100 ml) or μmol/l. But there is still disagreement about the AT concentration in normal human reference plasma (vide infra). An alternative, then, is to use units. Unfortunately, even AT units are used in various ways: Most often, one AT U is defined as the amount in one ml of reference plasma. But even 100 U/ml plasma, or units, referring to thrombin units inhibited, have been used.

Until the AT concentration (g/l or μmol/l) is known with greater certainty, it is most convenient to express results in per cent of a reference plasma. As AT may easily be denatured upon freezdrying, some freezdried reference plasma are unsuited (Kahlé et al, 1980), and frozen pooled plasma is probably to be preferred at present.

It is evident that the plasma concentration in normal individuals shows little variation (Ødegaard et al, 1976; Chan et al, 1979). With an SD of about 10 per cent the 'normal range' is 75–125 per cent.

The plasma concentration of human AT, as calculated from comparison with purified material is 19.6 ± 2.3 mg/ml (Collen et al, 1977; Chan et al, 1979). This is similar to the value calculated from the purification factor: 0.2 g/l or 3 μmol/l (Abildgaard, 1979). Other authors have suggested higher concentrations in normal plasma: 4.7 μmol/l (Harpel & Rosenberg, 1976) and 0.42 g/l (Heimburger, 1967). The last value is probably too high because of the partly inactivated nature of the purified material, which was compared with plasma.

Localization of AT in tissues

Immunofluorescence studies have demonstrated the presence of AT in the microvasculature of the lung and kidney and in the walls of the larger vessels (Lee et al, 1979). Lung tissue contains about 0.2 mg per g tissue, whereas liver, kidney and spleen contain less amounts of AT (Lee et al, 1979). AT was not detected in supernates from lymphocyte and monocyte cultures (Lee et al, 1979).

Immunoreactive AT may be demonstrated in fresh endothelial cells from human umbilical cord, and after culture AT is also found in the culture medium, suggesting synthesis of AT in endothelial cells (Chan & Chan, 1979). Despite strong evidence for synthesis of AT in hepatocytes, only weak reaction to AT antibody has been found in them (Lee et al, 1979).

Metabolism of AT

Studies with radiolabelled AT indicate a half-life of 2.69 ± 0.36 days in a combined group of controls and patients with vascular disease (Collen et al, 1977). In agreement with the demonstration of tissue AT, these workers demonstrated that the intravascular fraction in the controls was 0.45 ± 0.05. Whereas turnover of AT was in the normal range in patients with venous thrombosis not treated with heparin, the half-life was shortened (2.13 ± 0.08 days) in patients with thrombosis treated with heparin (Collen et al, 1977). In dogs, the intravascular fraction has been estimated to 0.5, and fractional breakdown to 0.51 by Reeves et al (1980).

Based on the finding of convariation between AT and haptoglobin, it has been suggested that AT is an acute phase reactant (Hedner & Nilsson, 1973). Clinical studies, however, have shown normal or only slightly elevated AT in patient groups with inflammatory disease (except conditions which are clearly connected with subnormal AT concentration) (Abildgaard et al, 1970; Ødegård & Teien, 1976).

In experimental inflammatory reaction in rabbits, Koj and Regoeczi (1978) demonstrated that the plasma half-life of AT was considerably shortened and synthesis rate of AT was increased threefold. Nevertheless, the AT plasma concentration remained steady at levels which were only marginally above the pretreatment values. These findings indicate that the balance between synthesis and consumption of AT is rather rigidly controlled. AT-thrombin complexes may be quantitated by immunoassay (Collen & Verstraete, 1979). Although it seems logical to assume that their presence in disseminated intravascular coagulation (DIC) will result in a reduced level of AT, studies in a few individuals with this condition showed little difference from that in normal plasma (Fagerhol & Abildgaard, 1972). Sas et al (1977) found that only one third of plasma samples from patients with DIC contained increased amounts of AT complexes. Recent animal studies have shown that such complexes are unstable in vivo, and that AT dissociated from a complex leaves the circulation at rates which are only marginally higher than those for native AT (Lam et al, 1979). The ratio of functional to immunological AT is increased in DIC (Abildgaard et al, 1970a; Gamba et al, 1980), and in pancreatitis without depressed AT, suggesting increased consumption balanced by increased synthesis (Philip et al, 1979). Endotoxin injection increases AT metabolism (Tanaka, 1979).

Acquired deficiency states

LIVER DISEASE
In cirrhosis of the liver, the AT concentration is often very low (Abildgaard et al, 1970; Hedner & Nilsson, 1973; Nagy et al, 1976). The AT concentration is usually much lower in chronic aggressive hepatitis than in the benign chronic hepatitis (Mannucci et al, 1973; Nagy et al, 1976). In biliary tract occlusion and primary biliary cirrhosis, normal AT concentrations have been found (Stormorken et al, 1976; Nagy et al, 1976). In acute viral hepatitis, moderately depressed levels are usually found (Stormorken et al, 1976). In haemolytic uraemic syndrome (HUS) of pregnancy, extremely low AT values have been found and it has been suggested that DIC may be pathogenetic for HUS (Brandt et al, 1980). AT synthesis is also decreased by l-asparaginase treatment (Conard et al, 1971).

KIDNEY DISEASE
AT is found in the urine when proteinuria is present, and there is an inverse correlation between the plasma AT level and the AT albumin clearance rates (Thaler et al, 1978; Kauffmann et al, 1978). In the nephrotic syndrome, the AT concentration is often low (Thaler et al, 1978; Kauffmann et al, 1978), but Jørgensen and Stoffersen (1979) found a normal mean AT concentration in 15 cases with an abnormally wide range. The frequent occurrence of renal vein thrombosis and other thrombotic complications in this syndrome (Older et al 1978) has been related to the tendency to low AT levels.

Hypercoagulation syndrome

DISSEMINATED INTRAVASCULAR COAGULATION (DIC)
This is a dreaded complication which most often arises in septic conditions, obstetric complications, polytraumatized patients, and, as a more subacute condition, in some

cases of malignancy. The common trigger appears to be liberation of thromboplastin in the blood and the term 'consumption coagulopathy' characterizes the decrease in platelets and clotting factors which, together with increased fibrinolysis, explains the bleeding defect. Lasch et al (1961) early described low AT levels both in clinical and experimental DIC. Immunoassays confirmed that DIC often leads to very low AT concentration (Abildgaard et al, 1970), and this has also been confirmed with amidolytic methods (Abildgaard, 1978; Schipper et al, 1978; Deutsch et al, 1979).

Experimental DIC may be prevented by AT infusion (Mann et al, 1969), and the clinical implication of this observation will be discussed later.

DEEP VENOUS THROMBOSIS (DVT)

In this condition the AT concentration is sometimes temporarily decreased. The frequency with which it is found, depends on the material and on the criteria. Lechner et al (1977) found an initial AT concentration below 78 per cent of normal in 27 of 290 patients with DVT. In 14, AT was temporarily decreased, whereas 13 patients had a congenital deficiency. Juillet et al (1978) found two congenital AT deficiencies and 25 patients with temporarily low AT levels during heparin treatment, in a study of 86 patients with extensive or recurrent DVT. In a study of 237 patients with DVT, an initial AT concentration below 70 per cent of normal was found in 10 individuals (4 per cent), and the level decreased further during heparin treatment (Holm et al, 1980). It is probable that when low AT concentration is found in DVT, it is either the result of an extraordinarily great AT consumption, or reflects a latent depression of the capacity for AT synthesis. In cases complicated by pulmonary embolism, the proportion of low AT is higher. In these patients, one also often finds some evidence of DIC, supporting the view that increased consumption of AT occurs. Thus de Boer et al (1979) reported low AT in six out of 15 patients with pulmonary embolism and in nine out of 45 with DVT.

Acute arterial thrombosis seems rarely to be associated with low AT. In diabetes mellitus with vascular complications, the AT concentration tends to be less than normal (Monnier et al, 1978), probably reflecting chronic DIC. In a group of patients with various arteriosclerotic diseases, cessation of warfarin treatment was followed by a significant decrease in the mean AT level, again pointing at low grade DIC in such conditions (Refvem et al, 1970). In cerebral thrombosis, normal AT values have been found (Panicucci et al, 1980; Mettinger et al, 1979).

POSTOPERATIVE CHANGES IN AT

The observation that DVT may occur in about 30 per cent of patients who undergo elective surgery has renewed the interest in the study of blood parameters that may signify thrombosis. Postoperatively, the AT concentration decreases, but in many patients no more than could be expected from the changes in hematocrit (Korvald et al, 1973; Bergström & Lahnborg, 1975). In hip surgery, the AT concentration decreases significantly more than in general surgery (Gitel et al, 1979) and Sagar et al (1976) and Wallenbeck et al (1979) reported that low AT was related to the occurrence of DVT. Intra-operative fall in AT is more pronounced in women on oral contraceptives (Sagar et al, 1976).

AT AND HORMONES

It was early found that use of contraceptive pills in the form of combined oestrogen-gestagen is associated with a reduced AT concentration (Fagerhol et al, 1970; von Kaulla & von Kaulla, 1970). With the introduction of lower oestrogen content, the fall in AT is less marked (Conard et al, 1974). The continuous low dose progestagen pill probably does not decrease the AT concentration. The relation between the reduced AT concentration and the tendency to thrombosis in users of combined pills has been much debated. AT is relatively more depressed in serum than in plasma, indicating increased in vitro consumption of AT. This might point to increased in vivo consumption as the cause of the subnormal plasma AT. Animal studies suggest, however, that oestrogen depresses AT synthesis, whereas cortisone increases the synthesis of AT (Takeda & Kobayashi, 1977). In a screening study involving about 25 000 women, the serum AT concentration appears to be a poor prognostic index to the occurrence of DVT, but the study led to the discovery of five cases of congenital AT deficiency (Fagerhol & Abildgaard, 1972). Anabolic steroids induce slightly elevated AT levels (Walker et al, 1975).

AT IN NEWBORNS

The AT concentration in newborns is about half that of adults, the mature level being reached at about 12 months (Teger-Nilsson, 1975). AT is gestational dependent, and infants with respiratory distress syndrome (RDS) show clearly subnormal levels, particularly when complicated by DIC or necrotizing enterocolitis (Hathaway et al, 1978).

THE DECREASE IN PLASMA ANTITHROMBIN DURING HEPARIN INFUSION

Blombäck et al (1963) found that the heparin cofactor activity decreased by 14 per cent after injection of heparin to healthy subjects. Marciiak and Gockermann (1977) showed that the decrease in AT may be considerable during heparin infusion to thrombosis patients, and this finding has been confirmed by several authors. In patients with liver cirrhosis, heparin injection did not cause a significant fall in AT under conditions that led to a 10 per cent decrease in normals and 20 per cent decrease in patients with severe renal disease (Teien, 1977), suggesting that the normal liver removes heparin bound to AT, and that this function is impaired in liver cirrhosis.

Particularly when the plasma AT concentration is decreased prior to start of heparin therapy (e.g. in congenital deficiency or liver diseases), a further fall in AT due to heparin may be harmful. In order to obtain adequate anticoagulation, the AT level should preferably be restored by infusion of AT or plasma.

Congenital deficiency

In the classical description of AT deficiency causing thrombophilia, Egeberg (1965) reported that the mean AT activity was about half the normal in the members of family Mi. The first thrombotic episode occurred between ten and 25 years of age, and was usually connected with inflammatory disease or trauma. Immunoassay showed that the affected members of the Mi family had about half the normal concentration of AT in plasma (Abildgaard et al, 1970). In the last ten years, families with AT deficiency have been described from many countries. The frequency with which AT deficiency is found among individuals with DVT varies. Johansson et al (1978) reports that at the Coagulation Laboratory in Malmö, Sweden, four families have been detected from about 2000 routine determinations of AT. Lechner et al (1977) reported 13 individuals with AT deficiency from nine families out of a material of 290 individuals with serious or recurrent DVT. In a material of 237 patients with DVT, no case of congenital deficiency was found (Holm et al, 1980). Ødegård et al (1976) found one congenital deficiency among 396 presumably healthy employees. It is not known if the varying frequency of AT deficiency reported reflects geographical variation, or mainly differently selected populations but the condition may be common in gipsies (Sas et al, 1980). Based on the finding of five congenital deficiencies out of 25 000 pill users, a frequency of 1:5000 was suggested (Fagerhol & Abildgaard, 1972). Most often, the detection of a single case of AT deficiency leads to the detection of several affected family members. Occasional AT deficient individuals seem to represent mutations, as the condition can neither be detected in parents nor offspring, and liver disease is not present.

The typical individual has the post-thrombotic syndrome in one or both legs and may have experienced pulmonary embolism. This condition and mesenteric vein thrombosis are the most dangerous situations for these individuals (Dayan et al, 1978; Juillet, 1979). In family Ma the mean survival in members with thrombotic tendency was 55 years, and in members without history of thrombosis 65 years (Ødegård & Abildgaard, 1977).

Arterial thrombosis is apparently not much more common in AT deficiency than in the remaining population.

It is not known why some individuals with the deficiency may reach old age without experiencing thrombosis. In some cases, hyperlipidemia might have increased the tendency to thrombosis (Gyde et al, 1978).

Individuals with AT deficiency who have suffered from DVT should probably be treated with oral anticoagulants. In some families, warfarin treatment leads to a definite increase in AT values (Marciniak et al, 1974). This has not been the case in the five Norwegian families Mi, My, Ma, Mag and Be (Abildgaard, 1980).

Pregnancy is likely to produce DVT in affected members (Brandt & Stenbjerg, 1979). The child has a 50 per cent chance of inheriting the condition. As warfarin may be harmful to the foetus and subcutaneous heparin may cause a more severe depression of the AT concentration, prophylactic anticoagulant therapy should probably not be given prior to delivery unless there is a history of thrombosis. Individuals with AT deficiency should be informed about these risks.

After delivery, it is probably wise to administer heparin in order to reduce the risk of DVT. If symptoms of DVT occur despite prophylactic heparin, AT infusion appears the treatment of choice. In most cases where DVT occurs in the absence of pregnancy or delivery, heparin therapy followed by warfarin seems to be successful, but the heparin dosage should be higher than usual. In cases with insufficient heparin effect, AT infusion should be given. Warfarin treatment is highly efficient in preventing thrombosis and seems to carry very little bleeding risk in these individuals.

Nature of the AT deficiency: Subtypes
In most families with thrombophilia and AT deficiency, immunoassays and functional assays both show about 50 per cent of normal values in the plasma of the affected members. In contrast, Sas et al (1974) described a family in which immunoassay

showed normal AT quantity, but functional assays showed a subnormal AT activity. Direct evidence of an abnormal AT molecule with abnormally slow electrophoretic motility in the presence of heparin was later reported (Sas et al, 1975), and the abnormal molecule was called antithrombin III 'Budapest'. Additional cases, in which the AT deficiency results from a normal concentration of a defective molecule have been described (Brozovic & Hamlyn, 1978, Nagy et al, 1979; Wolf et al, 1979). Thrombophilic families showing low AT activity and concentration have been termed 'classical' AT deficiency or type 1 deficiency, whereas type 2 designates deficiency due to a functionally abnormal AT molecule which is present in normal concentration. Although type 1 deficiency appears to be much more common than type 2, the existence of the latter condition has favoured the use of activity assays rather than immunoassays for the detection of AT deficiencies.

Recently it has been shown that both these two main types of AT deficiency may be divided into subtypes. As regards type 2, this is not surprising, as one would expect that more than one molecular abnormality may cause a functional abnormality. Nagy et al (1979) and Wolf et al (1979) have described AT variants which appear to react normally with the thrombin alone, but lack the ability to be accelerated by heparin. As the existence of this abnormal AT in normal concentration appears to be related to a thrombotic tendency, the finding implies that endogenous heparin (or heparan sulphate) is involved in the inactivation of clotting enzymes in vivo. But Penner et al (1979) described a similar AT abnormality which was clinically silent.

Even the 'classical' or type 1 deficiency is heterogeneous. By crossed immunoelec-trophoresis it has been shown that some cases with 'classical' deficiency have AT molecules with abnormal motility in the presence of heparin (Gomperts et al, 1976; Sas et al, 1980). It is probable that with the use of more refined methods, such abnormalities may be demonstrated in families originally thought to represent the 'classical' or type 1 deficiency. Thus, the first family described with AT deficiency, family Mi of Egeberg (1965), was originally thought to have about half the normal AT activity as well as concentration (Abildgaard et al, 1970). Upon renewed examina-tion, it has been found that plasma of affected members, in addition to apparently normal AT molecules, contain molecules which have a different motility in the presence of heparin and also weaker immuno precipitate than the 'normal' AT molecule (McKay & Abildgaard, 1980). The existence of two populations of AT molecules in AT deficiency have also been described by Lane (1978) in type 2 deficiency. These findings suggest that the synthesis of AT is regulated by at least two gene systems, and that abnormalities in any of these may result in AT deficiency.

It has been mentioned previously that in some families with AT deficiency, treatment with oral anticoagulants results in considerably elevated AT (Marciniak et al, 1974; Nagy et al, 1979). At present it is not clear if these families represent a distinct entity.

Analysis of the structure of functionally deficient AT molecules will provide new knowledge on the molecular reaction between AT, heparin and the clotting enzymes.

Therapy with AT infusion
When very low AT levels coexist with DIC or acute thrombosis, it seems logical to administer AT concentrates, which may be prepared by large scale methods (Miller-Andersson et al, 1974; Wickerhauser et al, 1979).

Schipper et al (1978) gave AT, prothrombin complex and blood platelets to three patients with DIC and severe bleeding, and obtained normal haemostatic function. Good results have also been obtained in patients with DIC by Schramm & Marx (1980) and Egbring et al (1980). Although AT infusion can normalize the AT concentration, it is difficult to evaluate the clinical effect, and AT infusion to two patients with severe DIC did not prevent a fatal outcome (Anker et al, 1980). A cooperative study will probably be required to evaluate the clinical effect of AT infusion in DIC. Postpartum haemolytic uraemic syndrome has recently been treated with AT infusion with good results (Brandt et al, 1980). Infusion of AT to patients with cirrhosis and low grade DIC led to increased fibrinogen concentration (Schipper et al, 1979).

Congenital AT deficiency complicated by thrombosis (or DIC) appears to be a good indication for AT infusion. Several authors have observed a good clinical effect (Thaler et al, 1979; Schramm et al, 1980; Miller et al, 1980). Congenital AT deficiency has been treated with injection of 125 U AT, with AT concentration increasing from about 27 to 70 per cent (Schander et al, 1980).

Administration of AT to patients with fractured hips prevented the postoperative drop in AT, but the tendency to postoperative thrombosis was not influenced (Medén-Britth & Teien, 1979).

AT and blood platelets
Platelets are intimately involved in the activation of coagulation. The binding of factor Xa to platelets which protects Xa against AT (Miletich et al, 1978) has already been mentioned. The aggregation of blood platelets by thrombin is inhibited by AT which inactivates thrombin (Eika, 1971). It has recently been shown that congenital AT deficiency may be accompanied by abnormally reactive platelets (Carvalho et al, 1976; Tullis & Watanabe, 1978; Matsuo et al, 1979). The greater tendency to venous than to arterial thrombosis in most cases with the congenital deficiency suggests, however, that hyperactive coagulation rather than platelets is characteristic.

OTHER PHYSIOLOGICAL ANTICOAGULANTS

Relatively little is known about other endogenous inhibitors than AT and the glycosaminoglycans. The serine proteinase inhibitors of plasma tend to have rather wide specificity but varying affinity towards the various enzymes. α_2-macroglobulin (α_2-M) is a relatively weak thrombin inhibitor. α_1-antitrypsin and C-1 Inactivator also exert some in vitro anticoagulant activity which probably is of little in vivo significance. Recently, protein C has been shown to be identical to a coagulation inhibitor elicited by thrombin action, but the in vivo relevance of this anticoagulant enzyme is also unknown. It is probable that advances in the field of the initial activation of coagulation will be followed by the discovery of 'new' natural coagulation inhibitors.

α_2-macroglobulin
In contrast to other proteinase inhibitors, α_2-M binds enzymes without blocking their active site, permitting the cleavage of small molecular substrates. Following the demonstration that α_2-M inhibits the clotting activity of thrombin (Steinbuck et al,

1966), it was found that α_2-M accounts for about 25 per cent and AT for about 70 per cent of the total thrombin inhibiting activity of plasma (Abildgaard, 1967; Shapiro & Anderson, 1977; Josso et al, 1978). The molar concentrations in plasma of α_2-M and AT are of the same order of magnitude, but thrombin reacts much faster with AT than with α_2-M (Abildgaard, 1969). In contrast to AT, α_2-M did not prevent fatal DIC in chicken embryos (Mann et al, 1969).

It has recently been shown that heparin, while accelerating the thrombin AT reaction, prevents the binding between α_2-M and thrombin (Fischer et al, 1979). α_2-M apparently does not inhibit the other clotting enzymes, but binds plasmin and was for some time considered its main inhibitor. But later studies have shown that α_2-antiplasmin probably is a more important inhibitor (Müllertz, 1979). As the physiological activity of plasmin is opposed to that of thrombin, the resultant activity of α_2-M appears to be a moderate inhibition of both enzymes without much effect on the balance between coagulation and fibrinolysis. α_2-M has a broad enzyme binding spectrum and traps proteinases from leukocytes and exogenous proteinases. The enzyme-α_2-M complexes are rapidly removed from the circulation and then degraded (for reviews, see Harpel & Rosenberg (1977) and Starkey (1979)).

In DIC and other conditions with increased proteolysis, low α_2-M concentrations are found. Congenital deficiency of α_2-M with normal haemostasis has recently been reported (Bergqvist & Nilsson, 1979).

α_1-antitrypsin

α_1-antitrypsin may inactivate thrombin at slow rates, provided initial thrombin concentration is high, but the effect is much weaker than that of AT and α_2-M. In vitro studies also suggest that α_1-antitrypsin has some inhibitory effect on the clotting enzymes of the intrinsic pathway. As individuals with α_1-antitrypsin deficiency have normal thrombin inhibiting activity in plasma and do not show a special tendency towards thrombosis, these in vitro anticoagulant effects appear to have little physiological relevance.

C-1 Inactivator

This protein inhibits factor XIa and XIIa in vitro. Individuals with C-1 Inactivator deficiency suffer from angioneurotic oedema and do not show evidence of hyper-coagulation, suggesting that this inhibitor is not anticoagulant in vivo.

Protein C

Stenflo (1976) isolated a vitamin K-dependent glycoprotein from bovine plasma which has structural similarities with the K-dependent clotting factors (Fernlund et al, 1978) and like these, is a zymogen. Proteolytic activation of protein C results in an enzyme which has anticoagulant effect in vitro and which is identical to the thrombin induced inhibitor (Marciniak, 1970) and to autoprothrombin II-A (Seegers et al, 1976).

Thrombin cleaves a peptide bond between residues 14 and 15 of the heavy chain of protein C, which now is activated. Activated protein C markedly prolongs the kaolin-cephalin clotting time of plasma, due to inactivation of clotting factor V (Kisiel et al, 1977), by the cleavage of peptide bonds in the factor Va molecule (Canfield et al, 1978). So far, the studies had been performed with bovine reagents, and bovine protein C proved inactive in human plasma. Human protein C, activated by human thrombin, was shown to prolong the partial thromboplastin time of human, but not of bovine plasma (Kisiel et al, 1979). This enzyme system thus shows considerable species specificity.

Coagulation factor V may be viewed as a cofactor in the prothrombin-thrombin conversion by factor Xa. It is well known that factor V is found in blood platelets, and it has recently been shown that factor Xa bound to factor Va on the platelet surface has a remarkable high catalytic activity in forming thrombin from prothrombin (Miletich et al, 1978). Activated protein C may destroy the factor Xa receptor in blood platelets and inhibit the binding of prothrombin to blood platelets (Stenflo & Dahlbäck, 1979). Conversely, factor Xa, when bound to blood platelets, prevents the proteolytic attack of activated protein C on the platelet. As protein C may be activated by thrombin formed in the prothrombin-platelet-factor Xa incubate, these results suggest that protein C may have a role as a regulator of prothrombin activation in vivo (Dahlbäck & Stenflo, 1980; Esmon et al, 1980). Thus activation of protein C may counteract to some extent the strong synergistic effect of blood platelets and factor Xa and indirectly facilitate factor Xa inactivation by AT. At present, no direct evidence of a physiological role of protein C is at hand. The concentration of protein C in disease is also unknown, but its biosynthesis is disturbed by oral anticoagulant treatment, and in view of its partial homology with clotting factors it is with all probability synthesized by liver cells.

CONCLUSION

A number of clotting factors are required for normal haemostasis, but bleeding tendency is usually not manifest unless the concentration of a coagulation factor is below 10 per cent of normal. AT is the only known physiological coagulation inhibitor in which a deficiency state leads to tendency to thrombosis. AT is the main inactivator of thrombin and factor Xa and also inactivates factors IXa, XIa and XIIa. These inactivation rates are roughly proportional to the AT concentration. A subnormal AT concentration will permit greater than normal activation in each of the sequential activation reactions. This probably explains why a moderately subnormal AT concentration may cause thrombosis. Possibly, the inhibitory effect of AT on some platelet reactions and the influence of endothelial AT contribute.

Congenital deficiency of AT may depend on quantitative (type 1) or various qualitative (type 2) defects or both. Profound acquired deficiency of AT is observed in severe liver disease and in DIC. Heparin therapy accelerates AT action, but the concentration of AT in the blood tends to fall.

Therapeutic infusion of AT has recently been performed in many patients. The clinical results in congenital AT deficiency complicated by thrombosis appear to be rewarding. Also in DIC the impression of the effect is favourable, but objective evaluation of the clinical results is more difficult to obtain.

α_2-M is a weak inhibitor of thrombin and plasmin and thus tends to inhibit both coagulation and fibrinolysis. The physiological effects of the other natural anticoagulants found in the blood is at present uncertain.

REFERENCES

Abildgaard U 1967a Puruification of two progressive antithrombins of human plama. Scandinavian Journal of Clinical and Laboratory Investigation 19: 190–195

Abildgaard U 1967b Inhibition of the thrombin-fibrin reaction by antithrombin III, studied by N-terminal analysis. Scandinavian Journal of Clinical and Laboratory Investigation 20: 207–216.

Abildgaard U 1968a Highly purified antithrombin III with heparin cofactor activity prepared by disc electrophoresis. Scandinavian Journal of Clinical Investigation 21: 89–91

Abildgaard U 1968b Inhibition of the thrombin-fibrinogen reaction by heparin and purified cofactor. Scandinavian Journal of Haematology 5: 440–453

Abildgaard U 1969a Inhibition of the thrombin-fibrinogen reaction by α_2-macroglobulin, studied by N-terminal analysis. Thrombosis et Diathesis Haemorrhagica (Stuttgart) 21: 173–180

Abildgaard U 1967a Purification of two progressive antithrombins of human plasma. Scandinavian Journal of Clinical and Laboratory Investigation 19: 190–195

Abildgaard U 1967b Inhibition of the thrombin-fibrin reaction by antithrombin III, studied by N-terminal analysis. Scandinavian Journal of Clinical and Laboratory Investigation 20: 207–216

Abildgaard U 1968a Highly purified antithrombin III with heparin cofactor activity prepared by disc electrophoresis. In: Abildgaard U (ed) Studies on the fibrinogen-fibrin conversion in human plasma Universitetsforlaget p. 89–91

Abildgaard U 1968b Inhibition of the thrombin-fibrinogen reaction by heparin and purified cofactor. Scandinavian Journal of Haematology 5: 440–453

Abildgaard U 1969a Inhibition of the thrombin-fibrinogen reaction by α_2-macroglobulin, studied by N-terminal analysis. Thrombosis et Diathesis Haemorrhagica (Stutgart) 21: 173–180

Abildgaard U 1969b Binding of thrombin to antithrombin III. Scandinavian Journal of Clinical and Laboratory Investigation 24: 23–27

Abildgaard U 1979 A review of antithrombin III. In: Collen D, Wiman B, Verstraete M (eds) The Physiological Inhibitors of Coagulation and Fibrinolysis, Elsevier/North-Holland Biomedical Press, 19–29

Abildgaard U 1980 Unpublished results

Abildgaard U, Fagerhol M K, Egeberg O 1970a Comparison of progressive antithrombin activity and the concentrations of three thrombin inhibitors in human plasma. Scandinavian Journal of Clinical and Laboratory Investigation 26: 349–354

Abildgaard U, Gravem K, Godal H C 1970b Assay of progressive antithrombin in plasma. Thrombosis et Diathesis Haemorrhagica (Stuttgart) 24: 224–229

Abildgaard U, Lie M, Ødegård O R 1977 Antithrombin (heparin cofactor assay with 'new' chromogenic substrates (S-2238 and Chromozym TH). Thrombosis Research 11: 549–553

Andersson L O, Barrowcliffe T W, Holmer E, Johnson E A, Sims G E C 1976 Anticoagulant properties of heparin fractionated by affinity chromatography on matrix-bound antithrombin III and by gel filtration. Thrombosis Research 9: 575–583

Anker E, Andersen R, Fagerhol M K, Abildgaard U, 1980 In preparation

Bergqvist, D, Nilsson I M 1979 A family with α_2-macroglobulin deficiency. Thrombosis Haemostasis 42: 219 Abstr

Bergström K, Lahnborg G 1975 The effect of major surgery, low doses of heparin and thromboemblolism on plasma antithrombin. Comparison of immediate thrombin inhibiting capacity and the antithrombin III content. Thrombosis Research 6: 223–233

Björk I, Larsson K 1980 Exposure to solvent of tyrosyl and tryptophanyl residues of bovine antithrombin in the absence and presence of high-affinity and low-affinity heparin. Biochemica et Biophysica Acta, 621: 273–82

Blombäck B, Blombäck M, Lagergren H, Olsson P 1963 The heparin cofactor activity in plasma and its relation to the anticoagulant effect of intravenously injected heparin. Acta Physiologica Scandinavica 58: 306–318

Blombäck M, Blombäck B, Olsson P, Svendsen L 1974 The assay of antithrombin using a synthetic chromogenic substrate for thrombin. Thrombosis Research 5: 621–632

de Boer A C, van Riel L A M, den Ottolander G J H 1979 Measurement of antithrombin III, α_2-macroglobulin and α_1-antitrypsin in patients with deep venous thrombosis and pulmonary embolism. Thrombosis Research 15: 17–25

Borsodi A, Machovich R 1979 Inhibition of esterase and amidase activities of α- and β-thrombin in the presence of antithrombin III and heparin. Biochemica et Biophysica Acta 566: 385–389

Bounameaux H, Duckert F, Walter M, Bounameaux Y 1978 The determination of antithrombin III. Comparison of six methods. Effect of oral contraceptive therapy. Thrombosis Haemostasis (Stuttgart) 39: 607–615

Brandt P, Jespersen J, Gregersen G 1980 Postpartum haemolytic-uraemic syndrome successfully treated with antithrombin III. British Medical Journal 1: 449

Brandt P, Stenbjerg S 1979 Subcutaneous heparin for thrombosis in pregnant women with hereditary antithrombin deficiency. The Lancet I: 100–101

Brozovic M, Hamlyn A M 1978 Thrombotic tendency and probable antithrombin III deficiency. Thrombosis Haemostasis 39: 778–779

Canfield W, Nesheim M, Kisiel W, Mann K G 1978 Proteolytic inactivation of bovine factor Va by bovine activated protein C. Circulation 57: supp II 210

Carvalho A, Ellman L 1976 Hereditary antithrombin III deficiency. The American Journal of Medicine 61: 179–183

Chan V, Chan T K 1979 Antithrombin III in fresh and cultured human endothelial cells: A natural anticoagulant from the vascular endothelium. Thrombosis Research 15: 209–213

Chan V, Chan T K, Wong V, Tso S C, Todd D 1979 The determination of antithrombin III by radioimmunoassay and its clinical application. British Journal of Haematology 41: 563–572

Chandra S, Bang N U 1977 Analysis of primary and secondary complexes between antithrombin III, thrombin, and factor Xa. In: Chemistry and Biology of Thrombin. Lundblad R L (ed) Ann Arbor Science, Michigan, p. 421–429

Chang T, Feinman R D, Landis B H, Fenton II J W 1979 Antithrombin reactions with α- and γ-thrombins. Biochemistry 18: 113–119

Collen D, Schetz J, de Cock F, Holmer E, Verstraete M 1977 Metabolism of antithrombin III (heparin cofactor) in man: effects of venous thrombosis and of heparin administration. European Journal of Clinical Investigation 7: 27–35

Collen D, Verstraete M 1979 Quantitation of thrombin-antithrombin III complex during coagulation of blood. In: Collen D, Wiman B, Verstraete M (eds) The Physiological Inhibitors of Coagulation and Fibrinolysis Elsevier/North-Holland Biomedical Press, p 35–38

Conard J, Salomon Y, Samama M 1974 Variations de l'antithrombine III chez les femmes sou contraception orale. Pathologie-Biologie (Paris) 22: 77–80

Conard J, Samama M 1978 L'Antithrombine III. La Revue de Médecine 42: 2343–2351

Conard J, Samama M, Bilski-Pasquier G, Bousser J 1971 Toxicité in vivo de la L-Asparaginase sur les faceteurs de la coagulation et en particulier sur l'antithrombine III. A propos de 25 observations. Coagulation 4: 195–201

Dahlbäck B, Stenflo J 1978 Binding of bovine coagulation factor Xa to platelets. Biochemistry 17: 4938–4945

Dahlbäck B, Stenflo J 1980 Inhibitory effect of activated protein C on activation of prothrombin by platelet bound factor Xa. European Journal of Biochemistry, in press

Damielsson Å, Björk I 1978 The binding of low-affinity and high-affinity heparin to antithrombin. Competition for the same binding site on the protein. European Journal of Biochemistry 90: 7–12

Danishefsky I, Zweben A, Slomiany B L 1978 Human antithrombin III. Carbohydrate components and associated glycolipid. The Journal of Biological Chemistry 253: 32–37

Dayan, L, Donadio D, David E, Huguet M 1978 Maladie thromboembolique familiale récidivante par déficit congénital en anti-thrombine III. La Nouvelle Presse médicale 7: 3229–3231

Deutsch E, Thaler E 1979 Acquired antithrombin III (At III) — deficiency in septicaemia. In: Schattauer F K (ed) Abstracts from VIIth International Congress on Thrombosis and Haemostasis 42: 375

Dombrose F A, Seegers W H, Sedenksy J A 1971 Antithrombin. Inhibition of thrombin and autoprothrombin C (F-Xa) as a mutual depletion system. Thrombosis et Diathesis Haemorrhagica (Stuttgart) 26: 103–123

Egbring R, Menche C H, Jacoby S, Klingemann H G, Hofmann A und U, Fuchs N, Heimburger K, Havemann K 1980 Vergleichende Antithrombin III-Bestimmungen bei Patienten mit akuten Leukämien, Septikämien, chronischen Leberkrankungen, Malignomen und Thrombosen und/oder Lungenembolien sowie vor und nach Antithrombin III-Konzentratgabe. Blut 40: 74–75

Egeberg O 1965 Inherited antithrombin deficiency causing thrombophilia. Thrombosis et Diathesis Haemorrhagica (Stuttgart) 13: 516–530

Eika C 1971 Inhibition of thrombin-induced aggregation of human platelets by heparin and antithrombin III. Scandinavian Journal of Haematology 8: 250–256

Einarsson R, Andersson L-O 1977 Binding of heparin to human antithrombin III as studied by measurements of tryptophan fluorescence. Biochemica et Biophysica Acta 490: 104–111

Esmon C T, Comp P C, Walker F J 1979 Functions for protein C. In: Eighth Steenboch Symposium. Suttie J W (ed) Vitamin K metabolism & vitamin K dependent proteins: Baltimore, University Park Press, p 72–83

Fagerhol M K, Abildgaard U 1970 Immunological studies on human antithrombin III. Influence of age, sex and use of contraceptives on serum concentration. Scandinavian Journal of Haematology 7: 10–17

Fagerhol M K, Abildgaard U 1972 Unpublished observations

Fagerhol M K, Abildgaard U, Bergsjø P, Jacobsen J H 1970 Oral contraceptives and low antithrombin III concentration. The Lancet I: 1175

Feinman R D 1979 Kinetics and mechanism of the antithrombinprotease reaction. In: Collen D, Wiman B, Verstraete M (eds) The physiological Inhibitors of Coagulation and Fibrinolysis Elsevier/North-Holland Biomedical Press, p 55–66

Fell C, Ivanovic N, Johnson S A, Seegers W H 1954 Differentiation of plasma antithrombin activities. Proceedings of the Society for Experimental Biology and Medicine 85: 199–202

Fernlund P, Stenflo J, Tufvesson A 1978 Bovine protein C: Amino acid sequence of the light chain. Proceedings of the National Academy of Sciences of the United States of America (Washington) 75: 5889–5892

Fish W W, Björk I 1979 Release of a two-chain form of antithrombin from the antithrombin-thrombin complex. European Journal of Biochemistry 101: 31–38

Fish W W, Orre K, Björk I 1979 Routes of thrombin action in the production of proteolytically modified, secondary forms of antithrombin-thrombin complex. European Journal of Biochemistry 101: 39–44

Fischer A M, Bros A, Ratowicz S, Josso F 1979 Heparin hinders thrombin inhibition by α_2-macroglobulin. Thrombosis Haemostasis (Stuttgart) 42: 9

Furugren B, Andersson L-O, Einarsson R 1977 Small-angle X-ray scattering studies on human antithrombin III and its complex with heparin. Archives of Biochemistry and Biophysics 178: 419–424

Gamba G, Fornasari P, Montani N, Biancardi M, Grignani G, Ascari E 1980 Plasma levels of protease inhibitors in acute myeloid leukemia at the onset of the disease and during antiblastic therapy. Thrombosis Research 17: 41–53

Ganrot P O 1969 Electrophoretic separation of two thrombin inhibitors in plasma and serum. Scandinavian Journal of Clinical and Laboratory Investigation 24: 11–14

Gerendas M 1960 Die Thrombininaktivierung als Enzymprozess. Thrombosis et Diathesis Haemorrhagica (Stuttgart) 4: 56–70

Gitel S N, Salvati E A, Wessler S, Robinson Jr H J, Worth M H 1979 The effect of total hip replacement and general surgery on antithrombin III in relation to venous thrombosis. Journal of Bone and Joint Surgery, American Volume 61 A: 653–656

Gitel S N, Wessler S 1975 Plasma antithrombin III: a quantitative assay of biological activity. Thrombosis Research 7: 5–16

Godal H C, Rygh M, Laake K 1974 Progressive inactivation of purified factor VII by heparin and antithrombin III. Thrombosis Research 5: 773–775

Gomperts E D, Feesey M, van der Walt J D 1976 Two dimensional immunoelectrophoretic studies in antithrombin III deficiency. Thrombosis Research 8: 713–718

Griffith M J, Kingdon H S, Lundblad R L 1978 Fractionation of heparin by affinity chromatography on covalently-bound human α-thrombin. Biochemical and Biophysical Research Communications 83: 1198–1205

Griffith M J, Kingdon H S, Lundblad R L 1979 Inhibition of the heparin-antithrombin III/thrombin reaction by active site blocked-thrombin. Biochemical and Biophysical Research Communications 87: 686–692

Grimmer Ø, Fagerhol M K 1977 Immunoelectrophoretic quantitation of antithrombin III. International Journal of Peptide and Protein Research 9: 85–90

Gyde O H B, Middleton M D, Vaughan G R, Fletcher D J 1978 Antithrombin III deficiency, hypertriglyceridaemia, and venous thrombosis. British Medical Journal 1: 621–622

Harpel P C, Rosenberg R D 1976 α_2-macroglobulin and antithrombin-heparian cofactor: modulators of hemostatic and inflammatory reactions. Progress in Haemostasis and Thrombosis 3: 145–189

Hathaway W E, Neumann L L, Borden C A, Jacobson L J 1978 Immunologic studies of antithrombin III heparin cofactor in the new born. Thrombosis Haemostasis (Stuttgart) 39: 624–630

Hatton M W C, Berry L R, Regoeczi E 1978 Inhibition of thrombin by antithrombin III in the presence of certain glycosaminoglycans found in the mammalian aorta. Thrombosis Research 13: 655–670

Hatton, M W C, Regoeczi E 1977 The inactivation of thrombin and plasmin by antithrombin III in the presence of Sepharoseheparin. Thrombosis Research 10: 645–660

Hedner U, Nilsson I M 1973 Antithrombin III in a clinical material. Thrombosis Research 3: 631–641

Heimburger N 1967 On the proteinase inhibitors of human plasma with especial reference to antithrombin. First International Symposium on Tissue Factors in the Homeostasis of the Coagulation-Fibrinolysis System, Florence

Hensen A, Loeliger E A 1963 Antithrombin III. Its metabolism and its function in blood coagulation. Thrombosis et Diathesis Haemorrhagica suppl 19: 1–84

Holm H A, Abildgaard U 1980 In preparation

Holmer E, Lindahl U, Bäckström G, Thunberg L, Sandberg H, Söderström G, Andersson L-O 1980 Anticoagulant activities and effects on platelets of a heparin fragment with high affinity for antithrombin. Thrombosis Research, in press

Holmer E, Söderström G, Andersson L-O 1979 Studies on the mechanism of the rate-enhancing effect of heparin on the thrombin-antithrombin III reaction. European Journal of Biochemistry 93: 1–5

Höök M, Björk I, Hopwood J, Lindahl U 1976 Anticoagulant activity of heparin: separation of high-activity and low-activity heparin species by affinity chromatograph on immobilized antithrombin. FEEBS Letters 66: 90–93

Howie P W, Prentice C R M, McNicol G P 1973 A method of antithrombin estimation using plasma defibrinated with Ancrod. British Journal of Haematology 25: 101–110

Jesty J 1978 The inhibition of activated bovine coagulation factors X and VII by antithrombin III. Archives of Biochemistry and Biophysics 185: 165–173

Jesty J 1979 Dissociation of complexes and their derivates formed during inhibition of bovine thrombin and activated factor X by antithrombin III. Journal of Biological Chemistry 254: 1044–1049

Johansson L, Hedner U, Hilsson I M 1978 Familial antithrombin III deficiency as pathogenesis of deep venous thrombosis. Acta Medica Scandinavica (Stockholm) 204: 491–495

Jordan R, Beeler D, Rosenberg R 1979 Fractionation of low molecular weight heparin species and their interaction with antithrombin. The Journal of Biological Chemistry 254: 2902–2913

Jørgenson K A, Stoffersen E 1979 Antithrombin III and the nephrotic syndrome. Scandinavian Journal of Haematology 22: 442–448

Jörnvall H, Fish W W, Björk I 1979 The thrombin cleavage site in bovine antithrombin. Febs Letters 106: 358–362

Juillet Y, Aiach M, Fiessinger J N, Leclerc M, Housset E 1978 Antithrombine III et thromboses veineuses. Semaine des Hopitaux de Paris 54: 1126–1129

Kahlé L H, Schipper H G, Jenkins C S P, Ten Kate J W 1978a Antithrombin III. I. Evaluation of an automated antithrombin III method. Thrombosis Research 12: 1003–1014

Kahlé L H, Jenkins C S P, Ali-Briggs E, ten Cate J W 1978b Antithrombin III. II. Comparison of different substrates and thrombin preparations. Thrombosis Research 13: 645–653

Kauffmann R H, Veltkamp J J, van Tilburg N H, van Es L 1978 Acquired antithrombin III deficiency and thrombosis in the nephrotic syndrome. The American Journal of Medicine 65: 607–613

von Kaulla E, von Kaulla K N 1967 Antithrombin III and diseases. American Journal of Clinical Pathology 48: 69–80

Kisiel W, Canfield W M, Ericsson L H, Davie E W 1977 Anticoagulant properties of bovine plasma protein C following activation by thrombin. Biochemistry 16: 5824–5831

Kisiel W 1979 Human plasma protein C. Isolation, characterization and mechanism of activation by α-thrombin. Journal of Clinical Investigation 64: 761–769

Koj A, Regoeczi E 1978 Effect of experimental inflammation on the synthesis and distribution of antithrombin III and α₁-antitrypsin in rabbits. British Journal of Experimental Pathology (London) 59: 473–481

Korvald E, Abildgaard U, Fagerhol M K 1974 Major operations, hemostatic parameters and venous thrombosis. Thrombosis Research 4: 147–154

Kurachi K, Fujikawa K, Schmer G, Davie E W 1976 Inhibition of bovine factor IXa and factor Xaβ by antithrombin. Biochemistry 15: 373–377

Lam L S L, Regoeczi E, Hatton M W C 1979 In vivo behaviour of some antithrombin III-protease complexes. British Journal of Experimental Pathology (London) 60: 151–160

Lane J L 1978 Some immunological investigations on antithrombin III 'Budapest'. British Journal of Haematology 40: 459–470

Lane J L, Biggs R 1977 The natural inhibitors of coagulation: Antithrombin III, heparin cofactor and antifactor Xa. In: Poller L (ed) 1977 Recent Advances in Blood Coagulation. Nr. 2 Churchill Livingstone, Edinburgh

Lane J L, Bird P, Rizza C R 1975 A new assay for the measurement of total progressive antithrombin. British Journal of Haematology 30: 103–115

Larsen M L, Abildgaard U, Teien A N, Gjesdal K 1978 Assay of plasma heparin using thrombin and the chromogenic substrate H-D-Phe-Pip-Arg-pNA (S-2238). Thrombosis Research 13: 285–288

Lasch H G, Rodriguez-Erdmann F, Schimpf K 1961 Antithrombin III und Anti-Blut, thrombokinase bei experimenteller Verbrauchskogululopathie. Klinische Wochenscrift 39: 645–647

Lechner K, Tahler E, Niessner H, Nowotny Ch, Partsch H 1977 Antithrombin-III-Mangel und Tromboseneigung. Wiener Klinische Wochenschrift 89: 215–222

Lee A K Y, Chan V, Chan T K 1979 The identification and localization of antithrombin III in human tissues. Thrombosis Research 14: 209–217

Li E H H, Fenton II J W, Feinman R D 1976 The role of heparin in the thrombin-antithrombin III reaction. Archives of Biochemistry and Biophysics 175: 153–159

Lindahl U, Bäckström G, Höök, M, Thunberg L, Fransson L-Å, Linker A 1979 Structure of the antithrombin-binding site in heparin. Proceedings of the National Academy of Sciences of the United States of America 76: 3198

MacGregor I R, Lane D A, Kakkar V V 1979 Evidence for a plasma inhibitor of the heparin accelerated inhibition of factor Xa by antithrombin III. Biochemica et Biophysica Acta 586: 584–593

Machovich R, Blasko G, Palos L A 1975 Action of heparin on thrombin-antithrombin reaction. Biochemica et Biophysica Acta 379: 193–200

Machovich R, Arányi P 1978 Effect of heparin on thrombin inactivation by antithrombin III. Biochemical Journal (London) 173: 869–875

Mann Jr L T, Jensenius J C, Simonsen M, Abildgaard U 1969 Antithrombin III: Protection against death after injection of thromboplastin. Science 166: 517–518

Mannucci L, Dioguardi N, del Ninno E, Mannucci P M 1973 Value of Normotest and antithrombin III in the assessment of liver function. Scandinavian Journal of Gastroenterology 8 supplement 19: 103–107

Marciniak E 1970 Coagulation Inhibitor elicited by thrombin. Science 170: 452–453

Marciniak E 1973 Factor Xa inactivation by antithrombin III: Evidence for biological stabilization of factor Xa by factor V — phospholipid complex. British Journal of Haematology 24: 391–400

Marciniak E, Farley C H, DeSimone P A 1974 Familial thrombosis due to antithrombin III deficiency. Blood 43: 219–231

Marciniak E, Gockerman J P 1977 Heparin-induced decrease in circulating antithrombin-III. The Lancet II: 581–584

Matsuo T, Ohki Y, Kondo S, Matsuo O 1979 Familial antithrombin III deficiency in a Japanese family. Thrombosis Research 16: 815–823

Medén-Britth G, Teien A 1979 Infusion of purified antithrombin III to patients with fracture of the neck of the femur. European Surgical Research 11: 289–295

Mettinger K L, Nyman D, Kjellin K G, Sidén Å, Söderström C E 1979 Factor VIII related antigen, antithrombin III, spontaneous platelet aggregation and plasminogen activator in ischemic cerebrovascular disease. Journal of the Neurological Sciences 41: 31–38

Miller-Andersson M, Borg H, Andersson L-O 1974 Purification of antithrombin III by affinity chromatography. Thrombosis Research 5: 439–452

McKay E J 1980 Immunochemical analysis of active and inactive antithrombin III. British Journal of Haematology, submitted for publication

Miletich J P, Jackson C M, Majerus P W 1978 Properties of the factor Xa binding site on human platelets. The Journal of Biological Chemistry 253: 6908–6916

Monnier L, Follea G, Mirouze J 1978 Antithrombin III deficiency in diabetes mellitus: Influence on vascular degenerative complications. Hormone and Metabolic Research (Stuttgart) 10: 470–473

Morawitz P 1905 Die Chemie der Blutgerinnung. Ergebnisse der Physiologie, biologischen Chemie und experimentellen Pharmakologie (Berlin) 4: 307–422

Müller N, Budde U, Schander M, Niesen M, Etzel F 1980 Zur perioperativen Substitutionstherapie bei angeborenem Antithrombin-III-mangel. Blut 40: 70–71

Müllertz S 1979 The primary plasmin-inhibitor, α_2-plasmin-inhibitor or α_2-antiplasmin. A review. In: Collen D, Wiman B, Verstraete M (eds) The Physiological Inhibitors of Coagulation and Fibrinolysis Elsevier/North-Holland Biomedical Press, p 87–101

Nagy I, Losonczy H, Pár A 1976 Heparin induced change of antithrombin III (AT III) activity in chronic active hepatitis and liver cirrhosis. Proceedings, Symposia and Round Table Conferences of the 10th International Congress of Gastroenterology, Budapest

Nagy I, Losonczy H, Szaksz I, Temesi C, Hergert K 1979 An analysis of clinical and laboratory data in patients with congenital antithombin III (AT III) deficiency. Acta Medica Academiae Scientiarum Hungaricae 36: 53–60

Nordenman B, Björk I 1978 Binding of low-affinity and high-affinity heparin to antithrombin. Ultraviolet difference spectroscopy and circular dichroism studies. Biochemistry 17: 3339–3344

Nordenman B, Nordling K, Björk I 1980 A differential effect of low-affinity heparin on the inhibition of thrombin and factor Xa by antithrombin. Thrombosis Research, 17: 595–600

Nordenman B, Nyströn C, Björk I 1977 The size and shape of human and bovine antithrombin III. European Journal of Biochemistry 78: 195–203

Ødegård O E, Abildgaard U 1977 Antifactor Xa activity in thrombophilia. Studies in a family with AT-III deficiency. Scandinavian Journal of Haematology 18: 86–90

Ødegård O R, Abildgaard U, Lie M, Miller-Andersson M 1977 Inactivation of bovine and human thrombin and factor Xa by antithrombin III studied with amidolytic methods. Thrombosis Research 11: 205–216

Ødegård O R, Fagerhol M K, Lie M 1976 Heparin cofactor activity and antithrombin III concentration in plasma related to age and sex. Scandinavian Journal of Haematology 17: 258–262

Ødegård O R, Lie M 1978 Simultaneous inactivation of thrombin and factor Xa by AT-III: influence of heparin. Thrombosis Research 12: 697–700

Ødegård O R, Lie M, Abildgaard U 1975 Heparin cofactor activity measured with an amidolytic method. Thrombosis Research 6: 287–294

Ødegård O R, Rosenlund B, Ervik E 1978 Automated antithrombin III assay with a centrifugal analyser. Hemostasis 7: 202–209

Ødegård O R, Teien A N 1976 Antithrombin III, heparin cofactor and antifactor Xa in a clinical material.

Thrombosis Research 8: 173–178

Older R A, Miller M D, Tisher C C 1978 Renal vein thrombosis. Complication of primary renal disease and the nephrotic syndrome. Journal of the American Medical Association 240: 1747–1748

Østerud B, Miller-Andersson M, Abildgaard U, Prydz H 1976 The effect of antithrombin III on the activity of the coagulation factors VII, IX and X. Thrombosis Haemostasis (Stuttgart) 35: 295–204

Owen W G, Penick, G D, Yoder E, Poole B L 1976 Evidence for an ester bond between thrombin and heparin cofactor. Thrombosis Haemostatis (Stuttgart) 35: 87–95

Panicucci F, Sagripanti A, Conte B, Pinori E, Vispi M, Lecchini L 1980 Antithrombin III, heparin cofactor and antifactor Xa in relation to age, sex and pathological conditions. Haemostasis, in press

Penner J A, Hassouna H, Hunter M J, Cockley M 1979 A clinically silent antithrombin III defect in an Ann Arbor Family. Thrombosis Haemostasis (Stuttgart) 42: 186 (Abstr.)

Petersen T E, Dudek-Wojciechowaska G, Sottrup-Jensen L, Magnusson S 1979 Primary structure of antithrombin-III (heparin cofactor. Partial homology between α_1-antitrypsin and antithrombin-III. In: Collen D, Wiman B, Verstraete M (eds) The physiological inhibitors of blood coagulation, Elsevier/North-Holland Biomedical Press p 19

Philip J A D, Walker I D, Davidson J F 1979 The ratio of functional: immunologic antithrombin III as an index of antithrombin consumption. In: Schattauer F K (ed) Abstracts from VIIth International Congress on Thrombosis and Haemostasis 42: 375

Piepkorn M W, Lagunoff D, Schmer G 1978 Heparin binding to antithrombin III: variation in binding sites and affinity. Biochemical and Biophysical Research Communications 85: 851–856

Piepkorn M W, Schmer G, Lagunoff D 1978 Isolation of high-activity heparin by DEAE-SEPHADEX and protamine-sepharose chromatography. Thrombosis Research 13: 1077–1087

Porter P, Porter M C, Shanberge J N 1967 Heparin cofactor and plasma antithrombin in relation to the mechanism of inactivation of thrombin by heparin. Clinica Chimca Acta 17: 189–200

Quick A J 1938 The normal antithrombin of the blood and its relation to heparin. American Journal of Physiology 123: 712–719

Reeve E B 1980 Steady state relations between factors X, Xa, II, IIa, antithrombin III and alpha-2 macroglobulin in thrombosis. Thrombosis Research, in press

Reve E B, Leonard B, Wentland S H, Damus P 1980 Studies with ^{131}I-labelled antithrombin III in dogs. Thrombosis Research, in press

Refvem O, Fagerhol M K, Abildgaard U 1973 Changes in antithrombin III levels following cessation of anticoagulant therapy. Acta Medica Scandinavica 193: 307–309

Rosenberg R D, Damus P S 1973 The purification and mechanism of action of human antithrombin-heparin cofactor. The Journal of Biological Chemistry 248: 6490–6505

Rosenberg R D, Jordan R E, Favreau L V, Lam L H 1979 Highly active heparin species with multiple binding sites for antithrombin. Biochemical and Biophysical Research Communications 86: 1319–1324

Rosenberg R, Lam L 1979 Correlation between structure and function of heparin. Proceedings of the National Academy of Sciences of the United States of America (Washington) 76: 1218–1222

Sas G, Blaskó B, Bánhegy D, Jákó J, Palos L A 1974 Abnormal antithrombin III/antithrombin III 'Budapest'/as a cause of a familial thrombophilia. Thrombosis et Diathesis Haemorrhagica (Stuttgart) 32: 105–115

Sas G, Köves A, Petó I 1977 Detection of antithrombin III/AT-III/complexes in 'hypercoagulable' and hyperfibrinolytic states. Thrombosis and Haemostasis (Stuttgart) 38: 164

Sas G, Pepper D S, Cash J D 1975 Further investigations on antithrombin III in the plasma of the patients with the abnormality of antithrombin III 'Budapest'. Thrombosis et Diathesis Haemorrhagica (Stuttgart) 33: 564–572

Sas, G, Petó I, Bánhegy D, Blaskó G, Domján G 1980 Heterogeneity of the 'classical' antithrombin III deficiency. Thrombosis and Haemostasis, 43: 133–136

Sagar S, Thomas D P, Stamatakis J D, Kakkar V V 1976 Oral contraceptives, antithrombin-III activity, and postoperative deep-vein thrombosis. The Lancet I: 509–511

Schander K, Niesen M, Rehm A, Budde U, Müller N 1980 Diagnose und Therapie eines kongenitalen Antithrombin-III-Mangels in der Neonatalperiode. Blut 40: 68

Schipper H G, Kahlé L H, Jenkins C S P, ten Cate J W 1978 Antithrombin III transfusion in disseminated intravascular coagulation. The Lancet II: 854

Schipper H G, Lamping R, Kahlé L, Ten Cate J W 1979 Antithrombin-III transfusion in patients with liver cirrhosis. Thrombosis Haemostasis 42: 327 Abstr.

Schmidt A 1892 Zur Blutlehre. F C W Vogel, Leipzig

Schramm W, Marx R 1980 Zur Behandlung thrombophiler Diathesen — Substitution mit Antithrombin-III-Konzentrat. Blut 40: 68–69

Scully M F, Kakkar V V 1977 Methods for semi micro or automated determination of thrombin, antithrombin, and heparin cofactor using the substrate, H-D-Phe-Pip-Arg-p-Nitroanilide 2 HC1. Clinica Chimica Acta 79: 595–602

Seegers W H, Novoa E, Henry R L, Hassouna H I 1976 Relationship of 'new' vitamin K-dependent protein C and 'old' autoprothombin II-A. Thrombosis Research 8: 543–552

Shapiro S S, Anderson D B 1977 Thrombin inhibition in normal plasma. In: Chemistry and Biology of Thrombin. Lundblad R L (ed) Ann Arbor Science, Michigan, p 361–374

Starkey P H M 1979 α_2-macroglobulin: A review. In: Collen D, Wiman B, Verstraete M (eds) The Physiological Inhibitors of Coagulation and Fibrinolysis Elsevier/North-Holland Biomedical Press, p 221–230

Stead N, Kaplan A P, Rosenberg R D 1976 Inhibition of activated factor XII by antithrombin-heparin cofactor. Journal of Biological Chemistry 251: 6481–6488

Steinbuch M, Blatrix C, Josso F L 1966 L'α_2-macroglobuline comme anti-thrombine progressive. Proceedings, XIth Congress of International Society of Haematology, Sidney 7

Stenflo J 1976 A new vitamin K-dependent protein. Purification from bovine plasma and preliminary characterization. The Journal of Biological Chemistry 251: 355–363

Stenflo J, Dahlbäck B 1979 Interaction between prothrombin and the platelet receptor for factor Xa inhibitory effect of protein C. In: Suttie J W (ed) Eight Steenbock Symposium, University Park Press p 89–95

Stormorken H, Ritland S, Baklund A 1976 Plasminogen, prekallikrein and antithrombin III in liver disease as assayed with synthetic chromogenic substrates. In: Okamoto S, Blombäck B (ed) Proceedings of ad hoc Discussion Group on Synthetic Substrates and Inhibitors of Coagulation and Fibrinolysis, Koyoto, p 41–46

Stürzebecher J 1977 Role of heparin in the interaction of serine proteinases with antithrombin III. Acta Biologica et Medica Germanica (Berlin) 36: 1893–1897

Takeda Y, Kobayashi N 1977 Antithrombin II responses in dogs to various stimuli. Thrombosis and Haemostasis (Stuttgart) 38: 164

Tanaka H, Hobayashi N, Takeuchi T, Takada M, Maekawa T 1979 Effect of endotoxin on kinetics of antithrombin III. Thrombosis Haemostasis 42: 374 Abstr.

Teger-Nilsson A C 1975 Antithrombin in infancy and childhood. Acta Pedriatica Scandinavica 64: 624–628

Teien A N 1977 Heparin elimination in patients with liver cirrhosis. Thrombosis and Haemostasis 38: 701–706

Teien A N, Abildgaard U, Höök M 1976 The anticoagulant effect of heparan sulfate and dermatan sulfate. Thrombosis Research 8: 859–867

Thaler E, Blazar E, Kopsa H, Pinggera W F 1978 Acquired antithrombin III deficiency in patients with glomerular proteinuria. Haemostasis 7: 257–272

Thaler E, Niessner H, Kleinberger G, Gassner A 1979 Antithrombin III replacement therapy in patients with congenital and acquired antithrombin III deficiency. In: Schattauer F K (ed) Abstracts from VIIth International Congress on Thrombosis and Haemostasis 42: 327

Thunberg L, Lindahl U, Tengblad A, Laurent T C, Jackson C M 1979 On the molecular-weight-dependence of the anticoagulant activity of heparin. Biochemical Journal 181: 241–243

Tullis J L, Watanabe K 1978 Platelet antithrombin deficiency. A new clinical entity. The American Journal of Medicine 65: 472–478

Villaneueva G, Danishefsky I 1978 Conformational changes accompanying the binding of antithrombin III to thrombin. Biochemistry 18: 810–817

Walker F J, Esmon C T 1979 The effect of prothrombin fragment 2 on the inhibition of thrombin by antithrombin III. Journal of Biological Chemistry 254: 5618–562

Walker I D, Davidson J F, Young P, Conkie J A 1975 Effect of anabolic steroids on plasma antithrombin III. α_2 macroglobulin and α_1 antitrypsin levels. Thrombosis et Diathesis Haemorrhagica (Stuttgart) 34: 106–114

Wallenbeck I, Bergqvist D, Hallböök T, Yin E T 1979 Xal (antithrombin III) activity in relation to postoperative deep vein thrombosis (DVT). Thrombosis Haemostasis 42: 385 Abstr.

Wickerhauser M, Williams C, Mercer J 1979 Development of large scale fractionation methods. VII. Preparation of antithrombin III concentrate. Vox Sanguinis (Basel) 36: 281–293

Weymouth F W 1913 The relation of metathrombin to thrombin. American Journal of Physiology 32: 266–285

Wolf M, Royer C, Lavergne J M, Larrieu M J 1979 A new variant of antithrombin III. Study of three related cases. Thrombosis Haemostasis 42: 186 Abstr.

Yin E T 1974 Effect of heparin on the neutralization of factor Xa and thrombin by the plasma alpha-2-globulin inhibitor. Thrombosis and Haemostasis (Stuttgart) 33: 43–50

7. The haemostatic plug

Jan J. Sixma

Introduction

Since it became evident towards the end of last century that haemostasis was brought about by the formation of occlusive plugs consisting of blood platelets much attention was paid to the formation and composition of these plugs. This resulted in a number of important studies between 1880 and 1900 and again since 1948 when the interest in blood platelets was revived. In a previous paper we have reviewed many of these studies and put them in framework of physiologic data derived from in vitro studies of platelet function (Sixma & Wester, 1977).

In the present paper I will review more recent observations regarding the haemostatic plug with particular emphasis on haemostasis in the uterus during menstruation which showed a number of interesting differences from haemostatic processes elsewhere.

Important new data have recently been gathered about the interaction of platelets with the vessel wall. Although an exhaustive treatment of all aspects of this area is impossible within the limitations of this chapter I will try to highlight the main issues.

Haemostasis in human skin

Almost the only tissue accessible in man to studies of the haemostatic process, is the skin. For these investigations either surgical excisions or punch biopsies of bleeding time wounds have been employed. The data prior to 1977 have been summarized in a previous review (Sixma & Wester, 1977). Here recent data on the morphology of the human skin (Wester et al, 1978; 1979) will be discussed.

Early haemostasis

The early haemostatic plug is characterized by firmly interdigitated degranulated platelets in the center of the plug. Degranulation of platelets starts as early as 30 seconds after the wound has been made and most platelets are degranulated at 3 minutes but occasionally one or even several platelets have retained all secretion granules.

The platelets are densely packed with distances of 10 to 60 nm between them. No fibrin is observed in the intercellular spaces but some floccular material is often seen and a dense line is often found between platelets in close contact. These dense lines have been reported previously (Hovig et al, 1967). They may represent condensation of the cell coat (White, 1970).

The peripheral part of the plug 3 minutes after the wound has been made, consists of platelet remnants appearing as large empty entirely translucent vesicles, containing few cell organelles of cytoplasmic matrix. These 'empty balloons' are obviously caused by leakage of intracellular contents through large holes in the membranes. The origin and nature of the lytic changes in the cell membrane are presently unknown. Similar changes were not observed in in vitro aggregates in which degranulation was observed (Sixma & Geuze, 1968) or in thrombi formed in a rotating tilted plastic tube.

Fibrin in the early haemostatic plug is only observed as tiny strands at the periphery of the plug between the empty balloons. At this location fibrin formation occurs relatively early probably via thrombin formation caused by activation of the extrinsic pathway by tissue thromboplastin.

Extensions of the haemostatic plug into blood vessels are regularly observed. The blood platelets in these extensions still contain most of their secretion granules. This may indicate that these platelets have accumulated recently perhaps after the vessel was occluded. This may be caused by continuous leakage of plasma through a yet permeable plug or by active migration of blood platelets which has been demonstrated in vitro (Lowenhaupt et al, 1977).

Fibrinous transformation
At 10 minutes after wounding degranulation has progressed and more electron dense material appears in intercellular spaces. Several platelets in the centre of the plug have decreased electron density. The peripheral rim of empty platelet remnants increases somewhat in size but this is more obvious at 30 minutes after a wound has been made. Small fibrin fibers are visible between these empty platelet vesicles and these have become quite thick strands at the periphery of the plug. Empty platelet vesicles are now also observed in the vessel lumen but no fibrin is observed here.

At 2 hours after the wound has been made considerable changes are observed. In large areas of the plug the platelets obtain rounded contours with few interdigitations. These platelets become empty and translucent. Inter-platelet distances increase up to 300 nm. Fibrin strands are observed between platelets in these areas (Fig. 7.1). Other parts of the plug are less transformed. Platelets are more interdigitated, less fibrin is present and the platelets have a normal electron density. In these areas platelets are occasionally seen that still contain secretion granules. Occasionally plugs similar to those at three and 10 minutes are observed. The plugs may have formed later due to rebleeding in the wound.

A striking feature of the wound at two hours is the strong infiltration with leukocytes into the wound but particularly around the blood vessel where cuff-like, sometimes even multi-layered accumulations may be observed up to distances of 200 μm from the wound.

On top of the wound a tough scab is formed consisting of air-dried proteins and red blood cells. This scab may have a function in the arrest of bleeding because it prevents haemostatic plugs to be torn away by slight accidental trauma.

The fibrinous transformation of the plug in human skin is in many regards similar to the changes occurring in mural thrombi experimentally produced in swine (Jørgensen et al, 1967). An important feature is the relatively late appearance of fibrin strands. Striking is also the absence of fibrin inside the vessel contrary to the popular belief of a consolidating fibrin-red cell mass behind the plug similar to what is observed in venous thrombi.

Haemostasis and inflammation
An underestimated feature of haemostatic plug formation is the important infiltration

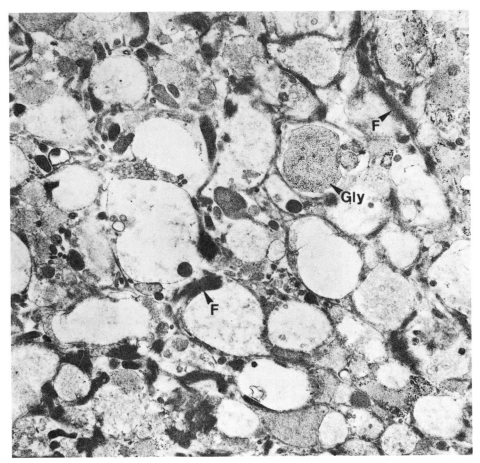

Fig. 7.1 Electron micrograph of a central part of the plug at 2 hours. Platelets exhibit rounded contours and are often empty. Platelets are loosely packed and much fibrin (F) can be seen between them. Gly, Glycogen. × 18 900.

with leucocytes, polymorphonuclears in particular. This infiltration may become so strong that close relationship between haemostasis and inflammation is suggested. Many in vitro data indicate that such an interrelationship indeed exists.

Platelets possess an active lipoxygenase system (Nugteren, 1975) and several of the products have chemotactic properties (Goetzl et al, 1977; Turner et al, 1975). Also two products of the prostaglandin metabolism in platelets, HTT and thromboxane B_2, (Goetz & Gorman, 1978) possess chemotactic activity. Platelets have also been reported to release a protein which requires the presence of complement factors C5 for activity (Weksler & Coupal, 1973).

The initial activation of the coagulation and fibrinolytic pathway is also directly linked to chemotaxis. Direct chemotactic activity has been postulated for kallikrein and plasminogen activator in blood (Kay & Kaplan, 1975). Some of this work should be re-evaluated with well characterized purified factors presently available. Further elucidation of the role of high molecular weight kininogen which circulates in a complex with prekallikrein is also of importance.

Chemotactic activity is not only the result of activation of the initial stages of the coagulation and fibrinolytic pathway but also of the action of thrombin and plasmin on fibrinogen. Fibrinopeptide B was demonstrated to have chemotactic activity and a fibrinogen degradation product as yet not identified, had a similar effect (Kay & Kaplan, 1975).

The chemotactic stimuli caused by the haemostatic process may be of importance in preventing infection in wounds. An alternative role was recently suggested when evidence was found that polymorphonuclear leukocytes might enhance endothelial regeneration and arterial healing (Fromer & Klintworth, 1975, 1976; Sholley et al, 1978).

Haemostasis in the uterus

Haemostatic plug formation in the uterus is of great importance. Increased menstrual blood loss is without doubt the single most important cause of iron deficiency anaemia and acceptability of contraceptive measures is strongly related to the amount of menstrual and intermenstrual bleeding caused by them.

Menorrhagia is also often the most important expression of a haemorrhagic disorder in women in the childbearing years particularly in von Willebrand's disease, Glanzmann's thrombasthenia and thrombocytopenia. The prolonged bleeding in these disorders indicates not only that platelets are involved in uterine haemostasis but also that fibrin formation is likely to play a role as indicated by the effectiveness of antifibrinolytic agents in menorrhagia (Nilsson & Rybo, 1967; Kasonde & Bonnar, 1975).

Until recently only curettage specimens from the first day of menstruation (Salvatore, 1969) and occasional chance observations on hysterectomy specimens (Bartelmez, 1941; Nogales et al, 1969) were available but recently a study was conducted in our laboratory involving systematic research of the time dependent changes in the haemostatic process in normal women (Christiaens et al, 1980a, b, and 1981). A number of interesting new data were obtained and pertinent differences from haemostasis elsewhere were identified that warrant inclusion in this review.

Premenstrual changes

Data from the premenstrual phase were first obtained from one hysterectomy specimen removed after three hours of premenstrual spotting. The vascular changes were then further confirmed in biopsy specimens of the premenstrual period (Christiaens et al, 1980b). No menstrual shedding was observed in the premenstrual phase but stromal disintegration had started in some places.

Vessel lesions with focal escape of red blood cells into the stroma were observed. The lesions were characterized by holes in the endometrium and interruptions in the basement membrane (Fig. 7.2). The most curious feature of these lesions was however the total absence of platelet adherence or accumulation although subendothelial collagen fibers were evidently exposed to the blood. Biopsies specimens of the premenstrual period indicated that such lesions were observed up to five days before a menstruation actually started.

Early menstruation (Shedding phase)

The compact layer of the endometrium was engorged with blood and this progressed

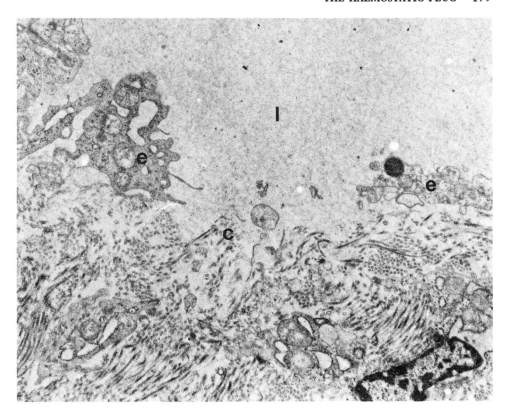

Fig. 7.2   (from Christiaens, G. C. M. L., Sixma J. J. and Haspels, A. A.: Morphology of haemostasis in menstrual endometrium. Brit. J. Obstet. Gynecol, 1980, 87: 428). Electron micrograph of a damaged vessel in the premenstrual uterus. The collagen (c) between two endothelial cells (e) is exposed to the luminal (l) content. (×9900).

towards deeper layers at later times. Part of the endometrium was shed into the cavity. Vessels ending on the shedding edge were filled with thrombi consisting of platelets and fibrin (Fig. 7.3). Alternating layers of fibrin and platelets were often observed giving an onion-skin like appearance to the thrombus indicating that blood had streamed along the thrombus. The platelets were fully degranulated and often converted into empty balloon-shaped vesicular platelet remnants. Fibrin was often present as thick bundles. Large amounts of polymorphonuclear cells were found near the plugs in the vessels and in the surrounding stroma. No platelet plugs or fibrin deposition was found outside the vessels. Shed tissue still contained blood vessels with occluding thrombi but extravascular fibrin was observed in this tissue (Christiaens, 1981).

The sample obtained at about 12 hours after the start of menstruation showed that most of the functional layer at this time was shed. The red cell extravasation was less and only small thrombi were observed. These thrombi consisted of platelets that were loosely aggregated and that still contained most of their granules.

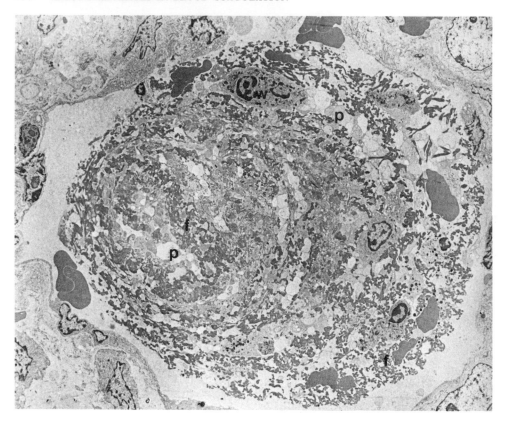

Fig. 7.3   (from Christiaens, G. C. M. L., Sixma, J. J. and Haspels, A. A.: Morphological aspects of menstrual bleeding. Possible influences of IUD. In: Medicated IUDs and polymeric delivery systems. Symposium Proceedings. Amsterdam 27–30 June 1979, abstract 43.)
Electron micrograph of a thrombus in the functional endometrium of a uterus removed 7 hours after the onset of bleeding. A layered structure of alternating fibrin fibers (f) and platelet remnants (p) is observed. w = white blood cell. (×1902.4)

Late menstruation
At 20 to 24 hours after the start of menstruation all tissue was apparently fully shed. Stromal disintegration and red cell extravasation was no longer observed. Small amounts of the functional layer remained. Occasionally some intra-vascular fibrin was observed but most vessels contained no thrombi. The vessels ending on the shedding margin were constricted and this may be responsible for the haemostasis.

Overall picture
From these observations conclusions may be drawn about the sequence of events. Menstruation starts with vessel lesions of unknown origin in which the haemostatic reaction is inhibited as evidenced by the lack of platelet accumulation. Platelet thrombi are only seen after tissue shedding has started. These thrombi differ from haemostatic plugs elsewhere in that they remain intravascular and lack the occlusive capsule form. In many vessels these thrombi are only partly occlusive. These thrombi are shed together with the surrounding stroma and new thrombi are formed

upstream. Gradually less strongly aggregated platelets and less fibrin deposition occurs and once shedding is completed, few thrombi are formed. Haemostasis may then be achieved by local vasoconstriction but this is far from certain.

The decreased tendency of platelets to adhere to stromal tissue particular in the early premenstrual phase and once shedding is completed are the most striking disparities with haemostasis elsewhere. It has been postulated that this diminished haemostatic reaction may be caused by high local concentration of inhibitory prostaglandins. In agreement with this notion is the clinical observation that inhibition of prostaglandin synthesis may improve haemostasis in the uterus (Guillebaud et al, 1978).

The lack of fibrin deposition outside the blood vessel may point to a role of the very active uterine fibrinolytic system (Rybo, 1966) which may remove all fibrine outside the vessel but is apparent but less active in shed tissue in the uterine cavity.

Interaction of platelets with the vessel wall

Two main factors regulate (determine) the interaction of platelets with the vessel wall. The *endothelial cell* forms a non reactive lining but also synthesizes substances inhibiting platelet vessel wall interaction. The *subendothelium* consisting of connective tissue and smooth muscle cells. This subendothelium may vary in composition and this may have a profound influence on platelet vessel wall interaction. Platelet vessel wall interaction is also dependent on the plasma protein composition and rheological influences.

Endothelium

Endothelial cells form a continuous single layer lining the blood vessels (for reviews see: Thorgeirsson & Robertson, 1978; Mason et al, 1977; Barnhart & Baechler, 1978). The cells are flat with the longitudinal axis parallel to the vessel. The length is 25–50 μ the breadth 10–15 μ and they vary in thickness from 0.1–3.0 μ. The luminal side is covered by a pronounced glycocalix; the basal side rests on a basement membrane or basement membrane like material.

Endothelial cells synthesize and secrete several components of the connective tissue on which they rest. Production of collagen type IV and III and of fibronectin is demonstrated (Howard et al, 1976; Jaffe et al, 1976; le Sage et al, 1979). Glycosaminoglycans are also synthesized and secreted (Buonassissi & Root, 1975; Busch et al, 1979) and these substances also compose the glycocalix. The most important glycosaminoglycan from endothelial cells is heparan sulphate (Busch et al, 1979) which is also the most important glycosaminoglycan in the glomerular basement membrane (Kanwar & Farquhar, 1979). The glycosaminoglycans are easily degraded by endoglycosidases but collagen may protect them against this and this may be important for the development of a basement membrane (David & Bernfield, 1979).

Endothelial cells also synthesize and release a number of substances that have a direct influence on the development of the haemostatic plug or thrombus. The most important one is prostacyclin (PGI_2) with which we will deal in the next paragraph. The other substances comprise plasminogen activator (Loskutoff & Edgington, 1977), an inhibitor of fibrinolysis (Dosne et al, 1978) and factor VIII-von Willebrand factor (Jaffe et al, 1974). The synthesis and release of the plasminogen activator is inhibited by the action of thrombin (Loskutoff, 1979). This may be of considerable importance in the development of a thrombus. The exact relation between the fibrinolytic inhibitor from endothelial cells and the fibrinolytic inhibitor demonstrated in muscular arteries (Noordhoek Hegt & Brakman, 1974) and their physiologic role require further study.

The factor VIII-VWF is only synthesized by megakaryocytes and endothelial cells (Jaffe et al, 1974: Jaffe & Nachman, 1975; Shearn et al, 1977). In plasma it is present as a series of poly-disperse aggregates (Von Mourik & Bolhuis, 1978; Bolhuis et al, 1981) with molecular weights of over 1 million daltons. The basic monomer has a molecular weight of 250 000 (Counts et al, 1978). The VIII-VWF synthesized by the vessel wall possesses ristocetin-cofactor activity and normal antigenicity but lacks coagulant activity. This coagulant activity is normally associated with the VIII-VWF. It is either synthesized elsewhere and combines with the VIII-VWF derived from the endothelium or it is present in precursor form in it but not exposed. The exact role of the endothelial VIII-VWF is not known. The bulk of the evidence indicates that it is the plasma VIII-VWF which has influence on the adherence of platelets to the vessel wall.

Endothelial cells also bind several substances on their surface which may play a role in the haemostatic and thrombotic process. One of these is the anti-protease α_2-macroglobulin (Becker & Harpel, 1976). Heparin is also bound to the endothelial cells probably by replacing heparan sulfate (Busch et al, 1979). Thrombin also binds to endothelial cells (Awbrey et al, 1975). This binding may have an effect because it removes thrombin from the circulation, but endothelial cells contract as a result of the stimulation by thrombin and this contraction although reversible may lead to cell damage as manifested by the leakage of ^{51}Chromium employed as cytoplasmic marker (Evensen, 1979). The stimulation by thrombin also leads to increased prostacyclin production (see below).

Apart from activity of substances involved in haemostasis, endothelial cells remove or degrade many other substances. Several of these are of importance for inflammatory processes. Among those are the activated complement factor C3a (Denny & Johnson, 1979) and histamine, serotonin and bradykinin (Johnson & Erdös, 1979).

PROSTACYCLIN 'PGI$_2$'

Perhaps the most important contribution of the endothelium to the prevention of thrombosis is the synthesis and release of the powerful prostaglandin-metabolite prostacyclin (PGI$_2$). The production of PGI$_2$ is however not the only factor which is responsible for the non-thrombogenecity of the endothelial cell lining. When PGI$_2$ production is completely blocked, endothelial cells are still less reactive for platelets than smooth muscle cells and fibroblasts (Fry et al, 1980). More and more evidence indicates that PGI$_2$ may play a central role in the pathogenesis of thrombosis and atherosclerosis and has a powerful on the normal haemostatic plug formation.

Synthesis and release. PGI$_2$ is produced by conversion of the endoperoxides PGG$_2$ and PGH$_2$ by the enzyme prostacyclin synthetase. PGI$_2$ has a short half life and is converted into the characteristic metabolite 6 oxo-PGF$_{1\alpha}$. Endoperoxides PGG$_2$ and PGH$_2$ are synthesized from arachidonic acid by cyclooxygenase. Arachidonic acid is derived from the membrane phospholipids through the action of a calcium dependent phospholipase A2 (for reviews see Moncada & Vane, 1979; Moncada & Amezcua,

1979; Samuelsson et al, 1978; Nalbandian & Henry, 1978; Marcus, 1978). In platelets a second pathway for arachidonic acid release has recently been detected. A diacylglycerol is split from phosphatidyl inositol in the membrane and this is degraded by a diglyceride lipase (Rittenhouse-Simons, 1979; Bell et al, 1979). This explains why only phosphatidyl-inositol provides arachidonic acid in the first minute of platelet stimulation. Phospholipase A2 is evidently activated later and arachidonic acid is then also relased from other phospholipids. In endothelial cells the existence of the phospholipase C-diglyceride lipase pathway has not been demonstrated yet. Endothelial cells are very efficient in converting endoperoxides into PGI_2 but only a small part of available arachidonic is converted into PGI_2. Because of this it was postulated at one time that endothelial cells might utilize endoperoxides produced by blood platelets. This has been disputed (Hornstra et al, 1978; Needleman et al, 1979), but recent studies employing optimal conditions indicate that this mechanism is indeed of importance (Marcus et al, 1980). Endothelial cells in culture produce a basic level of prostacyclin which is strongly increased after stimulation by thrombin, trypsin, the calcium ionophore A23187 and also by angiotensin II (Willems et al, 1978; Weksler et al, 1978; Gryglewski et al, 1979).

Continuous secretion and release of PGI_2 into the circulation has been postulated and this may explain why phosphodiesterases as dipyridamole have an effect in vivo, although they are only weak platelet function inhibitors in vitro (Moncada & Korbut, 1978) PGI_2 itself is the most potent platelet function inhibitor known and has also a vasodilating action. The effect on platelet receptors is mediated through the cyclic AMP system (Gorman et al, 1978; Tateson et al, 1977). PGI_2 produces a marked increase in platelet cyclic AMP. A small continuous PGI_2 level in plasma would produce an increase in cAMP in platelets and this effect would be strongly potentiated by an inhibitor of the phosphodiesterase responsible for the breakdown of cAMP. The notion of a sustained significant level of PGI_2 is disputed however (Haslam, 1979).

Balance with thromboxane A2. In platelets endoperoxides are converted into a number of minor prostaglandins PGE_2, $PGF_{2\alpha}$ and PGD_2 the latter of which is a relatively powerful platelet function inhibitor, but the main metabolic route is directed towards the very potent platelet aggregating substance thromboxane A_2. Thromboxane A_2 has also vasoconstricting properties. It has a very short half life and is degraded towards the inactive metabolite thromboxane B_2 which may have chemotactic properties.

The local balance between the production of PGI_2 and $ThxA_2$ may be of importance for the facilitation of haemostasis and thrombosis. This is suggested by the differential effect of aspirin which is an irreversible inhibitor of cyclooxygenase through acetylation of an active serine residu (Vane, 1971). The consequence of this is that endoperoxide production and thus thromboxane A_2 synthesis in platelets is irreversible blocked. Endothelial cells are able to synthesize new protein however and the inhibition by aspirin is abolished by the synthesis of new cyclooxygenase (Jaffe & Weksler, 1979). Continuous high doses of aspirin will block both PGI_2 and $ThxA_2$ production and this may lead to a thrombotic situation as demonstrated in rabbits (Kelton et al, 1978). Lower dosages of aspirin will block thromboxane synthetase and at a critical dose of administration inhibition of platelet function may occur with little or no impairment of PGI_2 production (Masotti et al, 1979) but these dosages are probably very small (Pareti et al, 1980). As a consequence of this aspirin will prolong the bleeding time at a low dosage but higher dosages may again lead to shortening of the bleeding time (O'Grady & Moncada, 1978) although this has not been found by all investigators.

The importance of PGI_2 for local haemostasis is also demonstrated by the influence of diets rich in fish oil on the bleeding time. These experiments stem from the observations that Eskimo's in Greenland suffer little from atherosclerotic disease and in general have prolonged bleeding times and diminished platelet aggregation (Dyerberg & Bang, 1979). The diet of these Eskimo's is rich in fish products and thus contains a high proportion of eicosa-pentaenoic acid instead of arachidonic acid. Eicosapentaenoic acid is precursor of prostaglandins of the PG_3 series. Thromboxane A_3 is either not formed or without any aggregation effect and PGI_3 may have a weak anti aggregating effect (Needleman et al, 1979). The effect of fish oil is already present after a few days on a 'mackerel diet' consisting of the unattractive mixture of smoked and boiled mackerel as only food. This led to a marked prolongation of the bleeding time and a decrease in platelet aggregation in all subjects (Siess et al, 1980).

Localization and regulation of PGI_2 production. PGI_2 production in the vessel wall is much higher at the luminal side than at the periphery (Moncada & Vane, 1979). In line with this endothelial cells produce more PGI_2 than smooth muscle cells (MacIntyre et al, 1978) although the latter do have an appreciable production (Baenziger et al, 1975) when compared to fibroblast which produce virtually no PGI_2. The production by smooth muscle cell only occurs in response to arachidonate or endoperoxide and is not stimulated by other material whereas as already mentioned PGI_2 production is stimulated by trypsin and the calcium ionophore A23187 (Weksler et al, 1978) and also by more physiologic compounds as thrombin (Weksler et al, 1978; Czervionke et al, 1979) and agiotensin II (Gryglewski et al, 1979). The latter observation may prove of interest for drug manufacture because it should be feasible to synthesize products stimulating PGI_2 synthesis but without effect on the blood pressure.

Important for the regulation of PGI_2 synthesis in situations in which platelets are interacting with exposed subendothelium near by is the observation that β-thromboglobulin binds to the endothelial cell and inhibits PGI_2 production (Hope et al, 1979). β-thromboglobulin is a tetrameric protein of 32 000 molecular weight, the amino-acid sequence of which is known (Begg et al, 1978). It is a platelet specific protein and is localized exclusively in α granules (Sander et al, 1980). On stimulation it is released in parallel with the platelet derived growth factor and platelet factor 4 and fibrinogen. The localization of the β-thromboglobulin effect is unknown. Corticosteroids also influence PGI_2 production by inhibiting arachidonic acid release by phospholipase A_2. A protein intermediate is involved in this inhibitory effect because no inhibition by hydrocortisone was observed when protein synthesis was inhibited beforehand (Flowers & Blackwell, 1979).

PGI_2 in disease. Regulation of PGI_2 synthesis may be disturbed in various diseases. Research in this area is only in its beginning and not many firm data are available yet. Decreased PGI_2 synthesis has been reported in thrombotic thrombocytopenic purpura (de Gaetano et al, 1979) a disorder characterized by many occlusive platelet thrombi in small vessels with thrombocytopenia due to platelet consumption.

Tranfusion of normal human plasma has been shown to be beneficial in many patients with this disorder (Byrnes & Lian, 1979). This may indicate that an unknown plasma protein may play a part in PGI_2 synthesis.

Decreased PGI_2 synthesis was also reported in diabetes mellitus and in atherosclerosis whereas increased PGI_2 synthesis was established in uremia. In the latter disorder this increased PGI_2 may contribute to the bleeding tendency but it is not solely responsible as demonstrated by the lack of effect of aspirin on the bleeding time (Remuzzi et al, 1977).

Interaction of platelets with subendothelium

INFLUENCE OF COMPOSITION OF SUBENDOTHELIUM

The nature and intensity of the response of platelets to damage to the vessel wall is dependent on the depth of the lesion. Minimal response with small thrombi and a final monolayer is encountered after removing the endothelial layer only. Deeper lesions lead to more extensive thrombus formation which becomes in many respects similar to the haemostatic plug formation described in the first part of this paper. One of the main reasons of this disparity in response is the difference in composition of various layers of the vessel wall. Only limited data are available but these already help explain the difference.

Composition of the subendothelium. The subendothelium consists of a basement membrane or basement membrane-like material on top of the internal elastic membrane. Most of the components of this subendothelium are synthesized by endothelial cells. The collagens synthesized here are collagen III and type A–B and IV (Howard et al, 1976; Jaffe et al, 1976; Sage et al, 1979). The glycoasminoglycans show a preponderance of heparan sulfate. Two characteristic glycoproteins have recently been recognized: *fibronectin*, a dimer with a molecular weight of 220 000 which is a nearly ubiquitous companion of collagen in reticulin fibers and which plays a part in cell-substrate adhesion and also in cell-cell attachment (Birdwell et al, 1978). The subject is reviewed by Yamada and Olden (1978). The second protein laminin with a molecular weight of 880 000 and subunits after reduction of 440 000 and 220 000 was recently purified from basement membrane in a mouse tumor. Studies employing antibodies indicate that it is an important component of the basement membrane (Timpl et al, 1979).

Reactivity of components of the basement membrane. Studies of the interaction of platelets with isolated compounds of the basement membrane have indicated that elastin and elastic microfibrils are without effect. Glycosaminoglycans have no direct effect but may interact with collagen and influence its behaviour. Of the collagen types collagen type III is definitely active in inducing platelet adhesion release and aggregation (Balleisen et al, 1979), (for a review of platelet collagen interaction see Beachey et al, 1979) whereas collagen type IV only induces adhesion but no aggregation and release. The activity of collagen type A–B is disputed (Balleissen et al, 1979). Some authors have found that it causes aggregation whereas others found that it was as inactive as collagen type IV (Trelstad & Carvalho, 1979). The role of the non-collagen proteins of the basement membrane is undecided. Digestion experiments with chymotrypsin and collagenase suggested that only collagen components were responsible for the reactivity of the vessel wall (Baumgartner et al, 1976; Barnhart & Chen, 1978) but studies in which non collagen protein complexes were directly investigated showed that they were more reactive than the collagens of the glomerular basement membrane (Huang & Benditt, 1978; Freitag et al, 1979). The apparent discrepancy between digestion experiments and experiments with isolated compounds may be explained by accepting that enzyme digestion may remove not only substances that are degraded but also materials closely associated with degraded substances.

Composition of deeper layers: products of the smooth muscle cell. The composition of deeper layers of the vessel wall is determined by the products synthesized by the smooth muscle cell (for a review see Burke & Ross, 1979). The collagens synthesized by smooth muscle cells in culture consist of collagens type I, III and A–B. Most authors report 30 per cent $\alpha 1$ (III) chains and about 70 per cent $\alpha 1$ (I) and $\alpha 2$ (I) chains (Layman et al, 1977; Mayne et al, 1978) but recently equal amounts of chains of collagen III and collagen I were found in fresh cells whereas the relative amount of collagen I increased after many passages (Mayne et al, 1979). Possibly the origin of the smooth muscle cell may also play a role because larger amounts of collagen I and less collagen III are encountered at the periphery of the vessel.

A recent study in which the response of platelets to collagen I, II and III was compared indicated that a similar reaction to the various components occurred and that they were similarly inhibited by antibodies (Balleissen et al, 1979).

As in the basement membrane, elastic tissue and elastin synthesized by the smooth muscle cell do not give rise to a platelet response (Naranayan et al, 1976). The glycosaminoglycans synthesized by the smooth muscle cell differ in composition from those produced by the endothelial cell. The most important glycosaminoglycan here is dermatan sulphate (60 per cent) followed by chondroitin sulphate A and C (10 to 20 per cent each) and less than 5 per cent hyaluronic acid (Wight & Ross, 1975; Burke & Ross, 1979). In the native form the glycosaminoglycans exist covalently bound to protein as proteoglycans (for a review see Indahl & Höök, 1979). A recent study showed that a proteoglycan complex with dermatan and chondroitin sulphate possesses anticoagulant properties and inhibits thrombin induced platelet aggregation but has no effect on no ADP or collagen induced aggregation (Vijayagopal et al, 1980).

IN VITRO PERFUSION STUDIES
Much has been learned about the interaction of platelets with the subendothelium by employing in vitro perfusions. For these studies a perfusion chamber was developed consisting of a central rod on which an everted piece of rabbit aorta was mounted. Most of these studies on this model have been performed by Baumgartner and his associates (for reviews see Baumgartner et al, 1976a, b; Tschopp et al, 1976). More recently this technique has also been applied to human blood vessels with very similar results (Tschopp et al, 1978; Sakariassen et al, 1979). The value of these studies is limited in this sense that blood vessels from which only the endothelium was removed were used for the studies. The model thus provides information on the interaction of platelets with the layer directly beneath the endothelium and the data are therefore of importance for the understanding of thrombogenesis rather than of haemostatic plug

formation. On the other hand the model has allowed the evaluation of a series of important variables that are also of relevance to haemostasis.

Blood platelets adhere to the subendothelium with pseudopodia or part of the membrane of a discoid platelet. These so called 'contact' platelets then spread along the subendothelium. This spreading is usually accompanied by a release reaction. Other platelets adhere to the first ones and small thrombi begin to form. Full coverage is in the case of normal blood usually attained after 10 minutes. Thrombus formation continues after this period but these thrombi are swept away by the blood stream and a single monolayer usually remains after about 40 minutes (Baumgartner et al, 1976a). This picture is very similar to what is obtained after limited removal of the endothelium in vivo (Stemerman, 1974). Fibrin formation is usually absent but it is observed at lower shear rates such as prevail in veins (Baumgartner, 1973).

The accumulation of blood platelets on the subendothelium is strongly dependent on the shear rate but also on the haematocrit. Little or no accumulation occurs in plasma whereas adhesion at a haematocrit of 40 is about 50 times as high.

Influence of plasma proteins

In Von Willebrand's disease adhesion of platelets to the connective tissue is disturbed. This leads to defective haemostatic plug formation (Hovig & Stormorken, 1974) which is corrected by transfusion with the factor VIII-Von Willebrand complex (VIII-VWF) (Kimura et al, 1979). In the perfusion chamber the effect of the von Willebrand factor appears to be on platelet adhesion (Tschopp et al, 1974) which is decreased in Von Willebrand's disease. The defect is stronger expressed at higher shear rates and the defect in Von Willebrand's plasma can be mimicked by antibodies against VIII-VWF (Baumgartner et al, 1980). Recent studies from our laboratory have indicated that human albumin solutions and dextran solution with an identical viscosity to plasma do have a low adherence similar to the plasma of patients with severe Von Willebrand's disease. In all these situations adhesion was fully corrected by addition of purified VIII-VWF to the perfusion fluid (Sakariassen et al, 1979). These data (Fig. 7.4) indicate that factor VIII-VWF is the only protein in plasma facilitating platelet vessel wall interaction. They also demonstrate that no inhibitory protein is present in plasma.

The mode of action of VIII-VWF in supporting platelet adhesion is uncertain. To elucidate this, double perfusion studies were performed in our laboratory in which a piece of human artery was first exposed to perfusion with a human albumin solution containing radiolabelled VIII-VWF, then rinsed and then subjected to perfusion with reconstituted blood containing ^{51}Cr-labelled platelets but no VIII-VWF. The amount of VIII-VWF bound to the subendothelium correlated well with the concentration in the first perfusion fluid and good correlation existed also between the bound VIII-VWF and the subsequently bound ^{51}Cr-platelets in the second perfusion. From these data we concluded that VIII-VWF first bound to the subendothelium and then facilitated platelet adherence. This was borne out in single perfusion studies in which we found that VIII-VWF binding to the subendothelium rapidly reached a plateau level and that the differences between adherence in normal plasma and Von Willebrand plasma was only noticeable after this time. Morphologic studies were thus performed at different time points and these indicated that VIII-VWF facilitated spreading rather than platelet adherence (Bolhuis et al, 1980). Further studies are

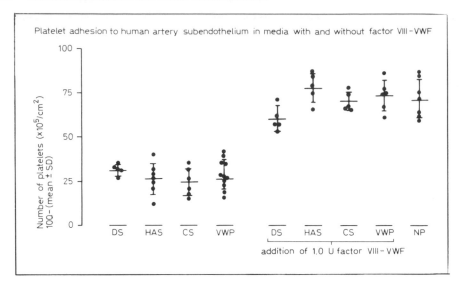

Fig. 7.4 Influence of plasma substitute and VIII-VWF on platelet adhesion. DS = Dextran 40 000 (3.3 per cent), HAS = human albumin solution (4.0 per cent); CS = supernatant plasma after cryoprecipitation; VWP = von Willebrand plasma (VIIIR: WF 1 per cent, VIII R: AG 15 per cent, VIII: C 15 per cent); NP = normal plasma. I.O.U. of factor VIII-VWF/ml was added to the indicated solutions (2.5 $\times 10^5$ platelets/μl).

certainly indicated to determine the components of the vessel wall to which VIII-VWF adheres and to elucidate which of the polydisperse series of molecular sizes of VIII-VWF has the ability to support platelet adhesion.

REFERENCES

Aparicio S R, Bradbury K, Bird C C, Foley M E, Jenkins D H, Clayton J K, Scott J S, Raga S M 1979 Effect of intrauterine haemostasis: a morphological study. British Journal of Obstetrics and Gynaecology 86: 314–324

Awbrey B J 1975 Binding of thrombin to human endothelial cells and platelets. Blood 46: 1046

Baenziger N L, Becherer P R, Majerus P W 1979 Characterization of prostacyclin synthesis in cultured human arterial smooth muscle cells venous endothelial cells and skin fibroblasts. Cell 6: 967–974

Balleisen L, Nowack H, Gay S, Timpl R 1979 Inhibition of collagen induced platelet aggregation by antibodies to distinct types of collagen. Biochemical Journal 184: 683–687

Barnes M J, MacIntyre D E 1979 Platelet reactivity of isolated constituents of the blood vessel wall. Haemostasis 8: 158–170

Barnhart M I, Baechler Ch A 1978a Endothelial cell physiology: perturbations and responses. Seminars in Thrombosis and Hemostasis 5: 50–86

Barnhart M I, Chen S T 1978b Vessel wall models for studying interaction capabilities with blood platelets. Seminars in Thrombosis and Hemostasis 5: 112–155

Bartelmez G W 1933 Histological studies on the menstruating mucous membrane of the human uterus. Contribution Embryology 142: 142–186

Baumgartner H R 1977 Platelet interaction with collagen fibrils in flowing blood I. Reaction of human platelets with α-chymo-trypsin-digested subendothelium. Thrombosis and Haemostasis 37: 1–16

Baumgartner H R, Muggli R 1976 Adhesion and aggregation: morphological demonstration and quantitation in vivo and in vitro. In: Gordon J L (ed) Platelets in biology and pathology. North Holland Publication Company Amsterdam Ch 1, p 23–60

Baumgartner H R 1973 The role of blood flow in platelet adhesion fibrin deposition and formation of mural thrombi. Microvascular Research 5: 167–179

Baumgartner H R, Tschopp T B, Meyer D 1980 Shear rate dependent inhibition of platelets adhesion and aggregation on collagenous surfaces by antibodies to human factor VIII Von Willebrand factor. British Journal of Haematology 44: 127–139

Baumgartner H R, Muggli R, Tschopp T B, Turitto V T 1976 Platelet adhesion, release and aggregation in flowing blood: effects of surface properties and platelet function. Thrombosis and Haemostasis 35: 124–138

Beachey E H, Chiang Th M, Kang A H 1979 Collagen-platelet interaction. International Reviews Connective Tissue Research 8: 1–23

Becker C G, Harpel P C 1976 $\alpha2$ macroglobulin on human vascular endothelium. Journal of Experimental Medicine 144: 1–9

Begg S, Pepper D S, Chesterman C N, Morgon F J 1978 Complete covalent structure of human β-thromboglobulin. Biochemistry 17: 1739

Bell R L, Kennerly D A, Stanford N, Majerus P W 1979 Diglyceride lipase: a pathway for arachidonate release from human platelets. Proceedings of National Academic Sciences USA 76: 3238–3241

Birdwell Ch R, Gospodarowicz D, Nickolson G L 1978 Identification, localization and role of fibronectin in cultured bovine endothelial cells. Proceedings of National Academic Sciences 75: 3273–3277

Blatt P M, Brinkhous K M, Culp H R, Krauss J S, Roberts H R 1976 Antihemophilic factor concentrate therapy in Von Willebrand disease. Journal of the American Medical Association 236: 2770–2772

Bolhuis P A, Sakariassen K S, Sander H J, Bouma B N 1981 The time dependent relation between binding of factor VIII-Von Willebrand factor at human arterial subendothelium and the attachment and spreading of platelets. J Clin Path (in press)

Buonassisi V, Root M 1975 Enzymatic degradation of heparin related mucopolysaccharides from the surface of endothelial cell culturels. Biochemica et Biophysica Acta 385: 1–10

Burke J M, Ross R 1979 Synthesis of connective tissue macromolecules by smooth muscle. International Reviews of Connective Tissue Research 8: 119–157

Busch C, Lyungman C, Heldin C M, Wasteson E, Öbrink B 1979 Surface properties of cultured endothelial cells. Haemostasis 8: 142–148

Byrnes J J, Lian E C 1979 Recent therapeutic advances in thrombotic thrombocytopenic purpura. Seminars in Thrombosis and Haemostasis 5: 199–215

Christiaens G C M L, Sixma J J, Haspels A A 1980a Morphology of menstrual bleeding. In: Hafez E S E, van Os W A A (ed) Progress in contraceptive delivery systems: i.u.d. pathology and management. MTP Press Lancaster, 3: 45–61

Christiaens G C M L, Sixma J J, Haspels A A 1980b Morphology of haemostasis in menstrual endometrium. British Journal of Obstetrics and Gynaecology 87: 425–439

Christiaens G C M L, Sixma J J, Haspels A A 1981 Morphology of shed tissue from menstrual blood. Am J Obst Gynec (in press)

Counts R B, Paskell S L, Elgee S K 1978 Disulfide bonds and the quaternary structure of factor VIII-VWF. Journal of Clinical Investigation 62: 702–709

Czervionke R L, Smits J B, Hoak J C, Fry G L 1979 Use of a radioimmunoassay to study thrombin-induced release of PGI_2 from cultured endothelium. Thrombosis Research 14: 781–786

David G, Bernfield M R 1979 Collagen reduces glycosaminoglycan degradation by cultured mammary epithelial cells: possible mechanism for basal lamina formation. Proceedings of National Academic Sciences 76: 786–790

Denny J B, Johnson A R 1979 Uptake of ^{125}J-labelled C3a by cultured human endothelial cells. Immunology 36: 169–177

Dosne A M, Dupuy E, Bodevin E Production of a fibrinolytic inhibitor by cultured endothelial cells derived from human umbilical vein. Thrombosis Research 12: 377–387

Dyerberg J, Bang H O 1979 Haemostatic function and platelet poly unsaturated fatty acids in eskimos. Lancet 2: 433–435

Evensen S A 1979 Injury to cultured endothelial cells: the role of lipoproteins and thrombo-active agents. Haemostasis 8: 203–210

Flower R J, Blackwell G J 1979 Anti-inflammatory steroid induce biosynthesis of a phopholipase A 2 inhibitor which prevents prostaglandin generation. Nature 278: 456–459

Fray G L, Czervionke R L, Hoak J C, Smith J B, Haycraft D L 1980 Platelet adherence to cultured vascular cells influence of prostacyclin (PGI_2). Blood 55: 271–275

Freytag J W, Dalrymple P N, Maguire M H, Strickland D K, Carraway K C, Hudson B G 1978 Glomerular basement membrane studies on its structure and interaction with platelets. Journal of Biological Chemistry 253: 9069–9074

Fromer C H, Gordon K, Klintworth M D 1975 Evaluation of the role of leucocytes in the pathogenesis of experimentally induced corneal vascularisation. American Journal of Pathology 81; 531–544

Fromer C H, Gordon K, Klintworth M D 1976 Evaluation of the role of leucocytes in the pathogenesis of experimentally induced corneal vascularisation. American Journal of Pathology 82; 157–170

de Gaetano G, Remuzzi G, Mysluexec M, Donati M B 1979 Vascular prostacyclin and plasminogen activator activity in experimental and clinical condition of disturbed haemostasis and thrombosis. Haemostasis 8: 300–311

Goetzl E J, Gorman R R 1978 Chemotactic and chemokinetic stimulation of human eosinophil and neutrophil-polymorphonuclear leucocytes by 12-L-hydroxy-5, 8, 10 heptadecatrienoic acid (HHT). Journal of Immunology 120: 520–531

Goetzl E J, Woods J M, Gorman R R 1977 Stimulation of human eosinophil and human eosinophil and neutrophil-polymorphonuclear chemotaxis and random migration by 12-L-hydroxy 5, 8, 10, 14, eicosa tetraenoic acid (HETE). Journal of Clinical Investigation 49: 179–183

Gorman R R, Bunting S, Miller O V 1977 Modulation of human platelet adenylate cyclase by prstacyclin (PGx). Prostaglandins 13: 377–388

Gorman R R, Fitzpatrick F A, Miller O V 1978 Reciprocal regulation of human platelet cAMP levels by thromboxane A2 and prostacyclin. Advances Cyclic Nucleotide Research 9: 597–609

Gryglewski R J, Korbut R, Splawinski 1979 Endogenous mechanisms which regulate prostacyclin release. Haemostasis 8: 294–299

Guillebaud J, Anderson A B M, Turnbull A C 1978 Reduction by mefenamic acid of increased menstrual blood loss associated with intra-uterine-contraception. British Journal of Obstetrics and Gynaecology 85: 53–62

Haslam R J 1979 Roles of cyclic nucleotides in the inhibition of platelet function by physiological and pharmacological agents. Thrombosis and Haemostasis 42: 86

Hohman W R, Shaw S T, Macaulay L, Moyer D L 1978 Ultrastructural hemostasis in response to vascular injury induced by intrauterine devices in human endometrium. Thrombosis Research 12: 1037–1050

Hope W, Martin T J, Chesterman C N, Morgan F J 1979 Human β thromboglobulin inhibits PGI_2 production and binds to a specific site in bovine aortic endothelial cells. Nature 282: 210–212

Hornstra G, Haddeman J, Don J A 1978 Some investigations into the role of prostacyclin in thromboregulation. Thrombosis Research 12: 367–374

Hovig T, Stormorken H 1974 Ultrastructural studies on the platelet plug formation in bleeding time wounds from normal individuals and patients with Von Willebrand's disease. Acta Pathologica et Microbiologica Scandinavica Supplement 248: 105–122

Howard B V, Macarak E J, Gunson D, Kefalides N 1976 Characterization of the collagen synthesized by endothelial cells in culture. Proceedings of National Academic Sciences USA 73: 2361–2364

Hoyer L W 1976 Von Willebrand's Disease. In: Spaet T (ed) Progress in Hemostasis and Thrombosis 3, Grune and Stratton, New York. p 231–287

Huang Th W, Benditt E P 1978 Mechanisms of platelet adhesion to the basal lamina. American Journal of Pathology 92: 99–108

Jaffe E A, Nachman R L 1975 Subunit structure of factor VIII-antigen by cultured human endothelial cells. Journal of Clinical Investigation 56: 698–702

Jaffe E A, Weksler B B 1979 Recovery of endothelial cell prostacyclin production after inhibition by low doses of aspirin. Journal of Clinical Investigation 63: 532–535

Jaffe E A, Hoyer L W, Nachman R L 1974 Synthesis of Von Willebrand factor by cultured human endothelial cells. Proceedings of National Academic Sciences USA 71: 1906–1909

Jaffe E A, Adelman B, Minick C R, Becker C G, Nachman R 1976 Synthesis of basement membrane collagen by cultured human endothelial cells. Journal of Experimental Medicine 144: 209–225

Johnson A R, Erdös E G 1977 Metabolism of vasoactive peptide by human endothelial cells in culture. Angiotensin converting enzyme (kininase II) and angiotensmase. Journal of Clinical Investigation 59: 684–695

Kanwar Y S, Farquhar M G 1979 Presence of heparan sulfate in the glomerular basement membrane. Proceedings of National Academic Sciences USA 76: 1303–1307

Kasonde J M, Bonnar J 1975 Aminocaproic acid and menstrual loss in women using intrauterine devices. British Medical Journal 4: 17–19

Kay A B, Kaplan A P 1975 Chemotaxis and Haemostasis, annotation. British Journal of Haematology 31: 417–422

Kelton J C, Hirsch J, Carter J 1979 Thrombogenic effects of high dose aspirin in rabbits. Journal of Clinical Investigation 62: 892–895

Kimura A, Bowie E J W, Campbell, Fass D N 1979 Willebrand factor in hemostasis in the in vitro bleeding time. Blood 54: 1347–1357

Layman D L, Epstein E H, Dodson R F, Titus J L 1977 Biosynthesis of type I and III collagen by culture smooth muscle cells from human aorta. Proceedings of National Academic Sciences USA 74: 671–675

Legrand Y J, Rodriquez-Zeballos A, Kartalis G, Fauvel F, Caen J P 1978 Adsorption of factor VIII antigen-activity complex by collagen. Thrombosis Research 13: 909–911

Lindahl U, Höök M 1978 Glycosaminoglycans and their binding to biological macromolecules. Annual Review of Biochemistry 47: 385–417

Loskutoff D 1979 Effect of thrombin on the fibrinolytic activity of cultured bovine endothelial cells.

Journal of Clinical Investigation 64: 329–332

Loskutoff D J, Edgington T S 1977 Synthesis of a fibrinolytic activator and inhibitor by endothelial cells. Proceedings of National Academic Sciences 74: 3903–3907

MacIntyre D E, Pearson J D, Gordon J L 1978 Localization and stimulation of prostacyclin production in vascular cells. Nature 271: 549–551

Marcus A J 1978 The role of lipids in platelet function: with particular reference to the arachidonic acid pathway. Journal of Lipid Research 19: 793–826

Marcus A J, Weksler B B, Jaffe E A, Broekman M J 1980 Synthesis of Prostacyclin (PGI$_2$) from platelet derived endoperoxides by cultured human endothelial cells. Journal of Clinical Investigation 66: 979–986

Mason R G, Sharp D, Chuang N Y K, Mahammad F 1977 The endothelium: roles in thrombosis and haemostasis. Archives of Pathology and Laboratory Medicine 101: 61–64

Masotti G, Galanti G, Poggesi L, Abbale R, Neri Serneri G G 1979 Differential inhibition of prostacyclin production and platelet aggregation by aspirin. Lancet II: 1213–1216

Mayne R, Vaile M S, Miller E J 1978 Characterization of the collagen chains synthesized by cultured smooth muscle cells derived from rhesus monkey thoracic aorta. Biochemistry 17: 446–452

Moncada S, Korbut R 1978 Dipyridamole and other phosphodiesterase inhibitors act as antithrombotic agents by potentiating endogenous prostacyclin. Lancet i: 1286–1289

Moncada S, Amezcua J L 1979 Prostacyclin, thrombocane A 2 interactions in haemostasis and thrombosis. Haemostasis 8: 252–265

Moncada S, Vane J R 1979 Arachidonic acid metabolites and the interactions between platelets and blood vessel walls. New England Journal of Medicine 300: 1142–1147

Mourik van J A, Bolhuis P A 1978 Dispersity of human factor VIII-Von Willebrand factor. Thrombosis Research 13: 15–24

Nalbandian R M, Henry R L 1978 Platelet-endothelial cell interactions metabolic maps of structure and actions of prostaglandins prostacyclin, thromboxane and cyclic AMP. Seminars in Thrombosis and Haemostasis 5: 87–111

Narayanan A S, Sandberg L B, Ross R, Layman D L 1976 The smooth muscle cell. III Elastin synthesis in arterial smooth muscle cell culture. Journal of Cell Biology 68: 411–419

Needleman Ph 1979 Prostacyclin in blood vessel-platelet interactions: perspectives and questions. Nature 279: 14–15

Needleman P, Wyche A, Raz A 1979 Platelet and blood vessel arachidonate metabolism and interactions. Journal of Clinical Investigation 63: 345–349

Needleman P, Raz A, Minkes M S, Ferrendelli J A, Sprecher H 1979 Triene prostaglandins: prostacyclin and thromboxane biosynthesis and unique biological properties. Proceedings of National Academic Sciences USA 76: 944–948

Nillson L, Rybo G Treatment of menorrhagia with an antifibrinolytic agent, tranexamic acid. Acta Ostetrica Gynecologica Scandinavica 46: 572–580

Nogales F, Martinez H, Parache J 1969 Abstossung und Wiederaufbau des menslichen Endometrium. Gynaekologische Rundschau 7: 292–312

Noordhoek Hegt V, Brakman P 1974 Histochemical study of an inhibitor of fibrinolyses in the human arterial wall. Nature 248: 75–76

Nugteren D H 1975 Arachidonate lipoxygenase in blood platelets. Biochemica Biophysica Acta 380: 299–307

O'Grady J, Moncada S 1978 Aspirin: a paradoxical effect on bleeding time. Lancet 2: 780

Pareti F I, D'Angelo A, Mannucci P M, Smith J B 1980 Platelets and the vessel wall: how much aspirin Lancet 1, 371–372

Ratlift N B, Gerrard J M, White J G 1979 Platelet leucocyte interactions following arterial endothelial injury. American Journal of Pathology 96: 567–580

Rauterberg J, Allain S, Brehmer U, Wirth, Hanes W H 1977 Characterization of the collagen synthesized by cultured human smooth muscle cells from fetal and adult aorta. Hoppe Seylers Zeitschrift für Physiologischen Chemie 358: 401–407

Remuzzi G, Cavenaghi A E, Mecca G, Donati M B, Gaetano de G 1977 Prostacyclin (PGI$_2$) and bleeding time in uremic patients. Thrombosis Research 11: 919–920

Rittenhouse-Simons S Production of diglyceride from phosphatidyl inositol in activated human platelets. Journal of Clinical Investigation 63: 580–587

Rybo G 1966 Plasminogen activations in the endometrium. Acta Obstetrica Gynecologica Scandinavica 45: 411–499

Sage H, Croudi E, Bornstein P 1979 Collagen synthesis by bovine aortic endothelial cells in culture. Biochemistry 18: 5433–5442

Sakariassen K S, Bolhuis P A, Sixma J J 1979 Adhesion of human blood platelets to human artery subendothelium is medicated by F VIII-VWF bound to subendothelium. Nature 279: 636–638

Sakariassen K S, Bolhuis P A, Sixma J J 1980 Platelet adherence to subendothelium of human arteries in pulsatile and steady flow. Thrombosis Research 19: 547

Salvatore C A 1969 Identification of fibrin in menstrual endometrium. American Journal of Obstetrics and Gynecology 103: 537–543

Samuelsson B, Goldyne M, Granström E, Hamberg M, Hammarström S, Malmsten C 1978 Prostaglandins and Thromboxanes. Annual Review of Biochemistry 47: 995–1029

Sandberg L B 1976 Elastin structure in health and disease. International Review of Connective Tissue Research 7: 159–210

Sander H J, Slot J W, Bolhuis P A, Sixma J J, Geuze J J, Pepper D S 1980 Immuno-electron microscopic localization of fibrinogen, platelet factor 4 and beta-thromboglobulin in ultra thin cryostat sections of human blood platelets. Submitted

Shearn S A M, Peake I R, Giddings J C, Humphrys J, Bloom A L 1977 The characterization and synthesis of antigens related to factor VIII in vascular endothelium. Thrombosis Research 11: 43

Sholley M M, Gimbrone M A, Cotran R S 1978 The effects of leucocyte depletion on corneal neo-vascularisation. Laboratory Investigation 38: 32–40

Siess W, Scherer B, Böhlig B, Roth P, Kurzmann I, Weber P C 1980 platelet membrane fatty acids, platelet aggregation, and thromboxane formation during a mackerel diet. Lancet 1: 441–444

Sixma J J, Geuze J J 1968 Degranulation of human platelets during ADP-induced aggregation, Vox Sang 15: 309–314

Sixma J J, Wester J 1977 The haemostatic plug. Seminars in Hematology 14: 265–299

Sixma J J, Christiaens G C M L, Haspels A A 1980 The sequence of events in the endometrial during normal menstruation. In: Proceedings of the symposium on steroid contraception and mechanisms of endometrial bleeding. Symposium 12–14 September Geneve. 86–106

Stemerman M B 1974 Vascular intima components: precursor in Thrombosis. In: Spaet Th (ed) Progress in Haemostasis and Thrombosis, 2, Grune and Stratton, New York, p 1–47

Stenman S, Vaheri A 1978 Distribution of a major connective tissue protein, fibronectin in normal human tissues. Journal of Experimental Medicine 147: 1054–1064

Tateson J E, Moncada S, Vane J R 1977 Effects of prostacyclin (PGx) on cyclic AMP concentrations in human platelets. Prostaglandins 13: 389–397

Thorgeirsson G, Robertson A L 1978 The vascular endothelium-pathobiologic significance. A review. American Journal of Pathology 93: 803–847

Timpl R, Rohde H, Robey P G, Reinard S I, Foidart J M, Martin G R 1979 Laminin — a glycoprotein from basement membranes. Journal of Biological Chemistry 254: 9933–9937

Trelstad R L, Carvalho A C A 1979 Type IV and Type AB collagens do not elicit platelet aggregation or the release reaction. Journal of Laboratory Clinical Medicine 93: 499–504

Tschopp Th B, Baumgartner H R 1975 Psychological experiments in haemostasis and thrombosis. British Journal of Haematology 31: 221–229

Tschopp Th B, Weiss H J, Baumgartner H R 1974 Decreased adhesion of platelet to subendothelium in Von Willebrand's disease. Journal of Laboratory Clinical Medicine 83: 296–300

Turner S R, Tainer J A, Lynn W S 1975 Biogenesis of chemotactic molecules by the arachidonate lipoxygenase system of platelets. Nature 257: 680–681

Vane J R 1971 Inhibition of prostaglandin synthesis as a mechanism of action for aspirin-like drugs. Nature New Biology 231: 232–235

Vijayagopal P, Radhakreslina Marthy R, Srinwasan S R, Berenson G S 1980 Studies of biologic properties from proteoglycans from bovene aorta. Laboratory Investigation 2: 190–196

Weksler B B, Ley C W, Jaffe E A 1978 Stimulation of endothelial cell prostacyclin production by thrombin, trypsin and the ionophore A 23187. Journal of Clinical Investigation 62: 923

Wester J, Sixma J J, Geuze J J, Veen van der J 1978 Morphology of the early haemostasis in human skin wounds. Influence of acetyl salicylic acid. Laboratory Investigation 39: 298–311

Wester J, Sixma J J, Geuze J J, Heynen H 1979 Morphology of the hemostatic plug in human skin wounds. Laboratory Investigation 41: 182–192

Wight Th N, Ross R 1975 Proteoglycans in primate arteries. Synthesis and secretion of glycosaminoglycans by arterial smooth muscle cells in culture. Journal of Cell Biology 67: 675–686

Willems Ch, Aken van W G, Peerscher-Prakke E M, Mourik van J A, Dutilh C, Hoor ten F 1978 Prostaglandin I_2 prostacyclin production by cultured human vascular endothelial cells in the absence of platelets. Journal of Molecular Medicine 3: 195–201

Yamada K M, Olden K 1978 Fibronectins-adhesive glycoproteins of cell surface and blood. Nature 275: 179–184

8. Hemophilia diagnosis and management: progress and problems

P. M. Mannucci

At present the future of patients with hemophilia A may be viewed with more optimism due to advances in diagnosis and management which have occurred in recent years. Hemophiliacs can now be recognized by simple methods even in relatively non-specialized laboratories and the detection of female carriers has greatly improved with the advent of newer techniques. A very recent and exciting development has been the possibility of performing prenatal diagnosis of hemophilia from fetal blood samples obtained by fetoscopy via a relatively simple but safe procedure. With respect to treatment problems, the greater availability of specific blood derivatives (cryoprecipitate and lyophilized concentrates) of improved purity has facilitated really effective control of hemorrhage. The advent of home care has markedly reduced the need for hospitalization through the early management of bleeding episodes. Finally, there are preliminary but encouraging reports suggesting that in some patients it is possible to use chemical compounds capable of increasing plasma factor-VIII coagulant activity (VIII:C) without the need for substitution therapy with plasma derivatives.

As a result of these developments, the hemophiliac is becoming a liberated, autonomous and fully active person capable of achieving the position he is entitled to expect from society. However, at a time when progress in hemophilia care is making so many important advances, a number of problems are still unresolved and others are now emerging against this optimistic background.

The development of an inhibitor specifically destroying VIII:C still makes home treatment impossible for most patients and renders hospital management at best difficult. It has been recognized recently that multitransfused hemophiliacs have a high incidence of abnormal liver function tests, and there is preliminary evidence that these are the expression of chronic active liver disease. Therefore, in considering advances in hemophilia diagnosis and management, this review must not be limited only to the highlights of these topics. Rather, it is also focused on the pitfalls which at present surround some aspects of hemophilia care.

ADVANCES AND PROBLEMS IN DIAGNOSIS

Diagnosing hemophilia with the activated partial thromboplastin time

Since its original description by Proctor and Rapaport (1961) the activated partial thromboplastin time (APTT) had been adopted increasingly as a screening test in the diagnosis of hemophilia. Being simple and more reproducible, the APTT has largely replaced methods such as the thromboplastin generation and thromboplastin screening tests in the majority of clinical laboratories. The numerous reagent kits for APPT, now available commercially, can detect easily patients with severe VIII:C deficiency.

It has been suggested, however, that some APTT techniques are more sensitive than others in detecting mild hemophilia in patients with no spontaneous abnormal bleeding who may nevertheless bleed excessively after surgery. In their comparison of five commercial reagents and one non-commercial reagent. Sibley et al (1973) showed that some methods were not sufficiently sensitive to VIII:C deficiency when the slope of VIII:C dose-response curve, obtained by diluting normal plasma with severely deficient plasma, was taken as an index of discrimination. These results, as well as those of the survey of the College of American Pathologists (Koepke, 1975), are somewhat at variance with the study of Babson and Babson (1974), who found five widely used APTT reagents were able to distinguish between pathological samples containing 20 U/dL VIII:C.

In order to clarify this important issue, a number of investigations were designed recently to assess whether commercial APTT reagents can detect critical degrees of factor-VIII deficiency. Unlike previous studies, the pathological samples tested in these recent trials were obtained from patients with mild hemophilia A, to avoid the artificial situation of diluting normal with VIII:C deficient plasma. Poller et al (1976), comparing the results of a series of collaborative exercises conducted in over three hundred hospitals in the United Kingdom and abroad, found that 97 per cent of participants using the standardized APTT reagent manufactured in their laboratory detected as abnormal a plasma containing 30 U/dL VIII:C.

The overall success-rate of 15 commercial reagents (63 per cent) was on the whole acceptable if one considers that 30 U/dL VIII:C are likely to be representative of the threshold between mild hemostatic failure and normality; and that all the laboratories (94 per cent) recognized as abnormal another plasma sample, more severely deficient in VIII:C (11 U/dL). This defect is definitely associated with some degree of abnormal bleeding and thus should not be missed by any APTT reagents. Unfortunately, when the performances of the commercial reagents were analyzed individually, a number of these gave an unacceptably high incidence of failure rates, i.e. they were unreliable for diagnostic screening. The results of Poller et al (1976) have been confirmed substantially by a similar multicenter study carried out by an Italian Study Group (1980). This survey was designed to assess whether 10 commercial APTT methods and Poller's reagent could detect two critical degrees of VIII:C deficiency (26 and 17 U/dL). All the APTT kits gave prolonged clotting times with the more severely deficient sample. With five reagents, at least one participating center obtained a result within the manufacturer's normal range when the 26 U/dL factor VIII sample was tested. This study has also demonstrated a considerable degree of variability between laboratories testing the same plasma samples with the same reagents. More uniform results were obtained reporting the ratios of VIII:C deficient to normal plasma clotting times instead of the actual clotting time values, suggesting that results from different laboratories might be more comparable if expressed as ratios rather than clotting time values.

In conclusion, despite the fact that a few APTT reagents fail to distinguish from normal plasma samples with VIII:C levels undoubtedly associated with bleeding symptoms, the majority of them can detect these defects and can also identify abnormalities which are of borderline clinical significance. Thus, the APTT appears to be a satisfactory simple measure in the screening of hemophiliacs although differences in performances between laboratories make uncertain the interpretation of the quantitative results obtained in different hospitals. Such a difficulty might be minimized if different laboratories were to use the same reference plasma and expressed the results in clotting time ratios of test to the given reference plasma and unsatisfactory reagents improved or eliminated.

Present status of carrier detection

The only women who can be identified as carriers with certainty are the daughters of a hemophilic father, mothers with a hemophilic son and a previous family history of hemophilia and mothers of more than one hemophilic son. In the strict sense, this statement is still valid because recent advances in laboratory methods, whilst providing better means to establish the probability favouring carriership, yet fail to give certainty.

An early methodological approach to the problem of detecting *possible carriers* (a mother with no previous family history and one hemophilic son, and women who have a hemophilic relative on the maternal side but no affected son) was made by assaying VIII:C levels in their plasma. The underlying assumption was that in these women such levels should be half of that of normal women since only one of the two X chromosomes in each somatic cell is normal. Although obligatory carriers taken as a group have lower average VIII:C activity than normal women, this approach is not satisfactory because the high degree of overlap between normals and carriers allows the detection of only 30 to 50 per cent of genetically proven carriers (Alagille & Prou-Wartelle, 1966; Ikkala, 1969). The problem of random inactivation of one of the two X chromosomes, the wide range of VIII:C levels encountered in normal women, as well as the inherent lack of accuracy of the biological VIII:C assays, are likely to account for the limitation of this approach.

A substantial advance in the field has been made with the introduction of a method pioneered by Zimmerman et al (1971a). This is established on the combination of the bioassay of VIII:C with the measurement of factor-VIII related antigen (VIII:RAg) by an electroimmunoassay based on the Laurell technique of electrophoresis. The background of this system is the observation that in severe hemophiliacs VIII:RAg is present in normal or increased amounts despite unrecordable VIII:C levels and that carriers have reduced plasma levels of VIII:C and normal or slightly higher than normal VIII:RAg. Since in normal women the level of VIII:C measured by bioassay is proportional to the concentration of VIII:RAg, the combined measurement of VIII:C and VIII:RAg has been proposed as a valuable approach to the problem of carrier identification. The validity of this method has been supported by the results of two studies conducted by Ratnoff and his colleagues (Zimmerman et al, 1971b; Bennett & Ratnoff, 1973), who were able to distinguish 92 to 95 per cent of obligatory carriers from normal women, only a negligible number of normal women being wrongly classified as carriers. The second study (Bennett & Ratnoff, 1973), conducted on plasma samples from a large series of subjects, provided the additional important information that half of the daughters of known carriers were identified as carriers, as would be expected on the basis of genetic probability. Subsequent investigations carried out in other laboratories have confirmed that identification of the carrier state is substantially improved by the combined use of VIII:C and VIII:RAg. However, the success rate of the majority of these studies was somewhat lower than the more than 90 per cent rate suggested by the initiators of this method. Bouma et al (1975), for example, were able to detect only 82 per cent of obligatory carriers; Rizza et al (1975), 73 per cent; Meyer et al (1975), 82 per cent. Also Zimmerman (1974), testing another large series of carriers, was less successful than in his original study.

There are, therefore, conflicting views on the success rate with which the carrier state can be established. It must be reiterated that an appropriate classification of all the obligatory carriers cannot be expected using a technique based on the discrepancy between VIII:RAg and VIII:C. Since the latter measurement is X chromosome dependent, extreme variations of the inactivation of the chromosome in somatic cells may result in normal amounts of VIII:C, making these carriers unidentifiable by the VIII:C/VIII:RAg method. If one considers that current data do not allow the identification of all the carriers, the differences in success rate between the initiators of the method (∼90 per cent) and subsequent investigators (∼80 per cent) were not so large as to justify the great controversy which developed in this field. All current data clearly indicate that the VIII:C/VIII:RAg method has substantially improved the possibility of carrier detection but the exclusion of this state is hazardous and as many as 10 to 20 per cent of carriers may be concealed as a result of the vagaries of X chromosome inactivation.

In the United States, public discussion on this issue led to a cooperative study sponsored jointly by the National Heart and Lung Institute (NIH) and the National Hemophilia Foundation and to a five-day laboratory workshop aiming to evaluate the reliability of current tests to identify carriers. Using their own procedures, five distinguished investigators in the field conducted their tests blindly in the same laboratory on the same blood samples drawn from 50 female subjects (normal and obligatory carriers). Their data were submitted to NIH statisticians for calculation and evaluation and the researchers decided to jointly author and publish the Workshop results (Klein et al, 1977). This exercise reached a number of important conclusions: overall correct classification ranged from 72 to 94 per cent, confirming in a controlled situation the different results of the previous individual studies. Differences between participants appeared to be related to variations in laboratory methods rather than to poor testing precision and to the varied statistical methods used by the investigators. In short, this prospective study confirmed the validity of the VIII:C/VIII:RAg method for detecting the carrier state of hemophilia A, suggesting strongly that each laboratory involved in genetic counselling should establish its own procedures and reference groups.

The state of the art of hemophilia carrier detection is summarized in a Memorandum (1977) produced by an international committee of expert hematologists, geneticists and biostatisticians convened under the joint auspices of the World Health Organization (WHO) and the World Federation of Hemophilia (WFH). The report discussed the methods for assaying VIII:C and VIII:RAg and dealt with statistical procedures used for distinguishing carriers from normal women. It explained in detail the procedures to be followed for calculating from the combined information derived from family pedigree and laboratory data the likelihood that a particular person might be a carrier. The report also produced a number of primary recommendations on the need for standardization of laboratory methods and the establishment in each country of at least one national laboratory with appropriate coagulation and genetic facilities to provide genetic counselling. Finally, a number of unresolved problems on which research should concentrate were suggested, i.e. the effect of pregnancy and oral estrogen intake on reliability of carrier detection, the projection of future prevalence of hemophiliacs and hemophilia carriers on the basis of more precise information on the incidence of hemophilia in various populations and the need to assess the problem of mild and moderate hemophilia carriers.

Prenatal diagnosis

One of the recommendations of the above report was support for research on prenatal diagnosis of hemophilia. Prenatal diagnosis aims to give the pregnant hemophilia carrier the choice of giving birth to a normal son and of avoiding the termination of pregnancy in 50 per cent normal male fetuses. It is encouraging to notice that so much progress has been made in this field since the original publication of the WHO-WFH report.

Amniocentesis carried out in the 14 to 15th week of pregnancy is now a simple method for determining fetal sex and is an essential step in prenatal diagnosis. The detection of sex through amniocentesis and fetal cell culture is a reasonably safe procedure and allows the identification of males. These stand a 50 per cent risk of having hemophilia if the mother is identified as a carrier, while half of the female children would be expected to be carriers. After sex determination, identification of the status of the individual male fetus at risk is based on techniques by which fetal blood samples can be assayed for the deficient clotting factor. A substantial contribution to this field has been the development of fetoscopy (Hobbins & Maloney, 1974), which has permitted the collection of fetal blood samples uncontaminated with maternal blood by puncturing placental vessels under direct vision. The method has been of great value in the detection of hemoglobinopathies (Alter et al, 1976), where the admixture of fetal samples with amniotic fluid does not affect fetal red cells analysis. Its application to the diagnosis of congenital plasma coagulation disorders seems to present formidable problems because amniotic fluid contains tissue thromboplastin which may induce a non-specific activation of clotting factor bioassays. In addition, such assays are not sensitive enough to compensate for the dilution of fetal blood induced by contaminating amniotic fluid. An exciting step forward has been the description of new radioimmunological methods of great sensitivity capable of detecting minute amounts of clotting factors in plasma and serum. These assays, whose specificity is unaffected by the presence of amniotic fluid, measure the antigenic determinants of VIII:C (VIII:CAg) which are greatly reduced or absent in the majority of hemophilia kindreds (Lazarchick & Hoyer, 1978; Peake & Bloom, 1978). Significantly, the antigenic determinants are also present, though reduced, in serum but absent from amniotic fluid. The comparative values of VIII:RAg to VIII:CAg allows an indirect estimation of dilution of the sample with amniotic fluid. Using this approach, Firshein et al (1979) have analyzed samples from six male fetuses at risk for severe hemophilia and found low concentrations of VIII:CAg but normal concentrations of VIII:RAg in three, whereas both the measurements were within the normal range in the remaining three. The diagnosis of severe hemophilia was subsequently confirmed with blood from the aborted fetuses whereas the remaining pregnancies proceeded to term and resulted in normal males.

Although these results are convincing and clear-cut, there are some problems which limit a wider application of this approach to prenatal diagnosis of hemophilia A. The antibody to VIII:CAg employed in this type of assay is obtained from multitransfused hemophiliacs (or from non-hemophilic subjects developing it spontaneously) and is not easily available in the particularly high titers which seem necessary for the assay. There is yet no convincing proof that different antibodies have similar reactivity with the antigenic determinant of VIII:C and thus the same diagnostic specificity. The method is not feasible in hemophilic families characterized by normal amounts of VIII:CAg in affected members (so called cross-reacting material or CRM-positive kindreds) and there is still some controversy about the frequency of polymorphism in hemophilia A. In addition, there are some unsolved technical problems in some centres for obtaining pure fetal blood samples. Contamination with maternal blood can be usually ruled out by simple methods such as the confirmations of a single, high modal MCV peak of fetal erythrocytes on a particle-size analyzer. However, amniotic fluid contamination remains a difficulty which cannot be simply solved by using VIII:RAg determination as an internal control and mathematical corrections based on the determination of fetal hematocrit. It may occur that the samples are so diluted with amniotic fluid (up to 38 fold or more) that the level of VIII:CAg in samples approximates the limit of sensitivity of the method.

Recently, a team of hematologists and gynecologists at King's College Hospital in London described a new approach which appears to avoid many of the drawbacks of the original method (Mibashan et al, 1979). By using a very small bore fetoscope and needle they have been able to obtain pure fetal blood with a high degree of safety around 19 weeks. Avoidance of contamination of fetal blood with maternal blood or amniotic fluid appears to be achieved by the adoption of certain special precautions in the sampling technique. One important point seems to be the choice for puncture of the largest fetal vessel that can be approached, namely one in the umbilical cord itself close to its placental insertion. Not only does this site provide a sample of better quality but it also appears less risky than the use of smaller fetal vessels. This procedure seem to eliminate contamination in 96 per cent of cases thereby allowing the performance of prenatal diagnosis on fetal plasma by a simple modification of the conventional VIII:C assay. Factor IX assay is used as an internal control to help rule out non-specific activation of the assay system (as well as a yardstick for hemophilia B diagnosis), and the immunoassay of VIII:CAg is an additional control. At the time of writing, the King's College Hospital Group have completed prenatal diagnosis in 39 fetuses at risk of hemophilia A (Mibashan et al, 1980). Twenty-eight fetuses were found to be normal with this method; such a proportion is greater than 0.5 because of the relative small size of the sample and the inclusion of a number of *possible* carriers among pregnant patients. Eighteen diagnoses were confirmed at birth and two after abortion for other medical reasons; pregnancy is continuing in the remaining eight cases. Hemophilia A was diagnosed in eleven fetuses: some were aborted and confirmed, others were aborted in other hospitals. All diagnostic fetal plasma samples were also assayed for VIII:CAg by Peake and Bloom (1978): two samples (one hemophiliac and one normal by VIII:C) appeared to be from CRM-positive kindreds and prenatal diagnosis relied on VIII:C assay only. Only one (normal) sample which was unusually difficult technically and was diluted 2.5 fold with amniotic fluid, had to rely on a normal VIII:CAg assay for prenatal diagnosis. These 39 cases were uncomplicated by any fetal loss so that 26 normal pregnancies could be scheduled for full term delivery. Therefore, this method appears to represent a substantial advance in the field although the success might be related to a particularly high expertise of the fetoscopist coupled with exceptional coordination with hematologists using more than one assay technique.

In summary, there seems to be little doubt that prenatal diagnosis is now feasible in pregnancies at risk for hemophilia. The technique appears to be extremely accurate and sufficiently safe for wider clinical application. Its standards of precision and coordination make its general availability in the near future unlikely. A few multinational reference centres appear to be the more reasonable immediate goal to be pursued, in order to concentrate the necessary specialized and elaborate expertise and to reduce the relatively high cost of these methods. This approach is already feasible within the countries of the EEC and appears to be justified by the small number of carriers who choose prenatal diagnosis with amniocentesis and fetoscopy (Ewans & Shaw, 1979). Research efforts should concentrate on the development of in vitro methods employing fetal cells accessible by amniocentesis. Unfortunately, the elusive nature of the site of synthesis of VIII:C makes this approach currently unrealistic.

ADVANCES AND PROBLEMS IN MANAGEMENT

DDAVP in the management of mild hemophilia

Patients with moderate and mild hemophilia A and von Willebrand's disease (VWD) have usually little exposure to blood products, which are administered only when surgery is undertaken. It has been shown that this situation results in a higher risk of these patients developing hepatitis after administration of concentrates (Kasper & Kipnis, 1972). Hence, an alternative to plasma derivatives would be a substantial advance in their management and several investigators have attempted to study pharmacological compounds capable of increasing VIII:C levels without the need of blood products. Drugs such as catecholamines, vasopressin derivatives and insulin are known to increase VIII:C (Ingram, 1961; Mannucci et al, 1972) but unpleasant side effects limit their potential clinical applications. 1-deamino-8-D-arginine vasopressin (DDAVP), a synthetic analogue of the antidiuretic hormone 8-arginine vasopressin, is well tolerated when infused intravenously in healthy human subjects. As shown by Mannucci et al (1975a) it produces a two-fold or greater increase in the activities related to Factor VIII/von Willebrand Factor (VIII:C, VIII:RAg and VIII:RCo, the factor needed for aggregation of washed platelet by the antibiotic ristocetin). Such an increase was also observed in patients with VWD and hemophilia A characterized by measurable plasma levels of Factor VIII/von Willebrand factor (FVIII/VWF) — related activities, whereas the drug is ineffective in severe hemophilia and VWD (Mannucci et al, 1976b). Poor knowledge of several aspects of FVIII/VWF biochemistry and physiology renders difficult the understanding of the mechanism(s) whereby DDAVP increases FVIII/VWF. The plasma rise of VIII:C, VIII:RAg and VIII:RCo is transient and appears so rapidly that increased synthesis is unlikely to account for it, endogenous release of autologous FVIII/VWF from storage sites appearing much more likely. Despite these limitations in our basic knowledge, in 1975 we initiated a clinical trial of the drug to assess whether autologous VIII:C was functionally effective in hemostasis. Dental extractions were thought to be a suitable clinical situation for a preliminary evaluation of the drug since any untoward bleeding can be observed continuously without the risk of complicating other surgical procedures by concealed hemorrhages. Dental surgery was safely carried out without plasma concentrates in patients with mild hemophilia and VWD, showing that autologous VIII:C released by DDAVP is at least as effective in achieving hemostasis as homologous VIII:C infused in concentrates (Mannucci et al, 1977a). Subsequently, the use of DDAVP was extended to patients undergoing major surgical operations such as tonsillectomy, thoracotomy, cholecystectomy, hysterectomy, colectomy, etc. (Mannucci et al, 1977a and b). To date, our experience has been based on the management of 29 patients (21 with mild to moderate hemophilia and eight with VWD), who were treated with DDAVP on 35 different occasions for dental extractions (15 cases), minor surgical procedures (3 cases), major surgery (6 cases) and spontaneous bleeding episodes (11 cases). The clinical outcome of this treatment confirms our previous reports and those of other investigators (Lowe et al, 1977; Ingram & Hilton, 1977; Menon et al, 1978; Theiss & Schmidt, 1978; Boulton & Smith, 1979) and demonstrates that DDAVP is a useful compound in the management of patients with hemophilia A and VWD characterized by measurable levels of FVIII/VWF related activities. Using a dosage of 0.3–0.4 μg/Kg DDAVP administered intravenously, a three to six-fold increase of VIII:C and a two- to four-fold rise of VIII:RAg and VIII:RCo can be expected in the recipient. Thus, the choice of DDAVP depends both on the baseline concentration of FVIII/VWF related activities and on the desirable levels maintained to treat a given bleeding episode or surgical procedure. It would be unrealistic for example, to use DDAVP to carry out a gastrectomy in a patient with baseline levels of 5 U/dL VIII:C, because the expected post-infusion concentrations of 20–25 U/dL are unlikely to be sufficient to deal with such a major surgical procedure. On the other hand, the same patient might benefit from the use of DDAVP for the management of a muscle hematoma, which is likely to be controlled when such VIII:C levels are attained in plasma. Similarly, the drug can be usefully adopted to carry out major surgery in patients with higher baseline concentrations of VIII:C such as, for instance, 20 U/dL.

As observed in our original study and confirmed by others (Mannucci et al, 1977a and b; Lowe et al, 1977; Theiss & Schmidt; Boulton & Smith, 1978) the extent of factor VIII response to DDAVP tends to decrease in some patients after repeated infusions, even though this occurrence is not constant and some patients respond equally well as after the first dose. It is not yet clear whether such 'resistance' is due to depletion of FVIII/VWF stores, or to the impairment of the release mechanism. Its occurrence, however, does not seem to be a major drawback in the management of patients with mild hemophilia and VWD undergoing surgery and needing a sustained increase of FVIII/VWF levels. We found that, once hemostasis has been firmly established at the time of surgery by DDAVP administration, the natural concentration of FVIII/VWF and the non-specific increase induced by surgery were sufficient to maintain hemostasis in the postoperative period in the majority of cases. The capacity of DDAVP to shorten the bleeding time in VWD is at present a matter of debate. In our first study conducted in a large series of non-bleeding patients with VWD (Mannucci et al, 1976b), at no time was the bleeding time substantially shortened following DDAVP administration. This failure was subsequently confirmed in treated patients, in whom it was paralleled by poor control of mucosal bleeding even though VIII:RCo was raised to normal levels. Such an observation is consistent with the view that the involvement of FVIII/VWF in primary hemostasis is not closely reflected by VIII:RCo, and suggests that in patients with VWD the 'bleeding time factor' is not released or made available by DDAVP in sufficient amounts to achieve a satisfactory control of mucosal bleeding. Perhaps the reason for the discrepancy between our own results and those reported elsewhere with respect to bleeding time changes (Menon et al, 1978; Theiss & Schmidt, 1978) are due to the fact that our template method provides a stronger challenge to primary hemostasis. This is suggested by the observation that the bleeding time is usually poorly controlled even after cryoprecipitate. (Mannucci et al, 1976). Another possibility is that different types of VWD respond differently to DDAVP: this is an interesting hypothesis which is presently being investigated in this laboratory.

Following our original report, Lowe et al (1977) gave cause for concern by showing that the antidiuretic properties of DDAVP induced severe water retention in a patient treated repeatedly following dental extraction. Subsequent experience has shown that water overload seems to be a rare complication of DDAVP treatment, and that it can probably be avoided by monitoring the patients and adopting a number of simple precautions (Ingram & Hilton, 1977). Nevertheless, removal of the antidiuretic affect with maintenance of the FVIII/VWF response appears a reasonable goal to be pursued, as shown by the preliminary results of Cort and Dodds (1979). Other reported side effects of DDAVP are of little clinical significance, e.g. a 20 to 40 per cent increase in heart rate and mild facial flushing unaccompanied by significant changes in blood-pressure. These side effects, possibly related to the peptide structure of the drug, are usually not disturbing and can be greatly reduced or avoided by extending the infusion time to 20 to 30 minutes.

A new important application of DDAVP had been recently proposed by Nilsson et al (1979). In a group of donors, treatment with DDAVP before blood drawing resulted in at least double the yield of VIII:C in the concentrate prepared from this plasma. More importantly, in vivo studies showed that infusion of post-DDAVP concentrates to patients with severe hemophilia A caused 2 to 3 times larger an increase in VIII:C than infusion of the same volume of control concentrates produced from untreated donors. Although it appears difficult to envisage that a substantial proportion of blood donors will accept to be injected with a drug before blood collection, these findings represent an important advance in the field of plasma fractionation and DDAVP might be adopted by the plasmapheresis centres supplying plasma to the pharmaceutical industry. Perhaps DDAVP might be more easily acceptable by donors if administered by intranasal application (Kobayashi, 1979). This route can be adopted to increase FVIII/VWF in normal subjects and in patients, although the response is less predictable than that produced by the i.v. route, probably due to the vagaries of drug absorption (Mannucci, 1980). In addition, three extensive studies have provided detailed informations on the effects of DDAVP in patients with mild hemophilia A and von Willebrand's disease; Ludlam et al (1980), Nilsson et al (1980) and Mannucci et al (1981).

In conclusion, the use of DDAVP has opened a new perspective in the management of FVIII/VWF deficiency states, showing that in some instances it is possible to treat patients without resorting to blood products. New compounds may soon become available with more potent activity, less side effects and a specific potential for increasing FVIII/VWF in plasma. It is likely that a number of cases of post-transfusion hepatitis might be avoided by wider adoption of DDAVP in mild hemophilia.

Prothrombin complex concentrates in 'resistant' hemophilia: the state of the art
The management of bleeding episodes in patients with inhibitors of VIII:C is still a major unsolved therapeutic problem. When the inhibitor titer is high enough, an increased dosage of clotting factor concentrates is usually not sufficient to neutralize the inhibitor and to achieve hemostatic levels of VIII:C in plasma. Treatment of bleeding episodes then becomes a formidable problem, which is difficult to manage even in specialized hemophilia centres. To reduce the inhibitor levels, plasmapheresis followed by high-potency concentrates has been used with some success (Edson et al, 1973). Measures such as these are, however, expensive, time-consuming and not without undesirable side effects. It is for these reasons that the use of prothrombin complex concentrates appears an interesting new approach to the management of patients suffering from hemophilia A complicated by the presence of VIII:C inhibitors in high titer.

These concentrates are either the products regularly used in the treatment of hemophilia B and other congenital deficiencies of the prothrombin complex clotting factors; or specially made preparations containing in controlled amounts the active principle(s) by-passing the need for VIII:C in the intrinsic coagulation system. The nature of such active principle(s) is still poorly understood, even though the alleged clinical effectiveness of 'regular' PCC is likely to be related to the presence of activated forms of Factor VII, IX and X. These views are supported by the observation that such PCC have apparently become much less effective in clinical practice since the manufactures have reduced the content of activated clotting factors with the purpose of decreasing the risk of thromboembolism (Penner & Kelly, 1977). Whether a given active clotting factor is more important than another in producing the clinical effect, is still a matter of uncertainty. More precise knowledge is of utmost importance, because the identification of the active principle would permit the preparation of specific concentrates devoid of unnecessary and potentially dangerous contaminants. This approach has been pursued by two pharmaceutical companies, who have attempted to prepare concentrates containing the active principle(s) in controlled conditions. The product manufactured in Austria contains a 'Factor Eight Inhibitor Bypassing Activity' (F.E.I.B.A.) of poorly defined nature, though some investigators tend to identify activated factor VII as the active principle (Mariani et al, 1979). According to the United States manufacturers of the preparation (alternatively designated Autoplex or Auto-Factor IX), the Factor VIII correctional activity is related to the presence of critical amounts of activated factors VII and X.

Despite limited basic knowledge, in recent years there have been several reports on the use of PCC in the management of bleeding episodes in 'resistant' hemophilia (see the review of Bloom, 1978). Varied results have been reported in conditions ranging from commonly occurring hemorrhages into joints and soft tissues to life threatening bleeding arising spontaneously or after surgery. In such cases it is often difficult to establish objective criteria and so avoid bias in the evaluation of results, because spontaneous resolution is not uncommon and in severe hemorrhagic episodes, additional therapeutic measures are frequently employed. To resolve this issue, there is a need for controlled clinical trials, which are currently being carried out in the United States and Holland. When it is considered that the effect of VIII:C concentrates in hemophiliacs with no inhibitor is so clear-cut that no clinical trial is ever needed, it is abundantly clear that effectiveness of the activated PCC is not as marked as that of VIII:C concentrates. This view is consistent with the conclusions of a multicentre survey of treated cases organized by the Subcommittee on Factor IX Concentrates of the International Committee for Thrombosis and Hemostasis (Blatt et al, 1980).

Whilst awaiting the results of ongoing clinical trials, a few tentative recommendations can be made on the basis of this survey and our own clinical experience. The use of PCC should be attempted in life-threatening conditions only when other therapeutic measures are not feasible or successful. Since little benefit can now be expected by the usual preparations of PCC, specially prepared fractions must be preferred. High doses of such fractions (80 to 100 arbitrary units per kilogram body weight) must be administered at frequent intervals (every 6 to 8 hours) because the majority of case reports suggest that lower doses and infrequent administration are less effective. A special attempt should be made to use activated PCC in conditions of external hemorrhages, such as open wounds or dental extractions. In these conditions, bleeding can be monitored continuously without the risk of complicating other surgical procedures by concealed hemorrhage and the effect of PCC might be objectively observed. It would be preferable to avoid the combined use of other hemostatic drugs such as the antifibrinolytic compounds tranexamic and ε-aminocaproic acid, although we believe that pharmacological inhibition of fibrinolysis alone cannot be responsible for the establishment of hemostasis.

Several reports have shown that PCC can elicit an anamnestic response of the inhibitor (Allain & Krieger, 1975; Mannucci et al, 1976a; Kasper & Feinstein, 1976) in some patients. Although the effect of PCC is independent of the inhibitor titer, such a complication is unwarranted because the increase in the inhibitor level may render more difficult the use of plasmapheresis and high potency VIII:C concentrates in case of PCC failure. According to a recent study by Lechner et al (1978), a rise of the inhibitor titer can be predicted in patients who show a marked inhibitor response after VIII:C concentrates (high responders), a low inhibitor level at the time of treatment and in those who are treated with large doses of PCC. Significant amounts of protein with VIII:CAg determinants were found in PCC (Onder & Hoyer, 1979). Although there is no proof that VIII:CAg is the substance eliciting the anamnestic response, it is reasonable to assume that the rise in VIII:C inhibitor titer is related to the presence of this protein. Other side effects are surprisingly rare following PCC. However, the danger of disseminated intravascular coagulation should always be considered (Stenbjerg & Jorgensen, 1978), especially following surgery and in patients with liver disease, hemorrhagic shock or trauma. The concomitant use of antifibrinolytic drugs might contribute an added risk which should be considered and perhaps avoided.

A group of investigators have included PCC in their original therapeutic scheme aimed to eradicate factor VIII inhibitors (Brackmann & Gormsen, 1977). The concept underlying this new therapeutic approach is that of inducing a state of immune tolerance by treating patients with large daily doses of VIII:C concentrates. After an initial rise due to anamnestic response which lasts 2 to 3 months, the inhibitor titer starts to decline until a complete disappearance is achieved which has lasted in some patients for several months. Although the majority of patients are being continued on VIII:C treatment even after the inhibitor has disappeared, a few of them are treated only on demand and the inhibitor has apparently not reappeared (Brackmann, 1979).

In this scheme, prevention of bleeding episodes during the phase of the anamnestic response is the concept underlying the use of PCC, although it is not ruled out that their administration might have a more specific role in the induction of immunological tolerance (Brackmann, 1979). This approach is new and ingenious. The formidable cost of the procedure might be justifiable if the details of the protocol and results become more generally available in a more extended published report, which is now urgently awaited. An important point which needs confirmation is whether continuous treatment is needed for maintaining the eradication of the inhibitor.

Lusher et al (1980) have recently reported the results of a multicenter trial comparing the therapeutic effectiveness of two commercial prothrombin-complex concentrates (Konyne and Proplex) in the management of acute hemarthroses occurring in patients with hemophilia A and inhibitors. Both the concentrates were judged effective in approximately half the episodes of acute bleeding treated, although the responses were not as good as responses to Factor VIII concentrates in hemophiliacs without inhibitors.

In conclusion, PCC are a useful new weapon in the management of the difficult situations so often encountered with haemophiliacs developing an inhibitor to VIII:C. Variations of clinical effectiveness of available preparations suggest the need of better standardization. This crucial problem is in turn related to the identification of the active principle(s), which is urgently needed for the production of more specific and effective products.

Liver disease in hemophiliacs

Hemophiliacs are undoubtedly the group of multitransfused patients exposed most frequently and for the longest period of time to the agent(s) implicated in post-transfusion hepatitis. The rate of exposure has probably increased since the wider use in the replacement therapy of highly-purified clotting factor concentrates which carry a higher risk of contamination, having been manufactured by pools of plasma from a large number of donors. The frequent exposure of hemophiliacs to hepatitis B virus (HBV) is well documented by the observed high incidence of positivity for HBV serologic markers. In recent series investigated with sensitive radioimmunoassays, the antibody to hepatitis B surface antigen (anti-HB$_s$) reaches an incidence very close to 100 per cent (Enck et al, 1979), whereas the prevalence of HB$_s$Ag appears to range from 4 to 9 per cent (see the review of Seef & Hoofnagle, 1976). Lack of availability of suitable markers renders difficult a detailed study on the exposure rate to non-A, non-B viruses. There is indirect but strong evidence, however, that they are contained in clotting factor concentrates and can be transmitted to hemophiliacs (Craske et al, 1975; Hruby & Schauf, 1978).

In the light of this information, the incidence of clinically manifested acute hepatitis is surprisingly low in hemophiliacs, ranging from 6 to 26 per cent. (Seef & Hoofnagle 1976). An important contribution to the understanding of hepatitis epidemiology has been provided by Kasper and Kipnis (1972) who showed that children, or mild hemophiliacs, who have had little exposure to blood products are at higher risk of developing clinical illness than multitransfused hemophiliacs. Clinical hepatologists, however, are well aware that in acute liver disease hepatitis is only the tip of the iceberg of clinical manifestations. The relatively low incidence of clinical illness associated with jaundice in hemophiliacs does not exclude the occurrence of asymptomatic hepatitis, nor the possibility that repeated and prolonged contact with viruses may cause chronic liver damage. Surprisingly, this problem was overlooked until 1975 when a study of 91 patients with severe hemophilia reported a high incidence of abnormal liver function tests (LFT) unaccompanied by overt liver disease (Mannucci et al, 1975b). The most frequent abnormalities were a moderate increase in both serum transaminases and bromsulphthalein retention, occurring in nearly half of the patients. Hypergammaglobulinemia was another common finding but the specific significance of this abnormality cannot be easily ascertained in patients continuously exposed to allogeneic antigens contained in blood, plasma and concentrates. The overall incidence of abnormality of tests exploring the synthetic capacity of the liver and biliary cell function was rather low, suggesting that liver involvement was not severe. Accordingly, all the patients were asymptomatic and only a minority of them showed mild to moderate liver enlargement or splenomegaly on physical examination (Mannucci et al, 1975b).

Following confirmation of these results in other series of patients (Hasiba et al, 1977; Hilgartner & Giardina, 1977), an important step-forward in understanding their clinical significance has recently been made through the availability of percutaneous liver biopsies, carried out by four groups of investigators in hemophiliacs presenting with persistently abnormal transaminases (Lesesne et al, 1977; Mannucci et al, 1978; Preston et al, 1978; Spero et al, 1978). The great majority of biopsies (95 per cent) provided histological evidence of chronic active liver disease (CALD), ranging from potentially regressive persistent hepatitis to severe cirrhosis. These studies were carried out in selected groups of patients undergoing biopsy because they presented elevations of transaminases lasting for one year or more. It cannot be ruled out, therefore, that these findings do not apply to the prevalent group of hemophiliacs showing normal or transiently elevated transaminases. To resolve this dilemma, Schimpf et al (1977) performed percutaneous liver biopsies in an unselected group of hemophiliacs taking advantage of the massive and prolonged substitution therapy given to cover procedures of major surgery. Although the observed incidence of CALD was lower (63 per cent) than in patients with persistently abnormal LFT, this important study demonstrates that CALD appears to be a frequent finding also in unselected multitransfused hemophiliacs and that minor forms of liver disease were present in the remaining 37 percent of the biopsied patients (Schimpf & Zimmerman, 1980). Since the magnitude of the problem has become apparent, clinicians have been confronted with the problem of searching for an acceptable solution. Both the approaches of prevention and treatment present formidable obstacles. First of all, it should be emphasized once again that hemophiliacs with CALD were surprisingly asymptomatic even in the presence of severe histologic abnormalities. Therefore, the use of corticosteroids in order to obtain the improvement in life-quality achieved in non-hemophiliacs with CALD appears to be unjustified. In general, the capacity of corticosteroids of stopping the evolution of CALD and prolonging survival is not well established, whereas it has been suggested that this treatment may worsen the condition of HB_sAg-positive patients (Plotz, 1975; Berk et al, 1976). Long-term corticosteroid treatment is associated with growth disturbances in children, and is likely to carry an increased risk of gastrointestinal bleeding in hemophiliacs. For these reasons, we have chosen to avoid corticosteroids in asymptomatic patients with CALD, until more clear-cut evidence of effectiveness becomes available from ongoing clinical trials carried out in non-hemophilic patients with CALD. It must be borne in mind that CALD might have an entirely different clinical course in hemophiliacs, who are characterized by a continuous re-exposure to infective agent(s) and by a peculiar immunological situation due to their repeated stimulations with allogeneic proteins. The natural history of CALD in hemophiliacs might now be elucidated by repeating biopsy at intervals of three to four years rather than by doing it in new patients.

The difficulties encountered in planning a rational treatment emphasize the priority of prevention. Needless to say, withdrawal or limitation of the present strategy of aggressive replacement therapy are not justified. Not only because this change would be accompanied by a consistent deterioration in the pattern of life of hemophiliacs, but also because it is unlikely to give the expected results. These views are supported by the findings of Hilgartner and Giardina (1977), who have related the incidence of abnormal liver function tests to the amount of concentrates given to the patients. Elevation of serum enzymes and the occurrence of HB_sAg and/or Ab were not remarkably different in patients on prophylactic or episodic treatment, even though the amounts of concentrates transfused in the latter groups was significantly lower.

Whether abnormal LFT are more frequent in patients treated with commercial concentrates rather than in these given only blood-bank cryoprecipitate from small pools of unpaid donors, is a matter of controversy (Count, 1976; Hasiba et al, 1977; Levine et al, 1977). Cryoprecipitate is a difficult material to handle, it shows variable potency from bag by bag and needs to be stored at $-20°C$. In contrast, freeze-dried concentrates are characterized by known potency, stability at $4°C$, ease in reconstitution and low risk of allergic reactions. These advantages make them preferable in home treatment, which is now considered by hemophiliacs the most effective form of management of which the withdrawal would not be acceptable. It must be also realized that in many countries hemophilia care is almost exclusively based on availability of commercial concentrates prepared by pooling plasma from thousands of donors. Leaving aside the complex ethical problem involved in this situation and the responsibilities of the countries who have not yet attempted to organize a modern national blood program, any solution to the prevention of post-transfusion liver disease in hemophiliacs should take into account that a deterioration of the pattern of life now assured by commercial concentrates would be unacceptable for these patients. The higher risk rate of children of developing hepatitis compared with that of multitransfused adults suggests an approach to CALD prevention which takes into account this situation. The rationale of this approach is also based on the fact that children are more likely to develop chronic persistence of HB_sAg, and that in them contact with the hepatitis virus is more often evolving towards CALD than in adults (Gerety & Schweitzer, 1977; Spero et al, 1979). Therefore, we have chosen to treat hemophiliacs under the age of six exclusively with an intensive regimen of blood-bank made cryoprecipitate, planning to switch them to treatment with commercial concentrates after this age. Although there is yet no proof that this treatment is safer in term of development of CALD, a close scrutiny of these patients for two years has shown that none of them developed LFT abnormalities and became HB_sAg positive. This seems at the moment the only realistic approach that can be proposed for the prevention of post-transfusion CALD in hemophiliacs.

In conclusion, post-transfusion liver disease in hemophilia is a formidable problem which is likely to be a primary challenge to clinicians, manufacturers of blood products, and virologists in the near future. Until substantial progress is made in these fields, the problem is unlikely to be solved. A better understanding of the clinical course of liver disease appears perhaps the most important research target in the next few years. To date, since there is no evidence of a high death rate from CALD in hemophiliacs, an approach based on the restriction of replacement therapy appears unjustified and probably ineffective.

A few notes on home care

In the preceding sections, an attempt has been made to summarize advances in hemophilia diagnosis and management. It is clear that, despite known and emerging problems, a more normal life can now be offered to the hemophiliac where previously it was a matter of fate and patients having to live with life-threatening and crippling conditions. The aims of modern treatment, however, cannot be only to improve life expectancy and avoid medical complications but also should be to prevent psychological and social handicaps. Home therapy makes these goals realistic. Home care aims to improve the condition and the quality of the life of the hemophiliac by placing most of the responsibilities for management of the disease on the patient and/or his family in conjunction with the staff of specialized hemophilia centres. In this approach it is essential to detect bleeding promptly, the hemophiliac being the only person able to do so before it becomes clinically obvious; and hence to stop bleeding at the earliest time by infusion of the missing clotting factor. Home care was initially developed in the United States (Britten, 1970; Rabiner & Telfer, 1970), where it is applied to nearly half of the hemophiliacs, and has subsequently spread in Europe. It seems to be the best way to provide adequate care to a large number of patients spread over a large geographical area in countries with few hemophilia centres. Wherever hematologists are willing to set up such a programme, lyophilized cryoprecipitate or concentrates must be available and hemophiliacs must be properly trained before home care can be instituted. A low social, economic and cultural background is not an insurmountable obstacle. The solution is more a question of adapting the training programme to the audience.

For the above reasons, home care seems to be the best system for providing hemophilia care in developing countries, in which the locally-made freeze-dried cryoprecipitate is a feasible prospect, as shown by the experience gained in Costa Rica (Cordero & Montero, 1975). The main thrust of developing countries should be the development of a national blood program based on unpaid donors. Cryoprecipitate production and the start of modern hemophilia care are simple by-products of such a program.

REFERENCES

Alagille D, Prou-Wartelle O 1966 Etude des condutrices d'hemophilie Sang 31: 797–806
Allain J P, Krieger G R 1975 Prothrombin complex concentrate in treatment of classical hemophilia with factor VIII antibody (letter). Lancet 2: 1203
Alter B P, Modell C B, Fairweather D 1976 Prenatal diagnosis of hemoglobinopathies: a review of 15 cases. New England Journal of Medicine 295: 1437–1443
Babson A L, Babson S R 1974 Comparative evaluation of a partial thromboplastin reagent containing a non-settling particulate activator. American Journal of Clinical Pathology 62: 856–860

Bennett B, Ratnoff O D 1973 Detection of the carrier state for classic hemophilia. New England Journal of Medicine 288: 342–345

Berk P D, Jones E A, Plotz P H 1976 Corticosteroid therapy for chronic active hepatitis. (editorial) Annals of Internal Medicine 85: 523–525

Blatt P M, Menache D, Roberts H R 1980 A survey of the effectiveness of prothrombin complex concentrates in controlling hemorrhage in patients with hemophilia and anti-factor VIII antibodies. Thrombosis and Hemostasis 44: 39–43

Bloom A L 1978 Clotting factor concentrates for resistant hemophilia. British Journal of Hematology 40: 21–27

Boulton F E, Smith A 1979 DDAVP and cryoprecipitate in mild hemophilia (letter) Lancet 2: 535

Bouma B N, Van Der Klaauw M M, Veltkamp J J, Starkenburg A E, Van Tilburg N H, Hermans J 1975 Evaluation of the detection rate of hemophilia carriers. Thrombosis Research 7: 339–350

Brackmann H H 1979 Personal communication

Brackmann H H, Gormsen J 1979 Massive factor-VIII infusion in hemophiliac with factor-VIII inhibitor, high responder (letter), Lancet 2: 933

Britten A F H 1970 A little freedom for the hemophiliac (editorial). New England Journal of Medicine 283: 1051–1052

Cordero R, Montero C 1975 Personal communication

Cort J H, Dodds W J 1979 Evidence for the existence of a factor VIII releasing factor from the brain released by the action of vasopressin-like cyclic nonapeptides. (abstract) Blood 54, supplement 1: 274

Count R B 1976 Serum transaminase and HB Ab in hemophiliacs treated exclusively with cryoprecipitate. In: Fratantoni J C and Aronson D L (ed) Unsolved therapeutic problems in hemophilia, DHEW Publication n. (NIH) 77–1089, Washington, DC, US Government Printing Office, p 77–81

Craske J, Dilling N, Stern D 1975 An outbreak of hepatitis associated with intravenous injection of factor-VIII concentrate. Lancet 2: 221–223

Edson J R, McArthur J R, Branda R F, McCullough J J, Chou S N 1973 Successful managements of a subdural hematoma in a hemophiliac with an anti-factor VIII antibody. Blood 41: 113–119

Enck R E, Betts R F, Brown M R, Miller G 1979 Viral serology (hepatitis B virus, cytomegalovirus, Epstein-Barr virus) and abnormal liver function tests in transfused patients with hereditary hemorrhagic diseases. Transfusion 19: 32–38

Evans D I K, Shaw A 1979 Attitude of hemophilia carriers to fetoscopy and amniocentesis (letter). Lancet 2: 1371

Firshein S I, Hoyer L W, Lazarchick J, Forget B G, Hobbins J C, Clyne L P, Pitlik F A, Muir W A, Merkatz I R, Mahoney M J 1979 Prenatal diagnosis of classic hemophilia. New England Journal of Medicine 300: 937–941

Gerety R J, Schweitzer I L 1977 Viral hepatitis type B during pregnancy, the neonatal period and infancy. Journal of Pediatrics 90: 368–373

Hasiba V W, Spero J A, Lewis J H 1977 Chronic liver dysfunction in multitransfused hemophiliacs. Transfusion 17: 490–494

Hilgartner M W, Giardina P 1977 Liver dysfunction in patients with hemophilia Scandinavian Journal of Hematology, supplementum 30: 6–10

Hobbins J C, Mahoney M J 1974 In utero diagnosis of hemoglobinopathies: technique for obtaining fetal blood. New England Journal of Medicine 290: 1065–1067

Hruby M A, Schauf V 1978 Transfusion related short-incubation hepatitis in hemophilic patients. Journal of American Medical Association 240: 1355–1357

Ikkala E 1960 Hemophilia. A study of its laboratory, clinical, genetic and social aspects based on known hemophiliacs in Finland. Scandinavian Journal of Clinical and Laboratory Investigation 12: Supplementum 46

Ingram G I C 1961 Increase in antihemophilic globulin activity following infusion of adrenaline. Journal of Physiology 156: 217–224

Ingram G I C, Hilton P J 1977 DDAVP in hemophilia (letter). Lancet 2: 721–722

Italian C.I.S.M.E.L. Study Group 1980 Activated partial thromboplastin time: a multicenter evaluation of commercial reagents in the diagnosis of mild hemophilia A and other coagulation defects. Scandinavian Journal of Hematology 25: 308–317

Kasper C K, Kipnis S A 1972 Hepatitis and clotting factor concentrates. (letter) Journal of American Medical Association 221: 510

Kasper C H, Feinstein D I 1976 Rising factor VIII inhibitor titers after konye factor IX complex (letter). New England Journal of Medicine 295: 505

Klein H G, Aledort L M, Bouma B N, Hoyer L W, Zimmerman T S, De Metz D L 1977 A co-operative study for the detection of the carrier state of classic hemophilia. New England Journal of Medicine 296: 959–962

Kobayashi I 1979 Treatment of hemophilia A and von Willebrand's disease patients with an intranasal dripping of DDAVP. Thrombosis Research 16: 775–780

Koepke J A 1975 The partial thromboplastin time in the CAP survey programme. American Journal of Clinical Pathology 63: 990–994

Lazarchick J, Hoyer L W 1978 Immunoradiometric measurement of the factor VIII procoagulant antigen. Journal of Clinical Investigation 62: 1048–1052

Lechner K, Nowotny C H, Krinninger B, Zegner M, Deutsch E 1978. Effect of treatment with activated prothrombin complex concentrate (FEIBA) on Factor VIII-antibody level. Thrombosis Haemostasis 40: 478–485

Lesesne H R, Morgan J E, Blatt P M, Webster W P, Roberts H R 1977 Liver biopsy in hemophilia A. Annals of Internal Medicine 86: 703–707

Levine P H, McVerry B A, Attock B, Dormandy K M 1977 Health of the intensively treated hemophiliac, with special reference to abnormal liver chemistries and splenomegaly. Blood 50: 1–9

Lowe G, Pettigrew A, Middleton J, Forbes C D, Prentice C R M 1977 DDAVP in hemophilia (letter). Lancet 2: 614–615

Ludlam C A, Peake I R, Allen B, Davies B L, Furlough R A, Bloom A L 1980 Factor VIII and fibrinolytic response to Deamino-8-D-Agenine-Vasopressin in normal subjects and dissociate response in some patients with haemophilia and von Willebrand's disease. British Journal of Haematology 45: 499–511

Lusher J M, Shapiro S S, Polascak J E, Rao A V, Levine P H, Blatt P M 1980 Efficacy of prothrombin-complex concentrates in hemophiliacs with antibodies to Factor VIII. A multicenter therapeutic trial. New England Journal of Medicine 303: 421–425

Mannucci P M 1980 Unpublished observations

Mannucci P M, Gagnatelli G, D'Alonzo R 1972 Stress and Blood Coagulation. In: Brinkhous K M (ed) Thrombosis: Risk Factors and Diagnostic Approaches. F K Schattauer, Stuttgart New York, p 105–113

Mannucci P M, Aberg M, Nilsson I M, Robertson B 1975a Mechanism of plasminogen activator and factor VIII increase after vasoactive drugs. British Journal of Hematology 30: 81–93

Mannucci P M, Capitanio A, Del Ninno E, Colombo M, Pareti F, Ruggeri Z M 1975b Asymptomatic liver disease in hemophiliacs. Journal of Clinical Pathology 28: 620–624

Mannucci P M, Bader R, Ruggeri Z M 1976a Concentrates of clotting factor IX (letter). Lancet 1: 41

Mannucci P M, Pareti F I, Holmberg L, Nilsson I M, Ruggeri Z M 1976b. Studies on the prolonged bleeding time in von Willebrand's disease. Journal of Laboratory and Clinical Medicine 88: 662–671

Mannucci P M, Ruggeri Z M, Pareti F I, Capitanio A 1977a 1-Deamino-8-D-arginine vasopressin: a new pharmacological approach to the management of hemophilia and von Willebrand's disease. Lancet 1: 869–872

Mannucci P M, Ruggeri Z M, Pareti F I, Capitanio A 1977b DDAVP in hemophilia (letter). Lancet 2: 1171–1172

Mannucci P M, Ronchi G, Rota L, Colombo M 1978 A clinicopathological study of liver disease in hemophiliacs. Journal of Clinical Pathology 31: 779–783

Mannucci PM, Canciani MT, Rota L, Donovan BS 1981 Response to Factor VIII/von Willebrand's factor to DDAVP in healthy subjects and patients with haemophilia A and von Willebrand's disease. British Journal of Haematology 47: 283–293

Mariani G, Romoli D, Salvitti C, Avvisati G, Hassan H J, Mazzucconi M G 1979 In vivo activation of the extrinsic pathway by F.E.I.B.A. (abstract). Thrombosis Haemostasis 42: 365

Menon C, Berry E W, Ockelford P 1978 Beneficial effect of DDAVP on bleeding time in von Willebrand's disease (letter). Lancet 2: 743–744

Methods for the detection of hemophilia carriers: a Memorandum. 1977. Bulletin of the World Health Organization 55: 675–702

Meyer D, Plas A, Allain J P, Sitar G M, Larrieu M J 1975 Problems in the detection of carriers of hemophilia A. Journal of Clinical Pathology 28: 690–695

Mibashan R S, Peake I R, Rodeck C H, Thumpston J K, Furlong R A, Gorer R, Bains L, Bloom A L 1980 Dual diagnosis of prenatal hemophilia by measurement of fetal factor VIII C and VIII C antigen. Lancet ii: 994–997

Mibashan R S, Rodeck C H, Thumpston J K, Edwards R J, Singer J D, White J M, Campbell S 1979 Plasma assay of fetal factors VIII and IX for prenatal diagnosis of hemophilia. Lancet i: 1309–1311

Nilsson I M, Walter H, Mikaelsson M, Vilhardt T 1979 Factor VIII concentrate prepared from DDAVP stimulated blood donor plasma. Scandinavian Journal of Hematology 22: 42–46

Nilsson I M, Holmberg L, Aberg M, Vilhardt M 1980 The release of plasminogen activator and Factor VIII after injection of DDAVP in healthy volunteers and in patients with von Willebrand's disease. Scandinavian Journal of Haematology 24: 351–359

Onder O, Hoyer L 1979 Factor VIII coagulant antigen in factor IX complex concentrates. Thrombosis Research 15: 569–572

Peake I R, Bloom A L 1978 Immunoradiometric assay of procoagulant factor-VIII antigen in plasma and serum and its reduction in haemophilia: preliminary studies on adult and fetal blood. Lancet 1: 473–475

Penner J, Kelly P 1977 Factor VIII inhibitors: therapeutic response to prothrombin complex concentrates (abstract). Thrombosis Haemostasis 38: 339

Plotz P H 1975 Asymptomatic chronic hepatitis (editorial). Gastroenterology 68: 1629–1630

Poller L, Thomson J M, Palmer M K 1976 Measuring partial thromboplastin time. An international collaborative study. Lancet ii: 842–846

Preston F E, Triger D R, Underwood J C E, Bardhan G, Mitchell V E, Stewart R M, Blackburn E K 1978 Percutaneous liver biopsy and chronic liver disease in hemophiliacs. Lancet 2: 592–594

Proctor R R, Rapaport S I 1961 The partial thromboplastin time with kaolin. A simple test for first stage plasma clotting factor deficiency. American Journal of Clinical Pathology 36: 212–219

Rabiner S F, Telfer M C 1970 Home transfusion for patients with hemophilia A. New England Journal of Medicine 283: 1001–1015

Rizza C R, Rhymes I L, Austen D E G, Kernoff P B A, Aroni S A 1975 Detection of carriers of hemophilia: a blind study. British Journal of Hematology 30: 447–456

Schimpf K L, Zimmermann K, Rudel J, Thanner G, Zeltsch P 1977 Result of liver biopsies, rate of icteric hepatitis and frequency of anti-HB$_s$ and HB$_s$-antigen in patients of the Heidelberg hemophilia centre (abstract). Thrombosis Haemostasis 38: 340

Schimpf K, Zimmermann K 1980 Hepatitishanfigkeit, serologische Befunde und Leberhistogie nach Therapie schwerer Hemorrhagischer Diathesen mit Gerinnungsfaktoren-Konzentraten. In: K Schimpf (ed) Fibrinogen, Fibrin and Fibrin Glue. Side Effects of Therapy with Clotting Factor Concentrates. F K Schattauer, Stuttgart and New York, p 229–308

Seef L B, Hoofnagle J 1976 Acute and chronic liver disease in hemophilia. In: Fratantoni J C & Aronson D L (ed) Unsolved therapeutic problems in hemophilia DHEW Publication n. (NIH) 77–1089, Washington, DC, US Government Printing Office, p 61–73

Sibley C, Singer J W, Wood R J 1973 Comparison of activated partial thromboplastin reagents. American Journal of Clinical Pathology 59: 581–586

Spero J A, Lewis J H, Van Thiel D H, Hasiba U, Rabin B 1978 Asymptomatic structural liver disease in hemophilia. New England Journal of Medicine 298: 1373–1378

Spero J A, Lewis J H, Fisher S E, Hasiba U, Van Thiel D H 1979 The high risk of chronic liver disease in multitransfused juvenile hemophilic patients. Journal of Pediatrics 94: 875–878

Stenjberg S, Jorgensen J 1978 Activated FIX concentrate (FEIBA) used in the treatment of hemophilic patients with antibody to FVIII. Acta Medica Scandinavica 203: 471–476

Theiss W, Schmidt G 1978 DDAVP in von Willebrand's disease. Repeated administration and behaviour of the bleeding time. Thrombosis Research 13: 1119–1123

Zimmerman T S, Ratnoff O D, Powell E E 1971a Immunologic differentiation of classic hemophilia (factor VIII deficiency) and von Willebrand's disease. Journal of Clinical Investigation 50: 244–255

Zimmerman T S, Ratnoff O D, Littell A S 1971b Detection of carriers of classic hemophilia using immunologic assay for antihemophilic factor (factor VIII). Journal of Clinical Investigation 50: 255–258

Zimmerman T S 1974 Quoted by Meyer et al 1975

9. Blood coagulation in animals other than man and animal models of human coagulation disorders

R. K. Archer

BLOOD COAGULATION IN VARIOUS ANIMALS

Here it is proposed to review some of the knowledge now available about how blood clots in animals other than man. By far the greatest amount of experimental work has been done with human blood while veterinary knowledge has lagged behind. However in recent years study has been much stimulated by the increasing use of animal blood products in human therapy. Besides this, animals are increasingly used as models with the intention of extrapolating results obtained with them to human use: a procedure which can be dangerous. So far there has been little attempt to study systematically blood coagulation in the 'simpler' animal with a view to casting light on the immense complexities of the systems now known in 'higher' animals and man. This field would seem likely to be exceedingly fertile.

Considering blood coagulation in animals as a whole, it is the extraordinary similarities rather than the differences which are striking. The changes seem to be of quantity rather than function. There are, of course, considerable species specificities and these are considered below. It is also necessary to guard against the confusion which has arisen from the use of the various synonyms for the same coagulation factors.

Many species have yet to be studied at all as to the mechanisms of blood, haemolymph or coelomic fluid clotting. Starting with invertebrates and working through the evolutionary tree towards primates and ungulates, some studies have been found and are considered from this evolutionary point of view and taking man as the ultimate to which each is to be compared and contrasted (Fig. 9.1).

Invertebrates

Regular circulation of a body fluid does not occur in animals more primitive than the brachiopods. Thus the coelomic fluid of the coelenterates does not circulate. However, the hamolymph found in worms and higher animals does circulate with increasing efficiency as the evolutionary tree is climbed. In the coelenterata the coelomic fluid is a mixture of sea water, some protein and metabolites. It does not clot (Gregoire & Tagnon, 1962). In echinoderms clotting does take place in one of three ways: by cell aggregation, by formation of a large coagulum or by enmeshment of cells in an extracellular network (Boolootian & Giese, 1959). In arthropods Gregoire (1970) has described how 'explosion corpuscles' undergo irreversible, instant changes which initiate plasma coagulation and occur locally in response to damage. This contrasts with the horseshoe crab (*Limulus polyphemus*) in which clottable protein is contained within cells, which is released following damage, to clot all the haemolymph in the animal. This coagulum rapidly retracts to a small plate over the damaged area so that the fluidity of the body fluid is restored (Solum, 1970). In the sand crab (*Ovalipes bipustulatus*) the amaebocytes contain a protein clottable with human thrombin. This protein is like human fibrinogen and the crab haemolymph contains a factor similar to human factor XIII (Madaras, Parkin & Castaldi, 1979).

Amongst the invertebrates, coagulation appears to be a relatively simple process without anything comparable to the enzyme cascade characteristic of the mammals. However, it does give the impression that it is none the less remarkably effective for the various animals in their normal surroundings.

Fish

A study of blood coagulation in fish was made by Doolittle and Surgenor (1962). These authors reviewed previous work and then described observations on the primitive cyclostomes, on the elasmobranchs and also on teleosts. The specimens were bled from the caudal vein by severing the tail and inserting a cannula into the vessel.

The whole blood-clotting time was less than one minute in the case of blackfish (*Tautoga onitis*) but longer with dogfish blood (*Mustelis canis*). Lamprey (*Petromyzon marinus*) blood did not clot well even after twenty-four hours, but if an aqueous tissue extract of lamprey were added, there was good clot formation within a minute. Indeed the plasmas of all these fish could be clotted quite rapidly in the presence of homologous tissue extract. This effect was greatest with the same species but was not completely specific in the sense that there was some effect in mixed systems.

Barium sulphate adsorption removed a factor essential for clotting, assumed to be prothrombin. With lamprey blood, considerably more barium sulphate was necessary to adsorb this component. Thrombin generation in the dogfish and blackfish was similar to that in man provided that concentrations of calcium over 30 mM were used instead of 8 mM as in the human system. In the lamprey, thrombin generation could not be measured unless tissue extract was added.

Assay of specific clotting factors was complicated by species specificity so that human plasmas deficient in one or another factor could not be used as substrates. Whilst the fish fibrinogens were readily clotted by mammalian thrombin, human fibrinogen was clotted only very slowly by lamprey thrombin.

Srivastava (1969) working in India found that the clotting time of local freshwater teleosts was inversely proportional to the number of thrombocytes present. Hougie (1972) examined Pacific salmon (*Oncorhynchus spp.*) which die after spawning with a marked coagulation defect. This defect is in many respects comparable to disseminated intravascular coagulation as it occurs in man.

Amphibians

The toad *Bufo marinus* Linn has been studied by Hackett and LePage (1961a and b). They bled these animals by cannulation of the bulbus arteriosus in pithed subjects obtaining some 5 to 8 ml from each.

Whole blood clotting time in glass at 25°C was about six to twelve minutes, but there was no clot after $2\frac{1}{2}$ hours in siliconed tubes. The clots formed were very friable and did not have the firm, fibrous structure of mammalian clots. Recalcified plasma clotted in about 25 seconds where the temperature was 20°C or more and was only slightly more rapid at 37°C. Leucocyte-rich plasma clotted rather more rapidly.

Homologous acetone-dried brain extract clotted the toad plasma in 22 seconds but aqueous extract in as little as 15 seconds. There was also a quite marked effect from toad leucocytes or their washings which suggests that these cells could act as an efficient toad thromboplastin.

Toad plasma absorbed with aluminium hydroxide lengthened the one-stage time considerably, but two-stage tests showed that thrombin was generated in proportion to the amount of unadsorbed plasma present. Bovine thrombin would clot toad plasma but had only about half the activity displayed when it was used in human plasma.

Toad plasma aged for several days clotted more slowly with calcium and this was not restored by alumina-adsorbed fresh toad plasma. Factor V activity was therefore not demonstrable.

Washed leucocytes were unable to restore the recalcified clotting time of alumina-adsorbed plasma so that it is unlikely that prothrombin was contributed by the cells. More prothrombin was consumed in a two-stage system when leucocytes were present, or when brain powder was added. There was a factor in toad serum which reduced the recalcification time of toad plasma but was unable to shorten the time of the same plasma with tissue extract in the system. This factor may be comparable to factor IX of man.

In a study of hibernating and active frogs (*Rana tigrina*), Ahmad et al (1979) found that there was prolongation of whole blood clotting time during hibernation, as has been reported for certain mammals and lizards. Perhaps the reduced tendency for coagulation is a real advantage to animals during hibernation whilst the ordinary course of blood circulation is much reduced leading to increased risk of intravascular coagulation.

Reptiles

The Australian sleepy lizard (*Trachydosaurus rugosus rugosus*) has been studied by Hackett and Hann (1967). They were bled, after intrathecal administration of pentobarbitone and opening the pectoral girdle, from an arterial trunk.

The whole blood-clotting time of this lizard was very long (over one hour). Natural plasma clotted in about 20 minutes, whilst recalcified plasma was no quicker (20 to 27 minutes). Treatment of the plasma with chloroform accelerated recalcification times, but no anticoagulant was recoverable from the chloroform. The addition of small quantities of chloroform-treated plasma to ordinary *Trachydosaurus* plasma did not accelerate the clotting time. The inhibitor was unaffected by protamine sulphate or toluidine blue, was unadsorbed by barium sulphate and did not inactivate lizard tissue extract incubated with it. The authors concluded that the anticoagulant was an antithrombin and a similar antithrombic activity was shown in a dozen or so other reptilia including a tortoise (*Chelodina longicollis*), a crocodile (*Crocodylus porosus*), several pythons (*Liasis spp.* and *Morclia spp.*), a skink (*Egernia cunninghami*), and a number of other lizards (*Tiliqua scincoides, Amphibolorus barbatus, Varanus acanthrus*). It would seem, then, that the reptiles have remarkably 'anticoagulated' blood but that this is quite appropriate for haemostasis in the relatively slow and sluggish lives that these creatures live inside their toughened integuments.

Birds

Most of the work on blood coagulation in birds has been done on the domestic fowl

(*Gallus domesticus*). The fowl was studied extensively by Wartelle (1957) who showed that the clotting time of whole blood was longer than that of man and that there were considerable differences in thromboplastin formation. Soulier, Wartelle and Ménaché (1959) extended the original findings of Wartelle and found that chicken plasma lacked both factor XI and factor XII. Bigland and Triantaphyllopoulos (1960) reinvestigated the whole blood-clotting time of chicken blood and found a mean time of 70 minutes (13 to 180 minutes). The authors accounted for this much longer time than those previously recorded by taking great care to avoid tissue trauma or damage to the vein wall. Where this damage did occur, shorter times were found. The addition of chicken thromboplastin produced clots in 13 seconds; of chicken thrombin in 30 seconds. It seems therefore that chicken haemostasis, which is certainly efficient, depends upon tissue thromboplastin and that intrinsic thromboplastin generation is weak or even absent. This is confirmed by Bigland (1964) who extended the study of chickens to include turkeys, wild pigeons, wild ducks and Japanese quail. In each case the whole blood-clotting times were very long (turkeys, 188 to 557 minutes; pigeons, 144 to 168 minutes; ducks, 47 minutes; quail, 32 minutes), but the bleeding times were short. In 25 chickens a mean bleeding time of 8 minutes was found, a figure within the normal human range.

It is interesting to note in passing that it was in 1934 that Dam described a haemorrhagic disease of chicks which started off the now extensive knowledge of vitamin K and the coagulation of blood: mammalian as well as avian.

Dorn and Muller (1965) investigated the one-stage times of chicken blood with various thromboplastins. They noted that only homologous thromboplastin permitted exact determinations both in the normal fowl and in birds whose clotting had been modified by vitamin K deficiency or sulphonamide drugs. Stopforth (1970) used homologous systems in domestic chickens and found that the effective haemostatic mechanisms depended mostly on the extrinsic clotting system, the development of blood thromboplastin being weak as compared to man. Factors V and VII were low or absent, though some factor X activity was demonstrated, but contact with glass surfaces did not activate this intrinsic system (Fig. 9.1).

Mammals
Amongst the mammals there are very large lacunae in our knowledge. I have not found, for instance, recent studies of the primitive egg-laying mammals and only one of the marsupials. Fantl and Ward (1957) worked on blood samples from two possums (*Trichosurus vulpecula, Pseudocheirus laniginosus*), a wallaby (*Wallabia bicolor*) and a tiger-cat (*Dasyurops maculatus*). They found that these marsupials all possessed the clotting factors recognized in other mammals. There was quite marked species specificity so far as brain thromboplastin in the one-stage test was concerned except that possum brain was equally quick with wallaby or tiger-cat plasma.

Of the placental mammals there remain a number of inadequately or quite unstudied orders (*Insectivora, Dermaptera, Chiroptera, Edentata* and *Sirenea*). Some examples from the other orders have been investigated and notes on these follow.

Cetaceans
Marine mammals were studied by Robinson, Kropatkin and Aggeller (1969). They used trained Atlantic bottle-nosed dolphins (*Tursiops truncatus*) and killer whales

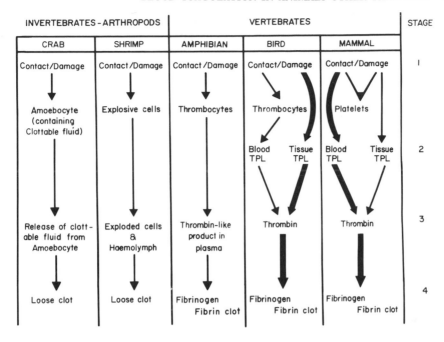

Fig. 9.1   Schematic representation of blood or haemolymph coagulation contrasted in invertebrates, amphibia, birds and mammals.

(*Orcinus orca*) and obtained blood samples from veins on the ventral surfaces of the flukes. There was no evidence of factor XII and the clotting time in glass or silicone was long (about 20 to 40 minutes). Factors VIII and V were high whilst VII and X were low in comparison with man, but for factor VII assay human tissue thromboplastin was used since no cetacean tissue was available.

Carnivores
It has been fairly clearly established that the coagulation system in dogs and cats is substantially similar to that of man. The various factors all appear to be present, although the partial thromboplastin times are considerably shorter in dogs than in man (Cade & Robinson, 1975).

Haemophilia A (antihaemophilic globulin or factor VIII deficiency) has been well documented in dogs (Archer & Bowden, 1959; Brinkhous & Graham, 1950; Didisheim & Bunting, 1964; Field et al, 1946; Graham et al, 1949; Howell & Lambert, 1964; Hutt et al, 1948; Parks et al 1964; Stormorken et al, 1965; Bellars, 1969) and a number of colonies have been established in which haemophilic dogs are bred and maintained (White & Holm, 1965). According to Parks et al (1964) female heterozygotes have factor VIII levels which are 50 per cent of normal and this can be corrected by transfusions. Graham and Barrow (1957) used haemophilic dogs to study the pathogenesis of the condition and concluded that it was exactly comparable to the human condition. Wagner et al (1957) investigated the effects of subcutaneous and intramuscular antihaemophilic globulin of bovine origin and found that higher blood levels of factor VIII were given for longer times after the intramuscular route was used. Middleton and Watson (1978) using silicaceous earth to perform activated clotting times found reasonable prolongation in coagulopathies whilst Byars et al (1976) found a larger normal range with diatomite as activator. Storb et al (1972) found that haemophilic beagles irradiated and grafted with normal canine marrow did not synthesise factor VIII.

The experiments of Hovig et al (1967) showed that induced bleeding in haemophilic dogs was prolonged as compared to normal, but with factor VII or factor IX deficiency prolongation was not observed.

Haemophilia B (Christmas disease, factor IX deficiency) was first reported in dogs by Mustard et al (1960). They described a number of line-bred Cairn terriers which had a haemorrhagic disorder both pathologically and genetically similar to human Christmas disease. Treatment of canine haemophilia B could be undertaken equally effectively with administration of normal dog serum (3 ml/kg) or plasma (4.36 ml/kg) (Mustard et al 1962). Ozge et al (1966) found that adrenaline injections at a dose less than 22 µg/kg caused an increase in blood levels of factors VIII and IX in normal dogs, but in Christmas disease dogs there was no effect on factor IX.

Von Willebrand's disease has been identified in dogs (Dodds, 1970), factor X deficiency (Dodds, 1973) and factor XI deficiency (Dodds & Kull, 1971). Factor VII deficiency has been found in beagles and well documented (Capel-Edwards & Hall, 1968; Garner & Conning, 1970; Poller et al, 1971; Spurling et al, 1972, 1974). The dogs are normally symptomless and the disorder is inherited as the homozygous state of a single autosomal factor as in man.

A general haemorrhagic syndrome in dogs can be induced by intravenous injection of thrombin (70 i.u./kg) (Girolami et al, 1966). In this condition, there are decreases in platelets, factors V, VIII and fibrinogen. The reaction of dogs to intravenous staphylococcal enterotoxin B was studied by Gilbert (1966) who found some alteration, as yet undefined, in the plasma clotting factors after four days. These two experiments form good examples of the sort of studies which can be made upon the coagulation mechanism of dogs, which are likely to be directly referable to man, but which could hardly be undertaken on human subjects.

In cats there is relatively little information. Cotter, Bremer and Dodds (1978) identified haemophilia in cats and Green and White (1977) described factor XII deficiency.

Rodents and lagomorphs

The smaller laboratory animals, rabbits, rats, mice and guinea pigs are all rodents and can conveniently be considered together. The coagulation mechanism of each is assumed to be, and the contrary has not as yet been demonstrated, comparable to that of man. All of these small rodents have been extensively used in experimental studies and some of the more recent of these are considered below.

RABBITS

Rabbits were used by Izak and Galewsky (1966) in a study of hypercoagulable states. Thromboplastin was injected intravenously and this caused intravenous thrombosis, but also profuse haemorrhages. This effect was not modified by administration of heparin where the heparin was administered after the thromboplastin.

MICE

Meier, Allen and Hoag (1961) studied the normal blood clotting of mice which was substantially similar to that of man except that there was more rapid loss of prothrombin activity after coagulation and there was a lower prothrombin concentration. The values were unaffected by strain or sex.

RATS

Clifton et al (1965) used rats in experiments on the prevention of traumatic bleeding with ellagic acid. The acid was administered intravenously at pH 7.5 and a concentration of 2×10^{-4}M, 1 ml per 100 g body weight. Where part of the tail was amputated immediately after administration of this material, blood loss was reduced from the control amount of 4.5 ml to about 0.3 ml

Waaler et al (1964) found that in germ-free rats there were lower factor VIII levels than in normally reared rats, but that factor V and fibrinogen levels were not different. Inversen and Waaler (1966) found that in rats there was no increase in factor VIII levels after exercise or after adrenaline injections. Caruso and Petrakis (1966) studied blood coagulation in 13 to 16 day mouse embryos. Blood was obtained by making a single deep cut in the neck of the foetuses. Adult mice were bled for comparison by section of the tail vessels. Both whole blood coagulation times and 'whole blood prothrombin times' were longer in the foetuses, especially the younger ones (13 days). The 'whole blood prothrombin time' was performed by adding a commercial thromboplastin (probably of rabbit origin) to whole blood in sodium citrate.

GUINEA-PIGS

Howard and Flute (1959) and Flute and Howard (1959) used guinea-pigs, in which scurvy had been induced by an ascorbic-acid-free diet, to investigate the coagulation defect repeatedly reported in scurvy of man. They found that in scorbutic guinea-pigs there was defective reaction to glass contact as compared with normal animals. Evidence was given to show that there was deficiency of both factor XII and also factor XI.

Primates

Hawkey and Symons (1966a) studied the blood coagulation of a number of monkeys. The animals were tranquillized before venepuncture. Thirteen species were studied (*Lagothrix lagotricha, Ateles ater, Cebus apella, C. capucina, Cercopithecus ascanius schmidti, C. patas, Cercocebus torquatus, Macaca mulatta, M. maurus, M. silenus, M. nemestrina, Papio anubis* and *Pan satyrus*). In each case the results obtained were within the generally accepted ranges for man and there were no important differences between the various monkeys. The results were apparently unaffected by differences in sex or age of the subjects. In a further paper (1966b) the same authors showed that there is, however, one important distinction between the blood coagulation system of non-human primates and man, since the former consistently showed longer clotting times with Russell's viper venom (RVV). This prolongation was apparent in all the species of primates examined, but it has not been reported as yet for any other mammal. The prothrombin times of the primates were normal so that deficiency of clotting factors was unlikely to explain the finding. Further, the presence of a venom-inhibitor was also excluded. By a two-stage sytem, the authors provisionally concluded that the defect was attributable to reduced reaction between monkey factor X activated by RVV and monkey prothrombin or that factor V was the limiting feature. Cooper and Sorensen (1969) examined the tree shrew (*Tupaia chinensis*) and also found ranges for the various assays within the normal human range. Shrew brain thromboplastin gave normal one-stage times, but with commercial rabbit brain preparations the times were about three times longer.

Ungulates
Coagulation studies of the ungulates have been made on pigs, cattle and horses. There are no major differences reported amongst the ungulates from human coagulation, but there are increasing reports of differences in quantities of various clotting factors. Some of the better established findings are given below.

PIGS
Thrombocytopenic purpura has been reported in pigs (Stormorken et al 1963; Saunders et al 1966). The disease appears to be caused by platelet antibodies, but it differs from that of man in that bleeding is not seen until the piglets are about a week old. Haemophilia has also been found in pigs (Muhrer et al 1965) but it differs from human or canine haemophilia A in that it responds to injections of plasma or serum by increase in the level of circulating factor VIII but without a reduction of bleeding. Muhrer et al (1965) suggested that the porcine disease may have some similarity to von Willebrand's disease of man.

Cornell et al (1972), Bowie et al (1973) and Owen et al (1974) extended studies of von Willebrand's disease in swine and were able to identify about half the carrier animals by assay of factor VIII provided a swine-only system was used.

SHEEP
Steel, Witzel and Blanks (1976) reported acquired factor X deficiency in sheep poisoned with bitterweed (*Hymenoxys odorata*).

CATTLE
It is interesting to recalle that Schofield (1924) described a haemorrhagic disease of cattle caused by eating spoiled sweet clover and this was, in a sense, the beginning of the dicoumarol-like anticoagulants (Campbell & Link, 1941; Stahmann et al 1941). There is another haemorrhagic syndrome of cattle which remains incompletely elucidated: this is the thrombocytopenic purpura which follows ingestion of bracken (Heath & Wood, 1958) and in which it is likely that there is either a thrombasthenia or a coagulation defect yet to be defined. Kociba et al (1969) identified factor XI deficiency in a cow, but generally speaking coagulation problems in cattle are a rarity.

HORSES
The coagulation mechanism of the horse has been subjected to several investigations (Bell et al 1955; Sjolin, 1956; Barkhan et al 1957; Fantl & Marr, 1958; Gardikas et al 1965; Abildgaard and Link, 1965). The consensus of these papers is that horse blood coagulation is similar to that of man, but that thromboplastin formation is somewhat slower. There appears to be a deficiency of factor VIII relative to man, but there is

some difference of opinion with regard to factor IX. Abildgaard and Link, Bell et al, Barkhan et al and Fantl and Marr maintained that factor IX was normal but Sjolin and Gardikas et al that it was reduced. There seems no doubt that thromboplastin generation differs somewhat from that of man and it may be that there is a reduction in factors XI and XII as suggested by Abildgaard and Link as a result of experiments with human plasmas deficient in one or other of these two factors.

It is certainly the case that haemostasis in the horse is effective and that naturally occurring coagulation disorders are rare. Haemophilia A has been recorded (Archer, 1961; Nossel et al, 1962; Sanger et al, 1964; Hutchins et al 1967; Archer & Allen, 1972) but these papers referred to only six individuals. Siblings of the subjects were not available for examination, although in these cases there was some evidence of unusual and early deaths amongst males of the same parentage. At the moment, comments on the inheritance of equine haemophilia cannot be made, although the dam of one of the propositi had a normal coagulogram.

A case of thrombocytopenic purpura in a horse has been described (Sorensen, 1963), but no details were given other than the platelet count (33 000 per mm^3). Ether anaesthesia has caused a reduction in the whole blood coagulation time of about 25 per cent according to Gabel (1963).

The species specificity of blood coagulation
The degree to which mixed experimental coagulation systems can yield meaningful results has yet to be determined. Certainly exciting figures can be obtained. The areas in which species specificity are most striking are thromboplastin (i.e. extrinsic coagulation) and thrombin-fibrinogen reactions. On the whole, other factors appear comparable but, as has been stated, they may differ in concentration or perhaps in activity.

It has been known for a long time that thromboplastin is species specific to some extent, but meaningful reports interpretable in current terminology are relatively few. A useful table of one-stage times was given by Didisheim et al (1959) where twelve species were checked by brain extracts from each against the plasmas of each. The variation of results is most marked, but   almost all cases the homologous system gave a result close to the human homologous system. Hawkey and Stafford (1961) reported interesting experiments with toad and human blood which showed that the species specificity at least of human thromboplastin depends upon the presence of both factors VII and X. Irsigler et al (1965) worked with human, bovine and chicken brain extracts and confirmed that the thromboplastins were species-specific. When a lipid extract of the thromboplastins was made by pyridin extraction the remaining protein was inactive as a thromboplastin for any species, but was reactivated by the addition of the lipid extract. However, full activity was only restored where the protein moiety of the reconstituted thromboplastin was derived from the same species as the plasma used as substrate.

Conclusions on comparative blood coagulation
Any review of blood coagulation in animals other than man must by its very nature be incomplete since our knowledge is so very uneven. However, it can be concluded that, on the whole, blood coagulation has more similarities than differences in the various species and that it is remarkably well adapted to the different forms of animal life

Table 9.1   A tentative summary of blood coagulation systems in various classes of animals.

	Factor	Mammals	Birds	Amphibians	Fish	Invertebrates
(I)	fibrinogen	X	X	X	X	(clottable protein)
(II)	prothrombin	X	X	X	X	(procoagulant)
(III)	thromboplastin	X	X	X	X	
(IV)	calcium	X	X	X	X	
V	(labile factor)	X	X			
VII	(stable factor)	X	X			
VIII	(A.H.G.)	X	X			
IX	(Christmas factor)	X	X	X		
X	(Stuart-Prower factor)	X				
XI	(Plasma thromboplastin antecedent)	X				
XII	(Hageman factor)	X				

(Note: the designation 'Factor VI' is not used)

(Table 9.1). For instance, the reptiles have slow, but efficient, coagulation which is quite appropriate. On the other hand, in birds there is little or no intrinsic thromboplastic activity, but a rapid and most effective extrinsic system.

Knowledge of the more primitive animals is very incomplete. It seems likely that a study in this field might not only be most fruitful in its own right but also quite likely to yield information of value to the better understanding of blood coagulation in man.

The changes reflected in evolutionary progress are of exceptional interest but, perhaps, not surprising. Feral animals with blood coagulation defects are unknown: presumably any that may occur are rapidly removed by predation and natural selection. Once animals are domesticated and thereby to a greater or lesser extent protected, coagulation defects become identifiable: so far most of all in dogs. It is also interesting that all animals examined need both cells of some sort and a body fluid in order to form a clot. The changes with increasing specialisation in evolution from this point of view are increasing gain in response attributable to relatively small damage to the vascular endothelium or default of body structure. Perhaps it is because one of the effects of human medicine includes the survival of the unfit for relatively long periods that man is the only animal to be troubled extensively by disorders of blood coagulation.

ANIMAL MODELS OF HUMAN COAGULATION DISORDERS

There is now available a substantial body of information about animal models of human disorders. There is a valuable registry of such models prepared by Jean Dodds (1977) which includes names and laboratory addresses of sources for most models. Where importation of animals across national borders is concerned, the anti-rabies laws, particularly of the United Kingdom, must be born in mind since periods of isolation in quarantine may be mandatory and subject to close control by the relevant government authority. There follows a review of some of the models now available which may well be very valuable in the study of certain human haemorrhagic diatheses (Table 9.2).

Table 9.2 Occurrence of defined coagulation disorders in vertebrates other than man. These disorders are inherited except where marked '(acquired)'.

Factor	Rabbits	Cats	Dogs	Pigs	Sheep	Cattle	Horses
(I) fibrinogen			variable				
(II) prothrombin							
(III) thromboplastin							
(IV) calcium							
V (labile factor)							
VII (stable factor)			no symptoms			severe (acquired)	fatal
VIII (A.H.G.)		variable	fatal				
(VIII) von Willebrand's disease	mild		mild	severe			
IX (Christmas factor)			variable		severe (acquired)		
X (Stuart-Prower factor)			fatal				
XI (plasma thromboplastin antecedent)			mild			very mild	
XII (Hageman factor)		no symptoms					

Factor VII deficiency

This condition has been repeatedly reported to occur naturally in dogs, but without increased tendency to bleed or other symptoms (Mustard et al 1962; Dodds et al 1967; Poller et al 1971; Spurling et al 1972). It appears that the condition occurs in beagles and is inherited as an autosomal recessive character. Indeed it was identified on routine screening of dogs used in pharmacological studies which had an unexplained prolongation of the one-stage time. The factor VII deficient canine plasma may be a useful reagent and, since the defect is quite widely spread, fairly readily available.

Factor VIII deficiency

Factor VIII deficiency has been reported in the cat, repeatedly in the dog and in the horse as reported above. In dog and horse the condition is severe so that maintenance of the stock is difficult. In the cat it is milder but control still requires periodic therapy with whole blood or plasma from normal cats.

von Willebrand's disease

von Willebrand's disease occurs in dogs, rabbits and pigs. In dogs the bleeding tendency is usually mild (Dodds, 1970, 1975) as also in rabbits (Benson & Dodds, 1977) whilst in pigs the bleeding is severe (Bowie et al 1973; Owen et al 1979).

Factor IX deficiency

Factor IX deficiency has been reported only in dogs (Mustard et al 1960, 1962a) and is a severe condition resembling the human disorder and requiring treatment with plasma from normal dogs. Double haemophilia (deficiency of both factors VIII and IX) has been reported (Brinkhous et al 1973) and is a very severe disease requiring special facilities for maintenance and treatment of the subjects.

Factor X deficiency

Factor X deficiency is a rare disorder of dogs (Dodds, 1973); the associated bleeding being severe or even lethal in puppies and young adults, but mild in mature adults.

Factor XI deficiency

Factor XI deficiency causes minor bleeding in dogs which can be difficult to control after surgery (Dodds & Kull, 1971). It also occurs in cattle (Kociba et al 1969; Gentry et al 1975) without serious bleeding and provides a valuable substrate plasma for assay of human and other animal plasmas for factor XI.

Factor XII deficiency

Factor XII deficiency has occurred in cats which do not show any haemorrhagic tendency (Green & White, 1977), the plasma being very low in factor XII activity.

Spontaneous disseminated intravascular coagulation

Spontaneous disseminated intravascular coagulation has been associated with infectious canine hepatitis (Wigton et al, 1976) and with bacterial sepsis in rhesus monkeys (Wing et al, 1978).

Resistance to Warfarin

Feral rats found to be resistant to Warfarin make good models both for studying vitamin K metabolism and for work on rodenticides. When on a vitamin K free diet, resistant rats require considerably more vitamin K to restore the blood coagulation to normal than do susceptible rats (Martin, 1973; Owen & Bowie, 1978). Vitamin K_1 metabolism is less susceptible to inhibition by Warfarin in resistant rats than in susceptible rats. This fact has been used by Martin et al (1979) to distinguish susceptibility from resistance to Warfarin in rats rapidly (within two days) and accurately.

REFERENCES

Abildgaard C F, Link R P 1965 Blood coagulation and haemostasis in thoroughbred horses. Proceedings of the Society for Experimental Biology and Medicine 119: 212–215

Ahmad N, Dube B, Agarwal G P, Dube R K 1979 Comparative studies of blood coagulation in hibernating and non-hibernating frogs (Rana tigrina). Thrombosis and Haemostasis 42: 959–964

Archer R K 1961 True haemophilia (Haemophilia A) in a thoroughbred horse. Veterinary Record 73: 338–340

Archer R K, Allen B V 1972 True haemophilia in horses. Veterinary Record 91: 655–656

Archer R K, Bowden R S T 1959 A case of true haemophilia in a labrador dog. Veterinary Record 71: 560–561

Barkhan P, Tomlin Sheila C, Archer R K 1957 Comparative coagulation studies on horse and human blood. Journal of Comparative Pathology 67: 358–368

Bell W N, Tomlin Sheila C, Archer R K 1955 The coagulation mechanism of the blood of the horse with particular reference to its 'Haemophiloid' status. Journal of Comparative Pathology 65: 255–261

Bellars A R M 1969 Hereditary disease in British Antarctic sledge dogs. Veterinary Record 85: 600–607

Benson R E, Dodds W J 1977 Autosomal factor VIII deficiency in rabbit: size variations of rabbit factor VIII. Thrombosis and Haemostasis 38: 380

Bigland C H 1964 Blood clotting times of five avian species. Poultry Science 43: 1035–1039

Bigland C H, Triantaphyllopoulos D C 1960 A re-evaluation of the clotting time of chicken blood. Nature 186: 644

Boolootian R A, Giese A C 1959 Clotting of echinoderm coelomic fluid. Journal of Experimental Zoology 140: 207–229

Bowie E J W, Owen C A, Zollman P E, Thompson J H, Fass D N 1973 Tests of hemostasis in swine: normal values and values in pigs affected with von Willebrand's disease. American Journal of Veterinary Research 34: 1405–1407

Brinkhouse K M, Davis P D, Graham J B, Dodds W J 1973 Expression and linkage of genes for x-linked hemophilias A and B in the dog. Blood 41: 577–585

Brinkhous K M, Graham J B 1950 Haemophilia in the female dog. Science 111: 723–724

Byars T D, Ling G V, Ferris N A, Keeton K S 1976 Activated coagulation time (ACT) of whole blood in normal dogs. American Journal of Veterinary Research 37: 1359–1361

Cade J F, Robinson T F 1975 Coagulation and fibrinolysis in the dog. Canadian Journal of Comparative Medicine 39: 296–298

Campbell H A, Link P K 1941 Studies on haemorrhagic sweet clover disease. IV The isolation and crystallization of the haemorrhagic agent. Journal of Biological Chemistry 138: 21–33

Capel-Edwards K, Hall D E 1968 Factor VII deficiency in the beagle dog. Laboratory Animals 2: 105–112

Caruso R, Petrakis N L 1966 Studies of the coagulation and prothrombin time in the mouse embryo. Thrombosis et Diathesis Haemorrhagica 16: 732–737

Clifton E E, Agostino D, Girolami A 1965 Prevention of traumatic bleeding by ellagic acid in rats. Proceedings of the Society of Experimental Biology and Medicine 120: 179–180

Cooper R G, Sorenson M W 1969 Blood coagulation in the tree shrew Tupaia chinensis. Laboratory Animal Care 19: 513–515

Cornell C N, Cooper R G, Muhrer M E, Garb S 1972 Effect of plasma and platelet concentrate infusions in factor VIII, platelet adhesiveness, and bleeding time in bleeder swine. Thrombosis et Diathesis Haemorrhagica 28: 431–439

Cotter S M, Brenner R M, Dodds W J 1978 Hemophilia A in three unrelated cats. Journal of the American Veterinary Medical Association 172: 166–168

Dam H 1934 Haemorrhages in chicks reared on artificial diets: a new deficiency disease. Nature 133: 909–910

Didisheim P, Bunting D L 1964 Canine hemophilia. Thrombosis et Diathesis Haemorrhagica 12: 377–381

Didisheim P, Hattori K, Lewis J 1959 Haematologic and coagulation studies in various animal species. Journal of Laboratory and Clinical Medicine 53: 866–875

Dodds W J 1970 Canine von Willebrand's disease. Journal of Laboratory and Clinical Medicine 76: 713–721

Dodds W J 1973 Canine factor X (Stuart-Prower factor) deficiency. Journal of Laboratory and Clinical Medicine 82: 560–566

Dodds W J 1975 Further studies of canine von Willebrand's disease. Blood 45: 221–230

Dodds W J 1977 First international registry of animal models of thrombosis and haemorrhagic diseases. Institute of Laboratory Animal Resources News 21: A1-A23

Dodds W J, Kull J E 1971 Canine factor XI (plasma thromboplastin antecedent) deficiency. Journal of Laboratory and Clinical Medicine 78: 746–752

Dodds W J, Packham M A, Rowsell H C, Mustard J F 1967 Factor VII survival and turnover in dogs. American Journal of Phyiology 213: 36–42

Doolittle R F, Surgenor D M 1962 Blood coagulation in fish. American Journal of Physiology 203: 964–970

Dorn P, Muller F 1965 Untersuchungen uber die thromboplastin-zeit-bestimmung mit homologen und heterologen thrombokinasen am normalen, vitamin K-arm ernahrten und sulfonamid-belasteten huhn. Zentralblatt für Veterinarmedizin 12A: 380–385

Fantl P, Marr A G 1958 The coagulation of horse blood. Journal of Physiology 142: 197–207

Fantl P, Ward H A 1957 Comparison of blood clotting in marsupials and man. Australian Journal of Experimental Biology and Medical Science 35: 209–224

Field R A, Rickard C G, Hutt F B 1946 Hemophilia in a family of dogs. Cornell Veterinarian 36: 285–300

Flute P T, Howard A N 1959 Blood coagulation in scorbutic guinea-pigs: a defect in activation by glass contact. British Journal of Haematology 5: 421–430

Gabel A A 1963 The effects of intravenous ether anesthesia on the blood of equine animals. American Journal of Veterinary Research 24: 993–996

Gardikas C, Kallinikou M, Kallinikos G 1965 Observations on horse blood coagulation. Scandinavian Journal of Haematology 2: 31–35

Garner R, Conning D M 1970 The assay of human Factor VII by means of modified Factor VII deficient dog plasma. British Journal of Haematology 18: 57–66

Gentry P A S, Lotz F 1975 Factor XI (plasma thromboplastin antecedent) deficiency in cattle. Journal of the Canadian Veterinary Medical Association 16: 160–163

Gilbert C F 1966 Effects of staphylococcal enterotoxin B on the coagulation mechanism and leukocyte response in beagle dogs. Thrombosis et Diathesis Haemorrhagica 16: 697–706

Girolami A, Agostino D, Clifton E E 1966 The effect of ellagic acid on coagulation in vivo. Blood 27: 93–102

Graham J B, Barrow E M 1957 The pathogenesis of hemophilia. An experimental analysis of the anticephalin hypothesis in hemophilic dogs. Journal of Experimental Medicine 106: 273–292

Graham J B, Buckwater J A, Hartley L J, Brinkhous K M 1949 Canine haemophilia. Observations on the course, the clotting anamoly and the effect of blood transfusions. Journal of Experimental Medicine 90: 97–111

Green R A, White F 1977 Feline factor XII (Hageman) deficiency. American Journal of Veterinary Research 38: 893–895

Gregoire C 1970 Haemolymph coagulation in arthropods. Symposia of the Zoological Society of London No 27 45–74

Gregoire C, Tagnon H J 1962 Blood coagulation. In: Florkin M, Mason H S (eds) Comparative biochemistry, Academic Press, New York, pp 435–482

Hackett E, LePage R 1961a The clotting of the blood of an amphibian, *Bufo marinus* Linn. I Prothrombin-thrombin and 'fibrinogen-fibrin' stages. Australian Journal of Experimental Biology and Medical Science 39: 57–66

Hackett E, LePage R 1961b The clotting of the blood of an amphibian, *Bufo marinus* Linn. II Blood thromboplastic activity. Australian Journal of Experimental Biology and Medical Science 39: 67–78

Hackett E, Hann C 1967 Slow clotting of reptile bloods. Journal of Comparative Pathology 77: 175–180

Hawkey C, Stafford J L 1961 Influence of serum factors on the species-specificity of tissue thromboplastin. Nature 191: 920–921

Hawkey C, Symons C 1966a Preliminary report of studies on platelet aggregation, blood coagulation and fibrinolysis in non-human primates. In: Some recent developments in comparative medicine. Symposia of the Zoological Society of London No 17, pp 213–228

Hawkey C, Symons C 1966b Coagulation of primate blood by Russell's viper venom. Nature 210: 141–142

Heath G B S, Wood B 1958 Bracken poisoning in cattle. Journal of Comparative Pathology 68: 201–212

Hovig T, Rowsell H C, Dodds W J, Jorgensen L, Mustard J F 1967 Experimental hemostasis in normal dogs and dogs with congenital disorders of blood coagulation. Blood 30: 636–668

Hougie C 1972 Coagulation changes in healthy and sick pacific salmon. Advances in Experimental Medicine and Biology 22: 89–102

Howard A N, Flute P T 1959 Defective blood coagulation in scorbutic guinea-pigs. Proceedings of the Nutrition Society 18: 32

Howell J McC, Lambert P S 1964 A case of haemophilia A in the dog. Veterinary Record 76: 1103–1105

Hutchins D R, Lepherd E E, Crook I G 1967 A case of equine haemophilia. Australian Veterinary Journal 43: 83–87

Hutt F B, Rickard C G, Field R A 1948 Sex-linked haemophilia in dogs. Journal of Heredity 39: 3

Irsigler K, Lechner K, Deutsch E 1965 Studies on tissue thromboplastin II. Species specificity. Thrombosis et Diathesis Haemorrhagica 14: 18–31

Iversen J G, Waaler B A 1966 The effect of adrenaline infusions and of muscular exercise upon the blood level of Factor VIII (antihaemophilic A factor) in the rat. Thrombosis et Diathesis Haemorrhagica 15: 29–35

Izak G, Galewsky K 1966 Studies on experimentally induced hypercoagulable state in rabbits. Thrombosis et Diathesis Haemorrhagica 16: 228–242

Kociba G J, Ratnoff O D, Loeb W F, Wall R L, Heider L E 1969 Bovine plasma thromboplastin antecedent (factor XI) deficiency. Journal of Laboratory and Clinical Medicine 74: 37–41

Madaras F, Parkin J D, Castaldi P A 1979 Coagulation in the sand crab (Ovalipes bipustulatus). Thrombosis and Haemostasis 42: 734–742

Martin A D 1973 Vitamin K requirement and anticoagulant response in the warfarin-resistant rat. Biochemical Society Transactions 1: 1206–1208

Martin A D, Steed L C, Redfern R, Gill J E, Huson L W 1979 Warfarin-resistance genotype determination in the Norway rat, Rattus norvegicus. Laboratory Animals 13: 209–214

Meier H, Allen R C, Hoag W G 1961 Normal blood clotting of inbred mice. American Journal of Physiology 201: 375–378

Middleton D J, Watson A D J 1978 Activated coagulation times of whole blood in normal dogs and dogs with coagulopathies. Journal of Small Animal Practice 19: 417–422

Muhrer M E, Lechler E, Cornell C N, Kirkland J L 1965 Antihemophilic factor levels in bleeder swine following infusions of plasma and serum. American Journal of Physiology 208: 508–10

Mustard J F, Basser W, Hedgardt G, Secord D, Rowsell H C, Downie H G 1962a A comparison of the effect of serum and plasma transfusions on the clotting defect in canine haemophilia B. British Journal of Haematology 8: 36–42

Mustard J F, Secord D, Hoeksemia T D, Downie H G, Rowsell H C 1962b Canine Factor-VII deficiency. British Journal of Haematology 8: 43–47

Mustard J F, Rowsell H C, Robinson G A, Hoeksema T D, Downie H G 1960 Canine haemophilia B (Christmas disease). British Journal of Haematology 6: 259–266

Nossel H L. Archer R K, Macfarlane R G 1962 Equine haemophilia: a report of a case and its response to multiple infusions of heterospecific AHG. British Journal of Haematology 8: 335–342

Owen C A, Bowie E J W 1978 Rat coagulation factors V, VIII, XI, and XII: vitamin K dependent. Haemostasis 7: 189–201

Owen C A, Bowie E J W, Fass D N 1979 Generation of factor VIII coagulant activity by isolated, perfused neonatal pig livers and adult rat livers. British Journal of Haematology 43: 307–315

Owen C A, Bowie E J W, Zollman P E, Fass D N, Gordon H 1974 Carrier of porcine von Willebrand's disease. American Journal of Veterinary Research 35: 245–248

Ozge A H, Rowsell H C, Downie H G, Mustard J F 1966 The effect of adrenaline infusions on blood coagulation in normal and haemophilia B dogs. Thrombosis et Diathesis Haemorrhagica 15: 349–364

Parks B J, Brinkhous K M, Harris P F, Penick G D 1964 Laboratory detection of female carriers of canine haemophilia. Thrombosis et Diathesis Haemorrhagica 12: 368–376

Poller L, Thomson J M, Sear C H J, Thomas W 1971 Identification of a congenital defect of factor VII in a colony of beagle dogs: the clinical use of plasma. Journal of Clinical Pathology 24: 626–632

Robinson A J, Kropatkin M, Aggeler P M 1969 Hageman factor (factor XII) deficiency in marine mammals. Science 166: 1420–1422

Sanger V L, Mairs R E, Trapp, A L 1964 Hemophilia in a foal. Journal of the American Veterinary Medical Association 144: 259–264

Saunders C N, Kinch D A, Imlah P 1966 Thrombocytopenic purpura in pigs. Veterinary Record 79: 549–550

Schofield F W 1924 Damaged sweet clover: the cause of a new disease in cattle simulating hamorrhagic septicaemia and blackleg. Journal of the American Veterinary Medical Association 64: 553–572

Sjolin K E 1956 Lack of Christmas factor in horse plasma. Nature 178: 153

Solumn N D 1970 Coagulation in limulus — some properties of the clottable protein of Limulus polyphemus blood cells. Symposia of the Zoological Society of London No 27: 207–216

Sorensen D K 1963 Primary idiopathic thrombocytopenic purpura. In: Bone J F, Catcott E J (eds) Equine medicine and surgery, American Veterinary Publications, Illinois, p 401–402

Spurling N W, Burton L K, Peacock R, Pilling T 1972 Hereditary Factor VII deficiency in the beagle. British Journal of Haematology 23: 59–67

Spurling N W, Burton L K, Pilling T 1974 Canine Factor VII deficiency: experience with a modified Thrombotest method in distinguishing between the genotypes. Research in Veterinary Science 16: 228–239

Srivastava A K 1969 Studies on the hematology of certain freshwater teleosts. V Thrombocytes and clotting of blood. Anatomische Anzeiger (Jena) 124: 368–374

Stahmann M A, Huebner C F, Link P K 1941 Studies on the haemorrhagic sweet clover diseases. V Identification and synthesis of the haemorrhagic agent. Journal of Biological Chemistry 138: 513–527

Steel E G, Witzel D A, Blanks A 1976 Acquired coagulation factor X activity deficiency connected with *Hymenoxys odorata* D C (compositae), bitterweed poisoning in sheep. American Journal of Veterinary Research 37: 1383–1386

Stopforth A 1970 A study of coagulation mechanisms in domestic chickens. Journal of Comparative Pathology 80: 525–533

Storb R, Marchioro T L, Graham T C, Willemin M, Hougie C, Thomas E D 1972 Canine hemophilia and hemopoietic grafting. Blood 40: 234–238

Stormorken H, Egeberg O, Austad R 1965 Haemophilia A in a Samojed dog. Scandinavian Journal of Haematology 2: 174–178

Stomorken H, Svenkerud R, Slagsvold P, Lie H, Lundevall J 1963 Thrombocytopenic bleeding in young pigs due to maternal isoimmunization. Nature 198: 1116–1117

Soulier J P, Wartelle O, Ménaché D 1959 Hageman trait and PTA deficiency; the role of contact of blood with glass. British Journal of Haematology 5: 121–138

Waaler B A, Gustaffsson B E, Hague A, Nilsson D, Amundsen E 1964 Plasma levels of various blood clotting factors in germfree rats. Proceedings of the Society for Experimental Biology and Medicine 117: 444–446

Wagner R H, Langdell R D, Richardson B A, Farrell R A, Brinkhous K M 1957 Antihemophilic factor (AHF): plasma levels after administration of AHF preparations to hemophilic dogs. Proceedings of the Society for Experimental Biology and Medicine 96: 152–155

Wartelle O 1957 Mecanisme de la coagulation chez la poule. L'étude des elements 'du complex prothrombique' et de la thromboplastino-formation. Révue d'Hématologie 12: 351–387

White J M, Holm G C 1965 Colony of hemophilic dogs. Science 150: 1766

Wigton D H, Kociba G J, Hoover, E A 1976 Infectious canine hepatitis: animal model for viral-induced disseminated intravascular coagulation. Blood 47: 287–293

Wing D A, Yamada T, Hawley H B, Pettit G W 1978 Model for disseminated intravascular coagulation: bacterial sepsis in Rhesus monkeys. Journal of Laboratory and Clinical Medicine 92: 239–251

10. Coagulation and malignancy

M. B. Donati   A. Poggi   N. Semeraro

More than a century ago Trousseau (1865) first described the frequent occurrence of vascular thrombosis in patients with cancer and Billroth (1878) noted thrombi in association with microscopic intravascular tumour deposits. Since these classical descriptions, many observations have strongly suggested the involvement of the haemostatic system in malignancy. First clinical studies have repeatedly demonstrated that malignant disease is associated with a high incidence of haemostatic disorders ranging from isolated abnormalities of laboratory tests to vascular thrombosis, haemorrhage or overt disseminated intravascular coagulation (DIC).

In addition, using histochemical, immunological or radioisotopic techniques, several investigators have found fibrin deposits in and around tumours leading to the assumption that blood coagulation plays an important role in tumour growth and metastatic processes. The mechanism by which malignant cells (or their products and secretions) interact with the various components of the haemostatic system has been the topic of extensive investigation during the past three decades (Donati et al, 1981).

The present review attempts to discuss first the available evidence on the occurrence of thromboembolic complications in malignancy and the underlying pathogenic mechanisms; in the second part, the most relevant interactions between cancer cells and factors of the haemostatic system will be discussed: these interactions are known mainly from investigations of in vitro systems and experimental models. Finally, the pharmacological modulation of the host's haemostatic system and its therapeutic implications in cancer growth control will be considered.

HAEMOSTASIS AND THROMBOSIS IN MALIGNANCY

Clinical conditions
Both haemorrhagic and thromboembolic complications are frequent in patients with malignant disease. However, the relative incidence and the clinical manifestations of these haemostatic disorders may vary according to the type of malignancy. In general, thrombotic disorders are more frequent in patients with solid tumours, whereas haemorrhage is one of the principal symptoms associated with leukaemias.

Solid tumours
Since the classical description by Trousseau (1865) mentioned above, the extensive study by Sproul (1938) revealed the high incidence (31 per cent) of thrombosis in patients with pancreatic cancer. Thereafter many other cases were reported to support the association between thrombosis (especially of the venous side), and solid cancers. Thromboembolic complications are most commonly observed in carcinomas (especially mucus-producing adenocarcinoma) of the various organs. They were the cause of

death in a high percentage of patients with cancer of the pancreas (around 50 per cent) and of lung, stomach, ovary and colon (between 20 and 50 per cent) (for references see Bick, 1978; Sack et al, 1977; Peuscher, 1980). These figures derive principally from post-mortem studies and it is questionable whether they are representative of in vivo events. In contrast, systematic studies of the frequency of clinical manifestations of thrombosis before and after the diagnosis of cancer have revealed some discrepancies. Some authors reported that clinical signs of thrombosis are relatively infrequent in patients with cancer, and occur in zero to 11 per cent (Anlyan, 1956; Miller et al, 1967; Slichter & Harker, 1974; Sun et al, 1979; Hoerr & Harper, 1957). However in the study by Lieberman et al (1961) venous thrombosis appeared to be the first symptom of malignancy in more than 50 per cent of all patients, the pancreas, lung and female reproductive tract being the original sites of cancer. Of the clinical characteristics of the thrombotic manifestations (Peuscher, 1980; Oster, 1976), thrombophlebitis migrans was most commonly observed. According to Durham (1955) its presence is usually pathognomic of advanced visceral carcinoma. This form is usually recurrent, superficial and involves multiple veins with rather unusual locations (upper extremities, neck, chest wall). Deep venous thrombosis, most often located in the veins of the leg, is less frequent but may occur in the absence of any predisposing factor (e.g. prolonged immobilization). Arterial thromboembolism has also been described in association with malignancies such as carcinoma of the pancreas and other types of cancer (Thompson & Rodgers, 1952; Al-Mondhiry, 1975; Siegman-Igra et al, 1977). In one study (Thompson & Rodgers, 1952) its incidence was in fact slightly higher (17 per cent) than that of venous thrombosis (13 per cent). It has been suggested that non-bacterial thrombotic endocarditis, which is often observed in patients with malignancy, may constitute a possible source of arterial emboli (Bryan, 1969; Rohner et al, 1967; Rosen & Armstrong, 1973; Waller et al, 1973).

Apart from the appearance of 'spontaneous' thromboembolism, other studies have shown that patients with cancer are at 'higher risk' for thrombosis when exposed to stimuli affecting the haemostatic system. For example, the incidence of deep vein thrombosis in patients undergoing surgery for cancer was about 40 per cent (Bick, 1978; Pineo et al, 1974), as compared to 12 per cent in patients without cancer who underwent comparable surgical procedures (Pineo et al, 1974). A bleeding tendency, isolated or in combination with thrombosis, has been reported in association with almost all types of solid tumours with a variable incidence (6 to 12 per cent) but it is especially common in the carcinoma of the prostate (Bick, 1978; Peuscher, 1980; Losito et al, 1977; Miller et al, 1967; Slichter & Harker, 1974; Sun et al, 1979). In contrast to thrombosis migrans and venous thrombosis, which sometimes appears as an early sign of malignancy, it has been suggested that severe bleeding may indicate the occurrence of wide-spread metastases (Rosenthal et al, 1963). Haemorrhagic diatheses may be mild clinically and present with easy and spontaneous bruising, purpura, ecchymosis, gingival bleeding, gastrointestinal, pulmonary or genitourinary haemorrhage and bruising at sites of invasive procedures. Life-threatening bleeding (intracranial or intraperitoneal) may also occur. Severe haemorrhagic symptoms are especially seen in widespread malignancy most notably of the prostate but also of the lung, stomach, colon, breast, ovary and in malignant melanoma (Peuscher, 1980; Bick, 1978).

Leukaemias

Haemorrhage is the most common haemostatic complication encountered in leukaemias (especially the acute forms) and other types of haematological malignancy. In acute leukaemia a haemorrhagic diathesis may precede other clinical or haematological symptoms in a high percentage (about 50 per cent) of patients (Lisiewicz, 1978; Rasche & Dietrick, 1977). Its incidence may even approach 80 to 90 per cent in acute promyelocytic leukaemia (Goodnight, 1974; Granlick, 1981). The development of the haemorrhagic syndrome is closely related to the evolution of the leukaemic process being more rapid and serious in patients with a highly malignant evolution. Although the bleeding localization varies greatly, epistaxis, gingival and skin haemorrhages are the most frequent; haemorrhagic lesions of the ocular fundus are also relatively common particularly in the later stages of the disease. Haemorrhage (intracranial, pulmonary, gastrointestinal) is also one of the major direct causes of death in patients with acute leukaemia.

In chronic myeloid leukaemia haemorrhagic complications do not usually represent a major clinical problem, are less frequently (about 25 per cent of patients) the primary symptoms of the process, are localized mainly to the skin and are less commonly the direct cause of death (Lisiewicz, 1978). In chronic lymphocytic leukaemia and in chronic monocyte leukaemia bleeding manifestations usually appear later in the clinical course of the disease. In contrast, in the initial stages of chronic lymphocytic leukaemia thrombotic signs are relatively frequent (thrombophlebitis of the deep and superficial veins or multifocal thrombosis) (Lisiewicz, 1978). Haemorrhagic symptoms may be seen with variable incidence in those more rare forms of leukaemia such as eosinophilic, basophilic and especially megakaryocytic leukaemia (Lisiewicz, 1978). An increased incidence of haemorrhagic and/or thromboembolic complications has long been observed in other myeloproliferative diseases, namely polycythaemia vera, where vascular accidents are detected in about 50 per cent of patients, and essential thrombocythaemia where bleeding is most commonly observed (Gunz, 1960; Lewis et al, 1972; Chievitz & Thiede, 1962; Wasserman & Gilbert, 1966).

Pathophysiological mechanisms

To define the mechanisms underlying the thromboembolic and/or haemorrhagic complications seen in cancer patients, the various components of the haemostatic system have been studied extensively.

A number of haemostatic abnormalities, including shortening of whole blood clotting time in silicone, shortened partial thromboplastin time and prothrombin time, elevated levels of one or more clotting factors, increased amounts of fibrinogen/ fibrin degradation products, presence of circulating fibrin monomers or fibrino-peptide A and reduced antithrombin III, have been reported in patients with malignant disease with or without clinically evident coagulation disorders (Bick, 1978; Brugarolas et al, 1973; Miller et al, 1967; Losito et al, 1977; Sun et al, 1979). The most consistent defect was increased platelet and/or fibrinogen turnover, which was also observed in patients with normal routine coagulation parameters. Interestingly, the latter changes were related not only to the presence of active malignant disease but also to the specific type and extent of disease (Lyman et al, 1978; Slichter & Harker, 1974). All these findings strongly suggest that in many patients with cancer intravascular activation of clotting takes place. This would render cancer patients highly susceptible to relatively minor events such as vascular stasis, infection, local trauma, surgical procedures and radio-or cytostatic therapy which may disturb the delicately balanced coagulation mechanism and favour the clinical manifestations of disordered haemostasis. When the process of intravascular coagulation is localized, it may become clinically manifest as thrombosis. On the other hand, when the trigger of blood clotting arises within or gains access to the circulation and is powerful enough, generalized or disseminated intravascular coagulation (DIC) will ensue with fibrin deposition in the microcirculation and consumption of platelets and clotting factors. DIC is one of the main pathogenetic mechanisms underlying the haemorrhagic diathesis in cancer patients (Lisiewicz, 1978; Bick, 1978; Peuscher, 1980). The most important laboratory abnormalities found in this condition include thrombocytopenia, decrease of the fibrinogen level and of the clotting factors (V, VIII, XIII, and others) and a decrease of antithrombin III.

Elevated levels of fibrinopeptide A, accelerated generation of fibrinopeptide A in vitro, the presence of fibrin monomers (as shown by positive ethanol gelation test or by other methods) and of fibrin(ogen) related antigens provide additional evidence for an activated clotting system and secondarily enhanced fibrinolysis. There are various mechanisms by which blood coagulation may be triggered in malignancy. Blood platelets may be activated by contact with cells from human or experimental tumours and by transformed cells: they subsequently aggregate and release their constitutents, as it has been shown both in vitro and in vivo (see later). Such platelet 'activation' might lead to unmasking or enhancement of the various platelet coagulant activities (Semeraro & Vermylen, 1977; Walsh, 1974) and thus contribute to blood clotting initiation. Mononuclear phagocytes (monocyte/macrophage cells) could play a similar role since they produce a procoagulant activity (tissue factor) in response to various stimuli (Niemetz et al, 1977; Semeraro, 1980) and it is well known that they are an intergral part of the lymphoreticular infiltrate of experimental and human tumours and may undergo functional changes upon contact with cancer cells (see later).

It is also recognized that most tumours undergo neovascularization; the potentially abnormal endothelial lining of the neoformed vessels might be responsible for activation of the contact system thus triggering blood clotting through the intrinsic pathway (Bick, 1978). The same mechanism is presumably elicited also by penetration of malignant cells into the vessel wall leading to destruction of the endothelium and exposure of subendothelial structures. The destruction of normal tissues during the natural course of tumour development and subsequent liberation of tissue thromboplastin is another possible trigger of blood coagulation via the extrinsic pathway (Bick, 1978). In pancreatic carcinoma the release of systemic trypsin, which has thrombin-like activity and activates several coagulation factors, is thought to play a major role (Bick, 1978). Although these relatively poorly defined mechanisms may be of importance in some particular types of cancer, blood clotting may also be initiated in malignancy, by the production of clot-promoting substances by the cancer cells themselves (see later).

Apart from various forms of DIC, the coagulation disorders seen in cancer patients may in some cases be attributed to other factors. In patients with acute leukaemia, they could be due to direct proteolysis of coagulation factors by granulocytic proteases released in plasma (Egbring et al, 1977). Other clotting defects observed in malignancy include deficiency of the prothrombin complex in patients with liver metastases (Bick, 1978; Soong & Miller, 1970), factor XIII deficiency, especially in patients with acute leukaemias (Rasche & Dietrich, 1977), dysfibrinogenaemia in patients with either primary hepatoma or metastases in the liver (Barr et al, 1976) and abnormal fibrin polymerization due to the presence of an inhibitory paraprotein in macroglobulinaemia (Perkins et al, 1970).

As far as platelets are concerned, both quantitative and qualitative abnormalities have been reported. Thrombocytopenia is a typical sign of acute leukaemia where it is considered a major cause of bleeding (Lisiewicz, 1978). It may occur independently of DIC mainly when the disease involves marrow or spleen, thus either limiting platelet production or increasing sequestration. Elevated platelet counts have also been reported in malignant disease and are especially common in many myeloproliferative disorders but they do not always correlate with the development of either thrombo-embolic or haemorrhagic complications (Bick, 1978; Lisiewicz, 1978). A number of functional platelet abnormalities (defective platelet aggregation in response to various aggregating agents, defective prostaglandin metabolism, defective platelet coagulant activities) may occur especially in myeloproliferative diseases and correlate better with the haemorrhagic tendency, than the platelet count (Cortellazzo et al, 1981). On the other hand, a close association between vascular occlusion and platelet hyperactivity has been suggested in myeloproliferative disorders (Cortellazzo et al, 1981). It must be stressed that the haemostatic abnormalities in cancer patients may also be influenced by non-specific factors, especially radio- and chemotherapy (Bick, 1978). These may contribute to bleeding mainly by causing thrombocytopenia (through bone marrow depression).

Other laboratory abnormalities observed during chemotherapy include: dysfibrino-genaemia induced by L-asparaginase treatment, platelet dysfunction, DIC associated with mithramycin and depression of vitamin K-dependent factors by actinomycin D (Bick, 1978).

Experimental models

Although much information on pathogenetic mechanisms can be derived from human malignancies, a number of interfering factors cannot be excluded; as mentioned before, these include the effects on haemostasis of concomitant bacterial infections, haemodynamic changes associated with major surgery, chemotherapy and radiotherapy. Moreover, different stage of the tumour, different tissue involvement by metastases and a number of other factors may render difficult the interpretation of results on haemostatic abnormalities in cancer patients. Animal models, studied in more standardized conditions, can partially contribute to overcome this problem. On the studies conducted so far, in experimental models, however, much criticism can be raised. In the past years, several long-term experiments have been carried out with allogenic instead of syngeneic tumours, leaving the possibility that uncontrolled immunological factors may have influenced the results. Moreover, most of the information on cancer procoagulants have been obtained in artificial models of tumour growth, such as haematogenous dissemination following intravenous (i.v.) injection of cancer cells. In these conditions, tumor emboli, rather than real metastases are formed, through a process which by-passes the first steps of local tumour invasion, i.e. development of cell proteolytic and/or migratory properties, detachment from the primary and penetration through the vascular walls into the circulation (Donati et al, 1977b).

Tumour cell-induced acute haemostatic changes
A rapid i.v. injection of Walker 256 Carcinosarcoma cells in allogenic rats has been described to induce an acute coagulopathy, characterized by an increase in plasma haemoglobin levels, a fall in peripheral platelet count, and a moderate reduction of plasma fibrinogen levels (Hilgard & Gordon-Smith, 1974). Sequestration of radio-labelled fibrinogen and platelets in the lungs of the same animals was also demonstrated. However, the lack of specificity of this reaction is indicated by the fact that the injection of dead cells or of particulate, inert, material can also induce the same coagulopathy (Hilgard, 1973). This could be due to activation of the coagulation cascade through the contact phase or to the introduction into the circulation of tissue-derived thromboplastic material. In our studies, we have shown that i.v. injection of cells obtained from Lewis Lung Carcinoma (3LL) in syngeneic mice induced a dose-dependent thrombocytopenia (Poggi et al, 1976). Moreover, reduction of fibrinogen levels and increase in fibrin(ogen) degradation products, with no changes in erythrocyte counts, were found, starting five minutes after the injection of 4×10^5 3LL cells (Poggi et al, 1977). These changes were rapidly reversible (within one hour); moreover, none of them could be observed at a later stage, when metastatic nodules to the lungs had grown (Donati et al, 1977b). Pretreatment of animals with platelet aggregation inhibitors (aspirin, ditazole) or with anticoagulants (warfarin, heparin) prevented these acute haemostatic changes (Donati et al, 1977b; Mussoni et al, 1978); it is however not yet clearly established whether the acute coagulopathy following the i.v. injection of cancer cells plays an important role in lodgement and subsequent lung colony growth.

Haemostatic changes during tumour growth
The involvement of the haemostatic system during the growth of experimental tumours has been considered only in a few models. Microangiopathic haemolytic anaemia, associated with chronic intravascular coagulation, has been shown to occur in rats bearing intramuscularly implanted, non disseminating Walker 256 Carcinosarcoma (Hilgard et al, 1973). Mild intravascular coagulation, with microangiopathic haemolytic anaemia, thrombocytopenia (mainly due to synthetic impairment) increased fibrinogen levels and enhanced fibrinogen turnover were found in association with the development of a spontaneously metastasizing tumour, the 3LL in syngeneic mice (Poggi et al, 1977). These changes were not abolished by chronic treatment with antiaggregating agents or anticoagulants and did not appear to have a clear pathogenic link to metastasis formation, since they were also observed in animals treated long-term with warfarin, in which metastatic growth was inhibited (Poggi et al, 1978). Moreover, although occurring mainly concomitantly with the growth of metastases, haemostatic changes in 3LL appeared rather closely related to the presence of the primary tumour. No changes were detected when lung metastases occurred in the absence of the primary, as in the artificial metastasis model, or in the spontaneous model after removal of the primary at adequate times after tumour implantation. These data suggest that the presence of the primary tumour singularly affect the host's haemostatic system. With regard to micro-

angiopathic signs, circulation of blood through the complex network of the primary tumour vasculature might lead to haemolytic anaemia; on the other hand, some inflammatory or toxic substance released from the primary could depress the platelet production. It has been suggested that the primary tumour could exert an inhibitory effect on the growth of metastatic nodules through a still undefined mediator (Yuhas & Pazmino, 1974); it is not known whether a similar mechanism could be operating towards blood platelet production.

A close association between thrombocytopenia, hyperfibrinogenaemia and the development of the primary tumour but not of metastatic nodules, is also suggested by some recent observations we have made with murine fibrosarcoma sublines with different metastatic potential: the same haemostatic changes were found in animals which had the same primary tumour weight but ranged from no metastases at all to various degrees of lung involvement (Delaini et al, 1981b). The limited experience so far available on the involvement of the host's haemostatic system in spontaneous metastasis models does not clarify whether differences in the changes observed depend on the host's reactivity or on specific cancer cell properties.

A closer association between cancer cell procoagulants and the development of intravascular coagulation can however be observed in some models of experimental leukaemias, such as the BNML, a myelomonocytic acute leukaemia of rats, where the appearance in the circulation of high counts of blasts, endowed with potent tissue-factor activity, coincided with laboratory signs of disseminated intravascular clotting (Mussoni et al, 1977; Donati et al, 1977a; Hilgard, 1977; Rasche et al, 1974). In all events different haemostatic changes can be observed in different experimental tumours: it may be of interest to mention some peculiarities of the two murine metastasizing tumours which have been more extensively characterized in this respect, the already mentioned 3LL and the JW sarcoma, a recently described tumour of Balb/c mice (Chmielewska et al, 1980a and b). Both tumours can give spontaneous metastases to the lungs, upon i.m. or s.c. implantation; however, 3LL secondary nodules are encapsulated and easily enucleated from the lungs whereas JWS metastases are infiltrating and difficult to distinguish from the surrounding tissue.

The survival of radiolabelled fibrinogen was decreased in 3LL, whereas it was normal in JWS; accordingly, fibrin was deposited at the tumour site in 3LL, not in JWS (Chmielewska et al, 1980a; Poggi et al, 1977). When tested in vitro, 3LL cells had a higher procoagulant and a lower fibrinolytic activity than JWS cells (Curatolo et al, 1979; Latallo et al, 1979). It is not known whether these properties could influence the different pattern of fibrin deposition and local invasiveness in the two models.

ROLE OF FACTORS OF THE HAEMOSTATIC SYSTEM IN CANCER CELL GROWTH AND DISSEMINATION

Fibrin at host-cancer cell interface

As already mentioned, fibrin deposits have been described in the immediate vicinity of many spontaneously arising tumours of lower animals and man (O'Meara, 1958; Hiramoto et al, 1960; Marrack et al, 1967; Poggi et al, 1977; Kodama & Tanaka, 1978); however, the extent of such deposits has been probably underestimated due to lack of techniques sensitive enough for their detection. The function of tumour-related fibrin has not yet been fully investigated, after O'Meara (1958) suggested for it a nutritional role. Essentially, two hypotheses have been put forward: (1) Fibrin would protect the primary tumour mass from escape of cells into the circulation and haematogenous dissemination. (2) fibrin would represent a biological barrier against host's cell defence mechanisms by retarding the diffusion of tumour antigens to host lymphoid tissues.

It has recently been shown that, out of two hepatocarcinoma lines in guinea-pigs, the one with higher invasive capacity had very little fibrin content (< 10 per cent of the tumour mass) which persisted without fibrous organization as the tumour grew progressively and invaded adjacent tissues; on the other hand, the tumour line with lower malignancy, developed, within hours after transplantation, a cocoon-like fibrin gel investment which represented more than 80 per cent of the tumour mass and underwent later a fibrous organization; the subsequent tumour destruction was attributed to ischaemic necrosis and widespread microvascular injury (Dvorak et al, 1979).

In the same animal species neovascularization, stimulation of inflammatory cell responses and, subsequently, fibroplasia could be induced by the subcutaneous implantation of fibrin. These data suggest that activation of the clotting and/or fibrinolytic systems by tumour cells may itself provide a sufficient stimulus to tumour angiogenesis without requiring a separate angiogenesis factor (Dvorak et al, 1979). On the other hand, fibrin has been described in the form of thrombi around embolic tumour cells by several authors (reviewed by Roos & Dingemans, 1979) after the first description of Wood (1958) in rabbit V_2 carcinoma. It has been proposed that fibrin (and/or platelet aggregates) around circulating tumour cells could favour their arrest and lodgement (Wood, 1958). Thus, fibrin may have opposing effects in different phases of the multistep process (Table 10.1) which leads from primary tumour growth

Table 10.1   Schematic sequence of events in metastasis from a primary tumour

1 — local growth
2 — detachment from primary tumour
3 — local invasion
4 — penetration into blood vessels
5 — transport in the circulation
6 — arrest and lodgement
7 — growth of metastastic nodules

to the appearance of distant metastases, since it could on one hand delay the detachment of cells from the primary, but enhance the trapping of circulating cells, on the other hand.

The cell surface component responsible for normal or abnormal interactions with fibrin is not yet well defined. Recently, interest has focused on *fibronectin*, a polymorphic glycoprotein found in vertebrate plasma and connective tissue, which represents the main surface-associated protein of fibroblasts and has been detected on macrophages, endothelial cells and platelets (Vaheri et al, 1978). It appears to be a crucial mediator of cell adhesion to collagen and can be cross-linked with fibrinogen on the cell surface by factor XIII. Transformed fibroblasts can synthesize fibronectin but cannot utilize it properly. It has recently been shown that fibronectin is involved in the binding of fibrinogen and fibrin to human fibroblasts and that such binding is defective in transformed cells (Colvin et al, 1979). This observation is in line with previous findings that transformation of fibroblasts is associated with loss of the cell capacity to interact with fibrin in a clot retraction system (Dolfini et al, 1976; Donati et al, 1978a). It has been proposed that the defective capability of transformed cells to utilize fibronectin contributes to their malignant behaviour in vivo (Chen et al, 1976).

Fibrin formation is conceivably brought about or influenced, at the local level, by a number of cancer and host cell activities among which are procoagulant factors, fibrinolytic activators and mediators which interact with platelet function, such as prostaglandins, and probably many others.

We shall first discuss cancer cell activities and then consider the contribution that macrophages, especially if activated in the tumour vicinity, may provide to fibrin formation and dissolution at the cancer cell-host interface.

Cancer cell procoagulant activities

It has long been known that procoagulant activity is present in malignant human tissues and in experimental tumours. About 20 years ago O'Meara (1958) first demonstrated that *human cancer tissues*, particularly carcinomas derived from different organs, consistently caused clotting (not followed by lysis) in normal diluted plasma in the presence of calcium ions. In contrast, normal tissue from the same organs only occasionally induced clotting which was followed by lysis. Subsequent studies (O'Meara & Thornes, 1961; Boggust et al, 1963; O'Meara, 1970; Svanberg, 1975; Sakuragawa et al, 1977) have essentially confirmed that human cancers (mostly tissue extracts) do, to varying degree, shorten the clotting time of recalcified autologous platelet-poor plasma. O'Meara (1970) further investigated the physicochemical properties of this 'cancer coagulative factor' and reported that it was acid, diffusible, and heat-labile; long-chain fatty acids associated with proteins, such as albumin, were proposed to be responsible for the procoagulant activity.

A similar procoagulant effect was found by several authors in experimental tumours (tissue homogenates, tissue extracts, single cell suspensions prepared from the tumor mass or from ascitic fluid or isolated in culture) and this property is reported to vary widely between different experimental tumours and different forms of the same tumour (Hilgard & Hiemeyer, 1970; Peterson & Zettergren, 1970; Holyoke & Ischihashi, 1966; Holyoke et al, 1972).

Although in most of the studies mentioned above the exact nature and mechanism of action of tumour procoagulant activity was not conclusively established, it was rather non-specifically called 'thromboplastic' because, as stated by Boggust et al (1968) 'it induces coagulation in recalcified citrated human plasma and is without direct action on fibrinogen alone or on citrated plasma before recalcification'. Since a similar procoagulant activity is obtained during extraction of several normal tissues, it was not at first clear why in cancer patients or in tumour bearing animals it should induce fibrin formation and deposition. Emphasis was placed mainly on the fact that thromboplastic activity is produced in greater amounts by malignant than normal tissues and that it can easily diffuse into its environment in contrast to normal tissue thromboplastin, of which little diffuses unless the tissue is damaged. Benign tumour extracts were virtually inert (O'Meara, 1958; Holyoke & Ichihashi, 1966). However, there is disagreement about quantitative differences between coagulant activities in malignant and normal tissues or in malignant and benign tumours. Svanberg (1975) reported that thromboplastic activity is present in similar amounts in benign and malignant human ovarian tumours although significantly more than that of normal ovaries. Holyoke et al (1972) have shown that cultured T-241 Lewis Sarcoma cells of mouse origin release thromboplastic activity, as measured by recalcification time of mouse plasma, into their culture medium. Moreover, cultured mouse embryo epithelial or muscle fibroblasts, with no demonstrable tumorigenic potential, released even more thromboplastic activity (per mg of total cell protein). In vitro trauma increased the release of thromboplastic activity from normal and tumour tissues. On the other hand, Gordon et al (1979) found there were no consistent *quantitative* differences between normal and malignant human tissues. More recent investigations have centred on the question of *qualitative* differences between procoagulants from normal and malignant tissues or from different malignancies with regard to the mechanism(s) triggering blood clotting.

Factor X activator activity

Pineo et al (1973, 1974) reported that partially purified mucin from secretions of non-purulent chronic bronchitis, ovarian cyst fluid and saliva, as well as extracts of mucin-producing adenocarcinomas initiated blood coagulation by direct factor VII-independent activation of coagulation factor X and suggested that this procoagulant might play a role in the coagulation disorders of patients with mucus-producing adenocarcinomas. Subsequently Gordon et al (1975) described a similar activity in extracts from human malignant tissues and from an experimental tumour (rabbit V_2 carcinoma). This activity appeared to be related to the presence in the extracts of a serine protease, called cancer procoagulant A (CPA), which was inhibited by diisopropyl fluorophosphate (DFP). Further studies by these investigators, comparing procoagulant activities in extracts of matched normal and malignant human tissue samples from the large intestine, breast, lung and kidney, showed that tumour extracts contained almost exclusively procoagulant activity with the two enzymatic characteristics of CPA (inhibition by DFP and lack of dependence on F VII) whereas extracts of normal tissues contained typical thromboplastin (F VII-dependent, insensitive to DFP) (Gordon et al, 1979). All these studies were performed using tissue extracts, so it was not clear whether procoagulant activity was actually derived from malignant cells.

In order to avoid any interference from connective tissue, muscle, vascular cells or other common contaminants of tumor masses, we have studied the procoagulant activity of cells from some experimental tumours isolated in culture or as single-cell suspensions from ascitic fluid (Curatolo et al, 1979; Colucci et al, 1980). Cells from 3LL (primary and lung metastases) Ehrlich Carcinoma ascites and JWS ascites markedly shortened the recalcification time of normal, factor VIII and factor VII-deficient but not of factor X-deficient human plasma. The same cells generated thrombin when mixed with a source of prothrombin and factor X, absorbed bovine serum (as a source of factor V), phospholipid and calcium chloride; thrombin formation in this assay was not influenced by the presence of factor VII (Curatolo et al, 1979). These findings strongly suggested that some cancer cells can directly activate coagulation factor X.

More direct evidence for this assumption was obtained in experiments in which cells generated factor Xa, as measured by a specific chromogenic substrate (S-2222), when incubated at 37°C with a source of factor X and calcium chloride. Whatever the method used, the procoagulant activity was present also in the supernatant of active cells. Cells from Sarcoma 180 and the control cell line NCTC-1-L929 were completely inactive in all test systems employed.

Recently, Gordon and Lewis (1978) have compared procoagulants in serum-free medium from matched normal and SV 40-transformed hamster embryo fibroblasts and found that procoagulant activity present in the latter had the enzymatic properties of CPA (DFP-sensitive serine protease activating factor X in the absence of factor VII) whereas the normal cells contained procoagulant activity similar to tissue thromboplastin.

Taken altogether, these studies demonstrate that some cancer cells and transformed cells produce a principle, most probably a serine protease, capable of directly activating coagulation factor X; they strongly suggest the existence of an alternative 'cellular' pathway in blood clotting initiation, distinct from both the intrinsic and extrinsic mechanisms.

It is worth mentioning that a weak coagulant activity directly activating factor X has been described in platelets from humans and some animal species (rabbit, rat, guinea pig) (Semeraro & Vermylen, 1977; Tremoli et al, 1977; Semeraro et al, 1979).

Tissue factor activity
Direct factor X activation does not appear to be the only pathway of blood clotting initiated by cancer cells; typical tissue factor, activating coagulation factor X through factor VII (extrinsic pathway), may indeed occur in some malignant cells. In man the paradigmatic example is the leukaemic cell (Gralnick & Abrell, 1973; Gouault-Heilmann et al, 1975; Sakuragawa et al, 1976; Gralnick, 1981). The production of tissue factor by circulating promyeloblasts in acute promyelocytic leukaemia has been regarded as the archetypal contribution of malignant cells to haemostasis and thrombosis (Gralnick & Tan, 1974). Isolated leukaemic promyelocytes have potent clot-promoting activity, found mainly in the granular fraction (Gralnick & Abrell, 1973). The thromboplastin-like nature of this activity was clearly established not only by the fact that it is demonstrable only in the presence of factor VII and is heat-labile (two properties shared by normal tissue extract activity) but also that it is antigenically related to brain tissue factor (Gralnick & Abrell, 1973; Gouault-Heilmann et al, 1975). The presence of tissue factor in leukaemic promyelocytes is consistent with the high incidence of the DIC syndrome in acute promyelocytic leukaemia.

As already mentioned, a clot-promoting activity with the characteristics of tissue factor (factor VII dependence) was also found in cells from an experimental leukaemia, rat BNML leukaemia (Mussoni et al, 1977a; Mussoni et al, unpublished). These findings are of interest in view of the fact that signs of intravascular activation of the clotting system were observed in BNML leukaemia bearing rats (Donati et al, 1977a). Finally, typical tissue factor was present in some solid tumours such as Walker 256 carcinosarcoma (Semeraro and Donati, 1981) and others (Khato et al, 1974).

Very recently, the procoagulant activity of tumour cell sublines from a murine fibrosarcoma (mFS6) have been characterized as tissue factor; among variants with different metastatic potential, the activity was 6 to 8 fold higher in those two which had no capacity to give metastases as compared with the parent line and the hypermetastasizing sublines (Colucci et al, 1981). This data would support the assumption that clot promotion within the primary tumour can reduce the escape of metastatic cells.

In conclusion, there are at least two pathways of blood clotting initiation by cancer cells (direct activation of factor X and extrinsic pathway) both requiring calcium ions

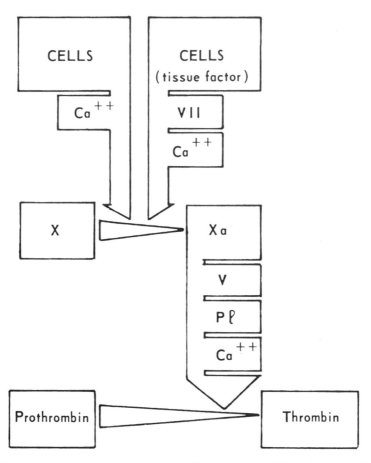

Fig. 10.1 Schematic representation of two pathways of blood clotting which can be triggered by cancer cells. Pl stand for phospholipids.

as schematically represented in Figure 10.1. The possible pathophysiological implications of cancer procoagulant activities are not yet well defined. It is also difficult to establish the relative importance of the two different pathways in favouring fibrin formation around tumours (Semeraro & Donati, 1981). As already mentioned, we found the same type of procoagulant in primary and metastases of 3LL and in cells from two other tumours, the JWS and Ehrlich carcinoma, which differ markedly as to their metastatic capacity (Curatolo et al, 1979; Colucci et al, 1980). Gordon and Lewis (1978) found no apparent correlation between the presence of the specific procoagulant activity (CPA) and tumorigenicity of transformed fibroblasts.

In conclusion, although the role of cancer procoagulants in malignancy remains unclear, tumour cells have become in recent years a unique tool to investigate the cellular contribution to fibrin formation.

Cancer cell fibrinolytic activity

Many tumour tissues are the source of both procoagulant and fibrinolytic activity, the extent of both being largely independent from each other, but varying from one tumour to another (Peterson, 1977; Roos & Dingemans, 1979; Astedt, 1981). There is no agreement so far whether malignant tissues do indeed produce higher amounts of fibrinolytic activity, than their normal or benign counterparts (Markus et al, 1980). The fibrinolytic activity released by most tumour tissues appears to be a plasminogen activator (PA), a serine protease which, in some human tumours, has been found immunologically identical to urokinase (Astedt & Homberg, 1976; Markus et al, 1980). Based on this observation, a radioimmunoassay has been developed, using monospecific anti-urokinase antibodies, to detect the PA release by human ovarian carcinomas, in an attempt to develop new markers of malignancy (Astedt, 1981). PA synthesis can be stimulated in normal cells by transforming agents, such as viruses, chemical substances, retinoids, carcinogenic promoters and physical carcinogens (Unkeless et al, 1973; Miskin et al, 1978). However, such a response is not limited to neoplastic or transformed cells; evidence is accumulating that PA production is the most widely distributed mechanism used by cells for generating localized extracellular proteolysis. The mechanism is typically associated with macrophage activation and response to inflammatory stimuli, and also with other processes such as follicle rupture at the time of ovulation, trophoblast implantation, myogenic differentiation and basement membrane metabolism, all processes accompanied by tissue remodelling and cell migration (Reich, 1978).

Even if PA is not exclusively produced by malignant cells, its possible role in the development of tumours is presently receiving considerable attention.

Cell lines with a long history in culture may loose the property to produce PA without losing tumorigenicity upon reintroduction into the host (Rifkin & Pollack, 1977). In contrast, the induction of PA production appears to be a consistent feature of freshly transformed cells, at least of fibroblasts and some epithelial cell lines (Gallimore et al, 1977). Such a phenomenon is not obligatorily linked to any other phenotypic change, although good correlation between PA production and loss of anchorage dependence has been observed (Pollack et al, 1974). It has very recently been shown that, in avian and mammalian fibroblasts, the synthesis of PA is induced by UV radiations and agents that inflict DNA damage (Miskin & Reich, 1980). Under these conditions, PA generation may accompany the induction of DNA repair enzymes. PA synthesis would be a response which, like neoplasia, is limited to cells which retain their capacity for DNA replication (Miskin & Reich, 1980).

As it may appear from the data mentioned above, an expanding volume of experimental work is being produced on the significance of PA as an expression of the transformed phenotype in cultured cell systems; comparatively little information is instead available on the significance of PA produced within experimental (or human) tumours in relation to their invasive growth and metastasis. It has been repeatedly proposed that tumours possessing a high PA activity should be able to digest surrounding fibrin and penetrate into the circulation much more easily than do tumours with less PA. However, the evidence for this assumption is as yet scanty.

No differences were observed between the PA activity of cells from primary and metastatic nodules of the 3LL (Mussoni et al, 1981; Whur et al, 1981). Moreover, results on the PA activity of sublines with different metastatic potential from B16 melanoma have given conflicting results (Nicolson et al, 1977; Hart, 1979; Wang et al, 1980) suggesting that the production of PA does not represent one of those cell properties consistently selected, in association with high metastatic capacity in tumour variants. The failure to find a clearcut correlation between PA and metastatic capacity could also be due to the fact that cell fibrinolytic activity may play opposing roles in the metastatic process favouring on one hand the detachment of cells from the primary and preventing or retarding, on the other hand the arrest of the same cells, when they are in the circulation.

Indirect support to this assumption is derived from studies with antifibrinolytic drugs in experimental tumours (Peterson, 1977), where primary tumour growth and subsequent spontaneous metastases were decreased, whereas lung nodule formation was enhanced, the former effect being presumably due to a decreased shedding of cells from the primary and the latter to microthrombus formation around intravascularly trapped tumour cells, a suggested prerequisite for development of metastases from trapped tumour cells.

Platelet-cancer cell interactions

The entry of tumour cells into the vascular compartment, the initial event in the genesis of blood borne metastasis, is the first opportunity for platelet-tumour cell interaction to occur. The mechanism(s) of such interaction and its significance in metastasis formation has been the topic of extensive investigation over the last years. Several authors have described the capacity of animal and human tumour cells and of transformed cells to aggregate platelets in vitro (Gasic et al, 1976, 1978a and b; Karpatkin & Pearlstein, 1981; Warren, 1978). The aggregation reaction is species-specific, may be accompanied by the release of serotonin and other constituents from the platelets, requires physiological concentrations of divalent cations and occurs after a variable lag period. More recent studies have shown that the aggregating activity of transformed cells and of different tumour cells is associated with cell membrane fragments (Hara et al, 1980a) or plasma membrane vesicles shed by these cells (Gasic et al, 1978b, 1981). The tumour cell-platelet interaction seems to occur in two sequential steps: the first is binding of tumour vesicles to platelets, which depends on the activation of the first four components of the complement system; platelet aggregation then ensues, probably due to generation of thrombin by the tumour vesicle-platelet complex (Gasic et al, 1981). The requirement of plasma factor(s) for the activity of a platelet aggregating material from transformed or tumour cells has been reported also by other investigators (Karpatkin & Pearlstein, 1981; Hara et al, 1980a). It must be stressed that there are tumour cells which do not cause either platelet aggregation or release of platelet constituents (Gasic et al, 1973, 1976). On the other hand, it has also been shown that cancer cells may be the source of platelet aggregation inhibitors, such as some prostaglandins (PGI_2, PGD_2) (Poggi et al, 1979; Fitzpatrick & Stringfellow, 1979). The role of these mediators in modulating cancer cell-platelet interactions remains to be defined.

In spite of these new pieces of information on the in vitro interactions between cancer cells and platelets, the problem remains whether they do occur consistently in vivo, how they do occur and in which way they could influence cancer cell dissemination.

There is some evidence that tumour cells may also adhere to and aggregate platelets in vivo (Hilgard, 1978; Gasic et al, 1978a; Warren, 1978). Human tumour cells associated with platelet masses have been demonstrated in the circulation of patients with metastatic dissemination of neoplastic disease (Warren, 1978; Ambrus et al, 1978). Much of our knowledge on platelet-cancer cell interactions in vivo derives however from experimental models. The i.v. injection of cells from certain tumours into animals results in a rapid thrombocytopenia, usually correlated with the number of cells injected.

Morphological examination of lung tissues has documented the presence of tumour cells accompanied by platelet masses in pulmonary vessels soon after i.v. administration; variable amounts of fibrin deposits are also seen, which may disappear after few hours (Dingemans, 1974; Chew & Wallace, 1976). A similar picture is observed in the liver vessels after injection of tumour cells in the portal veins (Dingemans, 1974; Warren, 1978; Roos & Dingemans, 1979).

The mechanism responsible for these phenomena is controversial. It has been proposed that blood platelets interact with tumour cells in the circulation and that platelet-tumour emboli are subsequently retained by different organs. This view is supported by the observation that tumour cells were frequently associated with platelet aggregates but there was no contact with the vessel wall nor any endothelial damage (Warren, 1978). Whether the platelet effect in vivo depends on the same tumour substance(s) producing platelet aggregation in vitro is unclear; in some instances, indeed, tumours inducing thrombocytopenia in vivo do not clump platelets in vitro (Gasic et al, 1973). It has also been suggested that platelet aggregates develop at the sites of tumour cell lodgement secondary to damage to the endothelium. This is supported by the classical microcinematographic investigations of Wood (1958), who, using the rabbit ear chamber, demonstrated, that cancer cells, shortly after their attachment to the endothelium, are surrounded by thrombotic material including platelets, red cells, and fibrin. Such a role of endothelium could also explain the thrombocytopenia and the accumulation of platelets in tissues induced by tumour cells lacking the capacity to aggregate platelets in vitro. It has been shown that anticoagulation of the animals before i.v. tumour cell challenge effectively prevents the acute platelet drop and may in some instances reduce the incidence and number of tumour colonies (Hilgard, 1978; Poggi et al, 1981b). These findings suggest that, at least in some experimental systems, thrombin generation may be responsible for the aggregation of platelets in the presence of tumour cells. This is further supported by the detection of fibrin(ogen) degradation products and fibrin monomers in the blood of animals injected with tumour cells (Poggi et al, 1977) as well as by ultrastructural studies showing the simultaneous presence of platelets and fibrin in the vicinity of intravascular Walker 256 cells shortly after their i.v. injection (Hilgard & Gordon-Smith, 1974; Hilgard, 1978).

Whatever the mechanism of tumour cell-platelet interaction in vivo, there are some observations suggesting a possible role for platelets in the pathogenesis of tumour cell metastasis. In some experimental models metastasis formation was greatly reduced when the animals were made thrombocytopenic by pretreatment with neuraminidase or antiplatelet antiserum (Gasic et al, 1968). In addition, a specific correlation could be made between the propensity of tumour cells for lung metastases (i.e. number of lung metastases per animal), their capacity to aggregate platelets in vitro and the extent to which thrombocytopenia decreased the number of lung metastases (Gasic et al, 1973). It is not clear why certain tumours do not aggregate platelets in vitro and do not decrease platelet numbers when injected into animals although previous induction of thrombocytopenia reduces the number of metastases which they form. Gasic et al (1973) have suggested that intravascular platelet aggregation produced by agents other than tumour cells (antigen-antibody complexes, aggregated IgG, viruses, endotoxins, etc.) may also play an important role as a contributory factor in metastasis formation. In fact, endotoxins can increase experimental metastases although this effect has not been related to their capacity to aggregate platelets (Gasic et al, 1973).

One must also consider that platelets, activated by whatever means, are the source of substances, such as prostaglandins, which, by modulating cellular cAMP levels, might be important in the control of tumour cell growth (Santoro et al, 1976). The platelet release reaction also leads to availability of one or more growth factors which are polypeptides able to stimulate growth and migration of fibroblasts and smooth muscle cells (Ross & Vogel, 1978). It has been suggested that also the growth of transformed or tumour cells may be influenced by platelet-derived mitogenic factors (Kepner et al, 1978; Hara et al, 1980b). Moreover, activated platelets release cationic proteins, serotonin and other amines active on vascular permeability (Nachman, 1978) which may influence cell transit towards extravascular areas. Thus, it would appear that, besides direct platelet-cancer cell interactions, removal of platelets (by inducing thrombocytopenia) or pharmacological inhibition of their function can reasonably be expected to influence primary or metastatic growth. Platelet aggregation inhibitors have indeed been reported to interfere with the development of metastases in some experimental models (Gasic et al, 1972; Kilenich et al, 1972; Ambrus et al, 1978). However the findings of different investigators are conflicting and do not allow to draw any definite conclusion on the role of platelets in metastasis growth.

Endothelium-cancer cell interactions
The two fundamental steps in the process of metastasis development are (1) the migration of cancer cells from the primary tumour into the vascular lumen (intravasation) and (2) the arrest of these tumour cells in the circulation with subsequent movement out of the vascular compartment (extravasation). In both instances cancer cells have to pass through the barrier between the extra- and intra-vascular compartments, i.e. the blood vessel wall. Although it is apparent that the interaction between endothelium and cancer cells is a focal point in the metastatic process, so far very little is known about it. In particular, the following points require clarification: (a) the morphological and functional characteristics of the vessel wall including the nature of endothelium and the presence or absence of damage to it; (b) the contribution made by the specific type of tumour cells; (c) the reaction of the blood to the tumour cell surface and the contribution of blood flow changes in cancer cell transport. As to the process of intravasation, the *structure of the circulatory bed* appears

of primary importance (Warren, 1978; Poste & Fidler, 1980). The capillary wall and small thin-walled venules, which offer relatively little mechanical resistance, are easily penetrated by tumour cells, whereas arterioles are rarely invaded. Within tumours, the often abnormal endothelial structure of the vessels (especially the marginal giant capillaries at the edge of the tumour) and the presence of areas with reduced oxygenation or overt necrosis preferentially favour penetration (Warren, 1981).

Active *tumour cell locomotion* also plays an important role in blood vessel invasion (Strauli & Weiss, 1978); this is further facilitated by the intrinsic pressure of expansive tumour growth and by the ability of some malignant cells to release tissue destructive enzymes (lysosomal hydrolases and collagenolytic enzymes) (Warren, 1981; Poste & Fidler, 1980). Following penetration of blood vessels, tumour cells are either transported passively in the bloodstream or remain at the site of vessel invasion where they proliferate and continue to shed emboli into the circulation. This may be exacerbated by intermittent changes in venous pressure, by turbulent alterations in blood flow and by movement or manipulation of the neoplasm during diagnostic tests or surgery. The presence of tumour cells in the circulation is necessary but certainly not sufficient to produce metastases (Poste & Fidler, 1980). Most tumour cells that enter the circulation, whether single or in clumps, are subject to destruction within the blood stream and only less than 1 per cent of the injected tumour cells survive to form metastases. The way in which circulating tumour emboli implant in supposedly normal tissues, and eventually form metastases, is at present poorly understood. Some degree of non-specific trapping and arrest of tumour cells in the circulation may occur simply as a result of mechanical factors. Blood capillaries with a diameter smaller than that of tumour emboli, may act simply as a sieve and thus arrest the tumour cells. The size and deformability of tumour cells, the diameter and distensibility of capillaries, the interactions of tumour cells with each other and with circulating host cells such as platelets (see above) and white cells are all relevant in this context (Roos & Dingemans, 1979; Poste & Fidler, 1980). However, there is increasing evidence that the specific properties of tumour cells themselves may be responsible for their arrest pattern. This evidence stems mainly from studies with experimental tumour sublines of differing metastatic potential (Poste & Fidler, 1980). Adhesion of tumour cells to the endothelium of the organ's capillaries, is thought to be a critical step in metastasis formation. Studies comparing the adhesive properties of two variant cell lines of B16 melanoma differing in their capacity to form lung metastasis have shown that the cells retained more easily in lung after i.v. injection have the capacity to adhere more strongly to dispersed lung cells and to 3T3 cell monolayers (Nicholson & Winkelhake, 1975; Winkelhake & Nicolson, 1976).

The interaction of tumour cells with vascular endothelium has been studied more directly in vitro utilizing cultured vascular endothelium cells which form a uniform cell monolayer, with intercellular junctions and underlying extracellular matrix (Kramer & Nicolson, 1979). In general, highly malignant or highly invasive cells in vivo were capable of firmly attaching to endothelial cells, causing morphologic changes such as rupture of intercellular junctions and retraction of endothelial cells with subsequent exposure of extracellular matrix, invading the endothelial cell monolayer and migrating under it. More recent studies indicate that endothelial basement membrane is a better substrate for adhesion of malignant tumour cells than the endothelial cells and that tumour cells with high metastatic potential adhere to the basement membrane more efficiently than cells with low metastatic potential (Poste & Fidler, 1980). In other experiments the in vitro manipulation of plasma membrane composition in B16 melanoma sublines of differing metastatic potential, led to changes in the metastatic behaviour in vivo. Thus when plasma membrane components from cells with a high capacity for lung colonisation were transferred to cells producing few pulmonary metastases, the latter acquired the ability to arrest in the lung capillary bed in significantly greater number than untreated cells (Poste & Fidler, 1980).

The actual contribution of the endothelium in the interaction with cancer cells is presently unknown in spite of the considerable information accumulated in recent years concerning its functional and biochemical properties. Damaged endothelial cells and exposed subendothelium will support platelet adhesion and aggregation. The subsequent platelet 'activation' might lead to unmasking or enhancement of platelet coagulant activities and thus contribute to blood clotting activation. Damage to endothelial cells and exposure of subendothelial structures might also provide a site for activation of the contact system of blood coagulation. Indeed, activation of the contact system may be promoted by some collagen preparations (Wilner et al, 1968). Recently it has been shown that cultured endothelial cells contain enzymes capable of cleaving and activating Hageman factor which, in turn, will activate factor XI and prekallikrein (Griffin & Cochrane, 1979). Furthermore, release of tissue factor by injured endothelial cells or other cells of the vascular wall (fibroblasts and smooth muscle cells) will activate the extrinsic coagulation pathway. Using a cell culture technique, Maynard et al (1977) showed that all three cell types occurring in blood vessels, namely endothelial cells, smooth muscle cells and fibroblasts have measurable tissue-factor activity. Endothelial cells had the lowest activity. Interestingly, the activity of undisturbed cells seemed to be in a 'protected state' and its full expression required cell disruption. The vascular endothelial cell is a major source of plasminogen activator, although the control mechanisms of activator release are still under investigation (Cash, 1978). Finally the vascular wall produces prostaglandin I_2 (prostacyclin) which is a potent antiaggregating and vasodilatory agent (Moncada & Vane, 1978).

How all these endothelial cell mediators influence the process of extravasation by tumour cells remains to be established. It has been shown that cells from several experimental tumours attach more readily to damaged vessel walls than to intact endothelium (Warren, 1978). Based on this and other studies a 'micro-injury hypothesis' has been put forward in metastasis formation. Briefly, blockade for varying periods of a microcirculatory unit by repeated showers of embolic tumour cells and subsequent injury of the capillary network gives rise to sites for preferential attachment of the circulating tumour cells (Warren, 1981). In the framework of this hypothesis the site and the composition of tumour emboli, which depend at least in part from the interaction of cancer cells with other blood components (platelets and other cells, fibrin) are of particular relevance. Following arrest and implantation in the vessel wall, tumour cells must exit from the vessel into the surrounding tissues. Extravasation of malignant cells is believed to involve mechanisms similar to those responsible for the initial intravasation. The observation that spontaneously metastatic B16 melanoma sublines produce high levels of type IV collagenase may be relevant in this context since type IV collagen is the predominant form of collagen in the basement membrane of capillaries (Poste & Fidler, 1980).

In summary, the processes of intravasation and extravasation are still poorly understood in their various steps. Vasoactive substances produced by platelets, leucocytes, endothelial cells and cancer cells themselves could also be important (see Prostaglandins).

Prostaglandins

Prostaglandins (PGs) consist of a large group of cyclic derivatives of C_{20} oxygenated unsaturated fatty acids and have been detected in virtually all cells and tissues of animals. They are considered to modulate a number of cellular reactions usually by altering the intracellular concentrations of cyclic AMP and calcium. However, interpretation of their role and function is complicated by the observation that different types of PGs can have opposing effects on the same systems, and that different concentrations of the same prostaglandin may have opposing effects on a single system, e.g. low concentrations of PGE_1 and PGE_2 have been found to stimulate growths of a lymphoid cell line, whereas high concentrations inhibited it (Karnali et al, 1979).

PGs, especially of the E series, have been found elevated in a large number of human and experimental tumours and may play a role in tumour promotion and in phenomena such as osteolysis and hypercalcemia associated with certain neoplasias (Seyberth et al, 1975). The interpretation of results presently available runs into two directions: (1) increased PGs synthesis would represent part of a homeostatic response directed to limitation of tumour growth; therefore, addition of exogenous PGs in vitro and in vivo will inhibit growth of tumour and of cancer cells in culture (Santoro et al, 1976). (2) PGs would be involved in the initiation and enhancement of tumour growth and, therefore, inhibition of PG synthesis will inhibit tumour growth.

As to the PG content of experimental and/or human tumours, the detection of elevated PG levels does not prove that the tumour cells are the actual source of the PGs. Macrophages and other leucocytic cells of the host may well contribute since they can produce high amounts of these mediators when stimulated by the presence of cancer cells (Pelus & Bockman, 1979).

In some experimental animal tumours, the immunological condition of the host, particularly the macrophage/lymphocyte system, is of crucial importance. PGs, especially of the E type, have potent immunodepressant activity, they inhibit mitogen-induced stimulation, cytolysis and antibody production by murine and human lymphocytes. Thus PGE produced by tumours may, be subverting the immunological system, inhibit the antitumour host defence mechanisms. This is part of the rational basis for the inhibitory effect on tumour growth of prostaglandin synthesis inhibitors, such as indomethacin or aspirin (Lynch et al, 1978).

Besides the above mentioned effects of PGs, evidence is accumulating that PGs would modulate blood flow through the tumour tissue, thus influencing extravasation of circulating tumour cells as well as vascular invasion. Indeed, blood vessel invasion by tumour cells is more frequently seen in inflamed tissue (Kim, 1979).

Mainly PGs of the E type have been so far described in cancer cells: recently a very potent platelet aggregation inhibitor has been found in tissues from two experimental tumours, the 3LL and the JWS (Poggi et al, 1979). This inhibitory activity was identified as prostacyclin (PGI_2) by various biological, pharmacological and chemical criteria, as well as by the use of a specific antiserum. In the 3LL model, the PGI_2 activity was higher in the metastatic lung than in the primary, but lower in isolated metastatic nodules than in normal lung tissue. The activity was also present in 3LL cells in culture, which were found devoid of macrophage contamination. In primary tissue and metastatic nodules of both 3LL and JWS the ability to generate PGI_2 correlated well with the relative distribution of cardiac output and appeared to modulate the response of the tumour vasculature to the vasoactive agent noradrenaline (Razcka et al, 1979; Quintana et al, 1979).

Moreover, experiments with B16 melanoma sublines have recently indicated that the highly metastatic line B16 F10 produces less PGD_2 than the moderately metastatic B16 F1 (Fitzpatrick & Stringfellow, 1979). Since PGD_2 is also a potent platelet aggregation inhibitor, it has been suggested that, the capability of the cells to interact with platelets through generation of PGD_2 could modulate the metastatic potential, at least in the model of lung colony growth (Fitzpatrick & Stringfellow, 1979).

Mononuclear phagocytes

It is widely accepted that mononuclear phagocytes (monocytes/macrophages) may be involved in the host defence against tumours either with non specific mechanisms or by cooperating with lymphocytes in a cell-mediated immune response. First of all, these cells are an integral part of the lymphoreticular infiltrate of experimental and human tumours (Evans, 1972; Gauci & Alexander, 1975; Wood & Gollahon, 1977; Haÿry & Totterman, 1978) and 'activated' macrophages have been isolated from some tumours (Mantovani, 1978; Russell et al, 1977). The relevance of the presence of these cells for tumour growth is debated. The number of macrophages found in tumour tissues was inversely correlated with the metastasizing capacity of tumour cells in some studies (Eccles & Alexander, 1974; Wood & Gillespie, 1975) but, in others, large numbers of these cells were associated with rapidly progressing tumours (Evans, 1972) and macrophages were even considered to favour tumour growth (Evans, 1978). In addition, Birsbeck and Carter (1972) reported that in a non-metastasizing lymphoma tumour macrophages were much more activated than in the metastasizing counterpart.

There is also evidence that neoplastic growth may be associated with profound changes in the functional state of mononuclear phagocytes. Macrophages from tumour-bearing mice and mononuclear phagocytes from cancer patients have been shown to be less responsive to chemotactic stimuli than cells from control populations (Synderman & Pike, 1976; Meltzer & Stevenson, 1978; Leb & Merrit, 1978).

Phagocytosis was altered in tumour bearing mice (Otu et al, 1977; North et al, 1976) and macrophage populations capable of host-mediated immunosuppression are present in animals with tumours (Kirchner et al, 1974). Finally, Pelus and Bockman (1979) demonstrated that macrophages from the spleen and peritoneal cavity of mice bearing progressively growing nonmetastasizing tumours possess a markedly enhanced capacity for the synthesis and release of PGE_2 and 6-keto-PGF_1 alpha (the stable metabolite of PGI_2). Augmented PG synthesis was found both in resting conditions and after nonspecific stimulation of macrophages with endotoxin, concanavallin A and zymosan. In this study, macrophages from normal and tumour-bearing mice were equivalent with respect to morphology, phagocytosis and nonspecific esterase staining. Moreover, Poleshuck and Strausser (1980) have shown that immunecomplex-induced prostaglandin production is increased in monocytes from cancer patients. Enhanced PG production may be a mechanism whereby macrophages can exert non-specific immunosuppressive activity in cancer patients and in tumour-bearing animals (Pelus & Bockman, 1979; Poleshuck & Strausser, 1980).

In the recent years considerable evidence has been accumulated on the close relationship between mononuclear phagocytes and the haemostatic system. Freshly isolated normal leucocytes have minimal if any, procoagulant activity. After appropriate in vitro or in vivo stimulation they generate a potent procoagulant which has been identified as tissue factor (Niemetz et al, 1977). The mononuclear phagocyte (monocyte/macrophage) is the cell primarily involved (Rivers et al, 1975; Edwards et al, 1979). Well known stimulating agents include bacterial endotoxin, phytohaemagglutinin, platelets and platelet membranes, antigen-antibody complexes, sensitized lymphocytes, adherence to various surfaces including vascular surfaces, renal dialysis membranes, C5 chemotactic fragment and C3b (Niemetz et al, 1977; Prydz et al, 1977; Rotherberger et al, 1977; van Ginkel et al, 1977; Muhlfleder et al, 1979). There is evidence that leucocyte procoagulant activity may play an important role in DIC induced by endotoxin, in experimental venous thrombosis and in fibrin deposition occurring in some inflammatory (particularly immunological) diseases (Lerner et al, 1977; Edwards & Rickles, 1978; Müller-Berghaus, 1978). Under adequate stimulation, macrophages are also capable of producing plasminogen activator (Unkeless et al, 1974) and the so-called platelet activating factor (PAF), a phospholipid mediator that causes aggregation of platelets and liberation of their inflammatory and vasoactive substances (Nencia-Huerta & Benveniste, 1979). PAF is also produced by IgE-sensitized basophils and by stimulated neutrophils (Lynch et al, 1979; Clark et al, 1979). Whether neoplastic growth and dissemination is associated with changes in these properties of mononuclear phagocytes represents a topic of considerable interest in order to define the contribution of these cells to fibrin deposition around the tumour as a part of their defence reaction.

PHARMACOLOGICAL APPROACHES

Experimental models
Most of the information so far available on the role of platelets and coagulation in cancer growth has been derived from studies with drugs influencing the haemostatic system of tumour-bearing animals. As already mentioned, the results are controversial, most probably due to differences in the experimental models used, in the period of treatment during tumour growth and in a number of other interfering factors, such as the animals' diet. Moreover, and most important, all the drugs which have been used in these studies, beside their specific effect on the haemostatic system, possess a number of other pharmacological activities which could by themselves influence cancer growth (Donati et al, 1977b; Poggi et al, 1981b).

Lung colonies and spontaneous dissemination
Some investigations have indicated that induction of hypocoagulability in animals prior to the intravenous injection of viable tumour cells reduced the number and incidence of lung nodule formation (Hilgard & Thornes, 1976). This effect was

ascribed to longer persistence of cells in the circulation in anticoagulated animals because of a better patency of the microcirculatory bed and impairment of tumour cell-fibrin emboli formation (Hilgard & Thornes, 1976; Griffith et al, 1978). However, as mentioned above, the approach of mimicking bloodborne metastases by intravenous injection of tumour cells into laboratory animals is highly artificial, since this model reflects only the final steps of dissemination (transport in blood and take by target organs), completely by-passing the initial phases which include detachment from the primary tumour and entry into the bloodstream. The clotting system may also play a role in these initial phases. For these and, probably, many other reasons, different results have been obtained when the same drugs were used in 'spontaneous' or in 'artificial' metastasis models. To summarize schematically the experience collected by several laboratories on drugs influencing the host's haemostatic system, one can conclude that anticoagulants (heparin and coumarin drugs), defibrinating enzymes and platelet aggregation inhibitors, share indeed some inhibitory effect on the 'artificial' metastasis model, whereas only coumarin drugs are really effective also in reducing 'spontaneous' metastasis growth (Poggi et al, 1981b; Hilgard, 1981).

Multiple drug effects

The supposed antitumor or antimetastatic activity of drugs modulating the host's haemostatic system, may be influenced by a number of other factors, due to the multiplicity of the pharmacological effects exerted by each drug. Indeed, possible modifications of cell metabolism or growth, or motility, changes in blood flow, of immune responses or prostaglandin metabolism have to be taken into account when evaluating the effect on tumour growth of many drugs primarily used to affect the haemostatic system. As an example, controversial results have been reported so far with platelet aggregation inhibitors in experimental models of dissemination (Hilgard & Thornes, 1976). Non-steroidal anti-inflammatory agents have been shown to reduce tumour growth in some experimental models (Lynch et al, 1978) whereas in other systems, they were completely ineffective (Hilgard et al, 1976; Mussoni et al, 1978) or even increased the tumour weight (Santoro et al, 1976).

It is difficult to reconcile these data, some of which have been obtained in different experimental models. It has to be considered, in any case, that these drugs act mainly as inhibitors of prostaglandin synthesis, not only in platelets where they prevent the generation of cyclic endoperoxides and thromboxanes (potent aggregating agents), but also in other cells, such as vascular cells, macrophages and tumour cells themselves (Flower, 1974). Changes in the pattern of prostaglandin generation by these cells may have important implications on tumour growth since some PGs are responsible for immunosuppression, changes in blood flow, response to inflammatory stimuli, anaphylactic type reactions and bone-resorbing activity of tumours (Easty & Easty, 1976; Karmali, 1980). Moreover, in view of the recent observations on PGI_2 and PGD_2 production by some tumour cells (Poggi et al, 1979; Fitzpatrick & Stringfellow, 1979) it is possible that treatment with aspirin or indomethacin might induce complex modifications in cancer cell-platelet interactions by inhibiting both platelet aggregation and the generation by cancer cells of potent platelet aggregation inhibitors.

On the other hand, *snake venom enzymes* have been repeatedly used to keep the animals defibrinated during growth of experimental tumours (Hilgard & Thornes, 1976). However, such agents could exert other effects potentially important for tumour growth, such as immunodepression. Indeed, both the primary humoral and the delayed type hypersensitivity reaction were depressed in mice defibrinated with either of two different batroxobin preparations (Anaclerio et al, 1980). This could account at least partially for the promotion of metastatic cancer growth observed in some experimental conditions when batroxobin was given chronically to 3LL bearing mice (Donati et al, 1978a). As a last example *coumarin compounds* have yielded the most consistent results in reducing primary and especially metastatic growth in rodent tumours (Hilgard, 1981; Donati & Poggi, 1980). However, also in this case, one may question the relevance of these results as an indication of the role of fibrin in metastasis formation. Warfarin could exert a direct cytotoxic effect or inhibit tumour cell motility and mitotic activity (Donati & Poggi, 1980; Hilgard, 1981). In our experiments, the antimetastatic effect of warfarin was closely associated with its anticoagulant activity. Experiments using the racemic form of warfarin and each of its resolved enantiomers showed that R-warfarin had almost no anticlotting activity in mice and did not modify the metastatic growth of 3LL, but the opposite was true for S-warfarin (Poggi et al, 1978). However, the observation that other anticoagulants (such as heparin) do not share with warfarin the same effect (Hilgard, 1981) would argue against the concept of warfarin's antimetastatic effect being mediated only by *plasma* anticoagulation. It has recently been proposed that, in the antimetastatic effect of warfarin, vitamin K-dependent proteins with a γ-carboxyglutamic acid mojety could be involved (Hilgard, 1977a). The cell changes induced by vitamin K deficiency, could, however, result again in reduction of the procoagulant activity of cancer or host cells and *cellular* anticoagulation could be important. Preliminary evidence for this effect has been obtained in the 3LL system.

As already mentioned, 3LL cells have a peculiar procoagulant activity (Factor X activating activity): this was found depressed in tumour cells or extracts harvested from animals treated long-term with warfarin or phenprocoumon (Poggi et al, 1981a, b; Hilgard, 1981). The warfarin's effect appeared to be reversed by administration of vitamin K and was also observed in mice chronically fed a vitamin K-deficient diet (Fig. 10.2). Thus, the factor X activator of 3LL cells could be a newly recognized vitamin K-dependent activity (Delaini et al, 1981a). In view of the unique anti-metastatic activity of coumarin anticoagulants, this may mean that, in order to achieve the control of metastasis formation, pharmacological modulation of the local cell's abilities to promote fibrin deposition is more important than systemic modifications of the host's haemostatic system.

Clinical applications

Histochemical, immunological and radioisotopic procedures have permitted detection of fibrin in human tumours (Marrack et al, 1967). Unfortunately, these interesting techniques have never been applied systematically in clinical studies to determine pathogenetic correlations. It is therefore not yet known whether anticoagulants interfere with fibrin deposition in human malignancy. Since most human malignancies kill by metastasis formation, their control could depend on ways of preventing or destroying embolic cells; anticoagulants could theoretically play a role in this process.

Reports on the effects of anticoagulants on human tumour cell growth are controversial. Most of the clinical studies have been conducted on relatively small numbers of patients and/or in non controlled conditions.

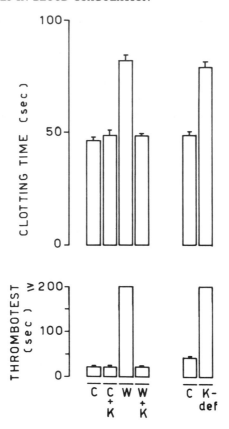

Fig. 10.2 Plasmatic and cellular anticoagulation in 3LL-bearing mice subjected to vitamin K deficiency or antagonism (chronic warfarin treatment) (Poggi et al, 1980a; Delaini et al, 1980b). Levels of plasma prothrombin complex factors are measured by Thrombotest and of 3LL procoagulant activity by the recalcification time in a test system devised to measure factor X activating activity (Curatolo et al, 1979). C = controls; W = warfarin-treated; K-def. = fed a vitamin K-deficient diet.

A wide variety of solid tumours have been treated with warfarin in addition to chemotherapy and/or immunotherapy (Thornes, 1974, 1975). Patients with advanced breast cancer, ovarian cancer and lymphosarcomas especially appeared to have prolonged survival times if treated with warfarin as an adjuvant. On the other hand, in patients with non-resectable lung cancer, heparin potentiated the tumour response to a combination of cytotoxic agents in some reports (Elias & Brugarolas, 1972; Elias et al, 1975) whereas it was ineffective in others (Edlis et al, 1976; Rohwedder & Sagastume, 1977). Warfarin anticoagulation as an adjunct to amputation has been recently reported to improve survival of patients with osteosarcoma (Hoover et al, 1978). Warfarin was started before operation and continued for up to six months postoperatively. The peroperative period appears to be the stage when anticoagulation could be useful. This is the time of maximal tumour manipulation due to needle or incisional biopsies and then operative resection, often with considerable trauma to the tumour before it is devascularized. It is an especially risky condition in view of the hypercoagulable state and diminished immunocompetence which accompanies surgical procedures under general anaesthesia. From available data (Hoover et al, 1978) it is reasonable to hypothesize that a significant percentage of metastases are actually initiated in the perioperative period. Clinical studies under way at present time aim at evaluating further the potential utility of modifying the coagulation/fibrinolysis balance during surgical removal of the primary tumour. Peroperative urokinase will be used (Hilgard, personal communication) on the basis of the concept that lysis of fibrin might prevent entrapment of tumour cells released during operation (Griffith et al, 1978). Moreover, a Veterans Administration Cooperative Study has been established to test the hypothesis that warfarin anticoagulation will modify the course of malignancy in man. The rational and experimental design of this trial in lung, colorectal, head and neck and prostate cancer have been recently published (Zacharski et al, 1979).

In another current study, immediately after surgery for head and neck cancer, patients start long-term treatment with RA 223, a pyrimidopyrimidine compound with platelet aggregation inhibitory activity; results on post-operative recurrence rate so far obtained appear of interest (Ambrus et al, 1978).

The need to treat acute leukaemias with anticoagulants is still debated (Thornes et al, 1972). In acute promyelocytic leukaemias, heparin has been proposed by some groups as prophylaxis of DIC expected during induction of remission (Gralnick et al, 1972; Drapkin et al, 1978).

Haemorrhage is one of the life-threatening complications of acute promyelocytic leukaemia; these patients are at great risk of bleeding when chemotherapy is started, presumably due to triggering of tissue factor release by the dying leukaemic promyelocytes.

Taken as a whole, studies with anticoagulants in cancer patients are fraught with a number of difficulties due to bleeding complications, differences in the individual response to anticoagulation, pharmacological interactions between concomitant treatments.

Further studies should be conducted on selected patients, with adequate medical and laboratory support, and according to criteria currently required for reliable clinical trials.

CONCLUSIONS

There is now sufficient experimental evidence that fibrin and platelets interact with cancer cells in vitro, and that haemostatic changes occur during tumour cell growth and dissemination. But a considerable gap still exists between the information available on in vitro 'artificial' systems such as cultured cells or tumour extracts and our knowledge of the in vivo significance of fibrin-cancer cell interactions. Besides the obvious interest of deeper studies to clarify pathogenic mechanisms, further basic and clinical research is warranted to support the present preliminary evidence on effectiveness of long-term anticoagulation in some selected conditions of human malignancies.

ACKNOWLEDGEMENTS

The authors's work mentioned in this review was supported by Contract 80.01621.96 of Italian National Research Council (Rome, Italy) and by Grant NIH PHRB-1RO1

CA L2765-01, National Cancer Institute, NIH, Bethesda, Maryland, USA. Anna Mancini, Graziella Scalvini and Vanna Pistotti helped prepare this manuscript.

REFERENCES

Al-Mondhiry, H 1975 Disseminated intravascular coagulation. Experience in a major cancer center. Thrombosis Diathesis Haemorrhagica 34: 181–193

Ambrus J L, Ambrus C M, Gastpar H 1978 Studies on platelet aggregation and platelet interaction with tumor cells. In: de Gaetano G, Garattini S(eds) Platelets: A multidisciplinary approach, Raven Press, New York, p 467–480

Anaclerio A, Ruggeri A, Poggi A, Spreafico, F, Donati M B 1980 In vivo and in vitro immunosuppressive effect of two batroxobin preparations in mice. Thrombosis Research 18: 253–258

Anlyan W G, Shingleton W W, Delaughter G D Jr 1956 Significance of idiopathic venous thrombosis and hidden cancer. Journal of American Medical Association 161: 964–970

Astedt B 1981 Plasminogen activator released from malignant ovarian tumours. In: Donati M B, Davidson J F, Garattini S (eds) Malignancy and the hemostatic system, Raven Press, New York, pp 83–88

Astedt B, Holberg L 1976 Immunological identity of urokinase and ovarian carcinoma plasminogen activator released in tissue culture. Nature 261: 595–597

Barr R D, Ouna N, Simpson J G, Bagshawe A F 1976 Dysfibrinogenaemia and primary hepato-cellular carcinoma. Quarterly Journal of Medicine 45: 647–659

Bick R L 1978 Alterations of hemostasis associated with malignancy: Etiology, pathophysiology, diagnosis and management. Seminars in Thrombosis and Haemostasis 5: 1–26

Billroth T 1878 Lectures on Surgical Pathology and Therapeutics, translated from the 8th ed. New Syndenham Society, London

Birbeck M S C, Carter R L 1972 Observations on the ultrastructure of two hamster lymphomas with particular reference to infiltrating macrophages. International Journal of Cancer 9: 249–257

Boggust W A, O'Brien D J, O'Meara R A Q, Thornes R D 1963 The coagulative factors of normal human and human cancer tissue. Irish Journal of Medical Sciences 477: 131–144

Boggust W A, O'Meara R A Q, Fullerton W W 1968 Diffusible thromboplastins of human cancer and chorion tissue. European Journal of Cancer 3: 467–473

Brugarolas A, Mink I B, Elias E G, Mittelman A 1973 Correlation of hyperfibrinogenemia with major thromboembolism in patients with cancer. Surgery and Gynecology 136: 75–77

Bryan C S 1969 Nonbacterial thrombotic endocarditis with malignant tumor. American Journal of Medicine 46: 787–793

Cash J D 1978 Control mechanism of activator release In: Davidson J F, Rowan R M, Samama M M, Desnoyers P C (eds) Progress in Chemical Fibrinolysis and Thrombolysis, Raven Press, New York, vol 3, p 65–75

Chen L B, Gallimore P H, McDougall J K 1976 Correlation between tumor induction and the large external transformation sensitive protein on the cell surface. Proceedings of the National Academy of Sciences 73: 3570–3574

Chew E-C, Wallace A C 1976 Demonstration of fibrin in early stages of experimental metastases. Cancer Research 36: 1904–1909

Chievitz E, Thiede T 1962 Complications and causes of death in polycythaemia vera. Acta Medica Scandinavica 172: 513–523

Chmielewska J, Poggi A, Janik, P, Latallo Z S, Donati M B 1980a Effect of defibrination with batroxobin on growth and metastasis of J E Sarcoma in mice. European Journal of Cancer 16: 919–923

Chimelewska J, Poggi A, Mussoni L, Donati M B, Garattini S 1980b Blood coagulation changes in JW sarcoma, a new metastasizing tumor in mice. European Journal of Cancer 16: 1399–1407

Clark P O, Hanahan D J, Pinckard R N 1979 Physiocochemical identity of platelet activating factor (PAF) isolated from human neutrophils and monocytes and rabbit neutrophils and basophils. Federation Proceedings 38: 1414

Colucci M, Curatolo L, Donati M B, Semeraro N 1980 Cancer cell procoagulant activity: evaluation by an amidolytic assay. Thrombosis Research 8: 589–595

Colucci M, Giavazzi R, Alessandri G, Semeraro N, Mantovani A, Donati M B 1981 Procoagulant activity of sarcoma sublines with different metastatic potential, Blood: 57

Colvin R B, Gardner P I, Roblin R O, Verderber E L, Lanigan J M, Mosesson M W 1979 Cell surface fibrinogen-fibrin receptors on cultured human fibroblasts. Association with fibronectin (cold insoluble globulin, LETS protein) and loss in SV40 transformed cells Laboratory Investigation 41: 464–473

Cortellazzo S, Colucci M, Barbui T, Dini E, Semeraro N 1981 Reduced platelet factor X activating activity; a possible contribution to bleeding complications in polycythaemia vera and essential thrombocythaemia. Haemostasis 10: 37–50

Curatolo L, Colucci M, Cambini A L, Poggi A, Morasca L, Donati M B, Semeraro N 1979 Evidence that cells from experimental tumours can activate coagulation factor X. British Journal of Cancer 40: 228–233

Delaini F, Colucci M, De Bellis Vitti G, Locati D, Poggi A, Semeraro N, Donati M B 1981a Vitamin K dependent procoagulant (factor X activating) activity in murine Lewis lung carcinoma cells. In press

Delaini F, Giavazzi R, De Bellis Vitti G, Alessandri G, Mantovani A, Donati M B 1981b Tumor sublines with different metastatic capacity induce similar blood coagulation changes in the host. Brit J Cancer (Jan)

Dingemans K P 1974 Invasion of liver tissue by blood-borne mammary carcinoma cells. Journal of the National Cancer Institute 53: 1813–1824

Dolfini E, Azzarone B, Pedullà D, Ottaviano E, de Gaetano G, Donati M B, Morasca L 1976 Characterization of human fibroblasts from cancer patients: loss of fibrin clot retractile activity after 'in vitro' spontaneous transformation. European Journal of Cancer 12: 823–825

Donati M B, Curatolo L, Borgia R, Baconi G, Morasca L 1978a Fibrin clot retraction by cultured human fibroblasts. In: de Gaetano G, Garattini S (eds) Platelets: a multidisciplinary approach, Raven Press, New York, p 149–158

Donati M B, Davidson J F, Garattini S (eds) 1981 Malignancy and the hemostatic system, Raven Press, New York: in press

Donati M B, Mussoni L, Kornblihtt L, Poggi A 1977a Changes in the hemostatic system of rats bearing L5222 or BNML experimental leukemias. Leukemia Research 1: 177–180

Donati M B, Mussoni L, Poggi A, de Gaetano G, Garattini S 1978b Growth and metastasis of the Lewis lung carcinoma in mice defibrinated with batroxobin. European Journal of Cancer 14: 343–347

Donati M B, Poggi A 1980 Malignancy and haemostasis. British Journal of Haematology 44: 173–182

Donati M B, Poggi A, Mussoni L, de Gaetano G, Garattini S 1977b Hemostasis and experimental cancer dissemination. In: Day S B, Myers W P L, Stansly P, Garattini S, Lewis M G (eds) Cancer Invasion and metastasis: biologic mechanisms and therapy, Raven Press, New York, p 151–160

Drapkin R L, Gee T S, Dowling M D, Arlin Z, McKenzie S, Kempin S, Clarkson B 1978 Prophylactic heparin therapy in acute promyelocytic leukemia. Cancer 41: 2484–2490

Durham R H 1955 Thrombophlebitis migrans and visceral carcinoma. Archives Internal Medicine 96: 380

Dvorak H F, Dvorak A M, Manseau E J, Wiberg L, Churchill W H 1979 Fibrin gel investment associated with line 1 and line 10 solid tumor growth angiogenesis, and fibroplasia in guinea pigs. Role of cellular immunity, myofibroblasts, microvascular damage, and infarction in line 1 tumor regression. Journal of the National Cancer Institute 62: 1459–1472

Easty G C, Easty D M 1976 Prostaglandins and cancer. Cancer Treatment Reviews 3: 217–225

Eccles S A, Alexander P 1974 Macrophage content of tumours in relation to metastatic spread and host immune reaction. Nature 250: 667–669

Edlis H E, Goudsmit A, Brindley C, Niemetz J 1976 Trial of heparin and cyclophosphamide (NSC-26271) in the treatment of lung cancer. Cancer Treatment Reports 60: 575–578

Edwards R L, Rickles F R 1978 delayed hypersensitivity in man: effects of systemic anticoagulation. Science 200: 541–543

Edwards R L, Rickles F R, Bobrove A M 1979 Mononuclear cell tissue factor: cell of origin and requirements for activation. Blood 54: 359–370

Egbring R, Schmidt W, Fuchs G, Havemann K 1977 Demonstration of granulocytic proteases in plasma of patients with acute leukemia and septicemia with coagulation defects. Blood 49: 219–231

Elias E G, Brugarolas A 1972 The role of heparin in the chemotherapy of solid tumors. Preliminary clinical trial in carcinoma of the lung. Cancer Chemotherapy Reports 56: 783–785

Elias E G, Shukla S K, Mink I B 1975 Heparin and chemotherapy in the management of inoperable lung carcinoma. Cancer 36: 129–136

Evans R 1972 Macrophages in syngeneic animal tumours. Transplantation 14: 468–473

Evans R 1978 Macrophage requirement for growth of a murine fibresarcoma. British Journal of Cancer 37: 1086–1089

Fitzpatrick F A, Stringfellow D A 1979 Prostaglandin D_2 formation by malignant melanoma cells correlates inversely with cellular metastatic potential. Proceedings of the National Academy of Sciences 76: 1765–1769

Flower R J 1974 Drugs which inhibit prostaglandin biosynthesis. Pharmacological Reviews 26: 33–67

Gallimore P H, McDougall J K, Chen L B 1977 In vitro traits by adenovirus-transformed cell lines and their relevance to tumorigenicity in nude mice. Cell 10: 669–678

Gasic G J, Boettiger D, Catalfamo J L, Gasic T B, Stewart G J 1978a Aggregation of platelets and cell membrane vesiculation by rat cells transformed 'in vitro' by Rous sarcoma virus. Cancer Research 38: 2950–2955

Gasic G J, Boettiger D, Catalfamo J L, Gasic T B, Stewart G J 1978b Platelet interactions in malignancy and cell transformation: functional and biochemical studies. In: de Gaetano G, Garattini S (eds) Platelets: a multidisciplinary approach, Raven Press, New York, p 447–456

Gasic G J, Catalfamo J L, Gasic T B, Avdalovic N 1981 In vitro mechanism of platelet aggregation by purified plasma membrane vesicles shed by mouse 15091A tumor. In: Donati M B, Davidson J F, Garattini S (eds) Malignancy and the hemostatic system, Raven Press New York, pp 27–36

Gasic G J, Gasic T B, Galanti N, Johnson T, Murphy S 1973 Platelet-tumor-cell interactions in mice. The role of platelets in the spread of malignant disease. International Journal of Cancer 11: 704–718

Gasic G J, Gasic T B, Murphy S 1972 Anti-metastatic effect of aspirin. Lancet 2: 932–933

Gasic G J, Gasic T B, Stewart C C 1968 Antimetastatic effects associated with platelet reduction. Proceedings of the National Academy of Sciences 61: 46–52

Gasic G J, Koch P A G, Hsu B, Gasic T B, Niewiarowski S 1976 Thrombogenic activity of mouse and human tumors: Effects on platelets, coagulation and fibrinolysis, and possible significance for metastases. Zeitschrift fur Krebsforschung 86: 263–277

Gauci C L, Alexander P 1975 The macrophage content of some human tumours. Cancer Letters 1: 29–32

Goodnight S H Jr 1974 Bleeding and intravascular clotting in malignancy: a review. Annals of the New York Academy of Sciences 230: 271–288

Gordon S G, Franks J J, Lewis B 1975 Cancer procoagulant A: a factor X activating procoagulant from malignant tissue. Thrombosis Research 6: 127–137

Gordon S G, Franks J J, Lewis B J. 1979 Comparison of procoagulant activities in extracts of normal and malignant human tissue. Journal of the National Cancer Institute 62: 773–776

Gordon S G, Lewis B J 1978 Comparison of procoagulant activity in tissue culture medium from normal and transformed fibroblasts. Cancer Research 38: 2467–2472

Gouault-Heilmann M, Chardon E, Sultan C, Josso F 1975 The procoagulant factor of leukaemic promyelocytes: demonstration of immunologic cross reactivity with human brain tissue factor. British Journal of Haematology 30: 151–158

Gralnick H R 1981 Cancer cell procoagulant activity. In: Donati M B, Davidson J F, Garattini S (eds) Malignancy and the hemostatic system, Raven Press, New York, pp 57–64

Gralnick H R, Abrell E 1973 Studies on the procoagulant and fibrinolytic activity of promyelocytes in acute promyelocytic leukaemia. British Journal of Haematology 24: 89–99

Gralnick H R, Bagley J, Abrell E 1972 Heparin treatment for the haemorrhagic diathesis of acute promyelocytic leukemia. American Journal of Medicine 52: 167–174

Gralnick H R, Tan H K 1974 Acute promyelocytic leukemia. A model for understanding the role of the malignant cell in hemostasis. Human Pathology 5: 661–673

Griffin J H, Cochrane C G 1979 Recent advances in the understanding of contact activation reactions. Seminars in Thrombosis and Hemostasis 5: 254–273

Griffith J D, Salsbury A J, White H 1978 Adjuvant fibrinolytic therapy following resection of colo-rectal cancer. Proceedings EORTC Metastases Project Group Meeting, London

Gunz F W 1960 Hemorrhagic thrombocythemia: a critical review. Blood 15: 706–723

Hara Y, Steiner M, Baldini M G 1980a Characterization of the platelet-aggregating activity of tumor cells. Cancer Research 40: 1217–1222

Hara Y, Steiner M, Baldini M G 1980b Platelets as a source of growth-promoting factor(s) for tumor cells. Cancer Research 40: 1212–1216

Hart I R 1979 The selection and characterization of an invasive variant of the B16 melanoma. American Journal of Pathology 97: 587–600

Häyry P, Tötterman T H 1978 Cytological and functional analysis of inflammatory infiltrates in human malignant tumors I. Composition of the inflammatory infiltrates. European Journal of Immunology 8: 866–871

Hilgard P 1973 The role of blood platelets in experimental metastases. British Journal of Cancer 28: 429–435

Hilgard P 1977a Experimental vitamin K Deficiency and spontaneous metastases. British Journal of Cancer 35: 891–892

Hilgard P 1977b Coagulation studies in the BNML rat leukemia. Leukemia Research 1: 175–176

Hilgard P 1978 Blood platelets and experimental metastases. In: de Gaetano G, Garattini S (eds) Platelets: A multidisciplinary approach, Raven Press, New York, p 457–466

Hilgard P 1981 The use of oral anticoagulants in tumour therapy. In: Donati M B, Davidson J F, Garattini S (eds) Malignancy and the hemostatic system, Raven Press, New York, pp 103–112

Hilgard P, Gordon-Smith E C 1974 Microangiopathic haemolytic anaemia and experimental tumour-cell emboli. British Journal of Haematology 26: 651–659

Hilgard P, Heller H, Schmidt C G 1976 The influence of platelet aggregation inhibitors on metastasis formation in mice (3LL). Zeitschrift fur Krebsforschung 86: 243–250

Hilgard P, Hiemeyer V 1970 Fibrinolysis, thromboplastin activity and localization of radioiodinated fibrinogen in experimental tumors. European Journal of Cancer 6: 157–158

Hilgard P, Hohage R, Schmitt W, Köhle W 1973 Microangiopathic haemolytic anaemia associated with hypercalcaemia in an experimental rat tumour. British Journal of Haematology 24: 245–254

Hilgard P, Thornes R D 1976 Anticoagulants in the treatment of cancer. European Journal of Cancer 12: 755–762

Hiramoto R, Bernecky J, Jurandowski J, Pressman D 1960 Fibrin in human tumors. Cancer Research 20: 592–593

Hoerr S O, Harper J R 1957 On peripheral thrombophlebitis. Its occurrence as a preventing system in malignant disease of pancreas biliary tract or duodenum. Journal of the American Medical Association 164: 2033

Holyoke E D, Ichihashi H 1966 The C3H/St/Ha mammary tumor. I. Thromboplastin content. Journal of the National Cancer Institute 36: 1049–1055

Holyoke E D, Frank A L, Weiss L 1972 Tumor thromboplastin activity 'in vitro'. International Journal of Cancer 9: 258–263

Hoover H C Jr, Ketcham A S, Millar R C, Gralnick H R 1978 Osteosarcoma. Improved survival with anticoagulation and amputation. Cancer 41: 2475–2480

Karmali R A 1980 Review: Prostaglandins and cancer. Prostaglandins and Medicine 5: 11–28

Karmali R A, Horrobin D F, Menezes J, Patel P 1979 The relationship between concentrations of prostaglandin A_1 E_1 E_2 and $F_{2\alpha}$ and rates of cell proliferation. Pharmacological Research Communications 11: 69–75

Karpatkin S, Pearlstein E 1981 The in vitro activity of platelet aggregating material (PAM) from SV-40 transformed mouse 3T3 fibroblasts. In: Donati M B, Davidson J F, Garattini S (eds) Malignancy and the hemostatic system, Raven Press, New York, pp 37–56

Kepner N, Creasy G, Lipton A 1978 Platelets as a source of cell-proliferating activity. In: de Gaetano G, Garattini S (eds) Platelets: A multidisciplinary approach, Raven Press, New York, p 205–212

Khato J, Suzuki M, Sato H 1974 Quantitative study on thromboplastin in various strains of Yoshida ascites hepatoma cells of rat. GANN 65: 289–294

Kim U 1979 Factors influencing metastasis of breast cancer. In: McGuire W L (ed) Breast cancer, vol 3, Plenum Press, New York, p 1–49

Kirchner H, Chused T M, Herberman R B, Holden H T, Lavrin D H 1974 Evidence of suppressor cell activity in spleen of mice bearing primary tumors induced by moloney sarcoma virus. Journal of Experimental Medicine 139: 1473–1487

Kodama Y, Tanaka K 1978 Thromboplastic and fibrinolytic activities of V_2 and V_7 carcinomas of rabbit, with special reference to fibrin deposition and thrombus formation in the tumors. Acta Pathologica Japonica 28: 279–286

Kolenich J J, Mansour E G, Flynn A 1972 Haematological effects of aspirin. Lancet 2: 714

Kramer R H, Nicolson G L 1979 Interactions of tumor cells with vascular endothelial cell monolayers: A model for metastatic invasion. Proceedings of the National Academy of Sciences 76: 5704–5708

Latallo Z S, Kowalska-Loth B, Chmielewska J, Teisseyre E, Raczka E, Kopec M 1979 A new approach to study factors from tumour cells which influence the clotting and fibrinolytic systems. In: Davidson J F, Cepelak V, Samama M M, Desnoyers P C (eds) Progress in chemical fibrinolysis and thrombolysis, Churchill Livingstone, Edinburgh, vol 4, p 411–415

Leb L, Merritt J A 1978 Decreased monocyte function in patients with Hodgkin's disease. Cancer 41: 1794–1803

Lerner R G, Goldstein R, Nelson J C 1977 Production of thromboplastin (tissue factor) and thrombin by polymorphonuclear neutrophilic leukocytes adhering to vein walls. Thrombosis Research 11: 11–22

Lewis S N, Szur L, Hoffbrand A L 1972 Thrombocythemia. Clinics of Haematology 1: 339

Lieberman J S, Borrero J, Urdaneta E, Wright I S 1961 Thrombophlebitis and cancer. Journal of The American Medical Association 177: 542–545

Lisiewicz J 1978 Mechanisms of hemorrhage in leukemias. Seminars in Thrombosis and Hemostasis 4: 241–267

Losito R, Beaudry P, Valderrama J C, Cousineau L, Longpré B 1977 Antithrombin III and factor VIII in patients with neoplasms. American Journal of Clinical Pathology 68: 258–262

Lyman G H, Bettigole R E, Robson E, Ambrus J L, Urban H 1978 Fibrinogen kinetics in patients with neoplastic disease. Cancer 41: 1113–1122

Lynch N R, Caster M, Astoin M, Salomon J C 1978 Mechanism of inhibition of tumour growth by aspirin and indomethacin. British Journal of Cancer 38: 503–512

Lynch J M, Lotner G Z, Betz S J 1979 The release of a platelet-activating factor by stimulated rabbit neutrophils. Journal of Immunology 23: 1219–1226

Mantovani A 1978 Effects on 'in vitro' tumor growth of murine macrophages isolated from sarcoma lines differing in immunogenicity and metastasizing capacity. International Journal of Cancer 22: 741–746

Markus G, Takita H, Camiolo S M, Corasanti J G, Evers J L, Hobika G H 1980 Content and characterization of plasminogen activators in human lung tumors and normal lung tissue. Cancer Research 40: 841–848

Marrack D, Kubala M, Corry P, Leavens M, Howze J, Dewey W, Bale W F, Spars I L 1967 Localization of intracranial tumors. Comparative study with 131-I-labeled antibody to human fibrinogen and neohydrin-230 Hg. Cancer 20: 751–755

Maynard J R, Dreyer B E, Stemerman M B, Pitlick F A 1977 Tissue-factor coagulant activity of cultured human endothelial and smooth muscle cells and fibroblasts. Blood 50: 387–396

Meltzer M S, Stevenson M M 1978 Macrophage function in tumor-bearing mice: Dissociation of phagocytic and chemotactic responsiveness. Cellular Immunology 35: 99–111

Mencia-Huerta J M, Beneveniste J 1979 Platelet-activating factor and macrophages. I. Evidence for the release from rat and mouse peritoneal macrophages and not from mastocytes. European Journal of Immunology 9: 409–415

Miller S P, Sanchez-Avalos J, Stefanski T, Zuckerman L 1967 Coagulation disorders in cancer. I. Clinical and laboratory studies. Cancer 20: 1452–1465

Miskin R, Easton T G, Reich E 1978 Plasminogen activator in chick embryo muscle cells: induction of enzyme by RSV, PMA and retinoic acid. Cell 15: 1301–1312

Miskin R, Reich E 1980 Plasminogen activator: Induction of synthesis by DNA damage. Cell 19: 217–224

Moncada S, Vane J R 1978 Prostacyclin, platelet aggregation and thrombosis. In: de Gaetano G, Garattini S (eds) Platelets. A Multidisciplinary Approach. Raven Press, New York, p 239–259

Muhlfelder T W, Niemetz J, Kreutzer D, Beebe D, Ward P A, Rosenfeld S I 1979 C 5 chemotactic fragment induced leukocyte production of tissue factor activity. A link between complement and coagulation. Journal of Clinical Investigation 63: 147–150

Müller-Berghaus G 1978 The role of platelets, leukocytes, and complement in the activation of intravascular coagulation by endotoxin. In: de Gaetano G, Garattini S (eds) Platelets: A Multidisciplinary Approach. Raven Press, New York, p 303–320

Mussoni L, Bertoni M P, Curatolo L, Poggi A, Donati M B 1977a 'in vitro' interaction of L5222 and BNML leukemia cells with fibrin. A preliminary report. Leukemia Research 1: 181–183

Mussoni L, Coen D, Balconi G, Delaini F, Donati M B 1981 Plasminogen activator activity of primary and metastatic cells of Lewis lung carcinoma. In: Davidson et al (eds) Progress in Fibrinolysis, vol 5, Churchill Livingstone, Edinburgh, in press

Mussoni L, Poggi A, de Gaetano G, Donati M B 1978 Effect of ditazole, an inhibitor of platelet aggregation, as metastasizing tumors in mice. British Journal of Cancer 37: 126–129

Mussoni L, Poggi A, Donati M B, de Gaetano G 1977b Ditazole and platelets. III. Effect of ditazole on tumor-cell induced thrombocytopenia and on bleeding time in mice. Hemostasis 6: 260–265

Nachman R L, 1978 The platelet as an inflammatory cell. In: de Gaetano G, Garattini S (eds) Platelets: A Multidisciplinary Approach. Raven Press, New York, p 199–203

Nicolson G, Birdwell C R, Brunson K W, Robbins J C, Beattie G, Fidler I J 1977 Cell interactions in the metastatic process: some cell surface properties associated with successful blood-borne tumor spread. In: Cash J W, Burger M M (eds) Cell and Tissue Interactions. Raven Press, New York, p 225–241

Nicolson G L, Winkelhake J L 1975 Organ specificity of blood-borne tumour metastasis determined by cell adhesion? Nature 255: 230–232

Niemetz J, Muhlfelder T, Chierego M E, Troy B 1977 Procoagulant activity of leukocytes. Annals of the New York Academy of Sciences 283: 208–217

North R J, Kirstein D P, Tuttle R L 1976 Subversion of host defense mechanisms by murine tumors. II. Journal of Experimental Medicine 143: 574–584

O'Meara R A Q 1970 Cancer research at Saint Luke's Hospital. Irish Journal of Medical Sciences 3: 59–65

O'Meara R A Q 1958 Coagulative properties of cancers. Irish Journal of Medical Sciences no. 394: 474–479

O'Meara R A Q, Thornes R D 1961 Some properties of the cancer coagulative factor. Irish Journal of Medical Sciences no. 423: 106–112

Oster M W 1976 Thrombophlebitis and cancer. A review. Angiology 27: 557

Otu A A, Russell R J, Wilkinson P C, White R G 1977 Alterations of mononuclear phagocyte function induced by Lewis lung carcinoma in C57BL mice. British Journal of Cancer 36: 330–340

Pelus L M, Bockman R S 1979 Increased prostaglandin synthesis by macrophages from tumor-bearing mice. Journal of Immunology 123: 2128–2125

Perkins H A, MacKenzie M R, Fundenberg HH 1970 Hemostatic defects in dysproteinemias. Blood 35: 695–707

Peterson H-I 1977 Fibrinolysis and antifibrinolytic drugs in the growth and spread of tumours. Cancer Treatment Reviews 1: 213–217

Peterson H-I, Zettergren L 1970 Thromboplastic and fibrinolytic properties of three transplantable rat tumours. Acta Chirurgica Scandinavica 136: 365–368

Peuscher F W 1980 Thrombosis and bleeding in cancer patients: A review. In: Peuscher F W The significance of Fibrinopeptide A in patients with cancer and venous thromboembolism. A thesis. Rodopi, Amsterdam, p 13–51

Pineo G F, Brain M C, Gallus A S, Hirsh J, Hatton M W C, Regoeczi E 1974 Tumors, mucus production, and hypercoagulability. Annals of the New York Academy of Sciences 230: 262–270

Pineo G F, Regoeczi E, Hatton M W C, Brain M C 1973 The activation of coagulation by extracts of mucus: A possible pathway of intravascular coagulation accompanying adenocarcinomas. Journal of Laboratory and Clinical Medicine 82: 255–266

Poggi A, Colucci M, Delaini F, Semeraro N, Donati M B 1981a Reduced procoagulant activity of Lewis lung carcinoma cell, from mice treated with warfarin. European Journal of Cancer 16: 1641–2

Poggi A, Dall'Olio A, Balconi G, Delaini F, de Gaetano G, Donati M B 1979 Generation of prostacyclin (PGI_2) activity by Lewis lung carcinoma (3LL) cells. Thrombosis Haemostasis 42: 339

Poggi A, Donati M B, Garattini S 1981b Fibrin and experimental cancer cell dissemination: Problems in the evaluation of experimental models. In: Donati M B, Davidson J F, Garattini S (eds) Malignancy and the Hemostatic System. Raven Press, New York, pp 89–102

Poggi A, Donati M B, Polentarutti N, de Gaetano G, Garattini S 1976 On the thrombocytopenia developing in mice bearing a spontaneously metastasizing tumor. Zeitschift Krebsforschung 86: 303–306

Poggi A, Mussoni L, Kornblihtt L, Ballabio E, de Gaetano G, Donati M B 1978 Warfarin enantiomers, anticoagulation and experimental tumour metastasis. Lancet 1: 163–164

Poggi A, Polentarutti N, Donati M B, de Gaetano G, Garattini S 1977 Blood coagulation changes in mice bearing Lewis lung carcinoma, a metastasizing tumor. Cancer Research 37: 272–277

Poleshuck L C, Strausser H R 1980 Immune-complex induced prostaglandin production by monocytes of normal human subjects and cancer patients. Prostaglandins and Medicine 4: 363–375

Pollack R, Risser R, Conlon S, Rifkin D 1974 Plasminogen activator production accompanies loss of anchorage regulation in transformation of primary rat embryo cells by simian virus 40. Proceeding of the National Academy of Sciences USA 71: 4792–4796

Poste G, Fidler I J 1980 The pathogenesis of cancer metastasis. Nature 283: 139–146

Prydz H, Allison A C, Schorlemmer H U 1977 Further link between complete activation and blood coagulation. Nature 270: 173–174

Quintana A, Raczka E, Donati M B 1979 Different reponses to noradrenaline (NA) of vascular tissues from two metastasizing tumours in mice. Thrombosis Haemostasis 42: 140

Rankin J H G, Jirtle R, Phernetton T M 1977 Anaomalous responses of tumor vasculature to norepinephrine and prostaglandin E_2 in the rabbit. Circulation Research 41: 496–502

Rasche H, Dietrich M 1977 Hemostatic abnormalities associated with malignant diseases. European Journal of Cancer 13: 1053–1064

Rasche H, Hoelzer D, Dietrich M, Keller A 1974 Hemostatic defects in experimental leukemia. Haemostasis 3: 46–54

Raczka E, Quintana A, Poggi A, Donati M B 1979 Cardiac output distribution in mice bearing Lewis lung carcinoma (3LL) or JW sarcoma (JWS), two spontaneously metastasizing tumours. Thrombosis Haemostatis 42: 142

Reich E 1978 Activation of plasminogen: A widespread mechanism for generating extracellular proteolysis. In: Ruddon R W (ed) Biological Markers of Neoplasia: Basic and Applied Aspects. Elsevier, New York, p 491–500

Rifkin D B, Pollack R 1977 Production of plasminogen activator by established cell lines of mouse origin. Journal of Cell Biology 73: 47–55

Rivers R P A, Hathaway W E, Weston W L 1975 The endotoxin-induced coagulant activity of human monocytes. British Journal of Haematology 30: 311–316

Rohner R F, Prior J T, Sipple J H 1966 Mucinous malignancies, venous thrombosis and terminal endocarditis with emboli. A syndrome. Cancer 19: 1805–1812

Rohwedder J J, Sagastume E 1977 Heparin and polychemotherapy for treatment of lung cancer. Cancer Treatment Reports 61: 1399–1401

Roos E, Dingemans K P 1979 Mechanisms of metastasis. Biochimica Biophysica Acta 560: 135–166

Rosen P, Armstrong D 1973 Nonbacterial thrombotic endocarditis in patients with malignant neoplastic diseases. American Journal of Medicine 54: 23–29

Rosenthal M C, Niemetz J, Wisch N 1963 Hemorrhage and thromboses associated with neoplastic disorders. Journal of Chronic Diseases 16: 667–675

Ross R, Vogel A 1978 The platelet-derived growth factor: Review. Cell 14: 203–210

Rothberger H, Zimmerman T S, Spiegelberg H L, Vaughan J H 1977 Leukocyte procoagulant activity. Enhancement of production in vitro by IgG and antigen-antibody complexes. Journal of Clinical Investigation 59: 549–557

Russell S W, Doe W F, McIntosh A T 1977 Functional characterization of a stable, noncytolytic stage of macrophage activation in tumors. Journal of Experimental Medicine 146: 1511–1520

Sack G H, Jr, Levin J, Bell W R 1977 Trousseau's syndrome and other manifestations of chronic disseminated coagulopathy in patients with neoplasms: Clinical, pathophysiolgic and therapeutic features. Medicine 56: 1–37

Sakuragawa N, Takahashi K, Hoshiyama M, Jimbo C, Matsuoka M, Onishi Y 1976 Pathological cells as procoagulant substance of disseminated intravascular coagulation syndrome in acute promyelocytic leukemia. Thrombosis Research 8: 263–273

Sakuragawa N, Takahashi K, Hoshiyama M, Jimbo C, Ashizawa K, Matsuoka M, Ohinishi Y 1977 The extract from the tissue of gastric cancer as procoagulant in disseminated intravascular coagulation syndrome. Thrombosis Research 10: 457–463

Santoro M G, Philpott G W, Jaffe B M 1976 Inhibition of tumour growth in vivo and in vitro by prostaglandin E. Nature 263: 777–779

Semeraro N 1980 Interactions of platelets, leukocytes, and endothelium with bacterial endotoxins: Possible relevance in kidney disorders. In: Remuzzi G, Mecca G, de Gaetano G (eds) Hemostasis, Prostaglandins, and Renal Disease. Raven Press, New York, p 99–115

Semeraro N, Colucci M, Vermylen J 1979 Complement-dependent and complement-independent interactions of bacterial lipopolysaccharides and mucopeptides with rabbit and human platelets. Thrombosis Haemostasis 41: 392–406

Semeraro N, Donati M B 1981 Pathways of blood clotting initiation by cancer cells. In: Donati M B, Davidson J F, Garattini S (eds) Malignancy and the hemostatic system, Raven Press, New York, pp 65–82

Semeraro N, Vermylen J 1977 Evidence that washed human platelets possess factor-X activator activity. British Journal of Haematology 36: 107–115

Seyberth H W, Segre G V, Morgan J L, Sweetman B J, Potts J T Jr, Oates J A 1975 Prostaglandins as mediators of hypercalcemia associated with certain types of cancer. New England Journal of Medicine 293: 1278–1283

Siegman-Igra Y, Flatau E, Deligdish L 1977 Chronic diffuse intravascular coagulation (DIC) in nonmetastatic ovarian cancer. Report of a case and review of the literature. Gynecologic Oncology 5: 92–100

Slichter S J, Harker L A 1974 Hemostasis in malignancy. Annals of the New York Academy of Sciences 230: 252–261

Snyderman R, Pike M C 1976 Defective macrophage migration produced by neoplasms: identification of an inhibitor of macrophage chemotaxis. In: Fink M A (ed) The macrophage in neoplasia, Academic Press, New York, p 49–55

Soong B C F, Miller S P 1970 Coagulation disorders in cancer. III. Fibrinolysis and inhibitors. Cancer 25: 867–874

Sproul E E 1938 Carcinoma and venous thrombosis: the frequency of association of carcinoma in the body or tail of the pancreas with multiple venous thrombosis. American Journal of Cancer 34: 566–572

Strauli P, Weiss L 1978 Cell locomotion and tumor penetration. Report on a workshop of the EORTC cell surface project group. European Journal of Cancer 13: 1–12

Sun N C J, McAfee W M, Hum G J, Weiner J M 1979 Hemostatic abnormalities in malignancy, a prospective study of one hundred eight patients. pt 1. Coagulation studies. American Journal of Clinical Pathology 71: 10–16

Svanberg L 1975 Thromboplastic activity of human ovarian tumours Thrombosis Research 6: 307–313

Thompson C M, Rodgers R L 1952 Analysis of the autopsy records of 157 cases of carcinoma of the pancreas with particular reference to the incidence of thromboembolism. American Journal of Medical Sciences 223: 469–475

Thornes R D 1974 Oral anticoagulant therapy of human cancer. Journal of Medicine 5: 83–91

Thornes R D 1975 Adjuvant therapy of cancer via the cellular immune mechanism or fibrin by induced fibrinolysis and oral anticoagulants Cancer 35: 91–97

Thornes R D, Deasy P F, Carroll R, Reen D, MacDonell J D 1972 The use of the proteolytic enzyme brinase to produce autocytotoxicity in patients with acute leukemia and its possible role in immunotherapy. Cancer Research 32: 280–284

Tremoli E, Donati M B, de Gaetano G 1977 Washed guinea-pig and rat platelets possess factor X activator activity. British Journal of Haematology 37: 155–156

Trousseau A 1865 Phlegmasia alba dolens. In: Clinique Médicale de l'Hôtel-Dieu de Paris, Balliére, vol 3, p 654–656

Unkeless J C, Gordon S, Reich E 1974 Secretion of plasminogen activator by stimulated macrophages. Journal of Experimental Medicine 139: 834–850

Unkeless J C, Tobia A, Ossowski L, Quigley J P, Rifkin D B, Reich E 1973 An enzymatic function associated with transformation of fibroblasts by oncogenic viruses. I. Chick embryo fibroblast cultures transformed by avian RNA-tumor viruses. Journal of Experimental Medicine 137: 85–111

Vaheri A, Ruoslahti E, Mosher D F (eds) 1978 Fibroblast surface protein, Annals of the New York Academy of Sciences, vol 312

Van Ginkel C J W, Van Aken W G, Oh J I H, Vreeken J 1977 Stimulation of monocyte procoagulant activity by adherence to different surfaces. British Journal of Haematology 37: 35–45

Waller B F, Knapp W S, Edwards J E 1973 Marantic valvular vegetations. Circulation 48: 644–650

Walsh P N 1974 Platelet coagulant activities and haemostasis: a hypothesis. Blood 43: 597–605

Wang B S, McLoughlin G A, Richie J P, Mannick J A 1980 Correlation of the production of plasminogen activator with tumor metastasis in B 16 mouse melanoma cell lines. Cancer Research 40: 288–292

Warren B A 1978 Platelet-tumor cell interactions; morphological studies. In: de Gaetano G, Garattini S (eds) Platelets: a multidisciplinary approach, Ravern Press, New York, p 427–446

Warren B A 1981 Cancer cell endothelial reactions: the microinjury hypothesis and localized thrombosis in the formation of micrometastases. In: Donati M B, Davidson J F, Garattini S (eds) Malignancy and the hemostatic system, Raven Press, New York, pp 5–26

Wasserman L R, Gilbert H S 1966 Complications of polycythemia vera Seminars in Hematology 3: 199–208

Whur P, Magudia M, Boston J, Lockwood J, Williams D C 1981 Plasminogen activator activity of cultured Lewis Lung Carcinoma cells measured by chromogenic substrate assay. British Journal of Cancer, 42: 305–13

Wilner G D, Nossel H L, Leroy E C 1968 Activation of Hageman factor by collegen. Journal of Clinical Investigation 47: 2608–2615

Winkelhake J L, Nicolson G L 1976 Determination of adhesive properties of variant metastatic melanoma cells to Balb/3T3 cells and their virus-transformed derivatives by a monolayer attachment assay. Journal of the National Cancer Institute 56: 285–291

Wood S 1958 Pathogenesis of metastasis formation observed in vivo in the rabbit ear chamber. Archives of Pathology 66: 550–568

Wood G W, Gillespie G Y 1975 Studies on the role of macrophages in regulation of growth and metastasis of murine chemically induced fibrosarcomas. International Journal of Cancer 16: 1022–1029

Wood G W, Gollahon K A 1977 Detection and quantitation of macrophage infiltration into primary human tumors with the use of cellsurface markers. Journal of the National Cancer Institute 59: 1081–1087

Yuhas J M, Pazmino N H 1974 Inhibition of subcutaneously growing line 1 carcinomas due to metastatic spread. Cancer Research 34: 2005–2010

Zacharski L R, Henderson W G, Rickles F R, Forman W B, Cornell C J, Forcier R J, Harrower H W, Johnson R O 1979 Rationale and experimental design for the VA cooperative study of anticoagulation (warfarin) in the treatment of cancer. Cancer 44: 732–741

11. Chromogenic substrates

Z. S. Latallo

INTRODUCTION

Traditionally, most of the tests employed in studies of factors participating in the coagulation and fibrinolytic systems have been end-point assays and have measured the rate of fibrin clot formation or dissolution, i.e. thrombin or plasmin activity respectively. This indirect way of measurement has made it necessary to elaborate highly complicated test systems especially for the assay of factors taking part in the coagulation cascade. Inevitably, problems in controlling many of the variables, accuracy, reproducibility and standardization, were inherent in this approach.

Recognition of the enzymatic nature of the various factors involved, and difficulties in isolating and standardizing their proper protein substrates promoted a search for synthetic substitutes.

The first step was made by Sherry and Troll (1954) and Troll et al (1954), who used arginine and lysine esters to assay thrombin and plasmin. Although quite sensitive to enzymes with esterolytic activities, the amino acid esters show very low specificity. Furthermore, their breakdown products, alcohol and free amino acid, are not convenient to measure. The introduction of benzoyl-arginine-β naphthylamide (BANA) by Reidel and Wunsch (1959) and benzoyl-arginine-p-nitroanilide (BAPNA) (Erlanger et al, 1961) provided a new type of substrate which, upon hydrolysis, released a chromophore group with distinctly different optical properties from the parent molecule. Colorimetric methods could be used, therefore, to follow the reaction, hence the name — chromogenic substrates.

Major progress in this area has been made in the last decade. It was initiated by the work of Blombäck's group on the sequencing of fibrinopeptides and of the thrombin cleavage site of fibrinogen molecule. It finally resulted in the synthesis of a short peptide composed of three amino acids to which p-nitroaniline (p-NA) was coupled at the C-terminal (Svendsen et al, 1972). Within a short time a whole series of similar chromogenic peptide substrates was synthesized. All have pNA as a chromophore, bound to arginine or lysine, and differ only in the two remaining amino acids. The selection of their amino acid composition and sequence was based either on imitation of the sequence around the peptide bond split by natural substrates (e.g. fibrinogen, prothrombin, plasma prekallikrein) or by trial-and-error studies on structure activity relationships (e.g. chromogenic substrates for plasmin, urokinase, glandular kallikrein). In order to avoid splitting by aminopeptidases, their N-terminal is protected by coupling a benzoyl-, carboxybenzoyl- or tosyl- group, or by substituting the L-form of N-terminal amino acid with its D-form. The latter procedure also increases the solubility 10–100 fold. All the other amino acids are in the L-form. More details concerning their design and structure-activity correlations can be found in the work of

Claeson et al (1979). An interesting approach to this problem based on mathematical analysis of experimental data was proposed by Pozsgay et al (1978).

A list of the currently commercially available chromogenic peptide substrates is presented in Table 11.1.

Table 11.1   List of chromogenic peptide substrates

Code	
S 2160	N-Benzoyl-L-phenylalanyl-L-valyl-L-arginine-p-nitroanilide.
S 2222	N-Benzoyl-L-isoleucyl-L-glutamyl-L-glycyl-L-arginine-p-nitroanilide. HCl.
S 2238	H-D-phenylalanyl-L-pipecolyl-L-arginine-p-nitroanilide 2 HCl.
S 2251	H-D-valyl-L-leucyl-L-lysine-p-nitroanilide HCl.
S 226	H-D-valyl-L-leucyl-L-arginyl-p-nitroanilide HCl.
S 2302	H-D-prolyl-L-phenylalanyl-L-arginyl-p-nitroanilide HCl.
S 2444	L-pyroglutamyl-L-glycyl-L-arginyl-p-nitroanilide HCl.
S 2227	H-D-glutamyl-L-glycyl-L-arginyl-p-nitroanilide HCl.
S 2337	H-Benzoyl-L-isoleucyl-L-glutamyl (γ-piperidyl)L-glycyl-L-arginyl-p-nitroanilide.
Chromozym TH	Tosyl-L-glycyl-L-prolyl-L-arginyl-p-nitroanilide HCl.
Chromozym PL	Tosyl-L-glycyl-L-prolyl-L-lysyl-p-nitroanilide HCl.
Chromozym PK	Benzoyl-L-prolyl-L-phenylalanyl-L-arginyl-p-nitroanilide HCl.
Chromozym TR	Carboxybenzoyl-L-valyl-L-glycyl-L-arginyl-p-nitroanilide.

Note: S- series products of Kabi Diagnostica, Stockholm
Chromozym- series products of Pentapharm, Basel distributed under various trade names: Chromozym TH etc./Boehringer, Mannheim/ chromothrombin etc./Stago, Paris/ chromorate TH etc. /Iatron, Tokyo/

Hydrolysis of all these substrates proceeds in a similar manner e.g.:

Tos-Gly-Pro-Arg-pNA $\xrightarrow{\text{enzyme}}$ Tos-Gly-Pro-Arg-OH + pNA

Physicochemical properties

ABSORPTION SPECTRUM

Absorption spectra of an intact chromogenic substrate and of free pNA released by enzymatic hydrolysis are compared in Figure 11.1.

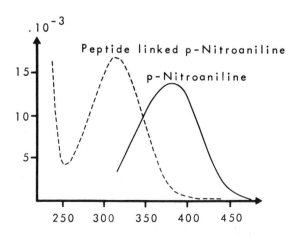

Fig. 11.1   Adsorption spectra of a chromogenic peptide substrate and of pNA, the product of its hydrolysis.

As can be seen from the graph the absorption spectrum of the intensely yellow pNA lies in the visible spectrum. At the wavelength of 405 nm it is still very high, whereas that of the colourless substrate is negligible. This wavelength has therefore been chosen for measuring the reaction rate. The value of extinction coefficient [$E_{405 nm} = 9.65 \times 10^3 \, mol^{-1} \, cm^{-1}$] for pNA was established as the result of collaborative work by the Subcommittee on Synthetic Substrates and Inhibitors of the International Committee for Haemostasis and Thrombosis (ICTH). It remains practically unchanged over a wide range of pH from about 3.0 to 10.5. Acidification below pH 3.0 (e.g. when precipitating the sample with TCA (trichloracetic acid) results in completely reversible loss of colour without having any effect on the intact substrate. In contrast, exposure of substrates to a pH above 10.5 results in a shift in absorbancy, again completely reversible.

SOLUBILITY

High solubility over a wide range of pH is one of the prerequisites of a good substrate since it allows the assay to be run under optimal conditions. This factor is taken into account in designing new substrates. Except for the first substrate produced, S-2160, and perhaps S-2222, the solubility of the remaining substrates is satisfactory. Table 11.2 contains data on solubility obtained from the manufacturers (Kabi, Stockholm; Pentapharm, Basel).

Table 11.2   Solubility of chromogenic peptide substrates

CODE	MW	Solubility mM/litre		pH	mol
		H$_2$O	TRIS/HCl		
S 2160	681.2	1.5	0.13	8.3	0.15
S 2222	741.3	6.0	2.0	8.3	0.25
S 2238	625.6	>10.0	5.0	8.3	0.15
S 2251	551.5	>40.0	10.0	7.4	0.15
S 2266	579.6	>40.0	5.0	9.0	0.05
S 2302	611.6	>10.0	5.0	7.8	0.05
S 2444	498.9	>10.0	3.0	8.8	0.05
S 2227	553.5				
Chromozym TH	662.6	>75.0			
Chromozym PL	634.7	>75.0			
Chromozym PK	702.9	>75.0			
Chromozym TR	644.7	>75.0			

Water is usually used as a solvent. It should be noted that the solubility decreases in the presence of salts. Since some of the substrates dissolve slowly it is advisable to prepare the solution on the day preceding the experiment. Ultrasonic treatment speeds up the process.

PURITY

It cannot be assumed that the commercially produced substrates are always 100 per cent pure, since this assumption has sometimes proved to be incorrect. This problem should be specified by the manufacturers. The label should clearly state the purity of the product. Meanwhile, a practical way of checking the molar concentration of the substrate is by measuring the OD of the product (pNA) after its complete hydrolysis with an excess of enzyme (assuming that only one substrate is present).

STABILITY

The stability of chromogenic peptide substrates is one of their most important features. The manufacturer's data are as follows.

dry state	+2 to +8	3 years
	+20 to +25	2 years
solution	+2 to +8	ca 6 months
	+20 to +25	ca 2 months
	+37	ca 24 hrs

Contamination of the solution with enzyme when pipetting, or with bacteria (from tested material or air) or exposure to strong light, has to be avoided. It is advisable to make stock solutions under aseptic conditions. An antibacterial agent, provided it does not interfere with enzyme action, should be added to the system if the reaction is to be carried out over a long period.

Kinetics of reaction

In spite of other advantages all assays based on natural protein substrates are in fact restricted to the measurement of end-point values. On the contrary, as already said, the use of synthetic chromogenic substrates permits us to follow very closely the whole enzymatic process. In order to take a full advantage of this, all basic rules of enzyme analysis should be strictly obeyed. In other words possession of a precisely defined substrate imposes the need for the utmost care in performance of a test as well as precise expression of result.

Small molecular size and good solubility of chromogenic substrates allows first of all to work on systems in which saturation of enzyme with the substrate is obtained. It is usually achieved when the molar ratio of the initial substrate concentration (s_0) to enzyme concentration (e) is equal or higher than $10^3:1$. The initial velocity (V_0) of the reaction is then described by the steady state rate equation:

$$V_0 = \frac{V_{max}}{1 + \dfrac{K_m}{S_0}} \tag{1}$$

A kinetic study could be easily carried out and therefore the values of V_{max} and the apparent Michaelis constant K_m calculated. Calculation of the catalytic constant k_{cat} is also possible but since

$$k_{cat} = \frac{V_0(1 + K_m/S_0)}{e} \text{ or } k_{cat} = \frac{V_{max}}{e} \tag{2}$$

it is necessary to know the molar concentration of the enzyme. Fortunately, the enzymes involved in blood coagulation and fibrinolysis are almost all serine proteases. Hence, the precise molar concentration of the enzymes could be also measured by titration of active center with p-nitrophenyl p-guanidinobenzoate (NPGB). When the k_{cat} value is established the molar concentration of enzyme (per litre) could be calculated using the following equation:

$$e = \frac{V_0(1 + K_m/S_0)}{k_{cat}} \tag{3}$$

It is of the utmost importance to recall that the values of the kinetic parameters K_m and k_{cat} depend very strongly upon the conditions (pH, temperature, etc) of the reaction and may differ greatly from substrate to substrate. They are also affected seriously if another substrate or an inhibitor is present in the system. Hence, their numerical values are useless if not accompanied by a detailed description of the conditions under which they were obtained.

Expression of the results
Experimental data are obtained in a form of optical density increase over a given period of time e.g. 1 minute at 405 nm wavelength and 1 cm light passway ($\Delta OD_{405\,nm}^{1\,cm}$/min). This value represents the reaction rate and, if the assay was carried out under steady state conditions, the initial velocity of reaction. The latter is directly proportional to the enzyme concentration in the system.

The ΔOD values obtained under standard conditions could be compared directly or converted into per cent activity of a given enzyme, activator or inhibitor using a calibration curve made under exactly the same conditions. For the expression of the amount of enzyme it is recommended, however, to use either molar concentration or the katal unit. If the k_{cat} and K_m values are established for a given set of reaction conditions and on the basis of precise titration of a standard enzyme preparation the amount of enzyme in a tested sample could be calculated from equation (3) and expressed in moles. This way is preferable since the resulting value can be compared directly with others obtained under different reaction conditions and using another substrate.

An alternative way, perhaps most commonly used, is to express the results in katal units. From definition, one katal unit (kat) is the amount of enzyme which hydrolyses one mole of substrate per second under standard conditions. It means that the kat value depends upon the conditions of the reaction: pH, temperature, ionic strength and most important substrate concentration, which theoretically should be, infinite. Expression in kat units is therefore valid only when the nature of substrate and exact reaction conditions are specified. An excellent review of these problems has been recently published by Christensen (1980). In practice, conversion into katal units is based on calculation of the initial velocity of substrate hydrolysis by measurement of the amount of product (pNA) formed in 1 second (mol/sec). If the OD increase is measured per minute, the value obtained should be divided by 60 and by the molar extinction coefficient of pNA (9.65×10^3). It should be multiplied by a dilution factor in order to express the activity of undiluted sample.

example:

       5 μl of plasma in a total volume of the system = 1 ml
       Dilution factor = 200
       Readings ΔOD/min = 0.12

$$\frac{0.12 \times 200}{9.65 \times 10^3 \times 60}$$

$$= \frac{24}{579\,000}$$

$$= 0.0000414 \text{ kat/litre}$$

$$= 41.4 \ \mu\text{kat/litre or } 41.4 \text{ nkat/ml}$$

Methods of assay

The intensely yellow colour of pNA makes it possible to detect its release with the naked eye. This allows for detection of the presence of various enzymes using different substrates in a large number of samples without using a spectrophotometer. If proper care is taken to avoid bacterial contamination the reaction can be carried on for 24 hours and allows even traces of activity to be detected. A quantitative screening of a large number of samples can also be done, e.g. by using an automatic Titertek Multiscan (Flow, Laboratories) which, using a vertical light path, measures absorbancies in 96 flat bottomed wells of a microtitre plastic plate in 60 seconds.

Immersion of polyacrylamide gel slabs after electrophoresis in substrate solution permits identification of active fractions. Similarly, the substrates can be used for histochemical work (Stemberger et al, 1978). In this type of study, as well as when dealing with very low activities, direct coupling of 4-dimethylaminocinnamaldehyde to pNA forms a complex with an intensive red colour (λmax = 570 nm), and produces an almost ten-fold increase in absorbancy value (Kwaan et al, 1978).

Kinetic assay

The most precise method for quantitative analysis is the measurement of the initial reaction rate. It consists of following absorbancy changes during the first few minutes of a reaction, usually with the aid of automatic recording device, and under carefully controlled optimal conditions. The temperature, usually 37°, should be kept constant using a thermostat, and all components of the test system should be prewarmed before mixing. Optimal pH and ionic strength are maintained with the correct buffer. An excess of substrate is of primary importance (see Fig. 11.4). Unfortunately these rules, especially the last one, are not always adhered to.

End-point assay

Alternatively, the end-point method can be employed. It is perhaps most popular in routine work when considerable numbers of assays are performed. This method is not to be recommended unless the same conditions are chosen as for initial rate measurements. The reaction rate at the highest expected enzyme activity then remains unchanged over a period exceeding the end-point. Usually the reaction is carried out for a short, exactly determined time, and stopped by the addition of concentrated acetic acid.

The problem of the blank sample also has to be taken into account. Usually, when relatively high values of absorbancy are obtained in the test sample the blank values which are rather low, are neglected. Nevertheless, hyperlipaemic plasma or plasma with an elevated bilirubin content may give rise to a considerable increase in OD, and thus lead to erroneous results.

However, providing all of the above restrictions are taken into account the results of both initial rate and end-point methods are in good agreement. The latter could be of considerable value when the material tested is not completely soluble (e.g. cell suspensions). In such a system we have used trichloracetic acid (TCA) to 10 per cent final concentration to stop the reaction and to precipitate proteins. After centrifugation the pH of the supernatant must be adjusted to neutral for optical density measurement at 450 nm. Alternatively, the above mentioned coupling with dimethylaminocinnamaldehyde (Kwaan et al, 1978) is performed directly after centrifugation and the sample read at 570 nm.

Both initial rate and end-point methods can be made automatic by appropriate setting of a programmed autoanalyzer.

Specificity
There is no doubt that the problem of the specificity of chromogenic substrates is of the utmost importance. It is inherent in the use of any kind of small substrate and has to be kept in mind in designing and interpreting enzymatic assays performed with these substrates. The very fact that the enzymes participating in blood coagulation and fibrinolysis are rather closely related serine proteases, specifically attacking arginyl- or lysylbonds, makes the problem even more acute. This is taken into account in designing new chromogenic peptide substrates. Introduction of the peptide part makes them much more selective. In fact some are, perhaps surprisingly, highly selective. Comparison of the activity of the main enzymes of interest (thrombin, X^a, plasmin, kallikreins, and urokinase) adjusted to the same molar concentration was performed by Claeson et al (1979) on seven substrates of the S-series using optimal conditions for each enzyme substrate combination. The results expressed in terms of ΔOD minute showed very low numerical values for the 'insensitive' substrates, giving a misleading impression of their specificity. Mattler and Bang (1977) studied the sensitivity of Chromozym PK to the above mentioned enzymes. However, instead of using a constant molar concentration they compared the enzymes at the concentrations equivalent to that of their content in plasma. The results indicated that under these conditions the ratio of plasma kallikrein to plasmin activity was 2:1.

Nevertheless, the data of Claeson et al (1979), as well as those of Mattler and Bang (1977) and ourselves, indicate that for practical purposes at least two substrates, namely S-2222 and S-2251, can be considered highly specific for factor X^a and plasmin respectively. The thrombin substrate S-2238 can also be considered fairly specific, provided plasmin and kallikrein interference are avoided.

In our own studies we have compared 14 enzymes on 12 substrates using the same conditions in all assays (see Table 11.3) with the enzyme concentrations constant, but adjusted in each case to give a convenient absorbancy reading on its 'proper' substrate (OD = 0.100 − 0.200/min). The results presented in Table 11.3 are expressed on a percentage basis, with the activity on the appropriate substrate taken as 100 per cent. The data which are to be compared horizontally only, show the relative sensitivity of all the substrates to each enzyme. This allows a ratio of activity towards various substrates to be established for a given enzyme. We found it of considerable help in identifying unknown activities of tested material, as well as in checking a purified enzyme preparation for cross contamination with other enzymes.

As can be seen, the substrate designed for plasma kallikrein S-2302 has the same sensitivity to streptokinase-plasminogen complex and to plasmin as does their correct substrate, S-2251. S-2302 also appears to be most sensitive to ecarin (EC — an enzyme isolated from *Echis carinatus* venom which specifically activates prothrombin).

Urokinase effectively attacks not only its proper substrates S-2227 and S-2444, but also Chromozyms PL and TH. Streptokinase-plasminogen complex hydrolyses S-2251 and S-2302 equally well. The latter, designed for plasma kallikrein is even more sensitive to human plasmin than the former. Interestingly enough the 2:1 ratio of activity of plasmin on Chromozym PL and S-2251 is reversed (1:2) for SK-

Table 11.3 Comparison of the sensitivity of various chromogenic peptide substrates to different enzymes

	S-2160	Chr PL	S-2251	Chr TH	S-2238	Chr PK	S-2302	S-2222	S-2337	S-2227	S-2444	Chr TRY
PLASMIN												
—porcine	7	100	48	19	13	7	58	·	11	··	7	6
—human	6	100	49	38	21	7	54	··		··	8	·
SK-PLG												
HUMAN	·	51	100	48	30	15	101		··	··	10	7
UROKINASE	·	61	·	46	17	·	·	7	22	64	100	19
FACTOR Xa												
BOVINE	·	··	·	85	·	·	39	88	100	··	9	18
THROMBIN												
HUMAN	6	16	·	94	100	·	·	·	8	·	·	26
EC-THROMBIN												
HUMAN	14	18	·	100	68	52	100	·	·	·	·	20
ECARIN	9	·	··	7	32	10	28	·	·	·	·	·
ANCROD	27	·	·	100	17	11	84	7	·	·	6	12
DEFIBRASE	7	·	··	10	100	·	·	·	·	6	·	·
PLASMA KALI-												
KREIN—human	·		·	25	18	29	100	·	n.d.	·	·	·
BRINASE	100	17	8	6	·	100	55	·	n.d.	·	·	·
PAPAIN	51	·	6	··	·	·	·	·	n.d.	·	·	·
TRYPSIN	18	20	··	71	47	··	14	100	n.d.	52	90	50

Results expressed in per cent of activity using proper substrate. One dot for 0–2 per cent, two dots for 2–5 per cent activity. Conditions: temp 37°C, buffer TRIS-HCl 0.05 M pH = 7.4, final concentration of substrates 0.4 mM.

plasminogen complex. In addition these two enzymes are quite active not only on S-2302, but also on the 'thrombin substrates' Chromozym TH and S-2238. Although slightly less sensitive, S-2222 is apparently more selective than the newly introduced S-2337. Whereas the activity of factor X^a activated human thrombin is almost the same on S-2238 and Chromozym TH, the respective ratios of EC-activated thrombin, Batroxobin and Ancrod on these two substrates differ greatly. According to Mattler & Bang (1977) S-2238 is equally sensitive to α and γ thrombin, whereas Chromozym TH and, especially, S-2160 appear to be capable of discriminating between the two forms of this enzyme.

Use of selective inhibitors to increase specificity
In practice, the problem of specificity could be solved in many cases by introducing appropriate inhibitors into the assay system. These inhibitors should selectively block the action of coexisting enzymes without affecting the one being tested. The inhibition should be non-competitive, fast and irreversible. An example of their application is provided by the results of an experiment with Chromozym TH. As shown in Table 11.3, Chromozym TH is highly sensitive to the majority of the enzymes subjected to analysis. Actually, one might consider it to be a universal substrate for coagulation and fibrinolytic studies. However, as indicated by the following experiment, it can be successfully used in a specific assay of a single enzyme in the presence of other enzymes. In this experiment samples of purified thrombin, plasmin and Factor X^a were assayed for their activity separately, after mixing all three together, and after the addition of the following inhibitors to the mixture: aprotinin, which blocks plasmin but not Factor X^a or thrombin; soyabean trypsin inhibitor (SBTI), which inhibits both plasmin and Factor X^a but does not affect thrombin; and in particular, purified hirudin, which exclusively inhibits thrombin only. Even the highest purity commercial preparations of hirudin also contain a strong plasmin inhibitor (Latallo et al, 1979). The results presented in Figure 11.2 indicate that with

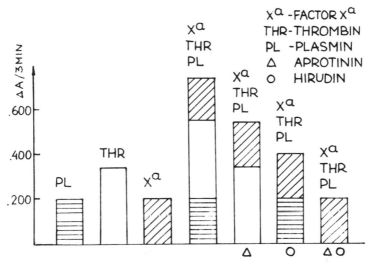

Fig. 11.2   Activity of plasmin (PL), thrombin (THR) and Factor X^a(X^a) measured with Chromozym TH. The first three bars from the left represent the activity of each enzyme alone, the following ones the activity of the mixture of the three, with aprotinin (Δ), pure hirudin (o) and both inhibitors added (Δo).

the use of these inhibitors it was possible to selectively quench other enzymes and to recover quantitatively the activity of a given one in the mixture.

Activity of immobilized enzymes

In contrast to natural protein substrates, the small size of the molecule enables peptide substrates to penetrate easily and to avoid the steric hindrance resulting from enzyme immobilization either to a solid artificial matrix or to a natural one e.g. the cell membrane. This allows for an easier detection and measurement of the activity of immobilized enzymes. It should be kept in mind, however, that the apparent activity of an immobilized enzyme assayed on chromogenic peptide substrates may be very different from that measured with protein substrates.

Activity of enzymes complexed with α_2-macroglobulin

Formation of an enzyme complex with α_2-macroglobulin may be considered as a particular form of immobilization. It is well known that many proteases are able to form such complexes. The reaction is considered to proceed in two steps; first, the splitting of a peptide bond(s) in α_2-macroglobulin molecule, and second, entrapping of the enzyme by conformational change. This results in an almost complete loss of activity towards HMW substrates, while the ability to hydrolyze small substrates (esters, peptides, etc.) is still retained. It has been claimed that in some cases this ability is even greatly increased (Nakamura et al, 1975).

Our own experience indicates the following:

1. The ability of enzymes involved in the blood coagulation-fibrinolytic system to form such complexes differs greatly.
2. The rate of complex formation appears to be related to enzyme specificity. Plasmin, which has the broadest specificity, is bound within about 15 minutes. Thrombin takes several hours, and urokinase (UK) even longer, while only small amounts of Factor X^a are bound overnight and it seems doubtful whether any streptokinase-plasmin complex reacts at all with α_2M. The apparent K_m values for free and α_2M bound plasmin are about the same (Dudek-Wojciechowska et al, 1980). In addition to these changes in ability of the enzymes to attack substrates of different molecular sizes, the susceptibility to attack by inhibitors is also affected by the formation of the enzyme-α_2-macroglobulin complex. As shown in Table 11.4 the activity of the plasmin-α_2 macroglobulin complex is practically unaffected

Table 11.4   Changes in the activity of the plasmin-α_2-macroglobulin complex depending upon time of incubation with various inhibitors (substrate: S-2251)

Inhibitor (final concentration)	Percent of the complex activity after incubation for			
	3 min	15 min	45 min	75 min
SBTI (200 μg/ml)	100	100	100	100
Aprotinin (200 KIU/ml)	100	57	42	39
OM 205 (10^{-5} M)	0	0	0	0

Activity of the complex + SBTI mixture after 1 min taken as 100 per cent by soyabean trypsin inhibitor (M.W. 23 000 daltons), whereas aprotinin (M.W. 6500 daltons) slowly penetrates the enzyme and N-α-dansyl-L-arginine-4 ethyl-piperdine amide-OM-205 (M.W. 502 daltons) inhibits it completely in less than 1 minute.

The use of chromogenic peptide substrates for measuring the α_2-macroglobulin concentration will be described in the methods section. Here, attention is drawn to the fact that when testing biological samples which might contain this protein, its possible interference with the results should be taken into account.

Standardization of enzymes

The high stability and solubility, well defined structure, and purity of the chromogenic peptide substrates allow optimal and perfectly reproducible assay systems to be established for measuring activity or concentration of various enzymes preparations. Hence, an obvious implication is the possibility of using these substrates as a basis for the preparation and control of reference enzyme standards. Such an approach is a logical one in view of the difficulties in preparing reproducible protein substrates. It has, however, been strongly criticized, especially in the case of the thrombin reference standard (Gaffney, 1979). Great discrepancies were observed when parallel clotting and amidolytic assays were performed on standard thrombin preparations presently in use. Further work in this area clearly indicated that these discrepancies could be accounted for by the fact that the standard preparations of thrombin contained other enzymes and, what is more important, varying amounts of different molecular forms of thrombin (Miller-Andersson & Seghatchian, 1978; Miller-Andersson et al, 1980). As already mentioned, S-2238 appears to be equally sensitive to α and γ thrombin (Mattler & Bang, 1977), whereas only the first one is able to clot fibrinogen.

One should be aware that similar discrepancies may occur in work with other enzymes. In general, it may be expected that partial degradation of an enzyme molecule will result in a more pronounced decrease in its ability to hydrolyze protein than the chromogenic peptide substrate.

All this does not exclude, in my opinion, the use of chromogenic substrate in the standardization of enzymes. On the contrary, by proper design of the assay (e.g. comparing the activity of the enzyme preparation on several substrates) it should be possible to establish the relative content of its various forms. More data concerning relative activity of isolated, pure forms of a given enzyme on different substrates are needed however.

It can be concluded that at present the synthetic substrates are perhaps too sensitive and not specific enough for enzyme standardization, or, alternatively, that the standard enzyme preparations are not good enough.

Design of assay system

All assays using chromogenic substrates eventually measure the activity of an enzyme. A direct assay of an enzyme in a purified form is relatively easy to design, but the possible presence of contaminating enzymes needs to be checked. For this purpose the preparation should be tested against various substrates and the effect of specific inhibitors evaluated. When samples of biological fluids are analyzed the possible presence of the enzyme-α_2-macroglobulin complex has to be taken into consideration. In such cases addition of a specific inhibitor of fairly large molecular size will not stop the reaction completely. Once the specificity of the test system is established, optimal conditions of pH, ionic strength and substrate concentration should be determined and strictly adhered to in subsequent work. The application of chromogenic substrates is, however, not only restricted to direct assays. In many instances indirect assays of enzyme inhibitors, proenzymes, activators and even reaction accelerators can be easily performed by measuring the activity of the residual or resulting enzyme. In such cases the problem of substrate specificity is not so acute, but others arise.

In assays of inhibitor, standard, well defined enzyme preparations are applied. An excess of enzyme is mixed with the sample to be tested and after incubation the remaining activity is measured. The amount of enzyme should be so adjusted to give convenient readings and a linear relationship over a wide range of inhibitor concentrations. The time of incubation must be long enough to allow completion of the inhibitory reaction, otherwise erroneous results will be obtained. Since the substrates are very sensitive, solutions of highly diluted enzymes are used. Hence there may be problems associated with a decline in their activity with time, as a result of adsorption onto glass and/or spontaneous autocatalytic degradation. In many instances it is necessary to keep the enzyme solution on ice, prewarming it just before use, and to add stabilizing agents (e.g. carbowax or glycerol). In all cases it is desirable to check the enzyme activity after each run of tests.

In this, as in all other assays, the sample to be tested should also be checked without enzyme for its spontaneous activity towards the substrate. If any is found it should be subtracted from the final result.

Assay of activators is performed in a similar way. A standard, highly purified proenzyme is used instead of enzyme, and the activity resulting from addition of the tested sample is measured. There must be a considerable excess of proenzyme in order to prevent its complete activation and to ensure a linear relationship over a wide range of activator concentrations. The time of incubation has to be carefully controlled. Checking for the presence of inhibitors in the tested material is also advised.

Assay of factors which merely accelerate activation such as Factor VIII or V, involves the presence in the test system of additional components, and the result depends upon the rates of various non-enzymatic and enzymatic reactions. Thus it is very difficult to control all the parameters and to set up optimal conditions.

Finally, I shall discuss the assay of proenzymes, which is perhaps the most popular and of the greatest interest to many laboratories. Optimal conditions for complete conversion have to be established, and interference due to the possible presence of inhibitors in the test sample excluded. The specificity of this assay depends largely on the type of activator used. Highly specific activators converting only the proenzyme being studied are preferred. Precision is enhanced by subtracting the amidolytic effect (if any) of the activator itself. Comparison with the results of direct assay of the active enzyme makes it possible to establish the proenzyme to enzyme ratio in the tested material. More details are discussed below.

Some technical remarks
The very high sensitivity of the substrates necessitates meticulous attention to all the conditions. As shown in Figure 11.3 proper cleaning of cuvettes can be of great importance, especially when different tests are being performed. Furthermore, our

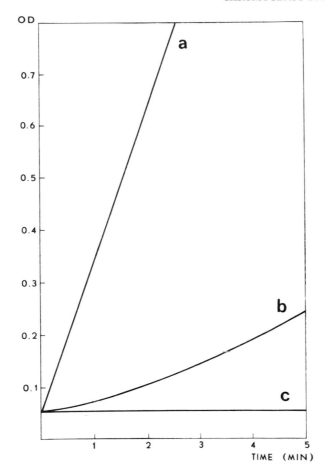

Fig. 11.3 Example of an error due to absorption of an enzyme onto the cuvette wall. OD changes recorded at 405 nm with time. Substrate S-2251. Sample (a) streptokinase-plasminogen complex, (b) purified plasminogen in the same cuvette which had been washed six times with buffer and distilled water, (c) same plasminogen preparation in the same cuvette but washed with 2 M urea in 0.2 M NaOH and distilled water.

experience indicates that some batches of disposable plastic cuvettes are defective. A slight change of their position in the cuvette holder (Beckman spectrophotometer, model 25) resulted in differences in readings of 0.120 OD units.

There is a tendency to minimize the total volume of sample for economic reasons. This involves dispensing very small, often microlitre, volumes of the system components and introduces the possibility of errors due to inaccuracy of volume measurements. Also, saving on highly priced substrates should not result in them being used at less than optimal concentration.

It is understandable that the use of end-point techniques can hardly be avoided when running a large number of tests. In such cases, however, careful control of the substrate concentration is necessary, since at higher activities, as illustrated in Figure 11.4, the reaction rate may deviate from a straight line. In many instances, the OD of the nonactivated-blank sample may be quite high due to its opacity or colour (e.g.

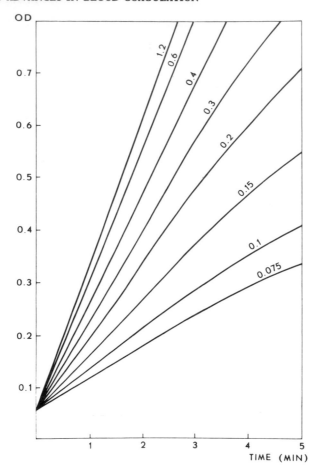

Fig. 11.4   Effect of substrate (S-2251) concentration on the rate of reaction with plasmin. Ordinate: OD at 405 nm, abscissa: time of reaction in minutes. Figures on the graph indicate the final concentration of the substrate in mM.

hemolysis, bilirubin), and has to be measured. On the other hand, it should be kept in mind that the formation of a clot, or slow precipitation, when recording the reaction rate may imitate amidolysis and lead to completely erroneous results. Parallel registration of OD changes at 500 nm, at which the pNA absorption is negligible, or stopping the reaction with acetic acid and checking the OD value after centrifugation of the sample, allows this source of error to be excluded.

PRACTICAL APPLICATION

A. Study of the coagulation system

THROMBIN AND FACTOR X[a]

These are the two enzymes of the coagulation system whose activities can be measured directly. It is seldom done in routine work except for the purpose of establishing control values in studies of antithrombin III and heparin (see below). Problems of standardization, especially in the case of thrombin, have already been discussed above.

Two substrates of about equal sensitivity, namely S-2238 and Chromozym TH, are in use for thrombin assay. Neither substrate is highly specific, although in contrast to the latter, the S-2238 is practically unsusceptible to Factor X^a. In fact it is a strong inhibitor of Factor X^a. Both substrates are more or less sensitive to some components of the plasmin and kallikrein system. Therefore, unless the possible presence of other activities in the test sample are excluded it is advisable to add aprotinin and/or soyabean trypsin inhibitor to the test system. The use of S-2160, originally developed for thrombin assay and used in earlier studies, has, because of its low specificity and sensitivity and very poor solubility, been abandoned in recent work in this area.

For Factor X^a, S-2222 appears to be the most specific substrate, but its solubility is relatively low. The newly introduced S-2337 is somewhat more sensitive to Factor X^a, but is to a small extent, sensitive to thrombin also. In systems in which generation of thrombin may occur, the addition of hirudin may be necessary. By using this inhibitor and aprotinin, Chromozym TH can be used for Factor X^a assay as well, since its sensitivity is comparable to S-2222 (see Table 11.3 and Fig. 11.2).

PROTHROMBIN

The methods elaborated for prothrombin assay differ mainly in respect of the activator and substrate used. Extrinsic pathway–thromboplastin (Bergstrom & Blomback, 1974; Witt, 1977), Russell's viper venom (Korsan-Bengsten, 1978) and some preparations of intrinsic activators as well as direct activation with Ecarin, an enzyme from *Echis carinatus* venom (Latallo, 1976; Latallo & Teisseyre, 1977; Witt & Hasler, 1978) have been used.

Principle: prothrombin $\xrightarrow{\text{activator}}$ thrombin $\longrightarrow$ substrate

Since the rate of thrombin formation depends upon the rates of the preceding reactions, the shorter the chain of these reactions, the more direct and precise the assay. Application of an assay system similar to the clotting prothrombin time test, but substituting for the amidolytic reaction rate measurement of fibrin clot formation provides an overall estimate of the prothrombin complex (Factor II, VII, X) and furthermore, is dependent on Factor V. In addition, rapid decrease in amidolytic activity is observed and thus the optimal incubation time may vary.

Curtailing the chain of reactions can be achieved by applying either activated Factor X or Ecarin as in the following systems elaborated in our laboratory (Latallo et al, 1980).

buffer: 0.05 M TRIS-HCl pH = 7.9
plasma sample diluted 1:50 in 0.05 M TRIS, 0.1M NaCl, 0.0129M Na citrate, pH = 7.9

method I:

0.1 ml Factor X^a(Kabi) 0.35 nkat/ml
0.1 ml cephalin Manchester Comparative Reagent (MCR) diluted 1:50 in buffer
0.1 ml 0.025 M $CaCl_2$
0.2 ml buffer
0.1 ml diluted plasma

incubation 5 min in 37°C
0.2 ml 2 mM substrate in H_2O

S-2238 substrate is used since it is not sensitive to Factor X^a. Chromozym TH can also be applied but in this case activity of X^a must be inhibited by the addition of soyabean trypsin inhibitor.

method II:

0.45 ml buffer
0.1 ml Ecarin (Pentapharm) 20 mU/ml
0.05 ml diluted plasma
incubation 5 min, 37°C
0.2 ml 2 mM Chromozym TH in H_2O

Chromozym TH is the preferred substrate since it is more sensitive to the Ecarin-thrombin (EC) and much less sensitive to Ecarin itself compared to S-2238.

The two methods of activation differ greatly in respect of the type of thrombin formed. EC-thrombin, when compared at an equal clotting potency to biothrombin, is about five times more active in hydrolysing chromogenic substrates than the latter (Latallo & Teisseyre 1977). It is not inhibited by hirudin and AT III-heparin unless the Ecarin is removed (Fulton et al, 1979).

The advantage of the Ecarin method lies in the fact that the activation is independent of other clotting factors and species specificity. Our observations indicate that Ecarin activates the prothrombin of man, ox, pig, sheep, goat, dog, rabbit, rat, mouse and chicken plasma. Thus, it can be conveniently used in animal studies and in testing various prothrombin preparations. On the other hand, since it is Ca^{2+} independent it appears to be less able to discriminate between native prothrombin and its variants, which are produced in the plasma of patients treated with oral anticoagulants. According to Ménaché et al (1975) and the recent studies of Malhotra (1978) it does convert dicoumarol-induced prothrombins (PIVKA — acarboxy forms). Nevertheless there is a surprisingly good correlation between the Ecarin assay and the prothrombin time test in plasma, especially in coumarin-treated patients on long-term anticoagulant treatment (Latallo et al, 1981). In spite of all the effort which has gone into substituting the prothrombin time assay by amidolytic methods further work in this area is necessary (Stormorken, 1979; Latallo et al, 1981).

FACTOR X

This factor can be easily assayed by the direct activation with RVV Russell's viper venom.

Principle: Factor X $\xrightarrow[Ca^{2+}]{RVV}$ Factor $X^a \longrightarrow$ substrate

Although the substrates S-2222 and S-2337 are fairly specific, the concentration of Factor X in plasma is not high enough to prevent interference of the OD measurement by fibrin clot formation (because of secondary thrombin activation).

Various assay systems have been elaborated (Aurell et al, 1978; Vinazzer, 1977, 1978; Witt & Hasler, 1978) using either RVV or the extrinsic pathway. In some, fibrinogen is first removed by Ancrod treatment of the plasma (Vinazzer, 1977, 1978).

Our experience (Latallo et al, 1981) suggest that by adding KCl to the system, secondary thrombin and eventual fibrin formation is prevented, without affecting Factor X activation by RVV. In our system the plasma sample is diluted 1 to 5 with the same TRIS citrate buffer as in methods I and II above.

0.35 ml buffer 0.15 M TRIS-HCl containing 1 M KCl
0.05 RVV (Wellcome) 0.1 mg/ml
0.1 ml CaCl$_2$, 0.025 M
0.1 ml diluted plasma

---

incubation 5 min, 37°C

0.2 ml 2 mM S-2337 or S-2222

Any thrombin generated in this system can be inhibited by the addition of hirudin. However, this is not necessary since, when tested with S-2238, the variations between various plasma samples are negligible. Hence, Chromozym TH could be used for this assay as well.

An interesting approach to assaying active Factor X^a in a patient's plasma, directly on S-2222 substrate, was proposed recently by Vinazzer (1978). For this assay, blood is collected in Na-citrate containing anti-AT III globulin in order to prevent Factor X^a inactivation.

FACTOR VII

Since no substrate sensitive enough to measure its activity directly is known at present, the assay of Factor VII is carried out using an indirect method.

$$\text{Principle: } X \xrightarrow[\substack{\text{thromboplastin} \\ Ca^{2+}}]{\text{VII}} X^a + EDTA \longrightarrow \text{substrate}$$

Addition of EDTA stops the reaction and the activity of the Factor X^a formed during a strictly determined time is taken as a measure of Factor VII activity.

The method recently described by Seligsohn et al (1978) appears to depend greatly upon the preparation of a purified Factor X (free of VII, II and active X^a) which should be present in excess. Our experience with a similar assay system indicates that it is a highly sensitive way of measuring the Factor VII level (Poller et al, 1981). It is of interest that although the method gives a good correlation with the clotting test for nonactivated plasma factor VII, neither kaolin nor cold activation increase the rate of chromogenic substrate hydrolysis (Seligsohn et al, 1978).

FACTOR VIII

Since it is not an enzyme, the problem of Factor VIII C assay involves setting up a rather complicated system in which various highly standardized components are used. The assay is based on the rate of Factor X activation and the conditions must be chosen so as to make it proportional to the Factor VIII C activity. An extensive review of the methodology approach can be found in recent work by Segatchian (1979).

FACTOR XII

None of the available substrates is sensitive enough to measure the activity of Factor XII directly. It is possible, however, to measure its activity via the resulting activity of kallikrein. Vinazzer (1978) proposed a system in which the sample of plasma is activated with kaolin, then incubated for 60 minutes at 37°C. This results in inactivation of the kallikrein formed, whereas XII^a remains unchanged. In the next step, the sample is incubated with a standard intact plasma, and the activity of kallikrein evolving in the system recorded. This author also proposed an assay for active XII^a in plasma, based on the same principle, except that the test sample is 'intact' (not activated with kaolin). It is crucial in these assays to avoid any activation of Factor XII when preparing the intact plasma.

PLATELET FACTOR 3

This factor, which participates in the activation of Factor X and II can be evaluated on the basis of its effect on both reactions (Sandberg & Andersson, 1980). We have recently worked out an assay of PF$_3$ (Harsfalvi et al, 1981) based on the following principle:

$$\text{Factor X}^a \xrightarrow[\text{Ca}^{2+}\ \text{V}]{\text{PF}_3} \text{Prothrombin} \longrightarrow \text{Thrombin}$$

reaction stopped with SBTI   S-2238

Purified Factor X^a and prothrombin are necessary, the latter in relative excess. PF$_3$ activity in 5 μl of PRP can be conveniently measured. This assay may be also useful in standardizing cephalin and in assessing the thromboplastic activity of various cells. In the latter two cases it is necessary to add diluted absorbed plasma as a source of Factor V.

INHIBITORS OF COAGULATION

Application of chromogenic substrates to study inhibitors of the clotting system has excited a rather wide interest. Several methods for the assay of AT III using thrombin and antifactor X^a-activity using Factor X^a have been developed.

Principles:

excess of thrombin $\xrightarrow{\text{inhibitor}}$ remaining thrombin $\longrightarrow$ substrate

excess of Factor X^a $\xrightarrow{\text{inhibitor}}$ remaining Factor X^a $\longrightarrow$ substrate

In most cases heparin is added to the test system to speed up the inhibitory reaction. It should be noted that various fractions of heparin have different effects on thrombin and on Factor X^a activity (Lane et al, 1979).

Critical analysis and review of the various methods using chromogenic substrates for the assay of thrombin and Factor X^a inhibitors and comparison of the results with clotting or immunological tests would go beyond the scope of this chapter. It has been recently the subject of various publications (Blomback et al, 1974; Odegard et al, 1976; Abildgaard et al, 1977; Odegard & Abildgaard, 1978; Abildgaard, 1979; Fareed et al, 1979; Teien, 1979). In my opinion these assays if properly controlled may provide very useful information not only on AT III activity, but also on some other not yet defined inhibitors.

Some methods (Teien et al, 1976; Mattler & Bang, 1977; Lane et al, 1979; Teien, 1979) were also elaborated for the assay of heparin primarily using the principle:

excess of Factor $X^a \dfrac{\text{heparin}}{\text{AT III}}$ remaining Factor $X^a \longrightarrow$ substrate

These methods appear to provide reliable and convenient ways of controlling treatment with high doses of heparin, but are perhaps not sensitive enough to measure the effect of low dose subcutaneous therapy. Interesting and useful information concerning the activity of different heparins and heparin-like substances have already been obtained (Lane et al, 1979). On the basis of the principle shown above, methods for antiheparins and for the assay of platelet factor 4 have also been worked out (Vinazzer, 1977a; Gjesdal, 1979; Lane et al, 1979).

B. Study of the fibrinolytic system

PLASMIN

Several chromogenic substrates are sensitive to the action of this enzyme. S-2251 is apparently most specific but Chromozym PL is about twice as sensitive. The latter as well as Chromozym TH and S-2302, can be conveniently used to measure plasmin activity, provided the presence of other enzymes is excluded, or appropriate inhibitors introduced into the system (application of commercial hirudin is not possible unless contaminating inhibitors of plasmin are removed). Similar problems to those found with thrombin will probably be encountered in the standardization of plasmin but the application of chromogenic substrates may eventually allow various forms or derivatives of this enzyme to be distinguished. All direct assays of plasmin in plasma actually measure the activity of plasmin-α_2-macroglobulin complex rather than free plasmin. The presence of this complex in circulating blood can be readily detected during thrombolytic therapy with SK or UK. Discrimination between free and α_2-macroglobulin bound plasmin could be achieved by adding SBTI or other inhibitors which inhibit only the free enzyme. However, the possible interference of kallikrein-α_2-macroglobulin complexes to which S-2302, Chromozyms TH and PK are sensitive, should be taken into account.

PLASMINOGEN

There are two methods for the assay of plasminogen: (a) by converting it into active plasmin with the use of UK or small amounts of SK and (b) by measuring activity of its complex with SK. The first reaction proceeds relatively slowly, and depends upon the type of plasminogen (Glu- or Lys-PLG). It would be very useful in the assay of the purified proenzyme to be able to distinguish between its native and degraded form. A procedure for discriminating between the two in plasma has been proposed by Scully & Kakkar (1978). It is based on the fact that addition of EACA or exposure to low pH (about 2.0) speeds up activation of Glu-PLG. Thus, comparing the results obtained with untreated and EACA or acid treated plasma, allows the ratio of Glu- and Lys-PLG to be determined. It should be borne in mind, however, that in untreated plasma, the fast acting α_2-antiplasmin binds at least part of the plasmin formed during the activation process. While the addition of EACA, or acid treatment, apparently changes the conformation of the PLG molecule and makes it more susceptible to activators, the latter procedure also destroys practically all of the inhibitors present in plasma.

The second way of assaying plasminogen consists in measuring the activity of its complex with SK. Plasminogen as well as plasmin, and even its derivative light B-chain, are able to form stoichiometric complexes with streptokinase. These complexes are enzymatic in nature but differ from plasmin. They are not inhibited by α_2-antiplasmin, the protease inhibitor contaminating hirudin preparations, or by SBTI. In contrast to plasmin SK complexes they have very low proteolytic activity toward fibrinogen and casein, but very high activity in converting plasminogen into plasmin. Their amidolytic activity is also high, but distinctly different from plasmin (compare the two activities on S-2251 and Chromozym PL in Table 11.3). An assay for plasminogen in plasma using a molar excess of SK has been proposed by Friberger et al (1978). Complete formation of the active complex of SK with native PLG in plasma in this assay takes at least 10 to 15 minutes. Our own results indicate that acid treatment of plasma results not only in much faster formation of the complex, but also in about a twofold increase in its activity (Latallo et al 1978). Consequently, we proposed a method for assaying the plasminogen in plasma in which plasma is acid treated prior to addition of an excess of SK (Latallo et al, 1978) as follows:

Acid treatment: 0.1 ml of citrated plasma + 0.2 ml of
0.1 M HCl incubated at 0°C for 15 min;
0.2 ml of 0.1 M NaOH is then added and the sample diluted
further with 1.5 ml of 0.15 M TRIS-HCl buffer pH = 7.4

Assay system: 0.1 ml of the above described plasma sample
0.6 ml of 0.15 M TRIS-HCl buffer pH = 7.4
0.1 ml of Streptokinase (10 000 u/ml) in 0.15 M NaCl

---

incubation for 5 min at 37°C

0.2 ml of 3.3 mM S-2251 in H_2O

This assay measures the total PLG content in plasma independent of the form (native or degraded) of proenzyme. If active plasmin is present in the system an appropriate correction should be applied.

It should be noted that the acid treatment of plasma allows the measurement of plasminogen in various animals using urokinase as an activator. According to our experience there is an excellent agreement between the above described amidolytic method and the caseinolytic assay.

PLASMINOGEN ACTIVATORS

Either direct or indirect (two stage procedure) can be used for the assay of plasminogen activators. Since SK is not an enzyme we have proposed that it is measured in the form of an SK-PLG complex (Latallo et al, 1979). Provided an excess of plasminogen (PLG) is present the activity of this complex is proportional to the amount of SK added. Hence, SK could be assayed after blocking plasmin and measuring the remaining activity of the complex.

Direct assay of urokinase (UK) can be performed using S-2227 substrate which is perhaps the most specific, or S-2444, which is more sensitive (Claeson et al, 1978; Latallo et al, 1979). Much less specific although of equal sensitivity with S-2227, are Chromozyms PL and TH. Any one of these can be used as long as purified UK preparations are assayed. Unfortunately none is sensitive enough to allow the direct reliable assay of UK in urine or plasma. A similar situation is encountered in the case of tissue activators of various origins. Even the newly developed S-2288 and S-2388, which were especially designed for this purpose are not sensitive enough. This is not to say that the direct assays of UK and tissue activators cannot be performed in biological samples but the problem is that their concentration is very low, and therefore, in order to obtain a significant increase in OD, the reaction with the substrate has to be carried out for between 30 minutes and several hours instead of 1–5 minutes. Hence, there is a danger of misinterpretation due to the interference of other proteases which could be present in biological samples. In such cases an indirect assay should be performed as well.

Principle: plasminogen $\xrightarrow{\text{activator}}$ plasmin $\longrightarrow$ substrate

This two stage procedure ensures the specificity of the assay and allows the study of the kinetics of the activation reaction. Highly purified plasminogen, free of plasmin, should be used in relatively high concentrations to provide enough substrate for the activator. The first activation reaction is usually carried out for the relatively long time of 30 to 60 minutes, whereas the second one, i.e. plasmin assay, for 1 to 5 minutes. Addition of fibrin to the activation mixture may speed up the reaction, especially in the case of a non-urokinase type of tissue activator.

PLASMIN INHIBITORS
Except for α_2-macroglobulin all others are assayed according to the following principle:

excess of plasmin $\xrightarrow{\text{inhibitor}}$ remaining free plasmin $\longrightarrow$ substrate

Any of the substrates used for plasmin assay can be used (see p. 268).

α_2-ANTIPLASMIN
The main inhibitor present in plasma is a very fast acting one. Its effect is measured immediately after mixing with plasmin. We have used the following assay system:

plasma: citrated PPP diluted 1:5 with 0.0129 M Na citrate in 0.15 M NaCl; buffer 0.15 M TRIS-HCl pH = 7.4
system: 0.1 ml diluted plasma
          0.5 ml buffer
          0.2 ml plasmin Kabi 0.3 CU/ml in 50% glycerol in 0.001 M HCl
          _____

          mix, after 10 seconds add
          _____

          0.2 ml 3.3 mM S-2251 in H_2O

Note: plasma and buffer should be prewarmed to 37°C, plasmin kept at room temperature at least 1 hour before the assay and its activity controlled at the end of the test run. Since platelets contain some antiplasmin they should be removed from plasma immediately after blood sampling. PPP samples can then be stored in the deep freeze without any apparent change in α_2-antiplasmin activity. A method for platelet antiplasmin assay on chromogenic substrates is presently being developed in our laboratory.

The values obtained either by the initial rate or end-point method (0.2 ml of glacial acetic acid added after 3 minutes) are calculated from the respective standard curves made from various dilutions of pooled normal plasma. A very similar assay system has been proposed by Teger-Nilsson et al (1977).

An overall estimate of α_2-antiplasmin and other plasma slow reacting inhibitors can be obtained by simply prolonging the plasma-plasmin interaction to 15 minutes (Latallo et al, 1978).

α_2-MACROGLOBULIN

α_2-macroglobulin assay is based on a different principle, namely on the fact that the enzyme-α_2-macroglobulin complex is active against chromogenic substrates but not inhibited by polypeptide inhibitors. The simplest procedure is a modification of the method of Ganrot (1966) using trypsin and SBTI and measuring the remaining trypsin-α_2-macroglobulin complex on S-2222 or other substrates sensitive to trypsin (see Table 11.3). We have used plasmin as an enzyme and aprotinin as the inhibitor (Latallo et al, 1948). In this case incubation for 15 minutes at 37°C was necessary to achieve complete formation of the complex. We subsequently observed that aprotinin, in contrast to SBTI, progressively inhibited the complex activity. Consequently the latter inhibitor is preferred (see Table 11.4).

C. Study of the prekallikrein-kallikrein system
Development in this area has been prompted to a large extent by the introduction of specially designed chromogenic substrates.

PLASMA KALLIKREIN ASSAY

Two substrates have been suggested for the assay of plasma kallikrein, namely S-2302 and Chromozym PK (Claeson et al, 1978; Amundsen et al, 1976). Unfortunately, neither is highly specific. As a matter of fact Chromozym TH, the universal substrate, could be used as well. Since the prekallikrein-kallikrein system is so tightly interlinked with the coagulation and fibrinolytic systems one should be aware in interpreting the results of possible interference due to activation of other than kallikrein enzymes. Addition of crude or commercial hirudin preparations containing, beside hirudin, substantial quantities of leech plasmin inhibitor which would block thrombin and plasmin, but not kallikrein, could be of considerable help in this respect. Another way of discriminating between kallikrein and other enzymes is to compare the relative ratio of activity using various substrates (see Table 11.3). Our observations indicate that highly purified kallikrein complexes with α_2-macroglobulin at a rather slow rate, whereas in plasma-containing medium the reaction appears to proceed much faster. Assay of kallikrein in the plasma sample will, therefore, measure both free and α_2-macroglobulin bound kallikrein. Comparatively fast activation of plasma prekallikrein by contact reaction on one side, and fast inactivation of kallikrein by C_1 esterase inhibitor on the other, makes it imperative to perform the assay immediately after blood withdrawal.

It should be mentioned that when testing various blood derived preparations (immunoglobulins, cryo-precipitates, fibrinogen) we have found a considerable, though varying, kallikrein or kallikrein-like activity, apparently due to the presence of the enzyme-α_2-macroglobulin complex in these preparations. All of the above observations are of a preliminary character. Further work in this area is necessary.

PREKALLIKREIN ASSAY
As in the case of plasminogen the problem of achieving complete conversion into the active enzyme, while at the same time avoiding inhibition by the inhibitors present in plasma sample, has to be dealt with.

Principle:

Factor XII $\xrightarrow{\text{surface}}$ Factor XII^a

Prekallikrein $\longrightarrow$ Kallikrein $\longrightarrow$ Substrate
HMW kininogen

Various agents are employed for Factor XII^a activation such as kaolin (Mattler & Bang, 1977), cephotest (cephalin + ellagic acid reagent, Nyco, Oslo) (Claeson et al, 1978; Egberg & Bergstrom, 1978; Stormorken et al, 1978) and dextran sulphate of 500 000 daltons M.W. (Kluft, 1977; Kluft et al, 1979; Witt & Hasler, 1978). If this reaction is performed in cold (0°C) and with diluted plasma inactivation of kallikrein by the inhibitors is practically negligible. Final values of kallikrein activity in normal plasma vary depending upon the procedure used. According to Mattler & Bang (1977), acid treatment of plasma prior to its activation with kaolin results in almost double value as compared to untreated plasma. The presence of HMW kininogen appears to be necessary in order to achieve complete activation of prekallikrein. Content of Factor XII in tested plasma should be at least more than 25 per cent of normal.

KALLIKREIN INHIBITORS
C_1 esterase inhibitor and α_2-macroglobulin are considered to be the two most important inhibitors of kallikrein in plasma (Gallimore & Fareed, 1979). Assay of the latter has been already described above. In contrast to α_2-macroglobulin, kallikrein complex inhibition by C_1 esterase inhibitor results in abolishing the amidolytic activity of the enzyme. In practice, for the study of kallikrein inhibition, two conditions have to be fulfilled. Namely, a good stable standard preparation of the enzyme has to be used, and its incubation with tested sample carried out to a completion of the inhibitory reaction. The inhibitory effect is then evaluated by measuring the amount of the remaining enzyme activity. It should be realized, however, that such a procedure is prone to some error since the remaining activity is represented by free as well as α_2-macroglobulin bound enzyme. Activity of the latter may, and probably does, as in the case of plasmin, differ from the former.

GLANDULAR KALLIKREIN
The substrate (S-2266) designed for glandular kallikrein assay is not sensitive enough to allow a short time assay. Determination of kallikrein in urine is therefore carried out by a prolonged reaction with the substrate. A sample of pooled urine from 24 hours collection should be mixed with 0.2 M TRIS-HCl buffer pH = 8.2, centrifuged and incubated with the substrate for 30 minutes at 37°C. After stopping the reaction with acetic acid, the sample is read at 405 nm. The blank value, which

contains in addition aprotinin, is subtracted from this value. In this way interference of other proteases not inhibited by aprotinin and of the colour of urine is prevented.

D. Other applications

Hitherto, production of chromogenic peptide substrates was centred primarily on those which have a arginyl- or lysyl-bond available for hydrolysis. This was mainly due to the fact that the blood proteases involved in coagulation and fibrinolysis specifically attack those bonds. It is purely a technical problem to design and synthesize different chromogenic peptides with other bonds available for enzymatic attack (e.g. tyrosyl-, valyl-, alanyl- etc.) and thus produce substrates for chymotrypsin, elastase or other enzymes. The work in this direction has already started and one should expect to have available a series of new substrates which will certainly find wide application in other fields of research and industry.

Several other applications should be mentioned besides the application discussed above. Namely, assays of thrombin-like preparations from snake venoms, trypsin in gastric juice, papain, brinase, proteases from haemolymph of Mediterranean crab or from hemocyte lysate of Limulus crab etc.

CONCLUDING REMARKS

This revue was concerned and primarily focused on the methodological aspects of the application of chromogenic substrates in the study of three enzymatic systems in blood, namely, clotting, fibrinolysis and kallikrein. In addition to those presented here detailed descriptions of a number of working procedures for the assay of various components of the three systems, are provided by the respective manufacturers. Several laboratory kits containing standardized reagents and working procedures were also introduced. Unfortunately, some of the kits were developed too hastily and are not as reliable as they should be.

Limitation of space does not allow the presentation and discussion of the results of studies concerning application of the methods described in clinical practice. Already, a considerable number of papers dealing with the diagnostic value of these methods for detection of disseminated intravascular coagulation, control of thrombolytic therapy with UK and SK, as well as laboratory control of treatment with oral anticoagulants have been published, and each new issue of periodicals, covering the field of blood coagulation, brings new work on chromogenic substrates. All this indicates that major steps forward in transition from test tube clotting time measurement to spectrophotometric assays are being made.

REFERENCES

Abildgaard U 1979 Antithrombin assays using chromogenic substrates. In: Scully M F, Kakkar V V (eds) Chromogenic peptide substrates, Churchill Livingstone, London, p 171–182

Abildgaard U, Lie M, Ødegard O R 1977 Antithrombin (heparin cofactor) assay with new chromogenic substrates (S-2238 and Chromozym TH). Thrombosis Research 11: 549–553

Amundsen E, Svendsen L, Vennerod A M, Laake K 1976 Determination of plasma kallikrein with a new chromogenic tripeptide derivative. In: Pisano J J, Austen K F (eds) Chemistry and Biology of the Kallikrein-Kinin System in Health and Disease. Fogarty Intern. Center Proceedings no 27, Washington, p 215

Aurell L, Simonsson R, Arielly S, Karlsson G, Friberger P, Claeson G 1978 Chromogenic peptide substrates for Factor X^a Haemostasis 7: 92–94

Bergström B, Blombäck M 1974 Determination of prothrombin with a reaction rate analyzer using a synthetic substrate. Thrombosis Research 4: 719–729

Blombäck M, Blombäck B, Olsson P, Svendsen L 1974 The assay of antithrombin using a synthetic chromogenic substrate for thrombin. Thrombosis Research 5: 621–632

Christensen U 1980 Requirements for valid assays of clotting enzymes using chromogenic substrates. Thrombosis and Haemostasis 43: 169-174

Claeson G, Aurell L, Karlsson G, Gustavsson S, Friberger P, Arielly S, Simonsson R 1979 Design of chromogenic peptide substrates. In: Scully M F, Kakkar V V (eds) Chromogenic peptide substrates, Churchill Livingstone, London, p 20–30

Claeson G, Friberger P, Knös M, Eriksson E 1978 Methods for determination of prekallikrein in plasma, glandular kallikrein and urokinase. Haemostasis 7: 76–78

Dudek-Wojciechowska G, Kopeć M, Latallo Z S 1980 Inhibition of the fibrinolytic system by a₂-macroglobulin. In: Davidson J F (ed) Progress in Fibrinolysis and Thrombolysis, vol V Churchill Livingstone, Edinburgh (to be published)

Egberg N, Bergström K, 1978 Studies on assays for plasma prekallikrein and for the monitoring of coumarol therapy. Haemostasis 7: 85–91

Erlanger B F, Kowosky N, Cohen W 1961 The preparation and properties of two new chromogenic substrates of trypsin. Arch. Biochem. Biophys. 95: 271

Fareed J, Messmore H L, Balis J U 1979 Current status of methodologies for antithrombin III and heparin with the advent of peptide chromogenic substrates. In: Scully M F, Kakkar V V (eds) Chromogenic peptide substrates, Churchill Livingstone, London, p 183–195

Friberger P, Knos M, Gustavsson S, Aurell L, Claeson G 1978 Methods for determination of plasmin, antiplasmin and plasminogen by means of substrates S-2251. Haemostasis 7: 138–145

Fulton A J, Dempster J, Prentice C R M 1979 Resistance of ecarin thrombin to inhibition by antithrombin III: a dual role for ecarin. Thrombosis Research 15: 143–155

Gaffney P J 1979 A critical evaluation of chromogenic substrates in standarisation. In: Scully M F, Kakkar V V (eds) Chromogenic peptide substrates, Churchill Livingstone, London, p 42–56

Gallimore M J, Fareid E 1979 Studies on human plasma inhibitors of plasmin, plasma kallikrein, trypsin, thrombin and urokinase using chromogenic substrate assays *ibidem*, p 248–261

Gjesdal K 1979 Platelet factor 4 and antiheparin activity in plasma *ibidem*, p 219–228

Harsfalvi J, Chmielewska J, Muszbek L, Latallo Z S (to be published)

Kluft C 1977 Assay for prekallikrein levels and prekallikrein in human plasma using dextran sulphate as a soluble activator. Thrombosis and Haemostasis 38: 20

Kluft C, Trumpi-Kalshoven M M, JIE AFH 1979 Crucial conditions for the determination of prekallikrein levels in plasma with chromogenic substrates. In: Scully M F, Kakkar V V (eds) Chromogenic substrates, Churchill Livingstone, London, p 84–92

Korsan-Bengsten K 1978 Bestimmung von Gerinnungsfaktoren mit chromogenen Substraten. In: Breddin H K (ed) Prostaglandine und Plattchenfunktion, Schattauer, Stuttgart-New York, p 217–226

Kwaan H C, Friedman R B, Szczecinski M 1978 Amplification of color yield of chromogenic substrates using p-dimethylaminnamaldehyde. Thrombosis Research 13: 5–14

Lane D A, MacGregor I, Scully M F, Kakkar V V 1979 Use of chromogenic substrates in the study of heparin heterogeneity: influence of platelet and plasma heparin neutralizing activity. In: Scully M F, Kakkar V V (eds) Chromogenic peptide substrates, Churchill Livingstone, London, p 206–218

Latallo Z S 1976 Specific assay of prothrombin. In: Proceedings of ad hoc Discussion Group on Synthetic Substrates and inhibitors of coagulation and fibrinolysis, ICTH, Kyoto

Latallo Z S, Teisseyre E 1977 Amidolytic assay of prothrombin activated with ecarin, a procoagulant from Echis carinatus venom. In: Witt I (ed) New methods for the analysis of coagulation using chromogenic substrates, de Gruyter, Berlin, New York, p 181–192

Latallo Z S, Teisseyre E, Lopaciuk S 1978 Assessment of plasma fibrinolytic system with use of chromogenic substrate. Haemostasis 7: 150–154

Latallo Z S, Teisseyre E, Raczka E 1979 Activators of plasminogen, measurement using chromogenic substrates. In: Scully M F, Kakkar V V (eds) Chromogenic peptide substrates, Churchill Livingstone, London, p 154–164

Latallo Z S, Thomson J M & Poller L 1981 An evaluation of chromogenic substrates in the control of oral anticoagulant therapy. Brit J. Haematology 47: 307–318

Malhotra Om P 1979 Purification and characterisation of dicoumarol-induced prothrombins III. Alumina ph 4.6 atypical (2-Gla) variant. Thrombosis Research 15: 449–463

Mattler L E, Bang N U 1977 Serine protease specificity for peptide chromogenic substrates. Thrombosis Haemostasis (Stuttg.) 38: 776–792

Ménaché D, Guilleir M-C, Boyer C, Casbron N 1975 Preliminary studies on human coumarin prothrombin. In: Hemker E C, Veltkamp J J (eds) Prothrombin and related coagulation factors Leyden University Press, p 759

Miller-Andersson M, Gaffney P J, Seghatchian M J 1980 Preparation and stability of a highly purified human thrombin. Thrombosis Research (to be published)

Miller-Andersson M, Seghatchian J 1978 Microheterogeneity in thrombin standards. Haemostasis 7: 113–120

Mussoni L, Raczka E, Chmielewska J, Donati M B, Latallo Z S 1979 Plasminogen assay in rabbit, rat and mouse plasma using the chromogenic substrate S-2251. Thrombosis Research 15: 341–349

Nakamura S, Ogata H, Takeo K, Kuwahara A, Suzuno R 1975 The effect of α_2-macroglobulin from bovine serum on bovine α-chymotrypsin. Hoppe-Seyler's Z. Physiol. Chem. 356: 677–692

Ødegard O R, Abildgaard U 1978 Antithrombin III: Critical review of assay methods. Significance of variations in health disease. Haemostasis 7: 127–134

Ødegard O R, Abildgaard U, Lie M 1976 Antifactor X^a activity measured with amidolytic methods. Haemostasis 5: 265–275

Poller L, Thomson Jean M, Bodzenta A, Easton A, Latallo Z S 1981 An assessment of an amidolytic assay for factor VII in the laboratory control of oral anticoagulants: in press

Pozsgay M, Gaspar R, Elodi P 1978 Method for designing peptidyl-p-nitroanilide substrates for trypsin. Acta Biochim. Biophys. Acad. Sci. Hung. 13: 185–189

Reidel A, Wunsch E 1959 N-benzoyl-arginin-naphtylamide als substrat zur quantitativen kolorimetrischen Bestimmungen von Trypsin. Zschr. Physiol. Chemie 316: 61

Sandberg H, Andersson L O 1980 A highly sensitive assay of platelet factor 3 using a chromogenic substrate. Thrombosis Res. (to be published)

Scully M F, Kakkar V V 1978 Method for the determination of plasminogen which discriminates between native and degraded plasminogen. Thrombosis Res. 12: 1201

Seghatchian M J 1979 The usefulness of chromogenic substrates in the diagnosis of haemophilia and control of blood products. In: Scully M F, Kakkar V V (eds) Chromogenic peptide substrates, Churchill Livingstone, London, p 102–118

Seligsohn U, Østerud B, Rapaport S I 1978 Coupled amidolytic assay for Factor VII: Its use with a clotting assay to determine the activity state of Factor VII. Blood 52: 978–988

Sherry S, Troll W 1954 The action of thrombin on synthetic substrates. J. Biol. Chem. 208: 95–105

Stemberger A, Blasini R, Wriedt-Lübbe I, Blümel G 1978 Chromogene Substrate zum histochemischem Nachweis gewebestandinger Enzyme. In: Breddin H K (ed) Prostaglandine und Plattchenfunktion, Schattauer, Stuttgart-New York, p 315–318

Stormorken H 1979 Advantages and disadvantages of assaying coagulation and fibrinolytic parameters using chromogenic substrates. In: Scully M F, Kakkar V V (eds) Chromogenic peptide substrates, Churchill Livingstone, London, p 32–39

Stormorken H, Baklund A, Gallimore M, Ritland S 1978 Chromogenic substrate assay of plasma prekallikrein. With a note on its site of biosynthesis. Haemostasis 7: 69–75

Svendsen L, Blombäck B, Blombäck M, Olsson P 1972 Synthetic chromogenic substrates for determination of trypsin, thrombin and thrombin-like enzymes. Thrombosis Res. 1: 267–278

Teger-Nilsson A C, Friberger P, Gyzander E 1977 Determination of a new rapid plasmin inhibitor in human blood by means of a plasmin specific tripeptide substrate. Scand. J. Clin. Lab. Invest. 37: 403–409

Teien A N, 1979 Assay of heparin using Factor X^a and a chromogenic substrate. In: Scully M F, Kakkar V V (eds) Chromogenic peptide substrates, Churchill Livingstone, London, p 196–205

Teien A N, Lie M, Abildgaard U 1976 Assay of heparin in plasma using a chromogenic substrate. Thrombosis Res. 8: 413–416

Troll W, Sherry S, Wackman J 1954 The action of plasmin on synthetic substrates. J. Biol. Chem. 208: 85–94

Vinazzer H 1977 Assay of factor X^a with a chromogenic substrate. In: Witt I (ed) New methods for analysis of coagulation using chromogenic substrates, de Gruyter, Berlin, New York, p 203–210

Vinazzer H 1977a Photometric assay of platelet factor 4 with a chromogenic substrate. Haemostasis 6: 283

Vinazzer H 1978 Diagnostik der intravascularen Aktivierung des Gerinnungsmechanismus mit Hilfe von chromogenen Substraten. In: Breddin H K (ed) Prostaglandine und Plattchenfunktion, Schattauer, Stuttgart-New York, p 309–313

Witt I 1977 Determination of plasma prothrombin with Chromozyn TH. In: Witt I (ed) New methods for the analysis of coagulation using chromogenic substrates, de Gruyter, Berlin, New York, p 155–179

Witt I, Hasler K 1978 Klinische Bedeuntung von Gerinnungsanalysen mit chromogenen Peptidsubstraten. In: Breddin H K (ed) Prostaglandine und Plattchenfunktion, Schattauer, Stuttgart-New York, p 227–242

12. Recent advances in the diagnosis of deep vein thrombosis and pulmonary embolism

Michael A. Bettmann   Edwin W. Salzman

It is now widely accepted that most pulmonary emboli arise from thrombi in the deep veins of the lower extremities and that both pulmonary embolism (PE) and deep vein thrombosis (DVT) are more frequent than is apparent clinically. Beyond these areas of agreement, controversies remain regarding the diagnosis of both of these diseases. This review will deal with recent developments in the diagnosis of pulmonary embolism and deep vein thrombosis and will consider their impact on questions of management and related disputed issues.

DIAGNOSIS OF DEEP VEIN THROMBOSIS

There is clear need for a simple, safe and accurate test for deep vein thrombosis for many reasons. Deep vein thrombosis cannot be diagnosed clinically with reliability, as has been shown in autopsy studies and studies employing contrast phlebography (Sevitt & Gallagher, 1961; Sevitt, 1969; Barnes et al, 1975; Bettmann & Paulin, 1977). The disease is common, particularly among patients at prolonged bed rest or those undergoing hip surgery or open urologic surgery. Recent studies utilizing labelled ^{125}I-fibrinogen have confirmed that the incidence of deep vein thrombosis is as great as had been documented in earlier post-mortem studies (Harris et al, 1975; Sevitt, 1969; Freiman et al, 1965). It is likely that more proximal and larger thrombi are more likely to propagate and embolize than are small thrombi. Kakkar et al (1969) showed that among surgical patients, most thrombi were confined to muscular calf veins, and many appeared to lyse spontaneously. The true occurrence of this disease and its natural history are not yet clear, but the disease is clearly common, with significant related morbidity and mortality. Until it is possible to uniformly prevent this disease in patients at risk, and predict the outcome once thrombi have formed, it is important to attempt to demonstrate deep vein (including muscular) thrombi in all locations and of all sizes, in all patients either at risk or clinically suspected of having deep vein thrombosis.

Contrast phlebography

The most accurate method available for the diagnosis of deep vein thrombosis is contrast phlebography. Radiographic visualization of veins was first used experimentally in 1910 by Franck and Alwens and in humans in 1923 by Berberich and Hirsch. Limitations at that time were the lack of resolution of the radiographic equipment and the toxicity of the contrast agents. With the introduction of tri-iodinated, fully-substituted contrast agents in the early 1950s the use of phlebography was facilitated and new techniques were introduced. Injection of contrast into the marrow cavity by puncture of the medial or lateral malleolus of the ankle (intraosseous phlebography) was undertaken, but was largely given up both because of the associated patient discomfort and the fear of causing fat emboli. Rogoff & DeWeese (1960) and others (Carlson, 1969) developed techniques for injecting contrast via needles placed in a vein in each foot. Tourniquets were left in place during the infusion of fixed amounts of contrast and overhead radiographs were exposed at intervals to demonstrate different portions of the deep venous system. Lea Thomas (1971) modified these techniques to achieve better vein detail. Following the lead of Bergvall (1971), Rabinov and Paulin described a technique which is currently probably the most widely used and is theoretically the most logical (1973).

One leg is studied at a time, as it is rarely necessary, given the usual clinical setting and the availability of non-invasive studies, to evaluate both lower extremities. Contrast agent is infused via a small-bore needle (23 gauge) placed in a dorsal pedal vein, either pointing cephalad in the region of the great toe or pointing caudad and placed more proximally and laterally. This allows good filling of the venous arcades in the foot, and consequently of all major deep and superficial veins. No tourniquet is used during the contrast infusion, as this may limit filling of muscular veins (which are thought to fill from the superficial system and are a common site of thrombus formation) and deep veins at the ankle level. Fluoroscopic monitoring is useful, since the capacity of the venous system varies markedly from individual to individual, and thus the amount of contrast necessary for adequate vein filling must be adjusted for each patient. Also, fluoroscopic monitoring of adequacy of filling permits a determination as to whether tourniquets should be applied or the needle re-positioned.

The patient is positioned foot-down about 45°, bearing weight on the contralateral foot, with minimal weight on the leg to be studied. This avoids artifacts caused by venous compression secondary to calf pressure or by contraction of calf muscles. 50–200 cc of contrast is infused, guided by fluoroscopy, and when adequate filling is obtained, overhead films are taken. If any questions remain after the films are examined, the study is repeated, with tourniquets, re-positioning of the needle, more rapid contrast infusion or steeper patient angulation.

The side effects of phlebography have been recognized for many years (Homans, 1942), but the true incidence has not been clear. Occasional episodes of extravasation of contrast at the puncture site have led to permanent damage to the foot (Lea Thomas, 1970), generally in patients with compromised arterial circulation. If care is taken during the injection to monitor for pain in the foot or other signs indicating extravasation, complications can be kept to a minimum.

The contrast agents most commonly used in the United States are 40 per cent or 45 per cent w/v sodium methylglucamine diatrizoate or iothalamate (about 200 m Eq I/ml). These dilute agents have been shown to decrease the discomfort experienced during the study, the incidence of a characteristic post-phlebography syndrome of pain, tenderness erythema of the low calf, and the incidence of post-phlebographic thrombosis (Bettmann & Paulin, 1977, Bettmann et al, 1980). The incidence of the post-phlebographic syndrome is about 30 per cent in patients with negative phlebograms (Albrechtsson & Olsson, 1976; Bettmann & Paulin, 1977), with standard, 60 per cent w/v contrast agents. By diluting the contrast with normal saline, the incidence of this complication can be lowered to 12 per cent in patients with negative phlebograms, without loss of sensitivity of the procedure (Bettmann & Paulin, 1977).

The described incidence of post-phlebographic thrombophlebitis after negative phlebograms ranges from 2.7 per cent in symptomatic patients (Athanasoulis, 1975) to 50 per cent at surgery for varicose veins (Cranley, 1978) to 62 per cent by isotopic tests (Albrechtsson & Olsson, 1979). In a study comparing the ionic contrast meglumine calcium metrizoate to the non-ionic metrizamide, Albrechtsson and Olsson (1979) found that no cases of thrombosis developed following the use of the latter, but the incidence with the former was 48 per cent. When standard 60 per cent w/v sodium meglumine diatrizoate was compared to the same agent at a concentration of 45 per cent w/v, the incidence of objectively documented thrombosis fell from 26 per cent to 9 per cent and of deep vein thrombosis from 12 per cent to 3 per cent (Bettmann et al, 1980). Other complications of phlebography, such as allergy-like reactions, are rare (3 per cent, Bettmann & Paulin, 1979), generally mild and readily treated.

The accuracy of contrast phlebography is very high but is limited by several factors. First, if there is vessel wall inflammation without thrombus formation, phlebography will show no abnormalities, though thrombi may form subsequently or may have been present and embolized (Webber et al, 1969; Kerrigan et al, 1974). Second, the minimum length or diameter of thrombi which can be recognized radiographically is about 2 mm. Third, accuracy may be diminished if the technique is not fastidious and if the interpretation does not follow strict criteria: that is, a fresh thrombus is indicated only by an intraluminal filling defect seen in more than one view (Fig. 12.1). Lack of filling of a vein and even abrupt termination of the contrast column are not definitive findings of acute DVT: they indicate merely that further effort must be made to define the veins. There is also some inter-observer variation with resultant loss of accuracy (McLachlan et al, 1979), but this appears to be less than with most diagnostic procedures. Because the iliac veins and the profunda femoris vein are not always well opacified, there may be additional loss of sensitivity. With careful technique, however, and a low threshold for performing catheter iliac phlebography, the effect of these limitations is small.

125I-Fibrinogen point count scanning

This test has proven extremely useful in deep vein thrombosis, both in establishing the diagnosis and in defining the epidemiology of the disease.

The technique, originated by Hobbs and Davies (1960) and refined by Flanc et al (1968) and Kakkar (1972), involves intravenous injection of 100 μCi of 125I-labeled fibrinogen after thyroid uptake is blocked by the oral administration of 100 mgm sodium iodide. The half life of 125I is long (60 days) but the energy of the gamma emission is low (35 Kv), so that imaging is not possible but relatively long follow-up point counting studies are. The duration of usefulness of labeled fibrinogen is about seven days, a function of the biological half life of the fibrinogen (about three days) and the long half life of 125I. If indicated, the labeled fibrinogen can be reinjected after the count density decreases. 'Scanning', actually point counting with a portable scintillation detector, is done at one or two day intervals. Counts over the heart are expressed as 100 per cent, and counts at eight points on each leg are expressed as percentages of this. The test is regarded as positive if the counts relative to precordial counts at any point are 15 per cent (using a four inch collimator [Browse, 1972]) or 20 per cent (using a two inch collimator [Harris et al, 1975; Kakkar, 1972]) greater than the same point on the other leg, an adjacent point or the same point on the previous examination, for at least 24 hours.

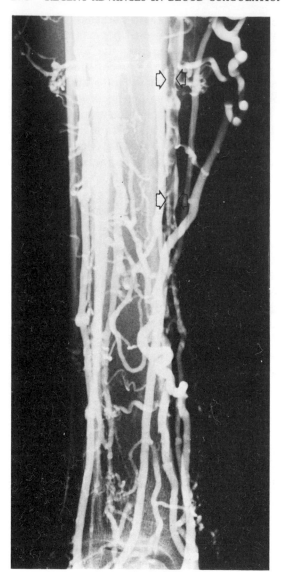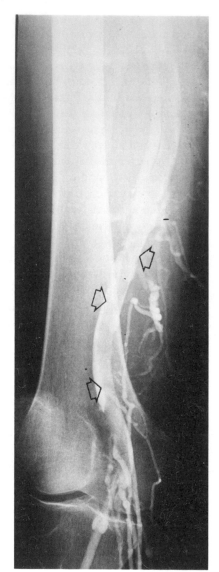

Fig. 12.1 Films from a contrast phlebogram, lower leg (a) and thigh (b), demonstrating thrombus extending from posterior tibial into popliteal and superficial femoral veins (arrows, ▷).

The advantages of this technique are that it is non-invasive but for the injection of isotope, simple to perform, safe, sensitive, relatively inexpensive, objective and easy to interpret. The method allows prospective monitoring of patients at risk of developing deep vein thrombosis, such as those undergoing elective surgery or at prolonged bed rest. In theory, it would allow documentation of propagation of thrombi, but in practice, whether because of clot dissolution or embolization, lack of propagation, or decreasing fibrin accumulation, this has not been possible (Kakkar et al, 1969; Hirsh, personal communication).

The drawbacks are both practical and theoretical. There is a theoretical risk of transmitting hepatitis, but this is not a problem if a carefully screened group of donors is used as a source for the fibrinogen. The study can evaluate the lower extremity only from ankle to mid-thigh because of background counts from blood and urine in the pelvic region and absorption of the low-energy gamma photons by the soft tissues of the thigh. Also, this technique does not allow discrimination among processes which lead to fibrin accumulation: i.e., labeled fibrinogen sequestration occurs not only in deep vein thrombi but also in incisions, ruptured popliteal (Baker's) cysts, cellulitis or hematomas. The ^{125}I-fibrinogen scan is of limited value in patients with symptoms suspected to be due to DVT, as these patients may have other causes for their symptoms or may have established thrombi which are no longer incorporating fibrin. The use of this test in patients suspected of having deep vein thrombosis is also compromised by the necessity of delaying therapy for 24 to 48 hours while waiting for a positive result. Anticoagulants cannot be given in the interim, as they would interfere with fibrin incorporation and thus render the test inaccurate. In a retrospective study, examining whether the usefulness of this test could be broadened, DeNardo et al (1977) showed that of studies ultimately regarded as positive, 67 per cent were positive at three-to-four hours after ^{125}I-fibrinogen administration and 98 per cent were positive at 24 hours. Unfortunately, this report does not deal with transiently positive results in tests which are ultimately negative (as many as 50 per cent of initially positive results [Kakkar et al, 1969]) and so does not justify a more rapid interpretation.

The accuracy of ^{125}I-fibrinogen scanning depends on the situation in which it is applied. It may be over 70 per cent accurate in patients with established acute thrombosis (Hirsh & Hull, 1978), but this is clearly not sufficiently reliable to mandate the sole use of this test. It is useful but limited in patients under-going elective hip surgery, as Harris et al (1975) showed that in these patients only 50 per cent of the thrombi demonstrable by phlebography were identified by scanning because of confusion caused by the surgical wound in the thigh. If the examination was considered interpretable only distant from the surgical wound, the scanning was 83 per cent accurate overall. In addition, there are a significant number of patients who develop positive scans despite negative phlebograms. This false positive rate of 25 to 30 per cent (Coe et al, 1978; Skillman et al, 1978) may actually reflect the greater sensitivity of the ^{125}I-fibrinogen test than contrast phlebography; nonetheless, there is no basis for treating patients unless thrombosis can be demonstrated. Other investigators report an overall accuracy of about 90 per cent compared to phlebography (Hirsh & Hull, 1978; Kakkar, 1972).

The overall accuracy of this technique, then, ranges from about 70 to 90 per cent, depending on the patient population studied. Lack of specificity, i.e. false positive studies, presents a greater problem than lack of sensitivity. This method may well be more sensitive than any other modality, and its role as a screening test in prospective studies, particularly in general surgical patients, is well established. However, the technique cannot be used by itself to confirm suspected deep vein thrombosis in most clinical settings.

Olsson and Albrechtsson (1980) reported a modification of the standard technique which produced more rapid results (62 per cent of tests positive one hour after injection, 71 per cent at 24 hours and 95 per cent at 48 hours) but unfortunately sacrificed specificity (48 per cent false positive rate). The modifications consisted of elevating the legs during counting to avoid venous pooling, elevating the entire patient feet up to allow inguinal evaluation, and assessing 12 points rather than eight on each leg. Although these modifications may lead to better sensitivity in the thigh, they do not provide any overall increase in specificity and thus do not seem to provide significant advantages.

Another recently reported modification may help to increase the specificity of this technique. By registering the X-ray photons produced by ^{125}I disintegrations, the depth localization of thrombi can be determined. In a preliminary study, this promising modification was reported to be as specific as phlebography in patients with positive standard ^{125}I-fibrinogen scans (Ulmsten et al, 1979).

Other alternatives include labelling of fibrinogen with ^{131}I or ^{123}I, and use of a ^{131}I-labeled anti-fibrinogen antibody. Both ^{131}I and ^{123}I disintegrate with the production of gamma photons of sufficient energy to allow imaging rather than counting, unlike ^{125}I which produces only low energy photons, and this difference might make the test useful in the upper thigh and pelvis. Unfortunately, ^{131}I, which is more readily available than ^{123}I, disintegrates with beta as well as gamma emissions and this markedly increases patient dose if the isotope is used for prolonged screening procedures. Furthermore, the study of Prescott et al (1978) indicates that ^{131}I-fibrinogen imaging of the low thigh and calf is only marginally better than point counting of these areas with ^{125}I-fibrinogen and that point counting of ^{131}I-fibrinogen also fails to reflect accurately ilio-femoral thrombosis.

[123]I provides the theoretical advantage of short half life (13.3 hours) and gamma emissions suitable for imaging. This short half life, however, would necessitate repeat injections if prospective screening, as is possible with ^{125}I, is to be performed. It has been possible to use this formulation to image thrombi 16 to 24 hours after injection with apparent accuracy (DeNardo & DeNardo, 1977), but no studies comparing this technique to contrast phlebography are available.

Impedance plethysmography
The theoretical basis for this technique is that in normal patients, venous volume in the extremities increases if there is a relative obstruction to outflow and decreases when this obstruction is released. Deep inspiration causes such an obstruction because of the pinchcock action of the diaphragm. Mullick, Wheeler and Songster (1970) applied this principle to the diagnosis of deep venous thrombosis using Ohm's Law, $R = V/I$, where R is electrical resistance (impedance), V is voltage drop and I is current. As blood is a conductor of electrical current, if blood volume (capacitance) increases, resistance decreases, and current at a constant voltage increases. If changes in current during maximal respiratory effort are recorded, there is a gradual rise with maximal inspiration and a rapid fall in current with expiration. In patients with occlusive thrombi in major deep veins, however, the theory holds that veins will be maximally distended and there will be little or no change in impedance with maximal inspiration and expiration.

The drawbacks to this technique as originally proposed were pointed out by Steer et al (1973). Calf vein thrombi and non-obstructing thigh vein thrombi may cause no alterations in the impedance pattern, because of the large capacity of the venous system and the normal interconnections and venous duplications. Further, this technique would not be reliable in patients with alterations of venous flow for reasons other than thrombosis, such as congestive heart failure, chronic venous insufficiency, large pelvic hematoma or marked lower extremity edema. Finally, the original technique depended to a large extent on patient cooperation, which was frequently incomplete.

Subsequent alterations in the technique have increased its usefulness. A large blood pressure cuff is applied to the thigh and is inflated above venous pressure, eliminating reliance on the patient's maximal inspiratory effort (Wheeler et al, 1974). The foot is elevated and the knee is flexed slightly, to allow free venous egress and relaxation of the leg muscles. Both the cuff size and inflation pressure are standardized: a 15 cm wide cuff is inflated to 40 cm of water (Hull et al, 1976). The cuff was originally inflated for 45 seconds and then released, but it was found that the discriminatory value of the test was increased if the cuff was kept inflated for two minutes (Hull et al, 1978). If sequential inflations and deflations are performed, rather than a single inflation for 45 seconds, specificity of diagnosis of proximal thrombi is increased 20 per cent and the sensitivity 10 per cent.

Muscle contraction may still cause artifacts which may be difficult to distinguish from abnormalities secondary to thrombi. This drawback can be eliminated if simultaneous electromyographic signals are recorded from the thigh (Biland et al, 1979).

Alterations in impedance with inflation and deflation of the cuff can be analyzed as recorded in several sequential cycles of inflation and deflation (Sasahara et al, 1979) (Fig. 12.2). The total fall in impedance can also be plotted against the rise in the first

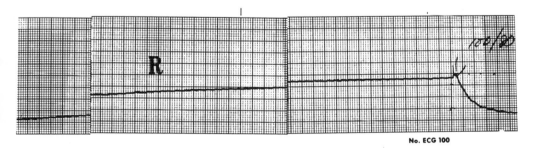

No. ECG 100

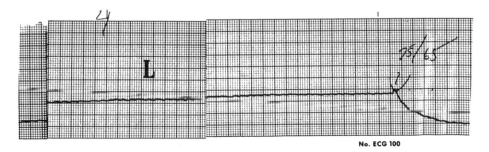

No. ECG 100

Fig. 12.2 Impedance plethysmography, single recording from right and left leg. Rising venous capacitance over three minutes following inflation of cuff to 45 mm Hg, and outflow over 3 seconds. Normal rise and fall in capacitance in both legs.

three seconds after deflation and a graph then constructed indicating a single point for each cycle. A discriminant line can be constructed: readings above indicate normal, below indicate deep vein thrombosis (Fig. 12.3).

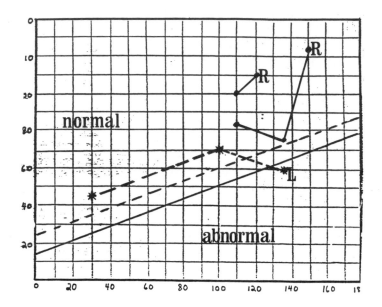

Fig. 12.3 IPG Scoring Graph: venous capacitance on horizontal axis (rise) and 3-second venous outflow on vertical axis. Below solid diagonal line is abnormal, above is normal. Second, 'discriminant' line above first identifies results which may be normal on first tracing but which are likely to become abnormal with repeated examinations. Right leg normal on five cycles. Left leg was initially normal but became abnormal on third cycle. Phlebography demonstrated DVT in left leg.

Although these modifications eliminate many of the drawbacks of this technique, only acute or subacute totally occlusive proximal thrombi are consistently detected. With these modifications, the accuracy of impedance plethysmography in the detection of thrombi in the popliteal or femoral veins is 85 to 97 per cent in comparison to contrast phlebography (Sasahara et al, 1979; Hirsh & Hull, 1978; Benedict et al, 1977). In contrast to ^{125}I-fibrinogen scans, the method appears to be less accurate when used prospectively for screening than it is in patients who present with symptoms suggestive of deep vein thrombosis. Unfortunately, while this technique is fairly sensitive and very specific for proximal occlusive thrombi, it remains inaccurate for thrombi at or below the knee. The clinical importance of thrombi confined to the calf is the subject of controversy. There is evidence that most post-operative thrombi which embolize begin in the muscular veins in the calf (Kakkar, 1969). There is evidence also that most of the deaths from pulmonary embolism occur within a few minutes of the incident (Coon & Coller, 1959), that pulmonary embolism is fatal in a significant fraction and number of patients (Hume et al, 1970) and that many patients with autopsy-proven deep vein thrombosis and pulmonary embolism had no clinical evidence of either process during life (Sevitt & Gallagher, 1961). Calf thrombi, from the evidence of Kakkar et al (1969) and Browse (1972), embolize in about 55 per cent of cases, usually causing few or no findings. Calf vein thrombi may propagate rapidly, however, in 12 hours or less, and the morbidity and mortality associated with embolization clearly increase with larger thromboemboli. Therefore, it does not appear to be logical to use impedance plethysmography by itself, either prospectively or in symptomatic patients. Its use in conjunction with other modalities, however, has been investigated and will be discussed subsequently.

Phleborrheography
This variant of impedance plethysmography uses pressure-sensitive cuffs to measure changes in volume of the lower extremity, rather than measuring alterations in electrical impedance (Cranley, 1975). The patient is positioned 10 to 15° feet down to distend the veins, and cuffs are placed around the abdomen (to measure normal respiratory waves), thigh, calf, and foot. A distal cuff is rapidly inflated (to 100 mm Hg at the foot or 50 mm Hg at the calf) and released, and changes in volume over several cycles are recorded in a more proximal cuff.

Cranley (1975, 1978) believes this technique to be rapid, sensitive to large deep vein thrombi and reproducible. He reports that respiratory variations are damped by acute deep vein thrombosis but begin to return at two weeks, that the false positive rate with this method is 2 per cent and that this method identifies 75 per cent of thrombi confined to veins below the knee. This method appears to have many of the same advantages (low cost, accuracy for occluding ilio-femoral thrombi) and disadvantages (lack of sensitivity to non-occluding, muscular and calf thrombi) as electrical impedance plethysmography. However, it has not been as thoroughly investigated.

Doppler ultrasound
This technique, introduced by Strandness et al (1967) and Sumner et al (1968), utilizes the Doppler principle: a sound wave encountering a stationary object will be reflected back at the same frequency, but a wave encountering a moving object will be reflected back at a different frequency, linearly related to the velocity of the object. The wave is produced by a piezo-electric crystal ultrasound transmitter with a frequency in the range of 5 MHz. The difference in frequency between the incident and reflected beams is recorded in a second crystal mounted adjacent to the first in a hand held transducer. The frequency difference is amplified to produce an audible sound, which is a reflection of both the velocity and the direction of flow.

The technique most often used is that of Barnes et al (1975) or Strandness (1977). The transducer is initially placed in the region of the inguinal ligament and the typical flow pattern of the femoral artery is located. The transducer is then moved medially and the femoral vein is identified. Normally, flow in the femoral vein decreases with inspiration and increases with expiration. The more distal veins are then evaluated by placing the transducer over each one in turn and compressing the leg distal to that point. This compression, in normals, causes an increase in flow, which is audible as a 'wooshing' noise. It is important to compare the results in one leg to the results at a similar point on the other leg. Deep vein thrombosis is indicated in the iliofemoral region by absence of the normal phasic pattern in response to respiration. Distally, thrombosis is indicated by absence of a velocity signal at an expected location or diminished augmentation with either distal compression or release of proximal compression.

The advantages of Doppler ultrasound are that it is rapid (an examination need take no more than 5 minutes) and non-invasive, and the necessary apparatus is not expensive. The examination can be repeated readily and, unlike impedance plethysmography, can be performed in patients with marked congestive heart failure or with leg casts.

The disadvantages include the major one of impedance plethysmography: this technique will reliably demonstrate only thrombi which obstruct the large deep veins. Furthermore, as no recording device is used, review of the results can be accomplished only by repeating the study. Finally, results are more subjective than with other methods and are more dependent on the experience of the examiner (Jacques et al, 1979).

As with the other modalities, it is important to consider the accuracy of Doppler ultrasound both in patients suspected of having deep vein thrombosis and those at risk for developing it. Surprisingly, the experiences with this technique as a prospective screening modality are limited and inconclusive (McIlroy, 1972; Milne et al, 1977). In patients studied because of the clinical suspicion of deep vein thrombosis, the accuracy in comparison to contrast phlebography has ranged from 62 per cent to 93.8 per cent (Johnson, 1974; Kiil & Miller, 1978; Barnes et al, 1976; Jacques et al, 1977). The reported sensitivity and specificity have also varied over a fairly wide range (Strandness, 1977). Barnes et al (1976) concluded that Doppler ultrasound is more accurate in diagnosing thrombi below the knee than is impedance plethysmography. Doppler does share with the latter method, however, the drawback of not demonstrating muscular vein thrombi, or, on occasion, large non-occlusive thrombi which may embolize (Kiil & Moller, 1978).

There have been promising recent reports of the diagnosis of arterial thrombi by gray-scale ultrasound (Dunnick et al, 1979). This imaging modality may also prove to be useful in patients suspected of having venous thrombosis, particularly in conjunction with other screening tests.

Thermography

The use of thermography is based on the clinical observation that the skin of the leg of a patient with deep vein thrombosis is warmer than normal. An infrared camera is used to record skin temperature photographically after the limbs are allowed to equilibrate to ambient temperature. The legs are elevated slightly to prevent venous pooling, and an anterior and sometimes a posterior view is obtained. The procedure takes 10 to 20 minutes. The Polaroid picture obtained demonstrates increased temperature as whiter areas and cooler zones as blacker areas.

When acute deep vein thrombosis is present, there may be increased arterial flow into the muscles which drain via the involved vein, possibly secondary to release of vasoactive amines (Hallböök & Ling, 1972; Cooke & Pilcher, 1974). Both increased temperature in the associated muscle groups and altered flow due to thrombosis lead to alterations in the normal thermographic pattern which have led to the development of empiric criteria for deep vein thrombosis (Cooke & Pilcher, 1974). Taking a 1.5°C elevation in temperature as the main criterion, thermography has been found about 90 per cent accurate in comparison to contrast phlebography in patients studied because of clinical suspicion of deep vein thrombosis (Bergvist & Hallböök, 1979). The accuracy was only 81 per cent, however, when thermography was compared to ^{125}I-fibrinogen scanning in post-operative patients. The specificity was 90 per cent in this group, but the sensitivity was only 62 per cent. Ritchie et al (1979) have proposed specific new criteria, with diagnostic patterns based on the muscle groups drained by each major vein group. The results of a clinical trial using these criteria are not yet available.

The major advantages of thermography are that it is totally non-invasive, can be repeated as often as desired, requires little patient cooperation, and has objective results suitable for detailed analysis.

The major drawbacks are that false positives may result from inflammatory conditions that are confused with deep vein thrombosis clinically, such as cellulitis or acute arthritis, particularly if the criterion of local temperature elevation is used. Some expertise is necessary to perform the thermographic scans and to interpret them. Proximal femoral and iliac thrombosis may be missed by this technique. Also, the necessary equipment is far more costly than that needed for most other non-invasive modalities, such as impedance plethysmography.

This technique has not been as thoroughly investigated as either impedance plethysmography or Doppler ultrasound. Further investigations comparing this modality to contrast phlebography are warranted.

Radionuclide diagnosis of deep vein thrombosis

There are three basic approaches to the use of radionuclides in this area: identification of forming thrombus, radionuclide phlebography, and thrombus scintigraphy. The first of these has been of major clinical and experimental importance, in the form of ^{125}I-fibrinogen point count scanning. The second and third approaches have been introduced more recently.

Radionuclide phlebography

This approach uses mainly ^{99m}Tc, an excellent isotope for gamma camera imaging, either as the sodium pertechnitate for flow studies, or complexed with human serum albumin or macroaggregated albumin (MAA), the form in which it is generally used for perfusion lung scans. Various techniques have been proposed, but there are not yet sufficient data to allow a choice among them. A theoretical objection to the use of flow studies alone is that the volume of fluid containing the isotope and injected via a dorsal foot vein is small, and therefore even major vessel occlusions, if confined to one of a pair of veins, may not be evident. In practice, flow studies have been used to demonstrate major alterations in venous drainage patterns and subsequent static images have been employed to demonstrate isotope retention, presumably in thrombi. Why thrombi sequester the isotope is not clear (Webber, 1977).

The major advantages of radionuclide phlebography are its relatively non-invasive nature, its ready availability in most large medical centres and the production of reviewable results. Such studies can be performed as preliminaries to perfusion lung scans, producing additional information at little additional cost, since the site of injection of the isotope is immaterial to the lung scan. Further, injection of the isotope into a dorsal vein on each foot allows good visualization of both iliac veins and the inferior vena cava, an advantage over most other techniques.

To date, there are few objective data on the accuracy of radionuclide phlebography. In a series of 32 contrast phlebograms, Johnson (1974) reported 81 per cent sensitivity, 75 per cent specificity and 78 per cent accuracy in radionuclide studies using ^{99m}Tc sodium pertechnitate for flow studies and subsequent imaging. In a study by Henkin et al (1974), isotope phlebography with ^{99m}Tc-human albumin microspheres was 96 per cent sensitive and 96 per cent specific in 25 patients who underwent contrast phlebography. In an earlier study using the same isotope formulation, 34 limbs were evaluated by both contrast and radionuclide phlebography, and the latter was 90 per cent specific, 88 per cent sensitive and 89 per cent accurate. In another study correlating 25 radiographic and radionuclide studies, using ^{99m}Tc-macroaggregated albumin, Hayt et al (1977) attempted to identify acute thrombosis. In their hands, this technique was 84 per cent specific and 80 per cent sensitive. Finally, Webber (1977) used the same isotope preparation in a correlative study in 39 patients and showed 77 per cent specificity and 72 per cent sensitivity. All of these series are small, and they concern three different isotope preparations and several technical modifications. It is possible that radionuclide phlebography will play a significant role, particularly in patients suspected of having iliac or vena cava thrombosis. It is not likely to be useful for prospective screening, as it requires careful injections into the foot veins in a nuclear medicine unit, a procedure which is frequently time consuming. Whether this technique will be of value in patients suspected of having deep vein thrombosis remains to be seen, but with current methods, this is not one of the more promising approaches.

Thrombus scintigraphy
There is overlap between thrombus scintigraphy and identification of forming thrombus with ^{125}I-fibrinogen. These two techniques are considered separately, however, because ^{125}I-fibrinogen scanning has been extensively investigated, whereas thrombus scintigraphy using other agents and formulations is an evolving area in which clinical information is still forthcoming. Many radiopharmaceuticals have been prepared for evaluation of thrombi, both venous and arterial; these have been reviewed by Krohn and Knight (1977). Only those with promise or with which there is clinical experience will be discussed here.

Such agents can be separated into those which utilize elements that are incorporated into forming thrombi and those which use elements that aid thrombolysis. Thrombus-forming elements include fibrinogen, platelets, leukocytes and red blood cells, and the latter group includes plasminogen, plasmin, streptokinase and urokinase.

Fibrinogen as a thrombus imaging agent has been mentioned above; ^{123}I-fibrinogen appears promising, particularly in pelvic and thigh thrombi. ^{99m}Tc-labeled fibrinogen is theoretically useful, because of the lower dose, better imaging characteristics and ready availability compared to ^{123}I and ^{131}I. Harwig et al (1976) were able to achieve this labelling, but not without denaturation of a high percentage of the fibrinogen. More recently, Hale and Tucker (1978) reported a preparation which did not lead to denaturation and thus may be useful clinically.

In vivo labelling of erythrocytes with ^{99m}Tc-stannous pyrophosphate and diphosphonate has been used extensively in the evaluation of patients for gastro-intestinal bleeding (Winzelberg et al, 1979), and in radionuclide ventriculography (Chervu, 1979). There have been no reports of the use of this technique in detecting thrombi, either venous or arterial. This technique is convenient, rapid and of theoretical use in patients with actively forming thrombi, which are known to incorporate red blood cells. With normal red blood cell turnover and incorporation of these cells into thrombi, imaging would be expected to disclose areas in which count rates were higher than circulating background radioactivity; even minor differences can be utilized by computer enhancement of radioisotopic images. This technique would be simple and non-invasive but it would not be helpful in identifying established thrombi.

Leukocyte labelling has been useful in humans in identifying inflammatory processes (McDougall et al, 1977). The technique of labelling polymorphonuclear leukocytes with [111]Indium developed by Thakur et al (1977) does not impair the functional capabilities of these cells, and the isotope used has a long enough half life and satisfactory decay to allow gamma imaging. This technique has not yet been correlated with contrast phlebography, but it is of theoretical value as leukocytes, as well as erythrocytes and platelets, accumulate in forming thrombi.

Although venous thrombi consist primarily of fibrin strands and erythrocytes, it is clear that they also contain large, although variable, numbers of platelets. Thakur et al (1976) developed a method of labelling platelets with [111]Indium, using a lipid soluble complex with 8-hydroxyquinoline (Indium oxine). This method allowed high labelling efficiency and adequate platelet survival in rabbits and dogs, but not in humans (Wistow et al, 1978). However, Goodwin et al (1978) modified the technique, by labelling the platelets in plasma instead of saline, and this yielded platelets with survival times in the same range as platelets labeled with [51]Cr. Using these autologous labeled platelets, this group was able to achieve correlation in three patients with contrast phlebography-proven deep vein thrombosis, correlation with an abnormal lung scan in another patient and with an arterial thrombus demonstrated by angiography in two others.

Several other studies have evaluated autologous labelled platelets. Uchida et al (1974) labelled platelets with ^{99m}Tc, but imaging suggested sequestration, possibly related to damage to the platelets. McIlmoyle et al (1977), using autologous [111]Indium platelets, was able to image small pulmonary emboli in dogs one hour after they occurred with great accuracy. In animal models of thrombosis, others have evaluated the efficacy of this technique with respect to time. Grossman et al (1978) found that autologous [111]Indium labelled platelets in rabbits provided striking localization of both venous thrombi and sites of arterial wall damage six hours after the creation of vascular lesions. If the platelets were injected 24 hours after the lesions were produced, however, there was little localization. Similarly, when pre-clotted blood was injected (i.e., established thrombi), labelled platelets were not helpful in localization. Knight et al (1978) compared [111]Indium platelets and ^{125}I-fibrinogen in dogs with experimentally induced venous thrombosis and arterial wall damage. The labelled platelets were more accurate in demonstrating thrombi less than 24 hours old, but neither method was of value in older lesions. Riba et al (1979) used the same method to evaluate experimentally induced coronary artery thrombi in dogs, with the same results: thrombi imaged at two and 22 hours after induction were seen very well, but by 24 hours, satisfactory imaging could not be obtained. Autologous [111]Indium-labelled platelets were used successfully in three patients by Davis et al (1979). Autologous platelets were labelled with [111]Indium oxine in Tyrode's solution, rather than plasma or saline. Platelet survival in vivo was satisfactory. It was possible in three patients to demonstrate an ilio femoral venous thrombosis, a renal vein thrombosis and ulcerated carotid plaques, all confirmed with contrast studies.

The use of [111]Indium, which has a half life of 2.8 days, thus shows some clinical promise. Although only thrombi less than 24 hours old could be demonstrated in animal studies, this may not prove an insurmountable obstacle in humans as this agent may be administered and then imaged over the course of several days and thus may be appropriate for screening. Another important practical consideration, however, is that preparation of autologous [111]Indium-labelled platelets requires care, technical expertise and a minimum of two hours.

Imaging of thrombi with labelled thrombolytic compounds gives the theoretical advantage of visualizing all but very old thrombi. There have been several attempts to label plasminogen, and Harwig et al (1977) have been successful in labelling canine plasminogen with both ^{123}I and ^{131}I without loss of enzymatic activity. In dogs with experimentally induced venous thrombosis, labelled plasminogen led to higher thrombus-to-blood ratios than did ^{125}I-fribrinogen in thrombi two days or more in age. Labelling in younger thrombi was variable. Imaging of even small thrombi, rather than merely point counting, was possible using ^{123}I-plasminogen. Questions arise in regard to lack of uptake in occlusive thrombi and only 80 per cent accuracy with small thrombi, but this technique is promising. Wong et al (1979) developed a method for labelling bovine thrombin and streptokinase-activated human plasmin with ^{99m}Tc without loss of enzymatic activity. This method deserves in vivo evaluation.

Persson and Darte (1977) reported a technique of labelling porcine plasmin with ^{99m}Tc, with preservation of enzymatic activity, and were able to image thrombi in rabbits after the administration of 2 mCi. This preparation has been used clinically by Olsson et al (1980), in conjunction with ^{125}I-fibrinogen point count scanning and contrast phlebography. In 93 patients referred because of the clinical suspicion of deep vein thrombosis, 500 microCuries ^{99m}Tc-plasmin was injected and point counting was carried out 10 and 30 minutes after injection. The sensitivity at 30 minutes was 94 per cent and the specificity 56 per cent, results which compare favorably to the results with the ^{125}I-fibrinogen test at 24 to 48 hours. With their modification of the ^{125}I-fibrinogen test, which involves elevation of the leg and counting of 12 points rather than eight, these authors found a high degree of accuracy in the thigh and lower accuracy in the lower leg in both tests, a surprising discrepancy from most authors' experiences with ^{125}I-fibrinogen. In view of these results, one wonders if labeled plasmin can be used to diagnose thrombi of all ages, if accuracy depends on size and location of the thrombus, and whether imaging as well as point counting is feasible.

Both streptokinase and urokinase have been radio-labelled for thrombus scintigraphy. To date, results with both are disappointing. Stable, enzymatically-active forms of ^{99m}Tc-streptokinase and urokinase have been prepared. The former was reported by Persson and Kempi (1976) to have possible value in humans in the diagnosis of deep vein thrombosis. The latter has been reported (Asavavekinkul et al, 1977) to have marked diminution of fibrinolytic activity in vitro, and both these authors and Weir et al (1976) showed little utility for this compound in thrombus localization in humans. These preparations retain theoretical advantages, but further developments are necessary to achieve practical usefulness.

Pedal venous pressure

The measurement of pedal venous pressure has been examined as a reflection of the presence or absence of deep venous thrombi (Gerlock, 1977). In correlation with phlebography, this simple, relatively non-invasive approach has had a high incidence of both false positive and false negative results (Ellwood, 1979; Martin, 1979). It does not, therefore, appear to have value as either a screening or a diagnostic test.

DIAGNOSIS OF PULMONARY EMBOLISM

It has become clear that pulmonary embolism is a process which is more common than is clinically apparent, that clinical diagnosis of either the presence or absence of this process is inaccurate, and that treatment of pulmonary embolism is effective but not without risk. The diagnosis, despite recent progress, still presents a formidable challenge.

Clinical diagnosis

The incidence of clinical signs and symptoms has been carefully documented and correlated with the diagnosis provided by angiography in the Urokinase-Pulmonary Embolism Trial (Sasahara, 1973). Pleuritic pain, cough, apprehension, dyspnea, tachypnea, tachycardia, hemoptysis, an S_3 or S_4 gallop and a loud P2 all occur in patients with acute pulmonary embolism. Dyspnea occurs in over 90 per cent of the patients, and the triad of dyspnea, tachypnea and pleuritic pain in 70 per cent, but these symptoms and signs occur also in patients with other processes. The classical triad of pleuritic pain, dyspnea and hemoptysis occurs in only 28 per cent of patients with angiographically proven pulmonary embolism. Cardiac findings are similarly non-specific: signs of acute onset of right-sided heart failure or of a new $S_1Q_3T_3$ pattern on electrocardiography are strongly suggestive of pulmonary embolism but are also consistent with an acute myocardial infarction. ST-T changes on an electrocardiogram are frequent but are clearly not specific. None of these features is sufficient to confirm the diagnosis of pulmonary embolism.

The awareness of certain predisposing factors, more than any symptom or sign, serves the clinician as a warning flag. It is important to keep the possibility of pulmonary embolism in mind in elderly patients at prolonged bed rest, neurological or neurosurgical patients, patients with abdominal, open urologic or hip operations, patients with deep vein thrombosis and patients with thrombotic diatheses.

Laboratory studies

The most helpful laboratory test is the arterial oxygen pressure (PaO_2), which is diminished in 85 to 100 per cent of patients with acute pulmonary embolism (Robin, 1977; Szucs et al, 1971). There are, however, patients who maintain normal arterial oxygen tension levels in the face of pulmonary emboli, even massive ones (Sasahara, 1973). Conversely, there are many other causes for depressed blood oxygen levels, aging among them, which are independent of pulmonary embolism. Thus, arterial oxygen tension measurements can serve only a limited, screening function.

Serum creatinine phosphokinase is generally elevated in acute myocardial infarction but not in pulmonary embolism, so measurement may help to distinguish these two entities (Coodley, 1969). Serum lactic acid dehydrogenase has been reported to be elevated in 39 to 80 per cent of patients with acute pulmonary embolism (Sasahara, 1973; Szucs et al, 1971).

Fibrin split products and fibrin-fibrinogen degradation products are frequently elevated in deep vein thrombosis and are more elevated in pulmonary embolism, albeit transiently. Levels of these factors are not specific for pulmonary embolism, however, because elevations occur following any process which activates the fibrinolytic system (e.g., surgery, malignancy, renal or hepatic disease, collagen vascular disease). Also, levels may rapidly fall to normal following a pulmonary embolus (Light & Bell, 1979; Cooper, 1974; Rickman et al, 1973). Bynum et al (1979) investigated the use of fibrin/fibrinogen degradation products (FDP/fdp) and soluble fibrin complexes (SFC) in patients with deep vein thrombosis, pulmonary embolism, or clinical conditions with a high risk of pulmonary embolic disease. They found that levels were generally highest for both FDP/fdp and SFC in patients with pulmonary embolism, elevated but not to as great a level in patients with deep vein thrombosis, and elevated to a still lesser extent in high risk patients who apparently did not have either pulmonary embolism or deep vein thrombosis. They also noted that FDP/fdp was 82 per cent specific in separating patients with pulmonary embolism from those in the high risk group, SFC was 92 per cent sensitive in distinguishing these two groups, and taking the two tests together, specificity was 91 per cent and sensitivity 97 per cent. These results, however, deal with patients, who either had been proven to have a pulmonary embolism or who were at high risk but were presumed *not* to have had such an event. This introduces a bias which has yet to be evaluated. The authors suggest that these two serum measurements may play an important ancillary role, for example in patients in whom the clinical suspicion is low or in whom the clinical suspicion is high but pulmonary angiography is contraindicated. As with other modalities, these tests are not yet accurate enough to use as the sole basis for diagnosing pulmonary embolism or deep vein thrombosis.

To achieve greater sensitivity with a single test, Nossel et al (1979) developed a measurement of plasma fibrinopeptide A, the first cleavage product in the conversion of fibrinogen to the fibrin monomer by thrombin. Normal serum levels were established, and levels were found to be elevated in patients with venous thromboembolism and with other disease states (malignancy, fractures, uremia) (Yudelman et al, 1978; Kockum, 1976). Yudelman et al (1978) demonstrated that fibrinopeptide A levels were generally elevated in patients with symptomatic deep vein thrombosis or with pulmonary embolism and remained high or increased again if extension of pulmonary embolism occurred. Heparin treatment promptly reduced the values to normal. Unfortunately, the test is cumbersome and, as indicated, lacks specificity. Measurement of plasma fibrinopeptide A levels may be useful for screening in conjunction with other modalities, such as ^{125}I-fibrinogen uptake or perfusion lung scanning, particularly in symptomatic patients without other active processes such as recent surgery.

In a recent report, radioimmunoassay for fibrinogen/fibrin fragment E was evaluated. In asymptomatic, postoperative venous thrombosis, fragment E levels were significantly elevated, but levels were also elevated in post-operative patients without venous thrombi. In patients who presented with symptoms, values were significantly higher in those who had venous thrombosis than in those who did not, and also higher than in normal volunteers (Zielinsky et al, 1979). This test thus appears to have promise in symptomatic patients but not as a screening test in asymptomatic post-operative patients. The accuracy of this test in a large group of patients and its applicability in pulmonary embolism are as yet unknown.

Measurement of free double-stranded DNA in plasma has disclosed that in most normal subjects levels are negligible. In systemic lupus erythematosus, levels are elevated if there is active central nervous system involvement or systemic vasculitis (Steinman, 1979). In patients suspected of having acute pulmonary embolism, free plasma DNA was present in 83 per cent of 23 patients proven to have emboli and none of 49 patients without emboli. Specifically, free plasma DNA was not present in patients with obvious venous thrombosis, myocardial infarction or pneumonia (Sipes, 1978). This test needs evaluation and validation in a larger number of patients but the initial studies suggest that free plasma DNA may prove useful in confirming or ruling out acute pulmonary embolism in patients with positive or equivocal lung scans.

Routine radiographic studies

Most patients with proven pulmonary embolism have abnormal chest radiographs (93 per cent, Moses, 1974). However, many patients suspected of having pulmonary embolism but subsequently proven not to have this disorder also have abnormal chest radiographs (McNeil et al, 1976; Baron, 1972), so that in general this does not aid in discrimination. Lung infiltrates and pleural effusion occur in about 50 per cent of patients with pulmonary embolism (Moses, 1974). In characterizing the effusions, Bynum & Wilson (1978) noted that they usually followed close upon the symptoms, were generally small (less than 15 per cent of the thorax) and unilateral, and were associated with pleuritic pain. In 55 per cent, there was associated consolidation, presumably indicative of pulmonary infarction. 83 per cent of those with consolidation, as compared to 38 per cent of those without, had bloody effusions.

In summary, a normal chest radiograph is unusual in a patient with pulmonary embolism. The most common findings are an infiltrate or an effusion, and there is usually associated chest pain. In practical terms, the major uses of chest radiographs are: (a) for comparison with lung scans, (b) as a baseline, (c) to rule out associated abnormalities, such as florid congestive heart failure.

There have been reports on the use of transmission computed tomography in both clinical and experimental infarction, but the results with this modality to date are not encouraging. Pleural based wedge-shaped densities were demonstrated in several patients shown by other modalities to have had pulmonary embolism (Sinner, 1978). Experimentally, computerized tomography had very low sensitivity in depicting balloon-induced or clot induced occlusions, either with or without contrast enhancement (Grossman et al, 1979).

Radionuclide studies

Lung scans form the cornerstone for the diagnosis of pulmonary embolism, although the debate about this technique continues to rage. There are two somewhat disparate opinions concerning lung scans, both of which have some objective support: lung scans are considered either the most reliable practical technique currently available, or less reliable than frequently claimed. Using an approach derived from the best available studies, lung scanning is clearly a safe and dependable approach. Lung scanning has limitations, but unlike many diagnostic tests, these limitations are fairly well defined.

Perfusion lung scanning involves the intravenous injection of ^{99m}Tc-labeled microspheres or macroaggregated albumin. These particles are about 30 microns in diameter, sufficiently large to occlude approximately 0.1 per cent of pre-capillary arterioles. Experimental studies have shown that abnormal perfusion patterns will result from 92 per cent of emboli occluding vessels 2.1 to 3.0 mm in diameter, and from 100 per cent of occlusions of vessels 3.0 mm or greater in diameter (Alderson, 1978). The very high sensitivity of perfusion lung scans has been supported by a number of clinical studies, which have shown that a normal perfusion lung scan is not compatible with significant pulmonary embolism (Bell & Simon, 1976; Robin, 1977).

The specificity of perfusion lung scans, however, is clearly not as great, as many non-embolic pulmonary processes can alter regional perfusion. Four major categories other than occlusion cause alterations in perfusion: extraluminal vascular compression, as by tumor; bronchopulmonary anastomoses, as in inflammatory disease; increased vascular resistance, as in pneumonia or congestive heart failure; regional hypoxemia and reflex vasoconstriction, as in chronic obstructive pulmonary disease or asthma (McNeil & Bettmann, 1981). To improve the specificity of radionuclide lung scans, ventilation lung scanning was introduced in 1970. Ventilation scanning using [133]Xenon (or [127]Xenon) is performed just prior to or immediately after the perfusion scan. The advantage to performing the ventilation study after the perfusion study is that if the latter is normal, as it is in a high percentage of patients, the former is unnecessary, an approach that saves both time and expense. Conversely, [133]Xenon has a half life of 5.3 days and a gamma emission of 80 kev, and it is eliminated via respiration, so the dose that can be given and the nature of the images are not optimal. If the ventilation study is performed after the perfusion study, there is additional degradation of the ventilation image by the emissions of the remaining ^{99m}Tc, probably leading to some loss of resolution (Biello, 1979). Nonetheless, most centers perform ventilation studies only subsequent to perfusion studies which are not clearly normal. An additional theoretical limitation of ventilation studies is that compensatory bronchoconstriction may occur following acute pulmonary embolism, generating an area of diminished ventilation in an area of diminished perfusion. This indisputably occurs in animals, but, since it appears to last for less than one hour, it is not thought to present a practical problem (Robinson et al, 1973; Alderson, 1976). Scans are obtained during first-breath inhalation or equilibrium and then during washout phase. A significant practical problem is that [133]Xenon ventilation studies require that the patient be able to breath-hold for 20 to 30 seconds to allow sufficient time for equilibration and imaging.

The applications of lung scans are well-defined: perfusion studies should be obtained in all patients suspected of having had pulmonary embolism, and ventilation scans are probably indicated in all of these patients who are able to co-operate except those who have unequivocally normal perfusion scans. Comparison then must be made with a good quality, recent chest radiograph. Interpretation involves evaluation of the size and number of perfusion defects, concordance or lack of concordance of perfusion defects with ventilation defects, and correspondence of scan abnormalities to the chest radiograph. Finally, correlation with the clinical status of the patient and the suspected likelihood of pulmonary embolism must be made. This is done with the clear realization that the clinical diagnosis of pulmonary embolism is unreliable.

The accuracy of the final interpretation of lung scans has been the subject of heated debate. As there are no large studies which objectively compare clinical suspicion of pulmonary embolism, lung scans and pulmonary angiography, the question must at present be addressed with incomplete evidence. In a retrospective study (McNeil, 1980) of 169 patients, all of whom had perfusion scintigraphy and pulmonary angiography, 39 per cent (66 patients) also had ^{133}Xenon single breath ventilation studies. As with most studies, all of these patients underwent pulmonary angiography because of abnormal scans, so the study is biased towards patients with pulmonary emboli. All cases in which scan abnormalities matched radiographic abnormalities were termed 'indeterminate', a category further discussed below. Twenty-one per cent of the patients had indeterminate scans.

11 per cent of patients had a single perfusion defect: in this group, angiography disclosed emboli in 50 per cent of those with lobar defects, 33 per cent of those with a segmental defect and none of those with a subsegmental defect. If a single area of ventilation-perfusion mismatch was present, patients with lung and lobar defects had pulmonary embolism, and those with segmental defects did *not*.

In patients with multiple perfusion defects (68 per cent), if the defects were subsegmental, angiography was positive in 7 per cent; if segmental, positive in 58 per cent; if lobar, 81 per cent. If there was an associated ventilation mismatch, the percentage rose from 7 to 25 with subsegmental lesions, 58 to 95 per cent for segmental lesions and 81 to 100 per cent for lobar lesions. The presence of matched ventilation/perfusion defects was associated with *no* positive angiograms. The combination of both ventilation/perfusion matches and mismatches is common in patients with chronic obstructive lung disease, and is essentially an indeterminate pattern. Thus, if a patient suspected of pulmonary embolism has a normal chest radiograph, a perfusion scan which demonstrates segmental or lobar defects and a normal ventilation scan, the likelihood of pulmonary embolism is at least 95 per cent (Fig. 12.4).

The indeterminate scan has been evaluated by several authors. Overall, about 25 to 35 per cent of patients with indeterminate scans who undergo pulmonary angiography have emboli (Biello et al, 1979a; McNeil, 1980). Again, there is probably a bias, as many patients with indeterminate scans are not thought to have a high likelihood of having pulmonary embolism and therefore do not undergo angiography. In a study of 111 patients who had indeterminate scans and subsequent angiography, Biello et al (1976b) found that if there was a ventilation/perfusion mismatch and the radiographic abnormality was substantially smaller than the perfusion abnormality, 89 per cent of patients had embolism. If the perfusion abnormalities were similar in size to or smaller than the radiographic abnormalities, the probabilities of pulmonary embolism were 26 per cent and 7 per cent respectively. Another study of indeterminate scans (Fischer, 1979) indicated that if the perfusion defects were lobar or segmental, the probability of pulmonary embolism was higher than if they were subsegmental (20 to 30 per cent vs. 9 per cent). Both of these studies indicated that specific radiographic abnormalities alone or in combination did not help diagnose pulmonary embolism.

There are several new approaches to pulmonary scintigraphy which may be useful. Baum et al (1979) suggested that flow studies following the intravenous injection of ^{99m}Tc preparations may demonstrate the main pulmonary artery and its branches and

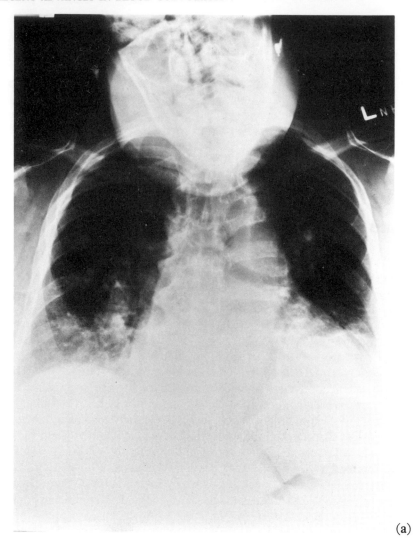

(a)

Fig. 12.4 Obese, sedentary 63 year old female with recent bouts of mild dyspnea and hypoxemia.
(a) Chest radiograph, frontal view: normal but for obesity and minor bibasilar fibrotic changes.
(b) ^{99m}Tc-MAA perfusion lung scan: frontal (top) and RPO (bottom) views demonstrate discrete defect conforming to anterior segment of right upper lobe, and possible defect in posterior segment as well.
(c) ^{133}Xenon ventilation scan: frontal projection after equilibration demonstrates normal ventilation.
(d) Pulmonary angiogram, right main pulmonary artery injection: Thrombus in branch to anterior segment of right upper lobe (open arrow) and probably non-occlusive thrombi in other major branches (solid arrows).

abnormalities in flow caused by pulmonary hypertension, occlusion or stenosis, and thus may be useful as an adjunct to routine perfusion scans. In dogs, it has been shown that the potent vasodilator isoproterenol usually leads to no alteration in perfusion of embolized areas, but it does lead to improved perfusion in experimental canine lobar pneumococcal pneumonia (Shepard et al, 1979). This study also indicated, however, that because of rapid partial dissolution of pulmonary emboli,

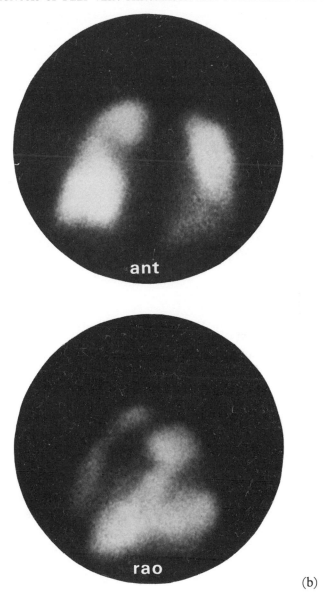

(b)

and perhaps because of reflex vasoconstriction in acute embolization, in some cases isoproterenol does improve perfusion following experimental embolization. An additional finding of this study was that the administration of isoproterenol improved cardiac output and decreased pulmonary vascular resistance, which suggests a possible therapeutic role for this medication.

[81]Krypton has been used for ventilation studies. Its short half life (13 sec) allows continuous inhalation and thus multiple projections, even in patients who are unable to cooperate. Because of the rapid decay, distribution is a reflection of ventilation only. As a result of the longer half-life of [133]Xenon, this isotope can only be used for a

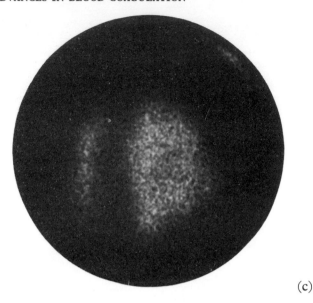

(c)

single inhalation and unless the patient is able to suspend respiration long enough to reach equilibration, only a single view can be obtained. Thus [81]Krypton would, in theory, be predicted to allow better image definition than [133]Xenon, but this remains to be demonstrated clinically (Fazio & Jones, 1975; Gorris et al, 1977; Gorris & Daspit, 1981).

$C^{15}O_2$ has recently been used for ventilation studies to aid in the diagnosis of pulmonary embolism. This cyclotron-produced isotope is inhaled and diffused across the pulmonary alveolar membrane. It is converted by erythrocyte carbonic anhydrase to $HC^{15}O_3$ and $H_2^{15}O_2$. The latter is distributed throughout the lungs, and is cleared by the capillaries at a rate proportional to the blood flow. Therefore, areas which have decreased flow because of embolism show delayed clearance of the $H_2^{15}O_2$ (Taplin et al, 1977). In a clinical comparison with the standard ventilation/perfusion studies and pulmonary angiography in 27 patients, Nichols and his colleagues (1978) showed that this technique was 87 per cent sensitive and 92 per cent specific. 56 per cent of the patients had angiographic evidence of pulmonary embolism. Sensitivity is probably about the same as standard ventilation/perfusion lung scintigraphy, but the specificity is much improved (92 per cent vs. 50 per cent in this series). There is one major drawback to this technique: the isotope $C^{15}O_2$ is cyclotron produced and is therefore available in only a few centers and is expensive. Further, careful consideration of patients with and without pulmonary embolism indicates that the accuracy of ventilation/perfusion scans combined with angiography in selected patients is at least as great as with $C^{15}O_2$ scans (Adelstein & McNeil, 1978). The physician is therefore once again faced with the question of whether this technique will be of any practical advantage compared to currently available methods.

Pulmonary angiography

Pulmonary angiography is the standard by which the accuracy of other techniques is measured, and it is widely accepted as the most accurate diagnostic test for pulmonary

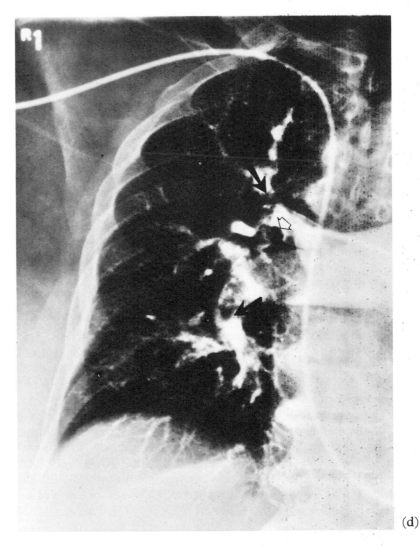

(d)

embolism short of post-mortem examination. Correlation with autopsy material has shown that pulmonary angiography is indeed very accurate (Dalen, 1971), and several studies have demonstrated relatively little inter-observer variation in the interpretation of angiograms (Bell & Simon, 1976; Sasahara et al, 1973). Other studies have shown that, as with contrast phlebography of the lower extremity, there is a limit of resolution for pulmonary angiography, and certain small emboli will not be seen with the usual techniques (Bynum et al, 1979a). Selective right or left pulmonary artery injections, superselective or wedge injections, and magnification studies have all been recommended to improve the resolution and accuracy (Bynum et al, 1979; Doughtery et al, 1980; Orta et al, 1979; Moses et al, 1974). Novelline and his colleagues (1978) examined the question of accuracy from a different point of view in a retrospective study of patients with abnormal perfusion lung scans and no evidence of embolism on pulmonary angiography. None of these 167 patients developed evidence of pulmonary embolism-related morbidity or mortality in a six month follow-up. Of the 20 patients who died, 10 were autopsied and three had small pulmonary emboli which may well have formed after the angiogram. Thus, if good quality pulmonary angiography does not show embolism, it is safe to withhold treatment.

The safety of pulmonary angiography requires consideration. Morbidity is less than 1 per cent, usually in the form of ventricular arryhthmias, hypotension, in situ thrombosis or renal failure. Mortality is less than 0.5 per cent (Bell & Simon, 1971; Dalen et al, 1971). In one series of 310 angiograms, complications were one ventricular perforation, five ventricular arrhythmias and no deaths or permanent disabilities (Sasahara, 1973). Certain groups of patients are at greater risk: those with acute myocardial infarctions, marked right or left heart failure or pulmonary hypertension. In these patients, the study can be made safer by selectively injecting a main pulmonary artery segment or even a branch vessel supplying the area in which the perfusion scan was abnormal. This practice avoids the higher dose of contrast and the consequent cardiovascular alterations caused by injection of the main pulmonary artery. As a matter of practice, we perform only selective right or left main pulmonary injections in patients with pulmonary artery systolic pressures greater than 60 mm Hg. In patients with *mean* pressures greater than 60 mm Hg, only subselective injections are performed.

Contrast material plays an important role in cardiovascular, endothelial, renal and allergy-like complications. The contrast agents in current use in the United States are hypertonic, hyperviscous, tri-iodinated, fully substituted organic compounds, containing sodium and methylglucamine as cations. The iodine content is on the order of 370 mEq/ml. This type of contrast agent is free of significant side effects in the vast majority of patients: overall mortality is about one per 10 to 30 000 examinations (Witten, 1975; Shehadi, 1975). The incidence varies, as allergy-like phenomena occur in 1 to 20 per cent of patients and renal failure occurs very rarely in patients with normal renal function but commonly, perhaps universally, in patients who have compromised renal function. Azotemic diabetics are particularly likely to have worsening of renal function after the administration of contrast. In all patients with renal failure, worsening appears to be related to the volume of contrast, and return to baseline renal function is the rule (Milman & Stage, 1974; Port et al, 1974). Patients with renal failure, particularly those with congestive heart failure as well, should undergo pulmonary angiography only if care is taken to limit the volume of contrast material used to an absolute minimum.

Allergic-like reactions create anxiety in physician and patient alike. The incidence of these reactions is about 1.2 per cent in the general population (Witten, 1975) and the vast majority of these reactions consist of mild urticaria. The incidence is higher in patients with a history of allergies (5 to 10 per cent) and still higher in patients with a prior reaction to contrast agents (20 per cent). The occurrence of a sensation of heat and of nausea is still more common, but these reactions are related to the hypertonicity of contrast and are not significant. Severe reactions, such as marked bronchospasm or cardiovascular collapse, are very unusual and the treatment is clear and effective: intubation equipment should be at hand, and an intravenous needle or catheter should be in place. For bronchospasm or cardiovascular collapse with tachycardia, epinephrine (Adrenalin) is administered. For cardiovascular collapse with bradycardia, atropine is administered, 0.6 to 0.8 mgm intravenously. These measures coupled with volume replacement as dictated by blood pressure are virtually always successful.

The finite occurrence of allergy-like reactions, particularly those that are life threatening, has led some authors to suggest that no contrast studies should be carried out in patients who have had a prior reaction to contrast. This approach may lead to greater danger than judicious re-use of contrast, e.g., in patients with indeterminate lung scans who are given anticoagulants needlessly. Zweiman et al (1975) suggested that patients who have had a prior reaction to contrast agents be given glucocorticoids before subsequent studies, although there are no data available to support the efficacy of this approach. Lalli (1974) performed contrast urography on a group of nine patients who had experienced shock and loss of consciousness with prior contrast urography. Even without pre-medication with glucocorticoids, none of the patients in this group experienced a reaction to repeat urography using a standard contrast agent. Shehadi's large study (1975) demonstrated a higher incidence of contrast reactions in patients who had previous (although not life-threatening) reactions to contrast injection than in the general population, but the incidence was still only 20 per cent.

Cardiovascular and hematologic parameters are also altered by contrast material, but these changes are for the most part mild and transient. Contrast suppresses myocardial contractility, provides a heavy osmotic load and may cause rouleaux formation and platelet aggregation near the catheter tip (Fischer & Thomson, 1978; Morris et al, 1979; Cohn et al, 1973; Schultz et al, 1977; Zir et al, 1973; Gafter et al, 1979). Finally, as has been described in contrast phlebography, contrast material has a direct toxic effect on endothelium which may lead to thrombosis (Bettmann et al, 1980). This effect is important in contrast phlebography but has not been demonstrated to have clinical import in other vascular studies.

In the development of new contrast agents the emphasis has been on decreasing tonicity and viscosity, which can be accomplished by primary chemical alterations, as with metrizamide (Almen, 1972), and by dimeric formulations, as with Ioxaglate (Holm & Prestholm, 1979; Grainger, 1979). Holm and Prestholm (1979) demonstrated less discomfort and less hemodynamic effect when Ioxaglate was used in comparison to standard contrast agent (Urografin 60). Albrechtsson and Olsson (1979) used a modified 125I-fibrinogen test to monitor the incidence of thrombosis following phlebography, and found that it was dramatically lowered when metrizamide rather than a conventional ionic compound was used.

Technical advances in pulmonary angiography have occurred in recent years. Either the brachial or the femoral approach may be used; the latter appears to have certain advantages. Using the percutaneous femoral approach, it is possible to avoid a cutdown, visualize the inferior vena cava and easily accomplish selective pulmonary artery studies. With a venous sheath, it is possible, although not generally indicated, to begin the procedure with a catheter with only an end hole or with a balloon and thus record a complete set of right-sided pressures, including pulmonary capillary wedge pressure. This catheter is then removed and replaced with a multiple side-hole catheter which allows safe injection of large volumes of contrast with little fear of causing wall damage or significant catheter recoil. The same can be accomplished via a basilic vein, but the vein is invariably occluded following the procedure. While this is probably harmless, it is also in most cases unnecessary.

A mandatory part of pulmonary angiography is measurement of right atrial and main pulmonary artery pressures, as these affect the safety of the study for the patient, the site at which injection should be made (i.e., main pulmonary artery vs. selective studies) and the amount of contrast agent used.

Grollman et al (1970) described a pre-shaped 'pig-tail' catheter which was modified by Beachley et al (1980) to facilitate entrance into the pulmonary outflow tract, with or without a guide wire. Others have used balloon-tipped, flow directed catheters for segmental pulmonary angiography in critically-ill patients who have Swan-Ganz catheters in place for monitoring. These catheters have also been used in patients in whom main pulmonary artery or right or left pulmonary artery injections were not definitive (Dougherty et al, 1980; Orta et al, 1979; Bynum et al, 1979). These techniques have not been associated with complications.

In summary, pulmonary angiography is an accurate and safe procedure, which can be made even safer by the use of selective rather than main pulmonary artery injections, by careful attention to detail (angiographic, hemodynamic and clinical), and probably by the use of the newer non-ionic and dimeric contrast agents. With these details attended to, it is almost certainly safer to perform pulmonary angiography in patients with the clinical and/or scintigraphic suspicion of pulmonary embolism than it is to base a treatment decision on incomplete data.

REFERENCES

Adelstein S J, McNeil B J 1978 A new diagnostic test for pulmonary embolism: How good and how costly? (editorial) New England Journal of Medicine 299 (6): 305–307

Albrechtsson U & Olsson C G 1976 Thrombotic side effects of lower limb phlebography. The Lancet i: 723–724

Albrechtsson U, Olsson C G 1979 Thrombosis after phlebography: A comparison of two contrast media. Cardiovascular Radiology 2: 9–14

Alderson P O, Rujanavech N, Secker-Walker R H, McKnight R C 1976 The role of ^{133}Xe ventilation studies in the scintigraphic detection of pulmonary embolism. Radiology 120: 633–640

Almen T 1973 Metrizamide-A non-ionic water-soluble contrast medium. Acta Radiologica: Supplement 335

Asavavekinkul S, Forbes C D, McDougall I R 1977 Is ^{99}Tc-Urokinase a useful agent for detection of deep venous thrombosis? Clinical Nuclear Medicine 2 (7): 235–238

Athanasoulis C A 1975 Phlebography for the diagnosis of deep leg vein thrombosis. In: Fratontoni J, Wessler S (eds) Prophylactic therapy of deep vein thrombosis and pulmonary embolism. DHEW Publication No. (NIH) 76: 866 62–76

Baum, S, d'Avignon M B, Latshaw R F 1979 Radionuclide pulmonary arteriography. Clinical Nuclear Medicine 4 (11): 461–464

Barnes R W, Wu K K, Hoak J C 1975 Fallibility of the clinical diagnosis of venous thrombosis. Journal of American Medical Association 234 (6): 605–607

Barnes R W, Russell H E, Wu K K, Hoak J C 1976 Accuracy of doppler ultrasound in clinically suspected venous thrombosis of the calf. Surgery, Gynecology and Obstetrics 143: 425–428

Beachley M C, Tisnado J, Konerding K, Vines F S 1980 Alternate technique for pulmonary arteriography. American Journal of Roentgenology 134: 195–196

Bell W R, Simon T L 1976 A comparative analysis of pulmonary perfusion scans with pulmonary angiograms. From a national cooperative study. American Heart Journal 92: 700–706

Benedict K T Jr., Wheeler H B, Patwardhan N A 1977 Impedance plethysmography: correlation with contrast phlebography. Radiology 125: 695–699

Berberich J, Hirsch S 1923 Die Roentgenologische Darstellung der Arterien und Venen im Lebenden Menschen. Klinische Wochenschrift 49: 226

Bergvall U 1971 Phlebography in acute deep venous thrombosis of the lower extremity. Acta Radiologica Diagnosis 11: 148–166

Bergvist D, Hallböök T 1979 Thermography for diagnosis of deep vein thrombosis and screening of postoperative venous thrombosis. Thrombosis and Hemostasis 42 (1): 28 (ab)

Bettmann M A & Paulin S 1977 Leg phlebography: the incidence, nature and modification of undesirable side effects. Radiology 122 (1): 101–104

Bettmann M A, Salzman E W, Rosenthal D, Clagett P, Davies G, Nebesar R, Rabinov K, Ploetz J, Skillman J 1980 Reduction of venous thrombosis complicating phlebography. American Journal of Roentgenology 134: 1169–1172

Biello D R, Mattar A G, Osei-Wusu A, Alderson P O, McNeil B J, Siegel B A 1979 Interpretation of indeterminate lung scintigrams. Radiology 133 (1): 189–194

Biello D, Mattar A G, McKnight R C, Siegel B A 1979 Ventilation-perfusion studies in suspected pulmonary embolism. American Journal of Roentgenology 133: 1033–1037

Biland L, Hull R, Hirsh J, Milner M 1979 The use of electromyography to detect muscle contraction responsible for falsely positive impedance plethysmographic results. Thrombosis Research 14: 811–816

Browse N L 1972 The ^{125}I-fibrinogen test. Archives of Surgery 104: 160–163

Bynum L J, Wilson J E 1978 Radiographic features of pleural effusions in pulmonary embolism. American Review of Respiratory Diseases 117: 829–834

Bynum L J, Crotty C M, Wilson J E III 1979 Diagnostic value of tests of fibrin metabolism in patients predisposed to pulmonary embolism. Archives of Internal Medicine 139: 283–285

Bynum L J, Wilson J E, Christensen E E, Sorensen C 1979 Radiographic techniques for balloon-occlusion pulmonary angiography. Radiology 133 (2): 518–520

Carlson P A 1969 Phlebography of the lower extremity and the pelvic region. American Journal of Surgery 118: 632–636

Chervu L R 1979 Radiopharmaceuticals in cardiovascular nuclear medicine. Seminars in Nuclear Medicine 9 (4): 241–256

Coe N P, Collins R E C, Klein L A, Bettmann M A, Skillman J J, Shapiro R M, Salzman E W 1978 Prevention of deep vein thrombosis in urological patients: A controlled randomized trial of low dose heparin and external pneumatic compression boots. Surgery 83 (2): 232–234

Coel M N, Lasser E C 1971 A pharmacologic basis for peripheral vascular resistance changes with contrast media injections. American Journal of Roentgenology 111: 802–806

Cohn P F, Horn H R, Teichholz L E, Kreulen T H, Herman M V, Gorlin R 1973 Effects of angiographic contrast medium on left ventricular function in coronary artery disease. American Journal of Cardiology 32: 21–26

Coodley E L 1969 Enzyme profiles in the evaluation of pulmonary infarction. Journal of American Medical Association 207: 1307

Cooke E D, Pilcher M F 1974 Deep vein thrombosis: preclinical diagnosis by thermography. British Journal of Surgery 61: 971–978

Coon W W, Coller F A 1959 Clinicopathologic correlation in thromboembolism. Surgery, Gynecology and Obstetrics 109: 259–269

Cooper H A, Bowie E J W, Owen C A Jr. 1974 Evaluation of patients with increased fibrinolytic split products (FSP) in their serum. Mayo Clinic Proceedings 49: 654–657

Cranley J J 1975 Diagnostic tests for venous thrombosis. In: Vascular surgery, Volume II, Peripheral venous diseases, Cranley J J (ed), Harper and Row, Hagerstown Maryland, 59–78

Cranley J J 1975 Phleborrheography, Vascular surgery Vol II, Cranley J J (ed), Harper and Row, Hagerstown, Maryland, 79–95

Cranley J J 1978 Comparative value of tests for the diagnosis of venous thrombosis-invited commentary. World Journal of Surgery 2 (1): 36–38

Davis H H, Heaton W A, Siegel B A Mathias C J, Joist J H, Sherman L A, Welch M J 1978 Scintigraphic detection of atherosclerotic lesions and venous thrombi in man using indium-III labeled autologous platelets. Lancet 1: 1185–1187

Dalen J E, Brooks H L, Johnson L W, Meister S G, Szucs M M, Dexter L 1971 Pulmonary angiography in acute pulmonary embolism: Indications, techniques and results in 367 patients. American Heart Journal 81: 175–185

DeNardo S J, DeNardo G L 1977 Iodine-123-fibrinogen scintigraphy. Seminars in Nuclear Medicine 7 (3): 245–251

DeNardo G L, DeNardo S, Barnett C A, Newcomer K A, Jansholt A L, Carretta R F, Rose A W 1977 Assessment of conventional criteria for the early diagnosis of thrombophlebitis with the ^{125}I-firbinogen uptake test. Radiology 125: 765 768

Dougherty J E, La Sala A F, Fieldman A 1980 Bedside pulmonary angiography utilizing an existing Swan-Ganz catheter. Chest 77 (1): 43–46

Dunnick R H, Schuete W H, Shawker T H 1979 Ultrasonic demonstration of thrombus in the common carotid artery. American Journal of Roentgenology 133: 544–545

Ellwood R A, Lee W B 1979 Pedal venous pressure: Correlation with presence and site of deep-venous abnormalities. Radiology 131 (1): 73–74

Fazio F, Jones T 1975 Assessment of regional ventilation by continuous inhalation of radioactive krypton-81m. British Medical Journal 3: 673–676

Fischer H W, Thomson K R 1978 Contrast media in coronary arteriography: A review. Investigative Radiology 13: 450–459

Fischer K C, McNeil B J 1979 The indeterminate lung scan: Its characteristics and its association with pulmonary embolism. European Journal of Nuclear Medicine 4: 49–53

Flanc C, Kakkar V V, Clarke M B 1968 The detection of venous thrombosis of the legs using ^{125}I-labeled fibrinogen. British Journal of Surgery 55: 742–747

Franck O, Alwens W 1910 Kreislaufstudien am roentgenshirm. Muenchner Medizinische Wochenschrift 57: 950

Freiman D G, Suyemoto J, Wessler S 1965 Frequency of pulmonary thromboembolism in man. New England Journal of Medicine 272: 1278–1280

Gafter U, Greter D, Zevin D Catz R, Djaldetti M 1979 Inhibition of platelet aggregation by contrast media. Radiology 132 (2): 341–342

Gerlock A J Jr 1977 Measurement of pedal venous pressure: A screening procedure in the detection of deep-vein thrombosis and occlusion. Radiology 122: 673–676

Goodwin D A, Bushberg J T, Doherty P W, Lipton M J, Conley F K, Diamantic C I, Meares C F 1978 Indium-III-labeled autologous platelets for location of vascular thrombi in humans. Journal of Nuclear Medicine 19: 626–634

Goris M L, Daspit S G, Walter J T, McRae J, Lamb J 1977 Applications of ventilation lung imaging with [81m]krypton. Radiology 122: 399–403

Goris M L, Daspit S G 1981 Krypton 81 m ventilation scintigraphy for the diagnosis of pulmonary emboli. In press

Grainger R G 1979 A clinical trial of a new low osmolality contrast medium. British Journal of Radiology 52: 781–786

Grollman J H Jr, Gyepes M T, Helmer E 1970 Transfemoral selective bilateral pulmonary arteriography with a pulmonary-artery-seeking catheter. Radiology 96: 202–209

Grossman Z D, Wistow B W, McAfee J G, Subramanian G, Thomas F D, Henderson R W, Rohner R F, Roskopf M L 1978 Platelets labeled with oxine complexes of Tc-99m and In-Ill. Part 2. Localization of experimentally induced vascular lesions. Journal of Nuclear Medicine 19 (5): 488–491

Grossman Z D, Gagne G, Zens A, Thomas F D, Chamberlain C C, Singh A, Cohen W N, Heitzman E R 1979 Transmission computed tomography, Tc-99m MAA scintigraphy, and plain chest radiography after experimentally produced acute pulmonary arterial occlusion in the dog. Journal of Nuclear Medicine 20 (12): 1251–1256

Hale T I, Jucker A 1978 ^{99m}Tc-fibrinogen as a thrombus-imaging agent. (Correspondence) British Journal of Radiology 51: 139–140

Hallböök T, Ling L 1972 Resting blood flow in deep venous thrombosis of the leg. Acta Chirurgica Scandinavica 138: 581–584

Harwig S L, Harwig J F, Coleman R E, Welch M J 1976 In vivo behaviour of ^{99m}Tc-fibrinogen and its potential as a thrombus-imaging agent. Journal of Nuclear Medicine 17: 40–46

Harwig S L, Harwig J F, Sherman L A, Coleman R E, Welch M J 1977 Radioiodinated plasminogen: An imaging agent for pre-existing thrombi. Journal of Nuclear Medicine 18: 42–45

Harris W H, Salzman E W, Athanasoulis C A, Waltman A, Baum S, De Sanctis R, Potsaid M, Sise H 1975 Comparison of ^{125}I-fibrinogen count scanning with phlebography for detection of venous thrombi after elective hip surgery. New England Journal of Medicine 292 (15): 665–667

Hayt D B, Blatt C J, Freeman L M 1977 Radionuclide venography: Its place as a modality for the investigation of thromboembolic phenomena. Seminars in Nuclear Medicine VII (3): 263–281

Henkin R E, Yao J S T, Quinn J L III, Bergan J J 1974 Radionuclide venography (RNV) in lower extremity venous disease. Journal of Nuclear Medicine 15 (3): 171–175

Hirsh J & Hull R 1978 Comparative value of tests for the diagnosis of venous thrombosis. World Journal of Surgery 2: 27–38

Hobbs J T, Davies J W L 1960 Detection of venous thrombosis with ^{131}I-labeled fibrinogen in the rabbit. The Lancet 2: 134–135

Holm M, Praestholm J 1979 Ioxaglate, A new low osmolar contrast medium used in femoral angiography. British Journal of Radiology 52: 169–172

Homans J 1942 Thrombosis as a complication of phlebography. JAMA 119: 36–42

Hull R, Van Aken W G, Hirsh J 1976 Impedance plethysmographyusing the occlusive cuff technique in the diagnosis of venous thrombosis. Circulation 53: 696–700

Hull R, Taylor D W, Hirsh J, Sackett D L, Powers P, Turpie A G G, Walker I 1978 Impedance plethysmography: the relationship between venous filling and sensitivity and specificity for proximal vein thrombosis. Circulation 58: 898–902

Hume M, Sevitt S, Thomas D P 1970 Venous thrombosis and pulmonary embolism. Harvard University Press, Cambridge, Massachusetts

Jacques P F, Richey W A, Ely C A, Johnson G Jr 1977 Doppler ultrasonic screening prior to venography for deep vein thrombosis. American Journal of Roentgenology 129: 451–452

Johnson W L 1974 Evaluation of Newer Techniques for the diagnosis of venous thrombosis. Journal of Surgical Research 16 (5): 473–481

Kakkar V V, Flanc C, Howe C T, Clarke M B 1969 Natural history of postoperative deep vein thrombosis. The Lancet 2: 230–232

Kakkar V V 1972 The diagnosis of deep vein thrombosis using the ^{125}I-fibrinogen test. Archives of Surgery 104: 152–159

Kerrigan G N W, Buchanan M R, Cade J F, Regoeczi E, Hirsh J 1974 Investigation of the mechanism of false positive ^{125}I-labeled fibrinogen scans. British Journal of Hematology 26: 469–473

Kiil J, Møller J C 1978 Ultrasound and clinical diagnosis of deep vein thrombosis of the leg. Acta Radiologica Diagnosis 20 (2): 292–298

Knight L C, Primean J L, Siegel B A, Welch M J 1978 Comparison of In-III-labeled platelets and iodinated fibrinogen for the detection of deep venous thrombosis. Journal of Nuclear Medicine 19 (8): 891–894

Kockum C 1976 Radioimmunoassay of fibrinopeptide A-clinical applications. Thrombosis Research 8: 225–236

Krohn K A, Knight L C 1977 Radiopharmaceuticals for thrombus detection: Selection, preparation and critical evaluation. Seminars in Nuclear Medicine VII (3): 219–228

Lalli A F 1975 Urography, shock reaction and repeated urography. American Journal of Roentgenology 125 (1): 264–268 (editorial)

Lea Thomas M 1970 Gangrene following peripheral phlebography of the legs. British Journal of Radiology 43: 528–530

Lea Thomas L, McAllister V, Tonge K 1971 Simplified phlebography in deep venous thrombosis. Clinical Radiology 22: 490–494

Lea Thomas M, O'Dwyer J A 1977 Site of origin of deep vein thrombus in the calf. Acta Radiologica Diagnosis 18 (4): 418–424

Light R W, Bell W R 1974 LDH and fibrinogen-fibrin degradation products in pulmonary embolism. Archives of Internal Medicine 133: 372

Martin E C, Cohen L, Sawyer P N, Gordon D H 1979 Supine pedal venous pressure measurement in patients with venous disease. Radiology 131 (1): 75–77

McDougall I R, Baumert J E, Lantieri R L 1979 Evaluation of ^{111}In leukocyte whole body scanning. American Journal Roentgenology 133: 849–854

McIlmoyle G, Davis H H, Welch M J, Primeau J L, Sherman L A, Siegel B A 1977 Scintigraphic diagnosis of experimental pulmonary embolism with In-111-labeled platelets. Journal of Nuclear Medicine 18: 910–914

McIlroy R F 1972 The routine use of ultrasound for the diagnosis of postoperative deep-vein thrombosis in a district general hospital. British Journal of Surgery 59: 133–135

McNeil B J, Hessel S J, Branch W T, Bjork L, Adelstein S J 1976 Measures of clinical efficacy. III The value of the lung scan in the evaluation of young patients with pleuritic chest pain. Journal of Nuclear Medicine 17 (3): 163–169

McNeil B J 1980 Ventilation-perfusion studies and the diagnosis of pulmonary embolism. Journal of Nuclear Medicine. J B Lippincott 21: 319–323

McNeil B J, Bettmann M A 1981 The diagnosis of pulmonary embolism-1980. In Salzman E and Hirsh J (eds), Textbook of Hematology: in press

McLachlan M S F, Thomson J G, Taylor D W, Kelley M E, Sachett D L 1979 Observer variation in the interpretation of lower limb venograms. American Journal of Roentgenology 132: 227–229

Milman N, Stage P 1974 High dose urography in advanced renal failure. Acta Radiologica Diagnosis 15 (1): 104–112

Milne R M, Grifiths J M I, Gunn A A, Ruckley C V 1971 Post-operative deep venous thrombosis: A comparison of diagnostic techniques. The Lancet 2: 445–447

Morris T W, Francis M, Fischer H W 1979 A comparison of the cardiovascular responses to carotid injections of ionic and non-ionic contrast media. Investigative Radiology 14: 217–223

Moses D C, Silver T M, Bookstein J J 1974 The complementary roles of chest radiography, lung scanning and selective pulmonary angiography in the diagnosis of pulmonary embolism. Circulation 49: 179–188

Mullick S C, Wheeler H B, Songster G P 1970 Diagnosis of deep venous thrombosis by measurement of electrical impedance. American Journal of Surgery 119: 417–422

Negus D, Pinto D J Le Quesne L P, Brown N 1968 ^{125}I-labeled fibrinogen in the diagnosis of deep vein thrombosis and its correlation with phlebography. British Journal of Surgery 55: 835–839

Nichols A B, Cochavi S, Hales C A, Strauss H W, McKusick K A, Waltman A C, Beller G A 1978 Scintigraphic detection of pulmonary emboli by serial positron imaging of inhaled ^{15}O-labeled carbon dioxide. New England Journal of Medicine 299 (6): 279–284

Nossel H L, Yudelman I, Canfield R E, Butler V P Jr, Spanoudis K, Wilner G D, Qureshi G D 1974 Measurement of fibrinopeptide a in human blood. Journal of Clinical Investigation 54 (1): 43–53

Novelline R Z, Battarowich O H, Athanasoulis C A, Waltman A C, Greenfield A J, McKusick K A 1978 The clinical course of patients with suspected pulmonary embolism and a negative pulmonary arteriogram. Radiology 126: 561–567

Orta D A, Eisen S, Yergin B M, Olsen G N 1979 Segmental pulmonary angiography in the critically ill patient using a flow-directed catheter. Chest 76: 269–273

Olsson C G, Albrechtsson U, Darte L, Persson R B R 1980 ^{99m}Tc plasmin for rapid detection of deep vein thrombosis In press

Olsson C G, Albrechtsson U 1980 A modified ^{125}I-fibrinogen technique in suspected deep vein thrombosis. A comparison with plethysmography and phlebography. Acta Medica Scandinavica In press

Persson B R R, Kempi V 1975 Labelling and testing of ^{99m}Tc-streptokinase for the diagnosis of deep vein thrombosis. Journal of Nuclear Medicine 16 (6): 474–477

Persson B R R, Darte L 1977 Labelling plasmin with technetium-99m for scintigraphic localization of thrombi. International Journal of Applied Radiation and Isotopes 28: 97–104

Port F K, Wagoner R D, Fulton R E 1974 Acute renal failure after angiography. American Journal of Roentgenology 121: 544–550

Prescott S M, Tikoff G, Coleman R E, Richards K L, Armstrong J D Jr, Hershgold E L, McDaniel D C, Ganchan R P 1978 ^{131}I-labeled fibrinogen in the diagnosis of deep vein thrombosis of the lower extremities. American Journal of Roentgenology 131: 451–453

Riba A L, Thakur M L, Gottschalk A, Zaret B L 1979 Imaging experimental coronary artery thrombosis with indium-ill platelets. Circulation 60 (4): 767–775

Rickman F D, Handin R, Howe J P, Alpert J S, Dexter L, Dalen J E 1973 Fibrin split products in acute pulmonary embolism. Annals of Internal Medicine 79: 664–668

Ritchie W G M, Lynch P R, Stewart G J 1974 The effect of contrast media on normal and inflamed canine veins. Investigative Radiology 9 (6): 444–455

Ritchie W G M, Lapayowker M S, Soulen R L 1979 Thermographic diagnosis of deep venous thrombosis; anatomically based diagnostic criteria. Radiology 132 (2): 321–329

Robin E D 1977 Overdiagnosis and overtreatment of pulmonary embolism: The emperor may have no clothes. Annals of Internal Medicine 87: 775–781

Robinson A T, Puckett C L, Green J D 1973 Demonstration of small-airway bronchonstriction following pulmonary embolism. Radiology 109: 283–286

Rogoff S M, DeWeese J A 1960 Phlebography of the lower extremity. Journal of the American Medical Association 172: 1599–1606

Sasahara A A, Hyers T M, Cole C M, Ederer F, Murray J A, Wenger N K, Sherry S, Stengle J M 1973 The urokinase pulmonary embolism trial, a national cooperative study. Chapter 10: Clinical and electrocardiographic observations. Circulation 47 (4): 60–65

Sasahara A A, Sharma G U R K Parisi, A F 1979 New developments in the detection and prevention of venous thromboembolism. American Journal of Cardiology 43: 1214–1224

Schulze Von B, Riester P, Blanke D, Fees K, Lehnard G Die Wirkung trijodierter Roentgenkontrastmittel auf gerinnung Fibrinolyse und Thrombozyten. Arzneim-Forsch 27 (11): 2128–2133

Sevitt S, Gallagher N 1961 Venous thrombosis and pulmonary embolism: A clinico-pathological study in injured and burned patients. British Journal of Surgery 48: 475–489

Sevitt S 1969 Venous thrombosis in injured patients (with some observations on pathogenesis), in Sherry S and Brinkhous K M and Genton E (eds) *Thrombosis*, Washington, D.C., National Academy of Sciences 29–49

Shehadi W 1975 Adverse reactions to intravenously administered contrast media. American Journal of Roentgenology 124: 142–152

Shepard J W Jr, Hauer D, Sgroi V, Moser K M 1979 Effect of isoproterenol on distribution of perfusion in embolized dog lungs. Journal of Nuclear Medicine 20 (9): 950–955

Sinner W N 1978 Computed tomographic patterns of pulmonary thromboembolism and infarction. Journal of Computer Assisted Tomography 2: 395–399

Sipes J N, Suratt P M, Teates C D, Barada F A, Davis J S, Tegtmeyer C J 1978 A prospective study of plasma DNA in the diagnosis of pulmonary embolism. American Review of Respiratory Diseases 118: 475–478

Skillman J J, Collins R E C, Coe N P, Goldstein B S, Shapiro R M, Zervas N T, Bettmann M A, Salzman E W 1978 Prevention of deep vein thrombosis in neurosurgical patients: A controlled, randomized trial of external pneumatic compression boots. Surgery 83 (3): 354–358

Steer M L, Spotnitz A J, Cohen S I, Paulin S, Salzman E W 1973 Limitations of impedance phlebography for diagnosis of venous thrombosis. Archives of Surgery 106: 44–48

Steinman C R 1979 Circulating DNA in systemic lupus erythematosus. American Journal of Medicine 67: 429–435

Strandness D E Jr., Schultz R D, Sumner D S, Rushmer R F 1967 Ultrasonic flow detection. A useful technique in the evaluation of peripheral vascular disease. American Journal of Surgery 113: 311–320

Strandness D E Jr. 1977 Thrombosis detection by ultrasound, plethysmography and phlebography. Seminars in Nuclear Medicine VII (3): 213–217

Sumner D S, Baker D W, Strandness D E Jr. 1968 The ultrasonic velocity detector in a clinical study of venous disease. Archives of Surgery 97: 75–80

Szucs M M, Brooks H L, Grossman W, Banas J S Jr., Meister S G, Dexter L, Dalen J E 1971 Diagnostic sensitivity of laboratory findings in acute pulmonary embolism. Annals of Internal Medicine 74: 161–166

Taplin G V, Chopra S K, Elam D 1977 Imaging experimental pulmonary ischemic lesions after inhalation of a diffusible radioaerosol: concise communication. Journal of Nuclear Medicine 18: 250–254

Thakur M L, Welch M J, Joist J H & Coleman R E 1976 Indium-111 labeled platelets: Studies on preparation and evaluation of in vitro and in vivo functions. Thrombosis Research 9: 345–357

Thakur M L, Lavender J P, Arnot R N, Silvester D J, Segal A W 1977 Indium-111 labeled autologous leukocytes in man. Journal of Nuclear Medicine 18: 1014–1021

Ulmsten U, Bernstein K, Jacobson L, Mattson S, Astedt B 1979 New technique for localization of deep vein thrombosis. The Lancet 2: 962–963

Webber M M, Bennett L R, Cragin M, Webb R Jr 1969 Thrombophlebitis-demonstration by scintiscanning. radiology 92: 620–623

Webber M M 1977 Labeled albumin aggregates for detection of clots. Seminars in Nuclear Medicine VII (3): 253–261

Weir G J, Wentzel F J, Roberts R C, Sautter R D 1976 Visualization of thrombi with technetium-99m urokinase. The Lancet 2: 341–342, (ADT 963–963)

Wheeler H B, O'Donnell J A, Anderson F A Jr. and Benedict K Jr. 1974 Occlusive impedance phlebography. a diagnostic procedure on venous thrombosis and pulmonary embolism. Progress in Cardiovascular Disease 17: 199–205, 11–12

Winzelberg G G, McKusick K A, Strauss H W, Waltman A C, Greenfield A J 1979 Evaluation of gastrointestinal bleeding by red blood cells labeled in vivo with technetium-99m. Journal of Nuclear Medicine 20 (10): 1080–1086

Wistow B W, Grossman Z D, McAfee J G, Subramanian G, Henderson R W, Roskopf M L 1978 Labelling of platelets with oxine complexes of Tc-99m and In-111. Part I. In vitro studies and survival in the rabbit. Journal of Nuclear Medicine 19 (5): 483–487

Witten D M 1975 Reactions to urographic contrast media. Journal of American Medical Association 231: 974–977

Wong D W, Tanaka T, Mishkin R, Lee T 1979 In vitro assessment of Tc-99m labeled bovine thrombin and streptokinase-activated human plasmin: Concise Communication. Journal of Nuclear Medicine 20 (9): 967–972

Yao J S T, Henkin R E, Conn J Jr., Quinn J L III, Bergan J J 1973 Combined isotope venography and lung scanning. Archives of Surgery 107: 146–151

Yudelman I M, Nossel H K, Kaplan K L, Hirsh J 1978 Plasma fibrinopeptide a levels in symptomatic venous thromboembolism. Blood 51 (6): 1189–1195

Zielinsky A, Hirsh J, Hull R, Powers P, Turpie A G G, Han P 1979 Evaluation of radioimmunoassay for fragment E (Fg E) in the diagnosis of venous thrombosis. Thrombosis and Hemostasis 42 (1): 28 (ab)

Zir M, Carvalho A C, Harthorne J W, Colman R W, Lees R S 1974 Effect of contrast agents on platelet aggregation and ^{14}C-serotonin release. New England Journal of Medicine 291 (3): 134–135

Zweiman B, Mishkin M, Hildreth E A 1975 An approach to the performance of contrast studies in contrast material-reactive persons. Annals of Internal Medicine 83: 159–162

13. The clinical evaluation of antiplatelet drugs

Michael Gent

Introduction

The important role of platelets in the genesis of thrombi and the development of atherosclerosis is now well recognized. This, and the identification of drugs that suppress platelet function, has provided hope of significant developments in the prophylaxis of clinical thromboembolic disease. However, the potential of such drugs relates to their ability to interfere with platelet reactions which are associated with thrombosis and is dependent on the nature of the thrombogenic stimulus, which is likely to vary between patient groups. It is not yet possible to predict the clinical effectiveness of drugs from tests of platelet function, or from experimental models of thrombosis in animals; hence, their assessment must be based on the results of clinical trials using appropriate thromboembolic events as outcome measures.

There are increasing numbers of reports of clinical studies of the antithrombotic effect of platelet suppressing drugs. These have included case reports, retrospective studies and prospective trials with wide variation in design and quality. It is the purpose of this review to evaluate critically the available data as a basis for establishing the current status of platelet inhibiting drugs.

Platelet suppressing drugs

The interaction of platelets with exposed collagen leads to the sequential freeing of arachidonate, cyclic endoperoxides, and thromboxane A_2, a potent platelet aggregant and vasoconstrictor. Aspirin irreversibly acetylates platelet cyclo-oxygenase thus preventing the conversion of arachidonate to cyclic endoperoxides and hence blocking thromboxane A_2 synthesis. Aspirin also blocks synthesis by the cells of vessel walls of PGI_2 (prostacyclin), a platelet anti-aggregant and potent vasodilator. Aspirin in low doses will block platelet cyclo-oxygenase whereas much higher doses are required to block vessel wall cyclo-oxygenase (Masotti et al, 1979). Furthermore, platelets are incapable of synthesizing more cyclo-oxygenase (Roth & Majerus, 1977), but the cells of vessel walls have this capacity and therefore regain the ability to synthesize PGI_2 within hours following aspirin administration (Czervionke et al, 1979). Clinical and laboratory evidence suggests considerably greater antithrombotic effect in males by comparison to females (Harris et al, 1977; Kelton et al, 1978). Aspirin has been shown to inhibit experimental thrombosis in animals (Mustard & Packham, 1980).

Sulfinpyrazone, a uricosuric agent closely related to phenylbutazone, also inhibits platelet cyclo-oxygenase but, in contrast to aspirin, the effect is reversible and dependent upon the serum concentration (Ali & McDonald, 1978). Sulfinpyrazone may also inhibit PGI_2 synthesis by the vessel wall, but at the concentrations which can be achieved in vivo, the effect is minimal (Gordon & Pearson, 1978). Sulfinpyrazone protects endothelial cells (Harker et al, 1978) and prolongs shortened platelet survival time (Smythe et al, 1965). This drug inhibits experimental thrombosis in animals (Mustard & Packham, 1980).

The elevation of cyclic AMP in platelets decreases their adherence to damaged vessel walls and inhibits aggregation, release of granule contents, and shape change in response to aggregating and release-inducing agents (Mustard & Packham, 1978). Dipyridamole, initially introduced as a vasodilator, inhibits platelet phosphodiesterase, thereby decreasing cyclic AMP breakdown (Mustard & Packham, 1978). In experimental animals, dipyridamole inhibits platelet adherence to collagen (Cazenave et al, 1978), subendothelium (Kinlough-Rathbone et al, 1978), and artificial surfaces (Harker et al, 1979).

Clofibrate was initially developed for the management of hypercholesterolemia although it was subsequently found to be more effective in lowering triglycerides. The drug also inhibits collagen-induced platelet aggregation and the second phase of ADP or epinephrine-induced aggregation (Lin & Smith, 1976; Robinson & Le Beau, 1967).

Hydroxychloroquine is an antimalarial drug with anti-inflammatory effects. It inhibits platelet aggregation by ADP and collagen, as well as platelet release caused by low concentrations of collagen or thrombi; it does not prolong the bleeding time (Kinlough-Rathbone, 1976). However, its effect on platelet arachidonate metabolism is not known (Packham & Mustard, 1977).

Design of clinical trials

In a clinical trial there should be a clear statement of its objectives, together with a detailed description of the type of patient under study, the intervention being evaluated, the outcome measures, and the methods of analysis. There should be sufficient specification to allow replication of the study. Long-term trials, particularly secondary prevention studies in myocardial infarction and cerebral ischaemia, are complex and time-consuming. Hence, there is a need for considerable care in their design, execution and analysis if there is to be general credibility and acceptance of the findings.

A series of methodological standards has been developed for good research in this area (Genton et al, 1975; Genton et al, 1977; Peto et al, 1976; Sackett, 1975). These include the need to define precise and appropriate inclusion/exclusion criteria for the patients to be studied; to ensure that enough patients are available and included in the study to enable valid conclusions to be drawn; to allocate patients to their respective treatment groups by randomization following appropriate stratification, so as to generate groups which are likely to be comparable with respect to important clinical and demographic prognostic factors; to provide a concurrent control group with an identical-appearing placebo; to conduct the trial in a double-blind manner; to provide the respective treatment groups with the same care and attention, except for the agents being compared; and to monitor and enforce protocol adherence — these features acting to minimize potential bias in the execution of the study. Finally, the statistical analysis must include and assess appropriately the various outcome measures.

None of the studies included in this review is above criticism but the more important ones, particularly the major studies in myocardial infarction and cerebral ischaemia, do seem to meet most of the above methodological requirements. For example, all the latter studies were randomized and double-blind with appropriate controls, and generally included large numbers of patients. At the same time, it is clear from the number of concerns which have been raised following the publication of these studies that these methodological standards are not in themselves sufficient and there are at least two specific areas which need further attention. The first relates to the multiple analyses of data and their subsequent effect on levels of statistical significance, and the second concerns the omission of certain patients and outcome events from the primary analysis of efficacy.

In clinical trials of antiplatelet drugs, multiple analyses of the data can result from the repeated examination of the accumulating data over time (an ethical requirement in long-term studies); from there being several treatment groups to compare; from the analysis of specific sub-sets or clusters of various outcome measures (e.g. total mortality; cardiac mortality; myocardial infarction, fatal or non-fatal); and from the analysis of clinically cogent sub-groups of patients (e.g. males v females; patients with or without a previous infarction).

In such circumstances there is a strong possibility of spurious statistical significance occurring simply as a result of the many questions being asked of the data. Unfortunately, there is no simple rule for making appropriate adjustments in the final P-values, although it can be shown that if one makes a number of (statistically) independent analyses of the data, say five, then the significance level at which each test should be carried out is approximately 0.01 (i.e. 0.05/5) in order to be sure of maintaining an overall level of statistical significance equal to 0.05. This represents the most stringent situation.

Sub-group analyses are often referred to as 'retrospective analyses'. However, this is generally not the case since they often represent questions which were specifically identified at the start of the trial and the only concern, therefore, is to allow for the multiple tests in the assessment and interpretation of the resulting P-values. Retrospective analysis is an appropriate description only when it applies to a test that was stimulated by an examination of the data. When this happens, it is a hypothesis-generating and not a hypothesis-testing situation.

Despite care in the planning and conduct of trials there will be protocol failures; some patients will be entered into the study who are found subsequently not to meet the study entry criteria and there will be occasions when patients withdraw from study treatment. These protocol deviations raise a number of methodological concerns (Armitage, 1979; Gent & Sackett, 1979; Sackett & Gent, 1979; Schwartz & Lellouch, 1967).

There is one school of thought which says that once a patient is randomized he/she must be retained and any outcome events which occur from the point of randomization to the end of the study must be counted (Peto et al, 1976; Peto et al, 1977). The consequence of this policy is that there is no resulting bias in the subsequent statistical analyses but there is a loss of sensitivity because of the 'noise' due to protocol deviants which, in turn, will result in the need for significantly greater numbers of patients to be studied.

In order to increase the efficiency of their trials, the Anturane Reinfarction Trial Research Group (1978; 1980) and the Canadian Cooperative Study Group (1978) considered a somewhat different strategy.

They said that any patients entered into the study who did not satisfy the specific inclusion/exclusion criteria would be ruled ineligible. Secondly, specific rules were defined for which outcome events should count, and the conditions under which they would occur, when assessing the efficacy of the test treatments. The consequence of this policy was that outcome events that could not be influenced by treatment would be excluded and it was expected that these should occur equally in the respective treatment groups. Hence, the studies were expected to be more sensitive and would thus require relatively fewer patients; on the other hand, it was recognized that there was the *opportunity* for bias due to possible differences between treatment groups in such matters as compliance and drop-out rates, both of which might be related to the patient's clinical condition and/or trial medication. It is important that such rules be applied consistently to each patient without knowledge of which treatment group he is in.

There is no simple resolution to this particular controversy but hopefully continued debate will lead to further advances in the methodology of clinical trials.

Clinical evaluation of antiplatelet drugs

Coronary heart disease

The principal rationale for studying antiplatelet drugs in post myocardial infarction patients was based on the postulated roles of platelets in the development of the atherosclerotic plaque (Ross & Glomset, 1976) and in the etiology of myocardial infarction and cardiac death (Haft, 1979) but it now seems possible that some drugs may also confer benefit independent of their antiplatelet properties (Cuddy et al, 1980; Moschos et al, 1978; Moschos et al, 1979). Myocardial infarction can result from a thrombotic occlusion but Maseri et al (1978) have provided evidence that sustained coronary spasm, even in the absence of thrombosis, can result in myocardial necrosis. Moschos et al (1973) and Capurro et al (1979) have shown that platelets may also play a role in determining the extent of myocardial necrosis following coronary occlusion. Dipyridamole is also a direct vasodilator and such properties might lead to infarct size limitation (Roberts et al, 1980).

Elwood et al (1974) reported a randomized, double-blind study of aspirin (300 mg daily) in 1239 men with a recent myocardial infarction. There was an observed reduction in total mortality of 25 per cent after one year, but this was not statistically significant. However, for men whose qualifying infarction was less than six weeks prior to entry to the study there was a statistically significant reduction in mortality from 13.2 per cent in the placebo group to 7.8 per cent in the aspirin group. The corresponding mortality rates in men with less recent infarctions were 8.3 per cent and 8.8 per cent respectively. Side effects did not appear to be well monitored in this study.

The Coronary Drug Project Research Group (1976) reported on 1529 males who had a myocardial infarction some seven years previously and were randomized to aspirin (975 mg daily) or placebo. The observed 30 per cent reduction in mortality, from 8.5 per cent in the placebo group to 5.8 per cent in the aspirin group, was not statistically significant. Twice as many patients on aspirin (12.3 per cent) complained of stomach pain at some time.

Breddin (1977) randomly allocated 946 patients (80 per cent males), within six weeks of their MI, to aspirin (1.5 g daily), a placebo (making the assessment of the benefit of aspirin double-blind) or to phenprocoumon, and followed them for up to two years. There was little difference in total mortality but the coronary death rate (sudden death or fatal myocardial infarction) while not significantly different was only 4.1 per cent in the aspirin treated patients compared with 7.1 per cent in the placebo group. Nine of the 317 patients on aspirin had their treatment stopped because of haemorrhage compared with none out of 309 in the placebo group; the corresponding numbers stopping for stomach complaints were 20 and 12.

In the randomized trial by Elwood and Sweetnam (1979), most of the 1682 patients (85 per cent males) were admitted within one week of their qualifying infarction. Total mortality was reduced by 17 per cent in the aspirin (900 mg daily) group, a mortality of 12.3 per cent compared with 14.8 per cent in the placebo group. The corresponding reduction for total mortality plus non-fatal MI was 28 per cent; and for ischaemic heart disease mortality it was 22 per cent. None was statistically significant. Side-effects sufficient for the patient to withdraw from the study were only slightly higher in the aspirin group (30.9 per cent v. 28.8 per cent); eight patients on aspirin had a gastrointestinal bleed compared with four on placebo.

The Aspirin Myocardial Infarction Study Research Group (1980) recruited 4524 patients (89 per cent males) who had a documented myocardial infarction two to 60 months previously, and followed them for three years. The total mortality was 10.8 per cent in the aspirin group and 9.7 per cent in the placebo group. There were fewer non-fatal MIs in the aspirin group and the coronary incidence (coronary heart disease mortality or definite non-fatal MI) was 14.1 per cent in the aspirin group compared with 14.8 per cent in the placebo group.

There were significantly more side-effects reported in the aspirin group including each of constipation, heartburn, stomach pain, nausea/vomiting, haematemesis, black tarry stools, bloody stools, symptomatic gout, and symptoms suggestive of peptic ulcer, gastritis, or erosion of gastric mucosa.

The Persantine-Aspirin Reinfarction Study Research Group (1980) recruited 2026 patients (87 per cent males) with a documented myocardial infarction two to 60 months previously, who were followed for 41 months on average. Within the aspirin (975 mg daily) and aspirin (975 mg daily), plus dipyridamole (225 mg daily) groups, the total mortality, coronary heart disease mortality, cardiovascular mortality, and coronary incidence (coronary death or non-fatal MI) were each quite similar and consistently less than in the placebo group, but none was statistically significant. For coronary mortality and coronary incidence the rates were about 50 per cent lower in the aspirin plus dipyridamole group than the placebo group from 8 to 24 months of follow-up and were statistically significant by the study criteria; the corresponding reduction for the aspirin group was 30 per cent over this period of follow-up.

For the sub-group of 447 patients entered within six months of their qualifying infarction it was found that the mortality was 51 per cent less in the aspirin group and 44 per cent less in the aspirin plus dipyridamole group when compared to the placebo group (comprising only 95 patients). In contrast, for patients enrolled more than six months after their MI the mortality differences were very small.

The reported side-effects were similar between the two active treatment groups. In looking at alleged drug-related reasons for permanent or temporary discontinuation of study medication, the rates were much higher in the active treatment groups; reasons included stomach pain, heartburn, nausea/vomiting, and haematemesis, bloody stools and/or black tarry stools.

There have been other studies of aspirin, both prospective and retrospective, which are relevant. Elwood and Williams (1979) carried out a randomized double-blind trial in which 1705 patients (75 per cent males) with myocardial infarction were given a single dose of aspirin (300 mg) or a placebo on first contact with a general practitioner. They found no effect on the 28-day mortality. Hammond and Garfinkel (1975) found no connection between frequent or occasional use of aspirin at the start of a survey and subsequent death from coronary artery disease in a five year follow-up of over a million people (primarily being studied to find risk factors for cancer). These findings are at variance with those of an earlier retrospective study of selected hospitalized patients reported by the Boston Collaborative Drug Surveillance Group (1974) in which the frequency of aspirin ingestion in patients with acute myocardial infarction was compared with that for other diagnoses. It was observed that the incidence of regular aspirin ingestion was significantly lower in the myocardial infarction group, being only 0.9 per cent as compared to 4.9 per cent in the other group. A follow-up survey showed consistent results; the corresponding figures being 3.5 per cent and 7.0 per cent respectively. However, the possibility of selection bias is always a problem in retrospective studies of this nature, and the results can only be interpreted as suggestive. Finally, Hennekens et al (1978) compared aspirin use among 568 white men who had died of coronary artery disease and a similar number of living, age-matched, neighbourhood controls and found no evidence that regular aspirin intake prevented fatal infarction.

Apart from the Persantine-aspirin study discussed above, there is only one study with dipyridamole in post myocardial infarction patients. Gent et al (1968) compared the short-term effects of dipyridamole (400 mg daily) with placebo in 103 patients who had an episode of myocardial infarction of less than two weeks standing. There was no real benefit of dipyridamole in terms of reducing venous and arterial thromboembolic events, recurrent myocardial infarction or death over the next four weeks, but the number of patients studied was too small to allow satisfactory evaluation.

The Anturane Reinfarction Trial Research Group (1978) reported the initial findings of a trial in which patients were randomly allocated to sulfinpyrazone (800 mg daily) or placebo, 25–35 days after a myocardial infarction, and claimed a statistically significant reduction in cardiac mortality from 9.5 per cent per annum to 4.9 per cent. Patient accession was stopped at that time and although a benefit over the first few months seemed clear, the long-term efficacy and tolerability of sulfinpyrazone could not be established with the data at hand. The trial was therefore continued until all 1558 eligible patients (87 per cent males) had completed at least one year of follow-up. By that time the patients had been followed for 16 months on average and a second report appeared (Anturane Reinfarction Trial Research Group, 1980) in which an overall reduction of 32 per cent in cardiac mortality was reported ($P = 0.06$) which was due almost entirely to a 75 per cent reduction in sudden death over the first six months of treatment ($P = 0.003$), after which time there seemed to be no further benefit of treatment.

None of the observed differences in reported side-effects between the two treatment groups was statistically significant except for thromboembolic events, which favoured sulfinpyrazone.

Blakely and Gent (1975) had earlier reported a double-blind study of 291 institutionalized elderly men, with an average age of 72 years, who were randomly allocated to sulfinpyrazone (600 mg daily) or matching placebo and followed for up to four years. Death was the primary outcome and the cause of death was assessed by observers unaware of the patient's treatment. For a sub-group of 96 patients with a history of myocardial infarction before entry to the study there was a statistically significant reduction in deaths from vascular causes among those patients treated with sulfinpyrazone.

Two similar multicentre trials (Group of Physicians of the Newcastle-upon-Tyne Region, 1971; Research Committee of the Scottish Society of Physicians, 1971), evaluated clofibrate (1.8 g daily) in patients who had symptoms of angina or evidence of myocardial infarction, or both. In the Newcastle Study there was a significant overall reduction in sudden death and in all deaths in the clofibrate treated group. This trend was most pronounced in patients who had angina, either alone or in combination with myocardial infarction. In the Scottish Study there was no overall benefit of treatment but for patients with angina, a significant reduction both in sudden death and in total mortality was demonstrated. Both trials have been criticized (Feinstein, 1972; Friedewald & Halperin, 1972; Rahlfs & Bedall, 1973) on methodological aspects of both their design and analysis, and for the occurrence of matching problems with important prognostic factors.

The Coronary Drug Project Research Group (1975) in a study of more than 4000 post MI patients reported no benefit of clofibrate (1.8 g daily) in terms of either total mortality or cause-specific mortality, either for the whole group or for clinically cogent sub-groups of patients.

In a double-blind primary prevention trial of clofibrate (Committee of Principal Investigators, 1978) a selected group of over 10 000 male volunteers free of ischemic heart disease were randomized to clofibrate (1.6 g daily) or placebo and followed for up to eight years. There was a statistically significant risk reduction of 20 per cent in the overall frequency of major ischaemic heart disease, attributed almost entirely to non-fatal myocardial infarction. However, the total mortality was significantly higher in the clofibrate group (162 v 127), the excess deaths being related primarily to the liver, the biliary, and intestinal systems. The increased rate of cholecystectomy for gall stones in the clofibrate treated group was statistically highly significant.

SUMMARY OF CURRENT STATUS
The strongest evidence relating to the efficacy of aspirin comes from the six long-term secondary prevention studies in five of which there was an observed reduction in mortality with the use of aspirin. None of these six individual observed differences in mortality was statistically significant. However, as Peto and Canner independently demonstrated in presentations at the first Annual Meeting of the Society for Clinical Trials in Philadelphia in May, 1980, the observed benefits in each of the six trials are statistically consistent with each other. It is valid to combine the unbiased information from one study with the (statistically independent) unbiased information from others and Peto showed that for cardiovascular death the pooled estimate of the risk reduction with aspirin is 16 per cent ($P < 0.01$); and for the outcome of first infarction, fatal or non-fatal, the pooled estimate of the risk reduction with aspirin is 21 per cent, with an approximate standard error of ± 4 per cent, and this is statistically highly significant ($P < 0.001$).

Questions remain about the best time to initiate treatment, about possible sex differences in response to aspirin and the choice of which dose of aspirin is optimal. However, it would be reasonable on the evidence currently available to conclude that aspirin (approximately 1 g daily) might result in a reduction in mortality of about 10 per cent. There are real side-effects of aspirin but these would seem relatively less important than its benefits.

A number of concerns have been raised about the Anturane Reinfarction Trial (Editorial, 1978a; Editorial, 1978b; Editorial 1980; Evans, 1978; Harnes, 1978; Sherry et al, 1978) relating primarily to the general strategy adopted for the exclusion of certain patients and events from the principal analysis of efficacy, to the multiple examinations of the data, and to the apparent switch of the study focus from cardiac death as the primary outcome event, to sudden death. In their response, members of the study Policy Committee have pointed out that the rules relating to the eligibility of patients and the disqualification of certain outcome events were established a priori, and applied consistently to individual patients, without knowledge of which treatment group they were in. Similarly, from the start of the study, deaths had been classified, without knowledge of treatment and according to specific criteria, as myocardial infarction, sudden, or other cardiac deaths, and it had always been the intention to analyse sudden deaths separately as one of several clinically cogent sub-groups of outcome. Even allowing for the multiple examinations of the data the observed reduction in sudden death at six months is statistically significant by conventional standards.

The finding that sulfinpyrazone reduces the rate of sudden death during the early post-infarction period implies that it may suppress the increased incidence of fatal arrhythmias that occur shortly after infarction. This thesis has received some support from subsequent animal studies by Moschos et al (1979).

The weight of evidence is in favour of sulfinpyrazone being of benefit, and well tolerated, but the findings will be more convincing and more readily accepted if they are confirmed by the Anturane Reinfarction Italy Study (ARIS) — a study of similar design to the Anturane Reinfarction Trial and expected to be published by mid-1981.

The evidence that the combination of dipyridamole plus aspirin is better than aspirin alone is not persuasive at this time. Unfortunately, the proposed PARIS II study will compare aspirin plus dipyridamole against a placebo and even if this treatment regimen is effective we will not know if the dipyridamole component is necessary.

The evidence that clofibrate influences the course of coronary artery disease is unimpressive and there are major concerns about its safety.

Cerebrovascular disease
Several investigators have provided evidence that platelet thromboemboli may be implicated in transient cerebral ischaemia. Fisher (1959), Russell (1961) and Ashby et al (1963) reported white bodies passing through the retinal arterial circulation in patients during episodes of amaurosis fugax. Gunning et al (1964) have demonstrated the presence of platelet fibrin thromboemboli in the cerebral and retinal blood vessels at autopsy in patients with a prior history of cerebral or retinal ischaemia. In addition, platelet containing material has often been observed in the ulcerative lesions of extracranial vessels at the time of operation.

Harrison et al (1971) found a marked reduction in the number of attacks of transient blindness when two patients were treated with aspirin. Mundall et al (1972) also reported a case with transient blindness whose attacks disappeared when aspirin was given and recurred only when the aspirin was stopped temporarily.

Evans (1972) carried out a short-term, double-blind, randomized, crossover study of sulfinpyrazone (600 mg daily) in 20 patients with amaurosis fugax and reported a significant reduction in TIAs with treatment. This study was limited to the effect of treatment on symptomatology and did not address the more important clinical endpoints of stroke or death; and there was also some question about the accuracy of his diagnosis of amaurosis fugax.

Dyken et al (1973) in reviewing their patient records identified 26 of 117 consecutive patients who satisfied specific criteria for the diagnosis of TIA. It was noted, in retrospect, that only two of 15 patients who had been taking aspirin (600 mg daily) had recurrences of TIAs compared with nine of 11 patients who did not take aspirin. This observed difference is striking but there is considerable potential for bias in retrospective studies.

In the study by Blakely and Gent (1975), 99 of the patients had a history of prior stroke, with or without coronary or peripheral arterial disease. Within this group, there was a statistically significant reduction in death from vascular causes among patients treated with sulfinpyrazone.

Clearly the above studies are limited but they did provide part of the rationale for two major clinical trials. In the first of these, the Canadian Cooperative Study Group (1978) reported a randomized, double-blind trial, in which 585 patients with threatened stroke were followed for 26 months on average, to assess the efficacy of aspirin (1.3 g daily) and sulfinpyrazone (800 mg daily), which were administered both singly and in combination. Aspirin was found to reduce the risk of continuing TIA, stroke or death by 19 per cent (P < 0.05) and that of stroke or death by 31 per cent (P < 0.05). Further, this benefit of aspirin was restricted to males for whom the risk of stroke or death was reduced by 48 per cent (P < 0.005) whereas there was no observed benefit for females. For sulfinpyrazone, no risk reduction of ischaemic attacks was observed and the observed 10 per cent risk reduction in stroke or death was not statistically significant. Although there was a trend towards an increased effect when aspirin and sulfinpyrazone were combined, this was not statistically significant.

In the second study, patients with a recent carotid TIA who were treated medically (Fields et al, 1977) or surgically (Fields et al, 1978) were separately randomized to aspirin (1.2 g daily) or placebo, and the primary outcome was defined as stroke-free survival with reduced TIAs during the first six months of follow-up. Among 178 medically treated patients, favourable outcomes were reported in 81 per cent of the aspirin treated group compared with 56 per cent in the controls; the corresponding figures among 125 surgically treated patients were 89 per cent and 76 per cent.

Two small randomized trials were unable to demonstrate a benefit of long-term treatment with either dipyridamole or clofibrate. In the first of these, Acheson et al (1969) evaluated the effects of dipyridamole (400 mg daily or 800 mg daily) in 153 patients with TIA or systemic stroke. They found no evidence of any effect on TIAs, ischaemic stroke or death at either dose level. However, the number of patients studied was small, the length of follow-up (one year) was short, and the incidence of stroke or death was low.

Acheson and Hutchinson (1972) later reported a small randomized study of the effect of clofibrate (1–2 g daily) in 95 patients with hypercholesterolemia and TIAs or stroke. This study was designed to determine the effect of reducing elevated cholesterol on the course of cerebrovascular disease; no differences were noted in the clinical outcomes although a reduction in cholesterol was obtained in the treated group.

A larger randomized trial in 532 men with completed stroke or TIA was carried out by the Veterans Administration Cooperative Study Group (1973). They reported a risk reduction in mortality of about 30 per cent with clofibrate (2 g daily), but an increased risk of stroke of about 50 per cent in the clofibrate group, with no effect on TIAs. Neither of the observed differences was statistically significant.

SUMMARY OF CURRENT STATUS

The one study with dipyridamole was too small to expect a definitive answer on its possible benefit. One of the studies with clofibrate was very inadequate in terms of patient numbers but the second and larger study did not offer any persuasive evidence that clofibrate is of benefit in cerebrovascular disease.

The Canadian study not only provided evidence of an overall benefit of aspirin in terms of reducing the incidence of stroke or death but also showed a striking 48 per cent reduction for males and no benefit for females. Fields' study was too small to expect to show a significant benefit of aspirin on the clinically important outcome of stroke or death. However, as reported in a critical review of this study and the Canadian Study (Gent, 1979), the observed risk reduction of stroke or death in the Fields' study was 47 per cent for males and 0 per cent for females, which is certainly confirmatory of the Canadian findings. Furthermore, this sex-related response to aspirin has been noted in other human studies (Harris et al, 1977; Hirsh et al, 1978; Linos et al, 1978) and confirmed in an animal study (Kelton et al, 1978) carried out specifically to test this hypothesis. The evidence of a sex-related response to aspirin, at these dosages, is thus very strong. The benefit of aspirin in men with threatened stroke is clearly demonstrated and, indeed, the U.S. Food and Drug Administration has now approved aspirin for men with this disorder.

At this time there is no real evidence that sulfinpyrazone is of benefit in cerebrovascular disease but it would be important to examine if there really is synergism between aspirin and sulfinpyrazone, as suggested by the data in the Canadian Study.

Valvular heart disease and prosthetic heart valves

Systemic arterial embolism remains a major problem in patients with valvular heart disease and in patients with prosthetic heart valves, despite improved design. Reduced platelet survival, which correlated with the observed frequency of arterial embolism, has been demonstrated in patients with substitute heart valves (Harker & Slichter, 1970; Weily et al, 1974) and in patients with mitral valve disease Steele et al, 1974). Both dipyridamole (Harker & Slichter, 1970) and sulfinpyrazone (Genton & Steele, 1977) have been shown to increase the shortened platelet survival towards normal in patients with valvular heart disease.

Sullivan et al (1971), in a double-blind trial in 163 patients with older model prosthetic heart valves, showed that adding dipyridamole (400 mg daily) to warfarin resulted in a striking reduction in embolism, from 14 per cent to 1.3 per cent, during one year of treatment. This finding was supported by the results of uncontrolled studies by Meyer et al (1971) and Arrants and Hairston (1972). Altman et al (1976) showed that combining aspirin (500 mg daily) with anticoagulants reduced the incidence of systemic embolism from 18 per cent to 5 per cent. Similarly, Dale et al (1977) in a randomized double-blind trial with 148 patients with aortic ball valve prostheses showed that aspirin (1 g daily) when combined with anticoagulants resulted in a reduction in systemic embolism from 14 per cent to 3 per cent over a two-year period.

Taguchi et al (1975), in a non-randomized controlled trial, reported that aspirin (3 g daily) in combination with dipyridamole (450 mg daily) reduced the incidence of systemic embolism after prosthetic heart valve replacement without concurrent anticoagulant therapy. In two retrospective surveys of patients with Bjork-Shiley valves, Bjork and Henze (1975) reported that a consecutive series treated with aspirin (1 g daily) plus dipyridamole (100 mg daily) did no better than untreated patients, and worse than patients on dicoumarol, and St John Sutton et al (1978) reported three times as much embolism among patients receiving dipyridamole (150 mg daily) compared with warfarin. Two other non-randomized studies (Dale, 1977; Moggio et al, 1978) suggested that aspirin was less effective than anticoagulants in preventing embolism.

SUMMARY OF CURRENT STATUS

It would appear that combining antiplatelet drugs with anticoagulants can be more efficacious than anticoagulants alone. Dipyridamole in combination with oral anti-coagulants is more effective in reducing systemic embolism in patients with rheumatic heart disease or prosthetic heart valves. Aspirin also appears to enhance the antithrombotic effect of oral anticoagulants but there is also some concern about increased bleeding. Antiplatelet drugs, without anticoagulants, do not appear to be effective.

Arterial thrombosis and arteriovenous shunt thrombosis

In spite of the established role of platelets in arterial thrombosis and arteriovenous shunt thrombosis, only a small number of studies with platelet-suppressing drugs have been reported in these disorders.

Hynes et al (1973) randomly assigned 150 consecutive patients having brachial artery catheterization to receive one of two doses of aspirin or a placebo 12 to 15 hours before the procedure. No benefit of aspirin was observed in terms of a reduction in the frequency of thrombi detected by either a balloon catheter or by a decreased pulse. Freed et al (1974) studied the effect of aspirin on the reduction of blood flow determined by oscillometry in children undergoing cardiac catheterization and reported no difference in outcome between the aspirin and placebo treated groups.

Andrassy et al (1974), in a randomized, double-blind trial of 92 patients with A-V fistulas, showed a significant reduction in shunt thrombosis, from 23 per cent to 4 per cent, during one month of treatment with aspirin (1.5 g daily). Zekert et al (1975) reported a randomized, double-blind trial of aspirin (1.5 g daily) in which they observed a four-fold reduction in graft occlusion following two weeks of treatment after iliac or femoral artery bypass grafting in 61 patients, but no apparent effect on the early outcome of endarterectomy in 137 patients. In yet another randomized, double-blind study (Ehresmann et al, 1977) aspirin (1.5 g daily) or placebo was given to 428 patients (94 per cent males) who had reconstructive surgery for chronic obliterative peripheral vascular disease. A significant benefit of aspirin was reflected in a 50 per cent reduction in occlusion. McEnany et al (1976) carried out a randomized trial to study the effects of aspirin, warfarin and placebo on aortocoronary vein graft patency rates. The preliminary report on 155 patients showed the graft patency rates were 84 per cent, 80 per cent and 70 per cent in the warfarin, aspirin and placebo groups respectively. These observed differences are not statistically significant.

Kaegi et al (1974) studied the effect of sulfinpyrazone in patients with arteriovenous shunts for haemodialysis. Fifty-two patients were randomly assigned to sulfinpyrazone (600 mg daily) or placebo for six months and efficacy was measured in terms of the total number of thrombi in each group (established by actual recovery of thrombus) as well as the number of patients with thrombi. There were significantly fewer patients who developed thrombi in the sulfinpyrazone group; furthermore, there was a four-fold difference in the number of thrombi per patient-month from 0.72 in the placebo group to 0.18 in the sulfinpyrazone group. The study was extended (Kaegi et al, 1975) with crossover at six months to the alternative therapy. The significant benefit of sulfinpyrazone was confirmed and this benefit was manifest within one week of treatment and was lost within one week of withdrawal of treatment.

Harter et al (1979) showed that aspirin (160 mg daily) also reduced shunt thrombosis in a randomized trial of 44 patients on chronic haemodialysis. Seventy-two per cent of 25 patients on placebo had thrombi over a five-month period compared with only 32 per cent of 19 patients on aspirin (P < 0.01).

In the study by Blakely and Gent (1975), 47 of the patients had a history of prior peripheral vascular disease but those numbers were too small to allow any meaningful assessment of efficacy.

Several reports have appeared on patients with thrombocytosis and intermittent arterial ischaemia. Vreekan and van Aken (1971) described a patient with recurrent painful toes who had associated thrombocytosis and spontaneous platelet aggregation. Dipyridamole (150 mg daily) was not effective but aspirin (300 mg daily) was associated with prolonged control of symptoms. Bierme et al (1972) observed benefit of aspirin (500 to 1000 mg daily) in three patients with thrombocytosis and painful fingers and toes. Preston et al (1974) also reported on six patients who experienced relief with aspirin, and Mundall et al (1972) described similar relief with aspirin for a single patient. Suggested benefit of aspirin was noted by Fitzgerald and Butterfield (1969) in a patient with Raynaud's disease and Wilding and Flute (1974) reported benefit with dipyridamole in two patients with postembolic upper-extremity ischaemia. Most of these observations were made without appropriate controls but are suggestive of a beneficial effect of aspirin in patients with thrombocytosis and ischaemic extremities.

SUMMARY OF CURRENT STATUS

Aspirin has not been shown to be of benefit either in reducing embolism following cardiac catheterization or preventing aortocoronary bypass graft occlusion. It has been shown to prevent A-V shunt thrombosis and is effective for syndrome of spontaneous aggregation and blue toes.

Sulfinpyrazone has been shown to prevent arteriovenous shunt thrombosis in chronic haemodialysis.

Geriatric population

The frequency of vascular disease and thromboembolic complication is high in institutionalized geriatric patients. In addition, the prospect for compliance in this group is good if medications are dispensed by medical personnel so that these patients are potentially well suited for inclusion in antithrombotic drug trials.

In the study by Blakely and Gent (1975), 125 of the institutionalized elderly men had no clear complications of arterial disease at entry to the study, whereas the remaining 166 patients had a previous history of one or more episodes of myocardial infarction, stroke or peripheral vascular disease. While there was no observed benefit of sulfinpyrazone in the former group, there was a significant reduction in total mortality in the second group among those treated with sulfinpyrazone. This benefit of treatment was even more marked when only deaths from vascular causes were assessed.

Heikinheimo and Jarvinen (1971) studied the effects of aspirin (1 g daily) on morbidity and mortality in a geriatric population. Of 430 subjects, 209 were randomly allocated to receive aspirin and the rest received placebo. There was no significant difference between the two groups in the incidence of hospitalization, morbidity from thromboembolic events, or mortality after one year of follow-up observation.

Venous thromboembolism

While the role of platelets in the development of venous thromboembolism is uncertain, the traditional view is that they occur as a result of fibrin deposition (Hirsh & Genton, 1974). This is supported by platelet and fibrinogen kinetic studies and the effectiveness of anticoagulants in the prophylaxis and treatment of venous thromboembolism. However, some histologic studies (Patterson, 1969; Sevitt, 1969; Freimann, 1972) report the presence of platelet aggregates at the apparent site of origin of venous thrombi, suggesting that platelets may take part in the initiation of venous thrombosis. Changes in platelet coagulant activity in patients with postoperative thrombosis (Walsh et al, 1974) and reduction in platelet survival in those with recurrent venous thrombosis (Steele et al, 1973) have been interpreted as supporting this view. It is possible, therefore, that platelet suppressing drugs may be of value in patients at risk of venous thrombosis, both in preventing the initial episode as well as possible recurrence.

Outcome events of interest include venous thrombosis and pulmonary embolism. These occur at unpredictable times in the high risk period and may be transient. All available diagnostic methods have some limitations as screening procedures (Kakkar, 1975). The clinical diagnosis of venous thrombosis lacks both sensitivity and specificity; this deficiency may thus mask a beneficial effect of the drug and produce a false-negative result. At the same time, a drug with anti-inflammatory properties may decrease clinical manifestations without affecting thrombosis and hence produce a false-positive result.

Isotopic fibrinogen-labelled leg scanning is readily repeatable and is sensitive and specific for distal leg-vein thrombosis. However, it is insensitive to thrombi in the iliac vein and the high femoral vein and it lacks specificity for femoral vein thrombosis when used to screen the operated leg in patients who have undergone hip surgery, because of the high background radioactivity produced by bleeding into this area. This is an acceptable end-point, however, in general surgery patients. Impedance plethysmography and ultrasound are noninvasive methods which are readily repeatable, are sensitive to occlusive thrombi in the popliteal or more proximal veins but are relatively insensitive to calf vein thrombi. Thus either of these methods is useful when combined with leg scanning. Venography is the most specific diagnostic method but it is invasive and cannot be repeated readily or at the bedside. The diagnostic methods used are therefore important in assessing the quality of reported studies in venous thrombosis. In addition, although specific criteria exist with each of these diagnostic procedures there is still a subjective element in their interpretation; hence, the results of these tests should be evaluated by someone unaware of the patient's treatment.

The clinical diagnosis of pulmonary embolism is also inaccurate. While the procedures are difficult to perform at frequent intervals, the combination of perfusion lung scanning and ventilation scans is relatively sensitive and specific for pulmonary embolism (Browse et al, 1974).

In considering the trials in venous thromboembolism, particular attention should be paid to the type and number of patients, the diagnostic procedures, the drug and its dose, and the use of randomization and double-blind procedures.

There have been several randomized trials in general surgical patients. The Medical Research Council Steering Committee (1972) reported on more than 300 patients who had received either aspirin (600 mg daily) or placebo. The incidence of DVT detected by leg scanning was very similar in the two treatment groups. Clagett et al (1975) studied 105 patients who took either aspirin (1.3 g daily) or were untreated. Phlebography was used to confirm the diagnosis of venous thrombosis in most of the patients with positive leg scans. There was a trend in favour of the aspirin group which was reported to be statistically significant after excluding four patients who had not received their aspirin.

Encke et al (1976) demonstrated little benefit of aspirin (990 mg daily) alone, but a four-fold reduction in venous thrombosis when combined with dipyridamole (100 mg daily), from 38 per cent to 10 per cent.

Weber et al (1971) assessed the relative efficacy of aspirin (1.5 g daily) in 450 surgical patients. There were significantly fewer cases of thrombosis in the aspirin group, but the findings are weakened by the lack of a placebo, the lack of blindness and the clinical diagnosis of outcomes. O'Brien et al (1971) using aspirin (2.4 g daily) in a small, non-randomized group of patients undergoing thoracotomy could not demonstrate any benefit on leg scan detected thrombosis.

Renney et al (1976) reported on 160 patients who had been randomly and equally allocated to aspirin (100 mg daily) plus dipyridamole (100 mg daily) or placebo. There was a statistically significant reduction in venous thrombosis detected by leg scanning from 32 per cent to 14 per cent.

Plante et al (1979) randomly allocated 146 abdominal surgery patients to aspirin (1 g daily) plus dipyridamole (150 mg daily), heparin or placebo. The platelet suppressing drugs were administered intravenously for three days and orally thereafter. The incidence in DVT detected by leg scanning was 7 per cent on heparin, 8 per cent on aspirin plus dipyridamole and 21 per cent on placebo, these differences being statistically significant.

Browse and Hall (1969) in comparing dipyridamole (400 mg daily) with placebo in a large number of patients found no difference between the two groups in the incidence of clinically detected venous thrombosis or pulmonary embolism. It is disconcerting that of 111 patients who did not complete the study because of alleged side-effects 102 were taking dipyridamole.

Carter et al (1971) reported that hydroxychloroquine (600 mg daily) significantly decreased the incidence of thrombosis in two separate studies. In the first study, 565 patients were randomly allocated to treatment or placebo but the study was not blind and the diagnosis of outcomes was based solely on clinical findings. In an extension of the trial in which venography was used to confirm thrombosis only 10 per cent of 50 patients had thrombosis in the treated group compared with 22 per cent of 45 patients in the control group. Unfortunately, this study was also unblinded and no assurance was given that the interpretation of the venograms was made by a blinded observer. Carter and Eban (1974) subsequently reported that an increased dose of hydroxy-chloroquine (800 mg daily) produced a significant reduction in the incidence of leg scan detected thrombosis from 50 per cent to 20 per cent in another open study of 202 patients.

There have been several randomized clinical trials in orthopaedic surgery patients. Zekert et al (1974) studied the effect of aspirin prophylaxis (1.5 g daily) in 278 patients with fractured hip. There were 9 deaths in the placebo group and 3 deaths in the aspirin group; the corresponding figures for fatal pulmonary embolism at autopsy were 8 and 1 — a statistically significant difference. Harris et al (1974) compared aspirin (1200 mg daily), warfarin, dextran and low-dose sub-cutaneous heparin in patients who underwent total hip replacement. With the exception of heparin, which was discontinued, no significant differences could be demonstrated in the number of patients with venous thrombosis diagnosed by phlebography. Soreff et al (1975) randomized 51 patients to either aspirin (200 mg daily) or placebo. Of the 35 patients on whom phlebography could be carried out 10 out of 21 patients on aspirin (47 per cent) developed thrombosis compared with five out of 14 patients on placebo (36 per cent). Clearly there is no significant benefit of aspirin.

Schondorf and Hey (1976) randomized 75 patients undergoing hip joint surgery to either aspirin (acetylsalicylic lysine; 450 mg intravenously daily), aspirin plus low dose heparin, or no treatment. The incidence of venous thrombosis detected by leg scanning was 16 out of 30 (53 per cent), eight out of 30 (27 per cent) and nine out of 15 (60 per cent) in the three groups respectively. The observed reduction with the combination therapy was statistically significant and there was no evidence of increased bleeding with this combination.

Harris et al (1977) reported a randomized double-blind study in 95 patients undergoing total hip replacement in which those receiving aspirin (1.2 g daily) had an incidence of venographically confirmed venous thrombosis of 25 per cent compared with 45 per cent in the placebo group. This protection, however, was limited to men. There was a striking 67 per cent reduction in the risk of venous thrombosis among men on aspirin compared with those on placebo; the corresponding reduction for females was only four per cent. When Hume et al (1978) carried out an identical study in 71 patients undergoing hip joint replacement they were not able to demonstrate an overall benefit of aspirin. However, when they separated the two sexes the observed reduction in the risk of thrombosis was found to be 50 per cent for males and there was no observed benefit in females. Hence these data are entirely consistent with those from Harris' study.

Hume et al (1977) reported two consecutive studies in a total of 81 patients undergoing elective hip joint reconstruction in which it appeared that aspirin (1.3 g daily) resulted in a significant reduction in (1) leg scan detected venous thrombosis from 50 per cent to 29 per cent and (2) extension of thrombosis confirmed by phlebography from 20 per cent to seven per cent. However, as the authors themselves point out, this evidence is only suggestive since the control group was not concurrent and it was not a blind study. Jennings et al (1976) reported on a series of 528 patients who underwent total hip replacement and were treated with aspirin (1.5 g daily). Seven of these patients had documented pulmonary emboli; there were no patients with fatal pulmonary emboli; and 34 had clinical evidence of deep vein thrombosis. These rates are all lower than the corresponding expected incidences but evidence from a simple descriptive study such as this is unconvincing by itself.

Dechavanne et al (1975) reported a study in patients undergoing hip replacement in which 60 patients were randomly and equally allocated to aspirin (1.5 g daily) plus dipyridamole (150 mg daily), low dose heparin or no treatment. The incidence of venous thrombosis detected by leg scanning was no different on aspirin plus dipyridamole (50 per cent) than in the control group (40 per cent). Silvergleid et al (1977) reported a randomized double-blind study in 60 patients undergoing hip replacement comparing a combination of aspirin (1.2 mg daily) plus dipyridamole (300 mg daily) with a control group. The rates of leg scan detected venous thrombosis was similar in the two groups, 40 per cent and 45 per cent respectively.

Morris and Mitchell (1977) reported a series of studies in patients with fractures of the femoral neck. In one study 48 patients were randomized into two equal groups one of which received dipyridamole (300 mg daily) and one which received no treatment; in a second similar study 64 patients were randomized but this time aspirin (900 mg daily) plus dipyridamole (300 mg daily) was the investigational drug regimen. Venous thrombosis was detected by leg scanning. The rates of thrombosis in the two control groups were both 67 per cent and the rates in the two treated groups were each 63 per cent. Clearly there is no demonstrable benefit of either aspirin or dipyridamole.

Chrisman et al (1976) compared the effects of hydroxychloroquine (600 mg daily) and placebo in a randomized double-blind trial in 80 patients with fractures or orthopaedic operations. The incidence of thrombosis detected by impedance plethysmography and confirmed by venography was reduced significantly from 60 per cent to 30 per cent. Hanson et al (1976) carried out a randomized, double-blind trial of hydroxychloroquine (600 mg daily) in 153 patients with fracture of the hip, pelvis or thoracolumbar spine, 98 of whom were treated surgically. A significant reduction in thromboembolic complications was reported but diagnostic methods and documentation of results weakens this claim. However, Hume et al (1977) were unable to demonstrate any benefit of this drug at a similar dosage in two randomized studies involving 81 patients undergoing elective total hip joint replacement. Similarly, Cooke et al (1977) could not demonstrate a benefit of hydroxychloroquine (1 g daily) in a randomized trial of 50 patients undergoing elective hip surgery.

McKenna et al (1976) reported on 32 consecutive patients undergoing elective knee surgery in half of whom deep vein thrombosis was detected by leg scanning and confirmed by venography. One of nine patients (11 per cent) who took aspirin regularly developed thrombosis compared with 20 in the remaining 23 patients (88 per cent). Following this observation, the same group (McKenna et al, 1980) randomized 43 patients undergoing elective knee surgery into one of four groups receiving either placebo, aspirin (975 mg daily), aspirin (3.9 g daily) or a pneumatic leg compression device. The rates of venous thrombosis in each of these groups, detected by leg scanning and confirmed by venography, were nine out of 12, seven out of nine, one out of 12 and one out of 10, respectively. These rates differ significantly and there is clear evidence of a benefit of high-dose aspirin and of the pneumatic compression device. It is significant that 36 of those 43 patients were female which suggests that high doses of aspirin may be necessary to reduce thromboembolism in women at high risk of developing this complication.

SUMMARY OF CURRENT STATUS

The evidence of the effectiveness of platelet suppressive drugs in the prophylaxis of venous thromboembolism is mixed and somewhat confusing. The results with aspirin following hip surgery or general surgery appear to be somewhat inconsistent but this may be explained by a possible sex-related benefit of aspirin. Most studies in venous thromboembolism included a majority of female patients who were not analysed separately and their inclusion in the overall analysis could possibly have masked a benefit in the males. In the study by Harris et al (1977) where the two sexes were analysed separately, there was a dramatic reduction in the risk of thrombosis among the males treated with aspirin and this benefit for males was confirmed by Hume et al (1978). It is probably reasonable, therefore, to conclude that the evidence for the benefit of aspirin in general surgery is presently inconclusive but that aspirin appears to be beneficial in males following hip surgery. The observed benefit of high doses of aspirin in females following elective knee surgery is interesting but needs to be confirmed.

The results for dipyridamole, either singly or in combination with aspirin, were generally negative but some of the studies were small, and larger, more carefully designed trials are required to establish the true efficacy of dipyridamole.

Hydroxychloroquine looks promising but design weaknesses in the studies by Carter and Eban (1974) and Hume et al (1977) leave room for doubt. A well-designed confirmatory study would be valuable.

REFERENCES

Acheson J, Hutchinson E C 1972 Controlled trial of clofibrate in cerebral vascular disease. Atherosclerosis 15: 177–183
Acheson J, Danta G, Hutchinson E C 1969 Controlled trial of dipyridamole in cerebral vascular disease. British Medical Journal 1: 614–615
Ali M, McDonald J W D 1978 Reversible and irreversible inhibition of platelet cycloxygenase and serotonin release by nonsteroidal anti-inflammatory drugs. Thrombosis Research 13: 1057–1065
Altman R, Boullon F, Ronvier J, Raca R, de la Fuente I, Favaloro R 1976 Aspirin and prophylaxis of thromboembolic complications in patients with substitute heart valves. Journal of Thoracic and Cardiovascular Surgery 72: 127–129
Andrassy K, Malluche H, Bornefeld H, Comberg H, Ritz E, Jesdinsky H, Mohring K 1974 Prevention of p.o. clotting of a.v. cimino fistulae with acetylsalicylic acid. Klinische Wochenschrift 52: 348–349

Anturane Reinfarction Trial Research Group 1978 Sulfinpyrazone in the prevention of cardiac death after myocardial infarction. The Anturane Reinfarction Trial. New England Journal of Medicine 298: 289–298

Anturane Reinfarction Trial Research Group 1980 Sulfinpyrazone in the prevention of sudden death after myocardial infarction. New England Journal of Medicine 302: 250–256

Armitage P 1979 Trials of antiplatelet drugs, some methodological considerations. Review Epidémiologic et Santé Publique 27: 87–90

Arrants J E, Hairston P 1972 Use of Persantine in preventing thromboembolism following valve replacement. The American Surgeon 38: 432–435

Ashby M, Oakley N, Lorentz I, Scott D 1963 Recurrent transient monocular blindness. British Medical Journal 2: 894–897

Aspirin Myocardial Infarction Study Research Group 1980 A randomized controlled trial of aspirin in persons recovered from myocardial infarction. Journal of the American Medical Association 243: 661–669

Bierme R, Boneu B, Guirand B Pris J 1972 Aspirin and recurrent painful toes and fingers in thrombocythaemia. Lancet 1: 432

Bjork V O, Henze A 1975 Management of thromboembolism after aortic valve replacement with the Bjork-Shiley tilting disc valve. Scandinavian Journal of Thoracic and Cardiovascular Surgery 9: 183–191

Blakeley J A, Gent M 1975 Platelets, drugs and longevity in a geriatric population. In: Hirsh J, Cade J F, Gallus A S, Schonbaum E (eds) Platelets, drugs and thrombosis, Karger, Basel, p. 284–291

Boston Collaborative Drug Surveillance Group 1974 Regular aspirin intake and acute myocardial infarction. British Medical Journal 1: 440–443

Breddin K 1977 Multicenter two-year prospective study on the prevention of secondary myocardial infarction by ASA in comparison with phenprocoumon and placebo. In: Boissel J P, Klimt C R (eds) Multicenter controlled trials: principles and problems, INSERM, Paris, p 79–92

Browse N L, Hall J H 1969 Effect of dipyridamole on the incidence of clinically detectable deep vein thrombosis. Lancet 2: 718–720

Browse N L, Clemenson G, Croft D N 1974 Fibrinogen-detectable thrombosis in the legs and pulmonary embolism. British Medical Journal 1: 603–604

Canadian Cooperative Study Group 1978 A randomized trial of aspirin and sulfinpyrazone in threatened stroke. New England Journal of Medicine 299: 53–59

Capurro N L, Marr K C, Aamodt R, Goldstein R E, Epstein S E 1979 Aspirin-induced increase in collateral flow after acute coronary occlusion in dogs. Circulation 59: 744–747

Carter A E, Eban R 1974 Prevention of postoperative venous thrombosis in legs by orally administered hydroxychloroquine sulphate. British Medical Journal 3: 94–95

Carter A E, Eban R, Perrett R D 1971 Prevention of postoperative deep venous thrombosis and pulmonary embolism. British Medical Journal 1: 312–314

Cazenave J-P, Packham M A, Kinlough-Rathbone R L, Mustard J F 1978 Platelet adherence to the vessel wall and to collagen-coated surfaces. In: Day H J, Molony B A, Nishizawa E E, Rynbrandt R H (eds) Thrombosis: animal and clinical models. Advanced medical biology vol 102, Plenum Press, New York, p 31–49

Chrisman O D, Snook G A, Wilson T C, Short J Y 1976 Prevention of venous thromboembolism by administration of hydroxychloroquine. Journal of Bone and Joint Surgery 58A: 918–920

Clagett G P, Schneider P, Rosoff C B, Salzman E W 1975 The influence of aspirin on postoperative platelet kinetics and venous thrombosis. Surgery 77: 61–74

Committee of Principal Investigators 1978 A co-operative trial in the primary prevention of ischaemic heart disease using clofibrate. British Heart Journal 40: 1069–1118

Cooke E D, Dawson M HO, Ibbotson R M, Bowcock S A, Ainsworth M E, Pitcher M F 1977 Failure of orally administered hydroxychloroquine sulphate to prevent venous thromboembolism following elective hip operations. Journal of Bone and Joint Surgery 59A: 496–500

Coronary Drug Project Research Group 1975 Clofibrate and niacin in coronary heart disease. Journal of the American Medical Association 231: 360–381

Coronary Drug Project Research Group 1976 Aspirin in coronary heart disease. Journal of Chronic Diseases 29: 625–642

Cuddy T E, Donen N, Karlinsky H, McManus J, Larson H 1980 Holter 24 hour recordings in post MI patients in double blind treatment with sulfinpyrazone. American Journal of Cardiology 45: 445

Czervionke R L, Smith J B, Fry G L, Hoak J C, Haycraft D L 1979 Inhibition of prostacyclin by treatment of endothelium with aspirin. Correlation with platelet adherence. Journal of Clinical Investigation 63: 1089–1092

Dale J 1977 Prevention of arterial thromboembolism with acetylsalicylic acid in patients with prosthetic heart valves. Proceedings of the VIth Congress of the International Society of Thrombosis and Haemostasis, Philadelphia

Dale J, Myhre E, Storstein O, Stormorken H, Efskind L 1977 Prevention of arterial thromboembolism with acetylsalicylic acid. A controlled clinical study in patients with aortic ball valves. American Heart Journal 94: 101–111

Dechavanne M, Ville D, Viala J J, Kher A, Faivre J, Poussset M G, Dejour H 1975 Controlled trial of platelet anti-aggregating agents and subcutaneous heparin in prevention of postoperative deep vein thrombosis in high risk patients. Haemostasis 4: 94–100

Dyken M L, Kolar O J, Jones F H 1973 Differences in the occurrence of carotid transient ischemic attacks associated with antiplatelet aggregation therapy. Stroke 4: 732–736

Editorial 1978a Sulfinpyrazone and prevention of myocardial infarction. Food and Drug Administration Drug Bulletin 8: 3

Editorial 1978b Sulfinpyrazone, cardiac infarction, and the prevention of death: a successful trial or another tribulation? British Medical Journal 1: 941–942

Editorial 1980 FDA says no to Anturane. Science 208: 1130–1132

Ehresmann V, Alemany J, Loew D 1977 Prophlaxe von Rezidivverschlussen nach Revaskularisation eingriffen mit acetylsalicylsaure. Medizinische Welt 28: 1157–1162

Elwood P C, Sweetnam P M 1979 Aspirin and secondary mortality after myocardial infarction. Lancet 2: 1313–1315

Elwood P C, Williams W O 1979 A randomized controlled trial of aspirin in the prevention of early mortality in myocardial infarction. Journal of the Royal College of General Practitioners 29: 413–416

Elwood P C, Cochrane A L, Burr M L, Sweetnam P M, Williams G, Welsby E, Hughes S J, Renton R 1974 A randomized controlled trial of acetyl-salicylic acid in the secondary prevention of mortality from myocardial infarction. British Medical Journal 1: 436–440

Encke A, Stock C, Dunke H O 1976 Doppelblindstudie zur postoperativen thrombose prophylaxe mit dipyridamol/acetylsalicylsaure. Chirurg 47: 670–673

Evans D W 1978 Anturane Reinfarction Trial. Lancet 2: 366–367

Evans G 1972 Effect of drugs that suppress platelet surface interaction on incidence of amaurosis fugax and transient cerebral ischemia. Surgical Forum 23: 239–241

Feinstein A R 1972 Clinical biostatistics XVIII. The clofibrate trials. Another dispute about contratrophic therapy. Clinical Pharmacology and Therapeutics 13: 953–968

Fields W S, Lemak N A, Frankowski R F, Hardy R J 1977 Controlled trial of aspirin in cerebral ischemia. Stroke 8: 301–316

Fields W S, Lemak N A, Frankowski R F, Hardy R J 1978 Controlled trial of aspirin in cerebral ischemia Part II, surgical group. Stroke 9: 309–319

Fisher C M 1959 Observations of the fundus oculi in transient monocular blindness. Neurology 9: 333–347

Fitzgerald D E, Butterfield W J H 1969 A case of increased platelet anti-heparin factor in a patient with Raynaud's phenomenon and gangrene treated by aspirin. Angiology 20: 317–324

Freed M D, Rosenthal A, Fyler D 1974 Attempts to reduce arterial thrombosis after cardiac catheterization in children: use of percutaneous technique and aspirin. American Heart Journal 87: 283–286

Freiman D G 1972 Surgical conditions as risk factors in the development of venous thrombosis. Milbank Memorial Fund Quarterly 50: 60–70

Friedewald W T, Halperin M 1972 Clofibrate in ischaemic heart failure. Annals of Internal Medicine 76: 821–823

Gent A E, Brook C G D, Foley T H, Miller T N 1968 Dipyridamole: A controlled trial of its effect in myocardial infarction. British Medical Journal 4: 366–368

Gent M 1979 Recent intervention studies of platelet suppressant drugs in cerebral ischemia: methodological aspects. In: Tognoni G, Garrattini S (eds) Drug treatment and prevention in cerebrovascular disorders, Elsevier/North Holland Biomedical Press, Amsterdam, p 437–448

Gent M, Sackett D L 1979 The qualification and disqualification of patients and events in long term cardiovascular clinical trials. Thrombosis and Hemostasis 41: 123–134

Genton E, Steele P 1977 Platelet survival time — alteration with disease and drug treatment. In: Mitchell J R A, Domenet J G (eds) Thromboembolism, a new approach to therapy, Academic Press, London, p 104–122

Genton E, Gent M, Hirsh J, Harker L A 1975 Platelet-inhibiting drugs in the prevention of clinical thrombotic disease. New England Journal of Medicine 293: 1174–1178, 1236–1240, 1296–1300

Genton E, Barnett H J M, Fields W S, Gent M, Hoak J C 1977 XIV Cerebral ischemia: The role of thrombosis and of antithrombotic therapy. Stroke 8: 150–175

Gordon J L, Pearson J D 1978 Effects of sulphinpyrazone and aspirin on prostaglandin I_1 (prostacyclin) synthesis by endothelial cells. British Journal of Pharmacology 64: 481–483

Group of Physicians of the Newcastle Upon Tyne Region 1971 Trial of clofibrate in the treatment of ischemic heart disease. British Medical Journal 4: 767–775

Gunning A J, Pickering G W, Robb-Smith A HT, Russell R R 1964 Mural thrombosis of the internal carotid artery and subsequent embolism. Quarterly Journal of Medicine New Series XXXIII, 129: 155–195

Haft J I 1979 Role of blood platelets in coronary artery disease. American Journal Cardiology 43: 1197–1206

Hammond E C, Garfinkel L 1975 Aspirin and coronary heart disease: findings of a prospective study. British Medical Journal 2: 269–271

Hansen E H, Jessing P, Lindewald H, Ostergaard P, Olesen T, Malrer E I 1976 Hydroxychloroquine sulphate in prevention of deep venous thrombosis following fracture of the hip, pelvis or thoracolumbar spine. Journal of Bone and Joint Surgery 58A: 1089–1093

Harker L A, Slichter S J 1970 Studies of platelet and fibrinogen kinetics in patients with prosthetic heart valves. New England Journal of Medicine 283: 1302–1305

Harker L A, Hanson S R, Kirkman T R 1979 Experimental arterial thromboembolism in baboons. Mechanism, quantitation, and pharmacologic prevention. Journal Clinical Investigation 64: 559–569

Harker L A, Wall R T, Harlan J M, Ross R 1978 Sulfinpyrazone prevention of homocysteine — induced endothelial cell injury and arteriosclerosis. Clinical Research 26: 554A

Harnes J R 1978 Sulfinpyrazone after myocardial infarction. New England Journal of Medicine 298: 1258

Harris W H, Salzman E W, Athanasoulis C A, Waltman A C, de Sanctis R W 1977 Aspirin prophylaxis of venous thromboembolism after total hip replacement. New England Journal of Medicine 297: 1246–1249

Harris W H, Salzman E W, Athanasoulis C, Waltman A C, Baum S, de Sanctis R W 1974 Comparison of warfarin, low-molecular-weight dextran, aspirin and subcutaneous heparin in prevention of venous thromboembolism following total hip replacement. Journal of Bone and Joint Surgery 56: 1552–1562

Harrison M J G, Marshall J, Meadows J C, Russell R W R 1971 Effect of aspirin in amaurosis fugax. Lancet 2: 743–744

Harter H R, Burch J W, Majerus P W, Stanford N, Delmez J A, Anderson C B, Weerts C A 1979 Prevention of thrombosis in patients on hemodialysis by low-dose aspirin. New England Journal of Medicine 301: 577–579

Heikinheimo R, Jarvinen K 1971 Acetylsalicylic acid and arteriosclerotic-thromboembolic disease in the aged. Journal of The American Geriatrics Society 197: 403–405

Hennekens C H, Karlson L K, Rosner B 1978 A case-control study of regular aspirin use and coronary deaths. Circulation 58: 35–38

Hirsh J, Genton E 1974 Thrombogenesis, physiological pharmacology: a comprehensive treaty. In: Root W S, Berlin N I (eds) Physiological pharmacology, Academic Press, New York, p 99–133

Hirsh J, Blajchman M, Kaegi A 1978 The bleeding time. In: Platelet function testing, DHEW Publication No (NIH) 78–1087, Washington, p 1–12

Hume M, Donaldson W R, Suprenant J 1978 Sex, aspirin and venous thrombosis. Symposium on Care of the Critically Ill Orthopedic Patient. Orthopedic Clinics of North America 9: 761–767

Hume M, Bierbaum B, Kuriakose T X, Suprenant J 1977 Prevention of postoperative thrombosis by aspirin. The American Journal of Surgery 133: 420–422

Hynes K M, Gau G T, Rutherford B D, Kazmier F J, Frye R L 1973 Effects of aspirin on brachial artery occlusion following brachial arteriotomy for coronary arteriography. Circulation 47: 554–557

Jennings J J, Harris W H, Sarmiento A 1976 A clinical evaluation of aspirin prophylaxis of thromboembolic disease after total hip arthroplasty. Journal of Bone and Joint Surgery 58A: 926–927

Kaegi A, Pineo G F, Shimizu A, Trivedi H, Hirsh J, Gent M 1974 Arterio-venous shunt thrombosis. Prevention by sulfinpyrazone. New England Journal of Medicine 290: 304–306

Kaegi A, Pineo G F, Shimizu A, Trivedi H, Hirsh J, Gent M 1975 The role of sulfinpyrazone in the prevention of arterio-venous shunt thrombosis. Circulation 52: 497–499

Kakkar V V 1975 Deep vein thrombosis: detection and prevention. Circulation 51: 8–19

Kelton J G, Hirsh J, Carter C J, Buchanan M R 1978 Sex differences in the antithrombotic effects of aspirin. Blood 52: 1073–1076

Kinlough-Rathbone R L, Reimers H J, Mustard J F, Packham M A 1976 Sodium arachidonate can induce platelet shape change and aggregation which are independent of the release reaction. Science 192: 1011–1012

Kinlough-Rathbone R L, Groves H M, Cazenave J-P, Richardson M, Mustard J F 1978 Effect of dipyridamole and aspirin on platelet adherence to damaged rabbit aortas in vitro and in vivo. Federation Proceedings 37: 260

Lin C Y, Smith S 1976 The effect of halofenate and clofibrate on aggregation and release of serontonin by human platelets. Life Sciences 18: 563–568

Linos A, Worthington J W, O'Fallon W, Fuster V, Whisnant J P, Kurland L T 1978 Effect of aspirin on prevention of coronary and cerebrovascular disease in patients with rheumatoid arthritis. Mayo Clinic Proceedings 53: 581–586

Maseri A, L'Abbate A, Baroldi G, Chierchia S, Marzili M, Bellestra A M, Severi S, Parodi O, Bragini A, Distante A, Pesola A 1978 Coronary vasospasm as a possible cause of myocardial infarction. New England Journal of Medicine 299: 1271–1277

Masotti G, Galanti G, Poggesi L, Abbate R, Neri Serneri G G 1979 Differential inhibition of prostacyclin production and platelet aggregation by aspirin. Lancet 2: 1213–1216

McEnany M T, de Sanctis R W, Harthorne J W, Mundth E D, Weintraub R M, Austen W G, Salzman E W 1976 Circulation (Supplement): 124

McKenna R, Bachmann F, Kaushal S D, Galante J O 1976 Thromboembolic disease in patients undergoing total knee replacement. Journal of Bone and Joint Surgery 58A: 928–932

McKenna R, Galante J, Bachmann F, Wallace D L, Kaushal S P, Meredith P 1980 Prevention of venous thromboembolism after total knee replacement by high-dose aspirin or intermittent calf and thigh compression. British Medical Journal 1: 514–517

Medical Research Council (Report of the Steering Committee) 1972 Effect of aspirin on postoperative venous thrombosis. Lancet 2: 441–444

Meyer J S, Charney J Z, Rivera V M, Mathew N T 1971 Cerebral embolization: prospective clinical analysis of 42 cases. Stroke 2: 541–554

Moggio R A, Hammond G I, Stausel H C, Glenn W W L 1978 Incidence of emboli with cloth-covered Starr-Edwards valve with anticoagulation and with varying forms of angicoagulation. Journal of Thoracic and Cardiovascular Surgery 75: 296–299

Morris G K, Mitchell J R A 1977 Preventing venous thromboembolism in elderly patients with hip fractures: studies of low-dose heparin, dipyridamole, aspirin and flurbiprofen. British Medical Journal 1: 535–537

Moschos C, Escobinas A, Jorgensen O, Regan T 1979 Effect of sulfinpyrazone on survival following experimental non-thrombotic coronary occlusion. American Journal Cardiology 43: 372

Moschos C, B, Haider B, Cruz C D, Lyons M M, Regan T J 1978 Antiarrhythmic effects of aspirin during nonthrombotic coronary occlusion. Circulation 57: 681–684

Moschos C B, Lahiri K, Lyons M, Weisse A B, Oldewurtel H A, Regan T J 1973 Relation of microcirculatory thrombosis to thrombus in the proximal coronary artery: effect of aspirin, dipyridamole and thrombolysis. American Heart Journal 86: 61–68

Mundall J, Quintero P, Von Kaulla K N, Harmon R, Austin J 1972 Transient monocular blindness and increased platelet aggregability treated with aspirin. Neurology 22: 280–285

Mustard J F, Packham M A 1978 Platelets, thrombosis and drugs. In: Avery G S (ed) Cardiovascular drugs. Vol. 3, antithrombotic drugs, ADIS Press, Syndney, p 1–83

Mustard J F, Packham M A 1980 Are aspirin and sulfinpyrazone useful in the prevention of myocardial infarction, strokes or venous thromboembolism? In: Lasagna L (ed) Controversies in therapeutics, Saunders, Philadelphia, p 319–332

O'Brien J R, Tulevski V, Etherington M 1971 Two in-vivo studies comparing high and low aspirin dosage. Lancet 1: 388–400

Packham M A, Mustard J F 1977 Clinical pharmacology of platelets. Blood 50: 555–573

Paterson J C 1969 The pathology of venous thrombi. In: Sherry S, Brinkhous K M, Genton E (eds) Thrombosis, National Academy of Sciences, Washington, DC, p 321–331

The Persantin-Aspirin Re-infarction Study Research Group 1980 Persantin and aspirin in coronary heart disease. Circulation 62: 449–461

Peto R, Pike M C, Armitage P, Breslow N E, Cox D R, Howard S V, Mantel N, McPherson K, Peto J, Smith P G 1976 Design and analysis of randomized clinical trials requiring prolonged observation of each patient. I: Introduction and design. British Journal of Cancer 34: 585–612

Peto R, Pike M C, Armitage P, Breslow N E, Cox D R, Howard S V, Mantel N, McPherson K, Peto J, Smith P G 1977 Design and analysis of randomized clinical trials requiring prolonged observation of each patient. II: Analysis and examples. British Journal of Cancer 35: 1–39

Plante J, Boneu B, Vaysse C, Barret A, Gouzi M, Bierme R 1979 Dipyridamole — aspirin versus low doses of heparin in the prophylaxis of deep venous thrombosis in abdominal surgery. Thrombosis Research 14: 399–403

Preston F E, Emmanuel I G, Winfield D A, Malia R G 1974 Essential thrombocythaemia and peripheral gangrene. British Medical Journal 3: 548–551

Rahlfs V W, Bedall F K 1973 The effect of clofibrate: a comment on two published studies. Journal of Chronic Diseases 26: 817–820

Renney J T G, O'Sullivan E F, Burke P F 1976 Prevention of postoperative deep vein thrombosis with dipyridamole and aspirin. British Medical Journal 1: 992–994

Research Committee of the Scottish Society of Physicians 1971 Ischaemic heart disease: a secondary prevention trial using clofibrate. British Medical Journal 4: 775–784

Roberts A J, Jacobstein J G, Cipriano P R 1980 Effectiveness of dipyridamole in reducing the size of experimental myocardial infarction. Circulation 61: 228–236

Robinson R W, Le Beau R J 1967 Platelet adhesiveness and aggregation with chlorophenoxyisobutyric ester. American Journal Medical Science 253: 106–112

Ross R, Glomset J A 1976 The pathogenesis of atherosclerosis. New England Journal of Medicine 295: 369–377

Roth G J, Majerus P W 1977 Acetylation of prostaglandin synthetase by aspirin. In: Silver M J, Smith J B, Kocsis J J (eds) Prostaglandins in hematology, Spectrum Publications Inc., New York, p 345–360

Russell R W R 1961 Observations on the retinal blood vessels in monocular blindness. Lancet 2: 1422–1428

Sackett D L 1975 Design, measurement and analysis in clinical trials. In: Hirsh J, Cade J F, Gallus A S, Schonbaum E (eds) Platelets, drugs and thrombosis, Karger, Basel, p 219–225

Sackett D L, Gent M 1979 Controversy in counting and attributing events in clinical trials. New England Journal of Medicine 301: 1410–1412

Schondorf T H, Hey D 1976 Combined administration of low dose heparin and aspirin as prophylaxis of deep vein thrombosis after hip joint surgery. Haemostasis 5: 250–257

Schwartz D, Lellouch J 1967 Explanatory and pragmatic attitudes in therapeutic trials. Journal of Chronic Diseases 20: 637–648

Sevitt S 1969 Venous thrombosis in injured patients (with some observations on pathogenesis). In: Sherry S, Brinkhous K M, Genton E (eds) Thrombosis, National Academy of Sciences, Washington D C, p 29–49

Sherry S, Gent M, Mustard J F, McGregor M, Lilienfeld A, Yu P 1978 Sulfinpyrazone after myocardial infarction. New England Journal of Medicine 298: 1259

Silvergleid A J, Bernstein R, Burton D S, Tanner J B, Silverman J F, Schrier S L 1977 Aspirin-Persantin prophylaxis in elective total hip replacement. Thrombosis and Haemostasis 38: 166

Smythe H A, Ogryzlo M A, Murphy E A, Mustard J F 1965 The effect of sulfinpyrazone (Anturan) on platelet economy and blood coagulation in man. Canadian Medical Association Journal 92: 818–821

Soreff J, Johnsson H, Diener L, Goransson L 1975 Acetylsalicylic acid in a trial to diminish thromboembolic complications after elective hip surgery. Acta Orthopaedica Scandinavica 46: 246–255

Steele P, Weilly H S, Genton E 1973 Platelet survival and adhesiveness in recurrent venous thrombosis. New England Journal of Medicine 288: 1148–1152

Steele P, Weily H S, Davies H, Genton E 1974 Platelet survival in patients with rheumatic heart disease. New England Journal of Medicine 290: 537–539

St John Sutton M G, Miller G A H, Oldershaw P J, Paneth M 1978 Anticoagulants and the Bjork-Shiley prosthesis: experience of 390 patients. British Heart Journal 40: 558–562

Sullivan J M, Harken D E, Gorlin R 1971 Pharmacologic control of thromboembolic complications of cardiac-valve replacement. New England Journal of Medicine 284: 1391–1394

Taguchi K, Matsumura H, Washizu T, Hirao M, Kato K, Kato E, Mochizuki T, Takamura K, Mashimo I, Morifuji K, Nakagaki M, Suma T 1975 Effect of athrombogenic therapy, especially high dose therapy of dipyridamole, after prosthetic valve replacement. Journal of Cardiovascular Surgery 16: 8–15

Veterans Administration Cooperative Study Group 1973 The treatment of cerebrovascular disease with clofibrate. Stroke 4: 684–693

Vreeken J, van Aken W G 1971 Spontaneous aggregation of blood platelets as a cause of idiopathic thrombosis and recurrent painful toes and fingers. Lancet 2: 1394–1397

Walsh P N, Rogers P H, Marden V I 1974 Platelet anticoagulant activities and venous thrombosis after hip surgery. Transactions of the Association of American Physicians 87: 140–152

Weber W, Wolff K, Bromig G 1971 Postoperative thromboembolies prophylaxe mir colfaret. Therap Berichte 43: 229–293

Weily H S, Genton E 1970 Altered platelet function in patients with prosthetic mitral valves. Effects of sulfinpyrazone therapy. Circulation 42: 967–972

Weily H S, Steele P P, Davies H, Pappas G, Genton E 1974 Platelet survival in patients with substitute heart valves. New England Journal of Medicine 290: 534–537

Wilding R P, Flute P T 1974 Dipyridamole in peripheral upper-limb ischaemia. Lancet 1: 999–1000

Zekert F, Kohn P, Vormittag E, Piza F, Thien M 1975 Zur acetylsalicylsaure-prophylaxe von sofortverschulssen nach gefasschirurgischern eingriffen in Colfarit Symposium III Bayer, Cologne, p 109–119

Zekert F, Kohn P, Vormittag E, Poigenfurst J, Thein M 1974 Thromboembolie prophylaxe mit acetylsalicylsaure bei operationen wegen jufgelenknahar fraskruren. Monatschrifr der Unfallheikunde 77: 97–110

Index

A 23187, 15, 184
ABH platelet antigens, 9
actin
 -binding protein, 15
 G-, 13, 14
 heterogeneity, 13
 platelet attachment, 7
 polymerization, 15
α-actinin, 7, 13, 14, 43, 44
 function, 14, 15
 platelet receptor, 43, 44
activated partial thromboplastin time (APTT), 90
 and haemophilia diagnosis, 193–5
 kit reagents, 194
active glomerular disease, platelet aggregation, 57
adenylate cyclase, PGD_2 activation, 62
adhesion, platelet, 2, 3, 6, 9, 26, 187, 188
 and cancer cells, 244
 and myocardial infarction, 62
 Willebrand factor-mediated, 6, 26
ADP release and aspirin, 64
adrenalin and fibrinolysis, 129
afibrinogenaemia, 21
 defective protein, 46
agglutination, platelet, 2
aggregation, platelet, 2, 3, 9
 ADP-induced, 97
 arachidonate-induced, 48
 cancer cell, 240, 244
 collagen induced, 23
 complement factors, 101
 decreased, 52
 and drugs, 64
 epinephrine-induced, 3
 factor, 63
 and fibrinogen, 21
 inhibitor, 63
  from cancer cells, 245
 spontaneous, 54, 58
agnogenic myeloid metaplasia, 52
albinism, 47, 48
alloantigen PI^{AI}, platelet-specific, 7
Alport's syndrome, 46, 50
amaurosis fugax, 327
ε-aminocaproic acid, 126
 plasminogen activation, 127, 128
amniocentesis, 197
AMP cyclic
 phosphodiesterase inhibitors, 65, 66
 and platelet function, 19

anamnestic response, 203, 204
angina pectoris, 67
angiography
 allergy reactions, 310, 311
 contrast media, 310, 311
 pulmonary, 305, 306, 308–12
 safety, 310, 312
angiotensin II, 184
animals, blood coagulation in, 211–19
antibody, antiplatelet, 55
antigens
 PL^{AI} detection, 42, 43
 platelet, 9
α_2-antiplasmin, 100, 117, 127
 acquired deficiency and liver disease, 134
 chromogenic assay, 281, 282
 congenital deficiency, 130, 133, 134
 measurement, 133
 properties, 133
antithrombin, 151–66, 229
 activity in reptiles, 213
 assay results, 157, 158
 clotting assays, 156
 and clotting enzymes, 153, 154
 clotting factor inactivation, 154
 deficiency
  acquired, 159
  congenital, 161, 162
  subtypes, 162, 163
 factor X_a and heparin, 155
 and heparin, 152–5, 161
 and hormones, 161
 hypercoagulation syndrome, 159, 160
 immunoassays, 157
 metabolism, 158, 159
 neonatal, 161
 nomenclature, 151, 152
 plasma concentration, 158
 and platelets, 164
 postoperative changes, 160
 proteinase inhibitor, 151
 structure, 152
 synthesis regulation, 163
 synthetic chromogenic substances, 157
 therapy, 163, 164
 tissue localization, 158
 thrombin inactivation and heparin, 155, 156
 thrombin modified, 153
antithrombin II, 151
antithrombin III, 25, 117, 118
 slow inactivation, 151